Critical Care Nursing

DATE DUE

made
Incredibly
Easy!®

Fourth Edition

Critical Care Nursing

made Incredibly Easy!

Fourth Edition

Clinical Editor

David W. Woodruff, MSN, RN-BC, CNS, CNE, FNAP

Dean of Academic Affairs/Associate Professor
Chamberlain College of Nursing
Cleveland, Ohio

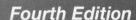 Wolters Kluwer

Philadelphia • Baltimore • New York • London
Buenos Aires • Hong Kong • Sydney • Tokyo

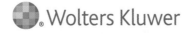

Executive Editor: Shannon W. Magee
Product Development Editor: Maria M. McAvey
Senior Marketing Manager: Mark Wiragh
Production Project Manager: Joan Sinclair
Design Coordinator: Elaine Kasmer
Manufacturing Coordinator: Kathleen Brown
Prepress Vendor: Absolute Service, Inc.

9 8 7 6 5 4 3 2 1

Printed in China

Library of Congress Cataloging-in-Publication Data

Critical care nursing made incredibly easy! / clinical editor, David W. Woodruff.—Fourth edition.
   p. ; cm.
 Includes bibliographical references and index.
 ISBN 978-1-4963-0693-7
 I. Woodruff, David W., editor.
 [DNLM: 1. Critical Care Nursing—methods—Handbooks. 2. Critical Illness—nursing—Handbooks. WY 49]
 RT120.I5
 616.02'8—dc23
                2015026774

LWW.com

Contributors

Maurice Espinoza, RN, MSN, CNS, CCRN
Clinical Nurse Specialist
University of California Irvine Healthcare
Orange, California

Ellie Z. Franges, MSN, RN, CRNP, CNRN
Nurse Practitioner
Neurosurgery
St. Luke's University Hospital & Health
   Network
Bethlehem, Pennsylvania

Wendeline J. Grbach, MSN, RN, CLNC, CHSE,
   CCRN Alumnus
Curriculum Developer for Simulation
   Education
UPMC Shadyside School of Nursing
Pittsburgh, Pennsylvania

Jodi L. Gunther, RN, MS, APN-CNS, CCRN-CSC-CMC
Certified Clinical Nurse Specialist
Adult Health, Physician Assistants & APNs
Elk Grove Village, Illinois

Anna Jarrett, RN, PhD, ACNP/ACNS, BC
Assistant Professor of Nursing
Eleanor Mann School of Nursing
Fayetteville, Arkansas

Kathryn L. Kay, MSN, RN, PCCN-CMC
Instructor of Nursing
Chamberlain College of Nursing
Cleveland, Ohio

Margaret J. Malone, RN, MN, CCRN
Registered Nurse
State University of New York Upstate
   Medical University
Syracuse, New York

Nicolette C. Mininni, RN, MEd, CCRN
Advanced Practice Nurse
UPMC Shadyside School of Nursing
Pittsburgh, Pennsylvania

Elizabeth Moots, MSN, RN
Adult Health Instructor
Chamberlain College of Nursing
Cleveland, Ohio

Carol A. Pehotsky, RN, BSN, MME
Assistant Director of Perioperative
   Education
Cleveland Clinic
Cleveland, Ohio

Susan M. Raymond, MSN, CCRN
Adjunct Faculty
University of Central Florida College of
   Nursing
Orlando, Florida

Previous edition contributors and consultants

Natalie Burkhalter, RN, MSN, FNP-BC,
ACNP-BC, CCRN

Maurice Espinoza, RN, MSN, CNS, CCRN

Ellie Z. Franges, MSN, RN, CRNP

Linda Fuhrman, RN, MS, ANP

Wendeline J. Grbach, MSN, RN, CCRN, CLNC

Jodi L. Gunther, RN, MS, APN-CNS,
CCRN-CSC-CMC

Anna Jarrett, RN, PhD, ACNP/ACNS, BC

Margaret J. Malone, RN, MN, CCRN

Nicolette C. Mininni, RN, MEd, CCRN

Carol A. Pehotsky, RN, BSN, MME

Susan M. Raymond, MSN, CCRN

Amy Shay, RN, MS, CNS, CCRN

Patricia A. Slachta, PhD, APRN, ACNS-BC,
CWOCN

Kathy Stallcup, MSN, RN, CCRN

Linda A. Valdiri, RN, MS, CCNS

Foreword

Critical care nursing transcends the walls of the intensive care unit and can include units as varied as emergency departments and postanesthesia care units. Nurses providing critical care treat patients with trauma, medical issues, surgical complications, and many other acute and life-threatening problems. Critical care nursing is holistic, dynamic, challenging, and interdisciplinary.

When critical care units began in the 1960s, the focus was on high-tech monitoring of critically ill patients, and although nurses still provide state-of-the-art monitoring, the focus of modern critical care is on achieving the best outcome for the patient and family. A holistic approach is necessary in order to manage ethical decisions, end-of-life decisions, family dynamics, and treatment options for chronic disease.

Critical care nursing is dynamic and challenging. Acutely ill patients have constantly changing needs and evolving health conditions that present many challenges for the critical care nurse including frequent assessments, computer and high-tech equipment literacy, and the need for continuous learning. Nurses, physicians, respiratory therapists, physical therapists, dietitians, and many other health care workers form a team in the critical care unit, ideally working in unison to provide coordinated interdisciplinary care.

In today's rapidly changing critical care environment, nurses need to clearly understand what they are doing and why. Education needs to be simple, understandable, and useful. I once had a professor tell me that if you really understand a concept, you can explain it to a child. That level of understanding takes simple yet complete education to achieve. *Critical Care Nursing Made Incredibly Easy* strives to achieve that outcome.

Chapters include critical care basics; holistic care issues; body system–based conditions; and hematologic, immune, and multisystem disorders. The updated content is expansive, and it includes applications to such specialized critical care arenas as rapid response teams and advanced life support measures. The spectrum of new information is timely and includes updates on moderate sedation; drug overdose; pressure ulcer management; and treating patients with specialized needs, such as elderly, pediatric, and bariatric patients.

The most important and necessary variable when transforming information to knowledge is comprehension. The signature of *Critical Care Nursing Made Incredibly Easy*, Fourth Edition, is the way in which the information is presented: clearly, directly, and simply. The unique writing style, color illustrations, witty characters, and clever icons—most notably, *Memory joggers*, which offer simple tricks to remember key points—create a reference that helps you to translate critical care nursing information into practice.

In addition, icons draw your attention to important issues:

Advice from the experts—offers tips and tricks for nurses and key troubleshooting techniques

Take charge!—focuses on potentially lethal situations and steps to take when they occur

Handle with care—identifies concerns and actions related to elderly, pediatric, and bariatric patients

Weighing the evidence—highlights research that guides practice

This book is perfect for nursing students preparing for critical care practice and practicing nurses preparing for clinical care and is a great adjunct for nurses preparing for the Critical Care Certification Exam (CCRN). Critical care nursing is a complex area of practice. In order to achieve your highest level, keep asking "why?" The goal is to keep learning and growing throughout your critical care career.

David W. Woodruff, MSN, RN-BC, CNS, CNE, FNAP
Dean of Academic Affairs/Associate Professor
Chamberlain College of Nursing
Cleveland, Ohio

Contents

Appendices and index

Chapter 1

Critical care basics

Just the facts

In this chapter, you'll learn:

♦ roles and responsibilities of the critical care nurse

♦ credentials for critical care nurses

♦ ways to work with a multidisciplinary team

♦ ways to incorporate clinical tools and best practices into your care.

What is critical care nursing?

Critical care nursing is the delivery of specialized care to critically ill patients—that is, ones who have life-threatening illnesses or injuries. Such patients may be unstable, have complex needs, and require intensive and vigilant nursing care.

Patients with illnesses and injuries commonly seen in intensive or critical care units (ICUs/CCUs) include:

- gunshot wounds
- traumatic injuries from such events as automotive collisions and falls
- cardiovascular disorders, such as heart failure and acute coronary syndromes (unstable angina and acute myocardial infarction [AMI])
- surgeries, such as abdominal aortic aneurysm repair and carotid endarterectomy
- respiratory disorders, such as acute respiratory failure and pulmonary embolism
- GI and hepatic disorders, such as acute pancreatitis, acute upper GI bleeding, and acute liver failure
- renal disorders, such as acute and chronic renal failure
- cancers, such as lung, esophageal, and gastric cancer
- shock caused by hypovolemia, sepsis, and cardiogenic events (such as after AMI).

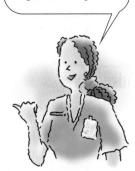

As a critical care nurse, you'll see the most critically ill or injured patients—those who are unstable, have complex needs, and require intensive and vigilant nursing care.

Meet the critical care nurse

Critical care nurses are responsible for making sure those critically ill patients and members of their families receive close attention and the best care possible.

Put your best foot forward and strive to deliver the best care possible to patients and their families.

What do you do?

Critical care nurses fill many roles in the critical care setting, such as staff nurses, nurse educators, nurse managers, case managers, clinical nurse specialists, nurse practitioners, and nurse researchers. (See *Role call.*)

Where do you work?

Critical care nurses work wherever critically ill patients are found, including:

- adult, pediatric, and neonatal ICU/CCUs
- coronary care and progressive coronary care units
- emergency departments
- postanesthesia care units.

What makes you special?

As a nurse who specializes in critical care, you accept a wide range of responsibilities, including:

- being an advocate
- using sound clinical judgment
- demonstrating caring practices
- collaborating with a multidisciplinary team
- demonstrating an understanding of cultural diversity
- providing patient and family teaching.

A critical care nurse is perfect for many roles. She can play a nurse manager, a nurse educator, a case manager, or another type of specialist.

Advocacy

An advocate is a person who works on another person's behalf. As a patient advocate, you should address the concerns of family members and the community whenever possible.

As an advocate, the critical care nurse is responsible for:

- protecting the patient's rights
- assisting the patient and his family in the decision-making process by providing education and support
- negotiating with other members of the health care team on behalf of the patient and his family
- keeping the patient and his family informed about the care plan
- advocating for flexible visitation
- respecting and supporting the patient's and his family's decisions

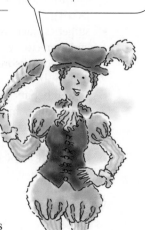

Role call

By filling various nursing and management roles, a critical care nurse helps promote optimum health, prevent illness, and aid coping with illness or death. Here are various capacities in which a critical care nurse may function (some require additional training, education, or advanced practice certification).

Staff nurse

- Makes independent assessments
- Plans and implements patient care
- Provides direct nursing care
- Makes clinical observations and executes interventions
- Administers medications and treatments
- Promotes activities of daily living

Nurse educator

- Assesses patients' and families' learning needs; plans and implements teaching strategies to meet those needs
- Evaluates effectiveness of teaching
- Educates peers and colleagues
- Possesses excellent interpersonal skills

Nurse manager

- Acts as an administrative representative of the unit
- Ensures that effective and quality nursing care is provided in a timely and fiscally sound environment

Case manager

- Manages comprehensive care of an individual patient
- Encompasses the patient's entire illness episode, crosses all care settings, and involves the collaboration of all personnel who provide care

- Is involved in discharge planning and making referrals
- Identifies community and personal resources
- Arranges for equipment and supplies needed by the patient on discharge

Clinical nurse specialist

- Practices as expert in evidence-based nursing
- Engages in mentoring, research, management, and systems improvement
- Participates in education and direct patient care
- Consults with patients and family members
- Collaborates with other nurses and health care team members to deliver high-quality care

Nurse practitioner

- Provides primary health care to patients and families; can function independently
- May obtain histories and conduct physical examinations
- Orders laboratory and diagnostic tests and interprets results
- Diagnoses disorders
- Treats patients
- Counsels and educates patients and families

Nurse researcher

- Reads current nursing literature
- Applies information in practice
- Collects data
- Conducts research studies
- Serves as a consultant during research study implementation

- serving as a liaison between the patient and his family and other members of the health care team
- respecting the values and cultures of the patient
- acting in the patient's best interest.

Stuck in the middle

Being a patient advocate can sometimes cause conflict between you and other members of the health care team. For example, when dialysis is ordered because of a patient's deteriorating renal status, you

One role of the critical care nurse is liaison between the patient and his family and the health care team.

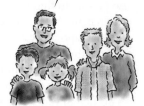

may need to contact the practitioner to relay the patient's request to decline this treatment.

It may also cause conflict between your professional duty and the patient's personal values. For example, the patient may be a Jehovah's Witness and refuse a blood transfusion. In this case, you should consult your facility's ethics committee as well as your facility's policies and procedures.

Clinical judgment

A critical care nurse needs to exercise clinical judgment. To develop sound clinical judgment, you need critical thinking skills. Critical thinking is a complex mixture of knowledge, intuition, logic, common sense, and experience.

Why be critical?

Critical thinking fosters understanding of issues and enables you to quickly find answers to difficult questions. It isn't a trial-and-error method, yet it isn't strictly a scientific problem-solving method, either.

Critical thinking enhances your ability to identify a patient's needs. It also enables you to use sound clinical decision making and to determine which nursing actions best meet a patient's needs.

Developing critical thinking skills

Critical thinking skills improve with increasing clinical and scientific experience. The best way for you to develop critical thinking skills is by asking questions and learning.

Always asking questions

The first question you should find the answer to is "What's the patient's diagnosis?" If it's a diagnosis with which you aren't familiar, look it up and read about it. Find the answers to such questions as these:

- What are the signs and symptoms?
- What's the usual cause?
- What complications can occur?

In addition to finding the answers to diagnosis-related questions, also be sure to find out:

- What are the patient's physical examination findings?
- What laboratory and diagnostic tests are necessary?
- Does the patient have any risk factors? If so, are they significant? What interventions would minimize those risk factors?
- What are the possible complications? What type of monitoring is needed to watch for complications?

> Here's a thought! Critical thinking fosters understanding and enables us to solve difficult problems.

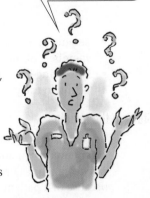

> Part of being a critical thinker is asking the right questions and digging to find the right answers.

- What are the usual medications and treatments for the patient's condition? (If you aren't familiar with the medications or treatments, look them up in a reliable source or consult a colleague.)
- What are the patient's cultural beliefs? How can you best address the patient's cultural concerns?

Critical thinking and the nursing process

Critical thinking skills are necessary when applying the nursing process—assessment, planning, intervention, and evaluation—and making patient care decisions.

Step 1: Assessment

To obtain assessment data:
- ask relevant questions
- validate evidence or data that has been collected
- identify present and potential concerns.
  Then be sure to analyze the assessment data and determine the nursing diagnoses. To do this, you must interpret the collected data and identify gaps. For example, if laboratory values are missing, call to obtain test results or schedule a test that wasn't performed.

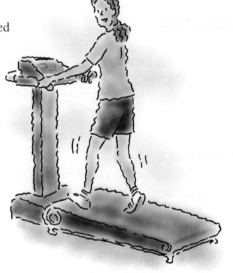

It's a workout for the mind. Applying the nursing process requires critical thinking.

Step 2: Planning

During the planning stage, critical thinking skills come in handy when considering how the patient is expected to achieve goals. During this stage, consider the consequences of planned interventions. This is also the time to set priorities of care for the patient.

Step 3: Implementation

During the implementation stage, use critical thinking to involve the patient and other members of the health care team in implementing the care plan.

Step 4: Evaluation

During the evaluation stage, use critical thinking to continually reassess, modify, and individualize care. Evaluation enables you to assess the patient's responses and determine whether expected outcomes have been met.

Caring practice

Caring practice is the use of a therapeutic and compassionate environment to focus on the patient's needs. Although care is based on standards and protocols, it must also be individualized to each patient.

Caring practice also involves:
- maintaining a safe environment
- interacting with the patient and his family in a compassionate and respectful manner throughout the critical care stay
- supporting the patient and his family in end-of-life issues and decisions.

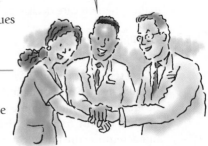

Critical care nurses are usually chief coordinators of a collaborative team of highly skilled professionals— pretty impressive, huh?

Collaboration

Collaboration allows a health care team to use all available resources for the patient. A critical care nurse is part of a multidisciplinary team in which each person contributes expertise. The collaborative goal is to optimize patient outcomes. As a nurse, you may often serve as the coordinator of such collaborative teams.

Two ways about it

Models of collaborative care include case management and outcome management:
- *Case management* consists of coordinating and organizing patient care in collaboration with the primary care practitioner.
- *Outcome management* uses a quality improvement process and team approach to manage patient outcomes.

Cultural awareness and sensitivity . . . it's all part of the patient equation in delivering high-quality care.

Cultural diversity

Culture is defined as the way people live and how they behave in a social group. This behavior is learned and passed on from generation to generation. Acknowledging and respecting patients' diverse cultural beliefs is a necessary part of high-quality care.

Keep an open mind

A critical care nurse is expected to demonstrate awareness and sensitivity toward a patient's religion, lifestyle, family makeup, socioeconomic status, age, gender, and values. Be sure to assess cultural factors and concerns and integrate them into the care plan.

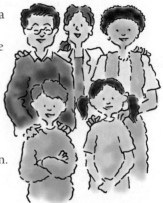

Education

As an educator, a critical care nurse is the facilitator of patient, family, and staff education. Patient education involves teaching patients and their families about:

- the patient's illness
- the importance of managing comorbid disorders (such as diabetes, arthritis, and hypertension)
- diagnostic and laboratory testing
- planned surgical procedures, including preoperative and postoperative expectations
- instructions on specific patient care, such as wound care and range-of-motion exercises.

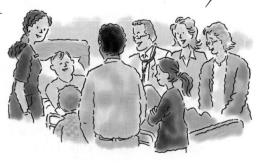

Critical care nurses are teachers, too. Their students include patients, family members, and other staff.

Staff as students

Critical care nurses also commonly serve as staff educators. Examples of staff teaching topics you may need to address include how to:

- use new equipment
- interpret diagnostic test results
- administer a new medication.

Becoming a critical care nurse

Most nursing students are only briefly exposed to critical care nursing. Much of the training required to become a critical care nurse is learned on the job.

Learning by doing

On-the-job training is central to gaining the extensive skills required by a critical care nurse. There are several ways to become trained as a critical care nurse.

One way . . .

Your facility may provide a critical care course. Such courses vary in duration from 1 to 3 months. The course consists of online learning modules or classroom lectures and clinical exposure to the critical care environment.

. . . or another

Your facility may also provide a competency-based orientation program for new critical care nurses. In a program such as this, you gain knowledge and experience while working in the ICU/CCU with a *preceptor* (a staff nurse or clinical nurse specialist with specialized training in critical care nursing) who provides guidance.

An orientation period allows the nurse time to acquire knowledge and the technical skills needed to work in the critical care environment. Such technical skills include working with equipment, such as cardiac monitoring systems, mechanical ventilators, hemodynamic monitoring devices, and intracranial pressure (ICP) monitoring devices. The nurse must also understand the actions of the various critical care medications she gives.

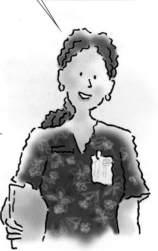

CCRN certification tells everyone you're highly skilled in a specialized area of nursing. A CCRN may be certified in adult, pediatric, or neonatal critical care.

Gaining credentials

The American Association of Critical-Care Nurses (AACN) is one of the world's largest specialty nursing organizations, with more than 80,000 members. The primary goal of the AACN is to enhance the education of critical care nurses.

Through AACN, you can become certified as a CCRN in adult, pediatric, or neonatal critical care. CCRN certification tells everyone you're a professional, with proficiency and skill in a highly specialized area of nursing. Many specialty nursing organizations offer certification. (See *Organizations offering certifications*.)

CCRN certification requires renewal after 3 years. Nurses can recertify by taking the examination again or by demonstrating continuing education in critical care nursing (by working 432 hours of direct bedside care and completing 100 continuing education hours during the certification period).

Help wanted

Certification isn't mandatory to work as a critical care nurse, but it's certainly encouraged. Many units prefer to hire nurses with certification because it means that they have demonstrated expertise and commitment to critical care nursing.

Safety first

The goal of any nursing certification program is to promote safe nursing care. CCRN certification is evidence that a nurse has demonstrated clinical excellence and recognizes the importance of patient safety. Certification validates the nurse's qualifications and specialized clinical knowledge.

What's in it for me?

For most nurses, the main reason for seeking CCRN certification is personal fulfillment, but there are other rewards as well. Many institutions reimburse nurses for taking the examination, and others offer monetary incentives to nurses with CCRN certification.

Organizations offering certifications

Here's a list of professional organizations that offer certifications of interest to critical care nurses.

- American Association of Critical-Care Nurses, *www.aacn.org*
- American Association of Neuroscience Nurses, *www.aann.org/cnrn/content /certification*
- American Board of Perianesthesia Nursing Certification, Inc., *www.cpancapa.org*
- American Nurses Credentialing Center, *www.nursingworld.org/ancc*
- Board of Certification for Emergency Nursing, *www.ena.org/bcen*
- Nephrology Nursing Certification Commission, *www.nncc-exam.org*

Nursing responsibilities

As a critical care nurse, you're responsible for all parts of the nursing process: assessing, planning, implementing, and evaluating care of critically ill patients. Remember that each of these steps gives you an opportunity to exercise your critical thinking skills.

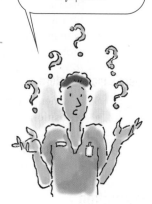

Critical care assessment involves constantly evaluating the patient's condition and monitoring equipment.

Assessment

Critical care nursing requires that you constantly assess the patient for subtle changes in condition and monitor all equipment being used. Caring for critically ill patients may involve the use of such highly specialized equipment as cardiac monitors, hemodynamic monitoring devices, intra-aortic balloon pumps, and ICP monitoring devices. As part of the patient assessment, you also assess the patient's physical and psychological statuses and interpret laboratory data.

Planning

Planning requires you to consider the patient's psychological and physiologic needs and set realistic patient goals. The result is an individualized care plan for your patient. To ensure safe passage through the critical care environment, you must also anticipate changes in the patient's condition. For example, for a patient admitted with a diagnosis of MI, you should monitor cardiac rhythm and anticipate rhythm changes. If an arrhythmia such as complete heart block develops, the treatment plan may need to be changed and new goals established.

What's the problem?

In planning, be sure to address present and potential problems, such as:
- pain
- cardiac arrhythmias
- altered hemodynamic states
- impaired physical mobility
- impaired skin integrity
- deficient fluid volume.

Implementation

As a nurse, you must implement specific interventions to address existing and potential patient problems.

A call to intervene

Examples of interventions include:
- monitoring and treating cardiac arrhythmias
- assessing hemodynamic parameters, such as pulmonary artery pressure, central venous pressure, and cardiac output
- titrating vasoactive drips
- managing pain
- monitoring responses to therapy.

There's more in store

Some other common interventions are:
- repositioning the patient to maintain joint and body functions
- performing hygiene measures to prevent skin breakdown
- elevating the head of the bed to improve ventilation.

Evaluation

It's necessary for you to continually evaluate a patient's response to interventions. Use such evaluations to change the care plan as needed to make sure that your patient continues to work toward achieving his outcome goals.

Multidisciplinary teamwork

Nurses working with critically ill patients commonly collaborate with a multidisciplinary team of health care professionals. The team approach enables caregivers to better meet the diverse needs of individual patients.

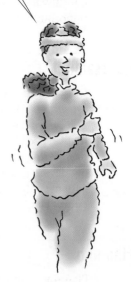

Gotta run! The wide range of interventions I perform really keeps me on the go!

The goal is holism

The goal of collaboration is to provide effective and comprehensive (holistic) care. Holistic care addresses the biologic, psychological, social, and spiritual dimensions of a person.

Team huddle

A multidisciplinary team providing direct patient care may consist of many professionals. Members commonly include:

- registered nurses
- doctors
- physician assistants
- advanced practice registered nurses (such as clinical nurse specialists and nurse practitioners)
- patient care technicians
- respiratory therapists and others. (See *Meet the team*, page 12.)

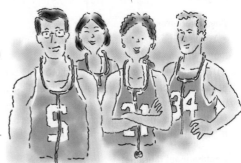

Everyone on the health care team contributes expertise. The goal is to provide effective holistic care.

Working with registered nurses

Teamwork is essential in the stressful environment of the ICU/CCU. The critical care nurse needs to work well with the other professional registered nurses on the unit.

The buddy system

It's important to have a colleague to look to for moral support, physical assistance with a patient, and problem solving. No one person has all the answers, but, together, nurses have a better chance of solving any problem.

Working with doctors

Patients in the ICU/CCU rarely have only one doctor. Most have an admitting doctor and several consultants, such as:

- a cardiologist
- a neurologist
- a pulmonologist
- an infectious disease specialist.

In addition, if you work in a teaching institution, you may also interact on a regular basis with medical students, interns, and residents who are under the direction of the attending doctor.

Coordinated efforts

Having a good professional working relationship with doctors involved in patient care is essential. In many cases, a nurse coordinates patient care among the many different specialists.

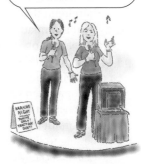

Teamwork requires a lot of coordination! It's so groovy when everything comes together.

Meet the team

Various members of the multidisciplinary team have collaborative relationships with critical care nurses. Here are some examples.

Patient care technician
- Provides direct patient care to critically ill patients
- Bathes patients
- Obtains vital signs
- Assists with transportation of patients for testing

Physical therapist
- Assesses muscle groups and mobility and improves motor function of critically ill patients
- Develops specialized care plan and provides care based on the patient's functional abilities and the disease process or physical injury
- Teaches gait and transfer training to patients and other health care team members

Occupational therapist
- Assesses a patient's activities of daily living
- Teaches the patient and his family methods for completing these tasks and achieving the discharge plan

Speech pathologist
- Assesses the critically ill patient's ability to swallow and develops a care plan with appropriate interventions
- Assesses for speech and language disorders
- Teaches techniques for dealing with swallowing impairment, communication methods for those with aphasia, and techniques to assist with auditory processing difficulties
- Works with health care providers to reinforce treatment

Wound-ostomy-continence nurse
- Assesses, monitors, and makes recommendations to the practitioner regarding the patient's skin integrity and bowel and bladder issues
- Helps to develop a treatment plan

Dietitian
- Monitors a critically ill patient's dietary intake
- Assesses the patient's daily caloric intake and reports deviations
- Devises meal plans to meet the practitioner-recommended needs for the patient
- Recommends dietary interventions

Pastoral caregiver
- Also known as a *chaplain*
- Meets patient's and family's spiritual and religious needs
- Provides support and empathy to the patient and his family
- Delivers patient's last rites if appropriate

Social services
- Assists patients and families with such problems as difficulty paying for medications, follow-up physician visits, and other health-related issues
- Assists patients with travel and housing if needed

Short and sweet

Because a doctor is available on the unit for only a short period, it's important that you accurately and succinctly convey important patient information to him during that time. When a doctor is visiting his patient on the unit, you need to relay assessment findings, laboratory data, and patient care issues in a concise report.

You'll often collaborate with doctors on patient care decisions; you may even suggest additional treatments or interventions that may benefit the patient. In addition, you need to know when it's important to call the doctor with a change in the patient's condition. Be sure to have important information at hand before you call. (See *Communicating effectively using SBAR*, page 14.)

Working with physician assistants

Physician assistants (PAs) are specially trained health care professionals who work under the supervision of a doctor. PAs conduct physical examinations, order tests and medications, assist in surgery, and have autonomy in medical decision making.

Typically, a PA helps the doctor care for patients in an ICU/CCU. You will need to have the same information available for a PA that you would for a doctor. You should also expect the PA to write orders for your patient, both independently and after consulting with the patient's doctor.

Working with advanced practice registered nurses

Advanced practice registered nurses—clinical nurse specialists (CNSs) and adult geriatric acute care nurse practitioners (AGACNPs)—are increasingly seen working in ICU/CCUs. An advanced practice nurse may be employed by a hospital and assigned to a specific unit or she may be employed by a doctor to assist in caring for and monitoring patients. The advanced practice nurse assists staff nurses in clinical decision making and enhances the quality of patient care, which improves patient care outcomes.

The roles of a lifetime

The traditional roles of a CNS are:
- clinician
- educator
- researcher
- consultant
- manager.

The CNS offers support and guidance to staff nurses as they care for patients. She assists with problem solving when complex care is necessary for patients and their families. In addition, the CNS may develop research projects dealing with problems identified on the unit. In some facilities, a CNS may be a case manager or outcomes manager.

On a role

An AGACNP fills the traditional roles of a nurse practitioner. These may include:
- conducting comprehensive health assessments
- diagnosing
- prescribing pharmacologic and nonpharmacologic treatments.

An AGACNP may also conduct research, manage care, and perform advanced procedures, such as removing chest tubes and inserting central lines.

Communicating effectively using SBAR

Because communication failures in health care can lead to errors and serious adverse events, health care professionals must pay close attention to communicating effectively. Consistent use of a structured communication tool, such as SBAR (situation, background, assessment, recommendation), improves the effectiveness of communications, provides a safer environment for patients, and promotes collegial relationships among health care team members.

SBAR is a communication tool for ensuring that the right information gets to the right person in the most clear, concise, and effective way. Each component of the tool seeks to answer a question:

Situation: What is going on at the present time?
This first step calls for a concise description of the current situation.

Background: What has happened in the past and is relevant to this situation?
In this step, you need to put the situation into context for the listener. Don't assume that the listener remembers the patient by giving only superficial information, such as a room number or any other brief information. However, limit the background information to only what is pertinent to the situation at hand.

Assessment: What do you think is happening?
This step summarizes your analysis of the situation after considering the data gathered in the background step. In the assessment step, your communication includes your concise assessment of the situation in a couple of sentences at most, the interventions you have started and the results so far, and your estimate of how serious the situation is and how quickly the receiver needs to act.

Recommendation: What do you think needs to be done?
Before ending the conversation, both parties must have an opportunity to clarify information and ask questions. To ensure that all information has been sent and received correctly, both parties should repeat the decisions made to resolve the problem. If they disagree about how to resolve the situation, they should use the SBAR tool again to make sure that all information about the situation has been sent and received. Always remember to stay calm and focused during the conversation to ensure that the information is received and sent accurately. Lastly, both parties should agree on the follow-up plan.

In the ICU/CCU, we're all packing the most efficient tools to get the job done.

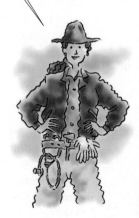

Working with patient care technicians

In many ICUs/CCUs, patient care technicians are members of the health care team. Generally, a patient care technician works under the supervision of a registered nurse to deliver patient care. The registered nurse is responsible for and delegates specific tasks to the patient care technician, which may include bathing and feeding patients, taking and recording vital signs, and performing such bedside testing as ECGs and blood glucose monitoring.

Working with respiratory therapists

A critical care nurse also commonly collaborates with a respiratory therapist in caring for critically ill patients.

Respiration-related roles

The role of a respiratory therapist is to monitor and manage the respiratory status of patients. To do this, the respiratory therapist may:
- administer breathing treatments
- suction patients
- collect specimens
- obtain arterial blood gas values
- manage ventilator changes.

In some cases, you may need to work closely with a respiratory therapist. For example, when weaning a patient from a ventilator, you're both responsible for monitoring the patient's response to ventilator changes and tolerance to weaning. You may also work closely with a respiratory therapist and others as a member of a rapid response team. (See *Understanding the rapid response team*, page 16.)

Clinical tools

The multidisciplinary team uses various tools to promote safe and comprehensive holistic care. These tools include clinical pathways, practice guidelines, and protocols.

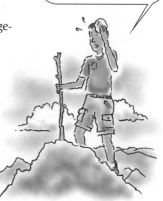

Oh, my! I must have taken a wrong turn at that last checkpoint. Better double-time it back to the ICU/CCU!

Clinical pathways

Clinical pathways (also known as *critical pathways*) are care management plans for patients with a given diagnosis or condition.

Follow the path

Clinical pathways are typically generated and used by facilities that deliver care for similar conditions to many patients. A multidisciplinary committee of clinicians at the facility usually develops clinical pathways. The overall goals are to:
- establish a standard approach to care for all providers in the facility
- establish roles for various members of the health care team
- provide a framework for collecting data on patient outcomes.

Take charge!

Understanding the rapid response team

In 2004, the Institute for Healthcare Improvement (IHI) encouraged hospitals to implement rapid response teams (RRTs). The use of RRTs was identified as an evidence-based, lifesaving strategy that would improve patient outcomes by preventing avoidable patient deaths outside the critical care areas.

Research has shown that a patient's condition can start to deteriorate about 6.5 hours before an unexpected critical event or actual cardiac arrest and that 70% of these events are preventable. Early recognition of warning signs of clinical deterioration and interventions by an RRT helps provide better outcomes for general medical-surgical patients and may also decrease the number of unnecessary transfers to a critical care unit.

Part of the team

An RRT can be called to a patient's bedside 24 hours a day, 7 days a week. Most RRTs consist of a structured group and usually include a critical care nurse, a respiratory therapist, and, possibly, a provider (physician or advanced practice registered nurse) who collaborates with the patient's nurse and intervenes. The RRT may be called on at any time a staff member becomes concerned about a patient's condition.

Criteria for activating the RRT vary, but most facilities have established evidence-based criteria to facilitate early identification of physiologic deterioration in adults and children. These guidelines help novice staff members determine if an RRT should be called for a bedside consultation.

Criteria for RRTs

Criteria may include:
- difficulty breathing, increased use of accessory muscles to breathe
- changes in respiratory rate—access for respiratory rate sustained at less than 10 beats/minute or greater than 30 beats/minute
- pulse oximetry readings less than 85% for more than 5 minutes not responding to oxygen therapy or escalating oxygen requirements
- new onset chest pain or chest pain not relieved with nitroglycerin
- hypotension with systolic blood pressure less than 90 mm Hg, not responding to I.V. fluid orders
- hypertension with systolic blood pressure greater than 200 mm Hg or diastolic blood pressure greater than 120 mm Hg
- bradycardia, sustained, less than 50 beats/minute
- tachycardia, sustained, greater than 130 beats/minute
- mottling or cyanosis of an extremity
- change in level of consciousness
- seizure
- stroke symptoms—changes in vision, loss of speech, weakness of an extremity
- sepsis or systemic inflammatory response syndrome (SIRS)
- bleeding into the airway
- uncontrolled bleeding from the surgical site or lower GI tract.

Tried and true

Pathways are based on evidence from reliable sources, such as benchmarks, research, and guidelines. The committee gathers and uses information from peer-reviewed literature and experts outside the facility.

Outlines and timelines

Clinical pathways usually outline the duties of all professionals involved with patient care. They follow specific timelines for indicated actions. They also specify expected patient outcomes, which serve as checkpoints for the patient's progress and caregiver's performance.

It's the responsibility of every nurse to stay up-to-date on the latest practice guidelines.

Practice guidelines

Practice guidelines specify courses of action to be taken in response to a diagnosis or condition. They reflect value judgments about the relative importance of various health and economic outcomes.

Practice guidelines aid decision making by providers. They're multidisciplinary in nature and can be used to coordinate care by multiple providers.

Let an expert be your guide

Expert health care providers usually write practice guidelines. They condense large amounts of information into easily usable formats, combining clinical expertise with the best available clinical evidence. Practice guidelines are used to:
- streamline care
- control variations in practice patterns
- distribute health care resources more effectively.

The evidence is in

Practice guidelines are valuable sources of information. They indicate which tests and treatments are appropriate. They also provide a framework for building a standard of care (a statement describing an expected level of care or performance).

Consider the source

Like research-based information, clinical guidelines should be evaluated for the quality of their sources. It's a good idea to read the developers' policy statement about how evidence was selected and what values were applied in making recommendations for care.

Protocols

Protocols are facility-established sets of procedures for a given circumstance. Their purpose is to outline actions that are most likely to produce optimal patient outcomes.

First things first

Protocols describe a sequence of actions a practitioner should take to establish a diagnosis or begin a treatment regimen. For example, a pain management protocol outlines a bedside strategy for managing acute pain.

Protocols facilitate delivery of consistent, cost-effective care. They're also educational resources for clinicians who strive to keep abreast of current best practices. Protocols may be either highly directive or flexible, allowing practitioners to use clinical judgment.

Input from experts

Nursing or medical experts write protocols, commonly with input from other health care providers. They may be approved by legislative bodies, such as boards of nursing or medicine in some states. Hospital committees may approve other types of protocols for various facilities.

Best practices

As new procedures and medicines become available, nurses committed to excellence regularly update and adapt their practices. An approach known as *best practice* is an important tool for providing high-quality care.

Best for all concerned

The term *best practice* refers to clinical practices, treatments, and interventions that result in the best possible outcomes for both the patient and your facility.

The best practice approach is generally a team effort that draws on various types of information. Common sources of information used to identify best practices are research data, personal experience, and expert opinion. (See *Research and nursing*.)

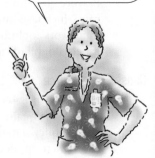

Simply put, the best practice results in the best possible outcomes for both the patient and your facility—and that's A-OK with me!

Critical care research

The goal of critical care research is to improve the delivery of care and, thereby, improve patient outcomes. Nursing care is commonly based on evidence that's derived from research. Evidence can be used to support current practices or to change practices.

Research and nursing

All scientific research is based on the same basic process.

Research steps

The research process consists of these steps:

1. **Identify a problem.** Identifying problems in the critical care environment isn't difficult. An example of such a problem is skin breakdown.
2. **Conduct a literature review.** The goal of this step is to see what has been published about the identified problem.
3. **Formulate a research question or hypothesis.** In the case of skin breakdown, one question is, "Which type of adhesive is most irritating to the skin of a patient on bed rest?"
4. **Design a study.** The study may be experimental or nonexperimental. The nurse must decide what data are to be collected and how to collect that data.
5. **Obtain consent.** The nurse must obtain consent to conduct research from the study participants. Most facilities have an internal review board that must approve such permission for studies.
6. **Collect data.** After the study is approved, the nurse can begin conducting the study and collecting the data.
7. **Analyze the data.** The nurse analyzes the data and states the conclusions derived from the analysis.
8. **Share the information.** Lastly, the researcher shares the collected information with other nurses through publications and presentations.

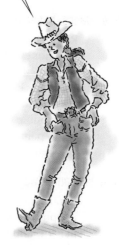

It seems there are more than *two* steps in this research process!

The best way to get involved in research is to be a good consumer of nursing research. You can do so by reading nursing journals and being aware of the quality of research and reported results.

Share and share alike

Don't be afraid to share research findings with colleagues. Sharing promotes sound clinical care, and all involved may learn about easier and more efficient ways to care for patients.

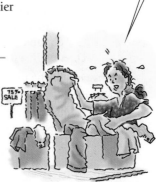

Well, I'm just following the book's advice . . . I read that shopping can be very therapeutic for busy nurses. Isn't this a way of being a good consumer of nursing research?

Evidence-based care

Health care professionals have long recognized the importance of laboratory research and have developed ways to make research results more useful in clinical practice. One way is by delivering evidence-based care.

Evidence-based care isn't based on tradition, custom, or intuition. It's derived from various concrete sources, such as:

- formal nursing research
- clinical knowledge
- scientific knowledge.

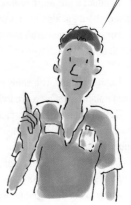

The number 1 goal of delivering evidence based care is to improve nursing care and patient outcomes.

An evidence-based example

Research results may provide insight into the treatment of a patient who, for example, doesn't respond to a medication or treatment that seemed effective for other patients.

In this example, you may believe that a certain drug should be effective for pain relief based on previous experience with that drug. The trouble with such an approach is that other factors can contribute to pain relief, such as the route of administration, the dosage, and concurrent treatments.

First, last, and always

Regardless of the value of evidence-based care, you should always use professional clinical judgment when dealing with critically ill patients and their families. Remember that each patient's condition ultimately dictates treatment.

Quick quiz

1. To work in an ICU/CCU, you must:
    A. have a baccalaureate degree.
    B. have certification in critical care nursing.
    C. use the nursing process in delivering nursing care.
    D. possess an advanced nursing degree.

Answer: C. The professional nurse uses the nursing process (assessment, planning, implementation, and evaluation) to care for critically ill patients.

2. Professional certification in critical care nursing allows you to:
    A. function as an advanced practice nurse.
    B. validate knowledge and skills in critical care nursing.
    C. obtain an administrative position.
    D. obtain a pay raise.

Answer: B. The purpose of professional certifications is to validate knowledge and skill in a particular area. Certification is a demonstration of excellence and commitment to your chosen specialty area.

3. The purpose of the multidisciplinary team is to:
    A. assist the nurse in performing patient care.
    B. replace the concept of primary care in the acute care setting.
    C. minimize lawsuits on the ICU/CCU.
    D. provide holistic, comprehensive care to the patient.

Answer: D. The purpose of the multidisciplinary team is to provide comprehensive care to the critically ill patient.

4. When alerting a doctor about a change in a patient's status, you need to:
    A. fax all of the vital signs to his office first.
    B. use a structured communication tool such as SBAR.
    C. ask for specific orders.
    D. delegate the phone call to the charge nurse.

Answer: B. Consistent use of a structured communication tool, such as SBAR, improves the effectiveness of communication and provides a safer environment for patients.

5. The easiest way to participate in research is to:
    A. be a good consumer of research.
    B. analyze related studies.
    C. conduct a research study.
    D. participate on your facility's internal review board.

Answer: A. Begin by reading research articles and judging whether they're applicable to your practice. Research findings aren't useful if they aren't incorporated into practice.

6. The purpose of evidence-based practice is to:
    A. validate traditional nursing practices.
    B. improve patient outcomes.
    C. refute traditional nursing practices.
    D. establish a body of knowledge unique to nursing.

Answer: B. Although evidence-based practices may validate or refute traditional practice, the purpose is to improve patient outcomes.

Scoring

☆☆☆   If you answered all six questions correctly, take a bow. You're basically a wiz when it comes to critical care basics.

  ☆☆   If you answered four or five questions correctly, there's no room for criticism. Your critical thinking skills are basically intact.

    ☆   If you answered fewer than four questions correctly, the situation is critical. Review the chapter and you'll be on the right pathway.

Suggested References

American Association of Critical-Care Nurses. (2011). *AACN PracticeAlert: Family presence: Visitation in the adult ICU*. Retrieved from http://www.aacn.org/wd/practice/content/practicealerts/family-visitation-icu-practicealert.pdf

Hardin, S. R., Bernhardt-Tindal, K., Hart, A., Stepp, A., & Henson, A. (2011). Critical-care visitation: The patients' perspective. *Dimensions in Critical Care Nursing*, *30*(1), 53–61.

Institute for Healthcare Improvement. (2014). *SBAR toolkit*. Retrieved from http://www.ihi.org/knowledge/pages/Tools/SBARToolkit.aspx

Leonard, M., Graham, S., & Bonacum, D. (2004). The human factor: The critical importance of effective teamwork and communication in providing safe care. *Quality Safe Health Care*, *13*, 185–190.

McHugh, M. D., Kelly, L. A., Smith, H. L., Wu, E. S., Vanak, J. M., & Aiken, L. H. (2013). Lower mortality in magnet hospitals. *Medical Care*, *51*(5), 382–388. Retrieved from http://www.ncbi.nlm.nih.gov/pubmed/23047129

Perrin, K. O. (2009). *Understanding the essentials of critical care nursing*. Upper Saddle River, NJ: Pearson/Prentice Hall.

Chapter 2

Holistic care issues

Just the facts

In this chapter, you'll learn:

♦ how illness affects family dynamics and family members' ability to cope

♦ issues that commonly affect critically ill patients and their families

♦ ways to assess and manage pain in critically ill patients

♦ important questions to consider when faced with ethical decision making

♦ concepts related to end-of-life decisions and how they're important to your care.

What is holistic health care?

Holistic health care revolves around a notion of totality. The goal of holistic care is to meet not just the patient's physical needs but also his social and emotional needs.

The whole is the goal

Holistic care addresses all dimensions of a person, including:
- physical
- emotional
- social
- spiritual.

Only by considering all dimensions of a person can the health care team provide high-quality holistic care. You should strive to provide holistic care to all critically ill patients, even though their physical needs may seem more pressing than their other needs.

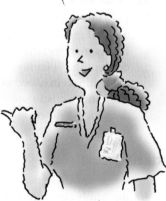

Here's the whole story about holistic health care.

The issues

The road to the goal of delivering the best holistic care is riddled with various issues (problems or concerns), including:
- patient and family issues
- cognitive issues
- pain control issues
- ethics issues.

Patient and family issues

A family is a group of two or more persons who possibly live together in the same household, perform certain interrelated social tasks, and share an emotional bond. Families can profoundly influence the individuals within them.

Family ties

A family is a dynamic system. During stress-free times, this system tends to maintain homeostasis, meaning that it exists in a stable state of harmony and balance. However, when a crisis sends a family member into a critical care environment, family members may feel a tremendous strain and family homeostasis is no longer maintained. The major effects of such imbalances are:
- increased stress levels for family members
- fear of death for the patient
- reorganization of family roles.

Unprepared for the worst

The family may be caught off guard by sudden exposure to the hospital environment, causing homeostasis to be disrupted. Family members may worry about the possible death of the ill family member. The suddenness of the illness may overwhelm the family and put it into a crisis state. The ramifications of the patient's illness may cause other family members to feel hopeless and helpless.

Circle out of round

When sudden critical illness or injury disrupts the family circle, the patient can no longer fulfil certain role responsibilities. Such roles are typically:
- financial (if the patient is a major contributor to the family's monetary stability)

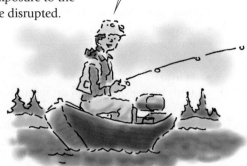

Holy mackerel (or maybe flounder)! Holistic care means that you may have to deal with several patient and family issues.

- social (if the patient fills such roles as spouse, parent, mediator, or disciplinarian).

One thing leads to another

A sudden shift in the patient's ability to bear family responsibilities can create havoc and a feeling of overwhelming responsibility for other family members.

Nursing responsibilities

Because a critical illness or injury greatly affects family members as well, be sure to provide care to the family as well as the patient. Members of the patient's family need guidance and support during the patient's hospital stay. The critical care nurse's responsibility to family members is to provide information about:
- nursing care
- the patient's prognosis and expected treatments
- ways to communicate with the patient
- support services that are available.

Slipping on emotional turmoil

The critically ill patient's condition may change rapidly (within minutes or hours). The result of such physiologic instability is emotional turmoil for the family.

The family may use whatever coping mechanisms they have, such as seeking support from friends or clergy. The longer the patient remains in critical care, however, the more stress increases for both the patient and his family. The result can be slow deterioration of the family system.

Step in and lend a helping hand

Because you're regularly exposed to members of the patient's family, you can help them during their time of crisis. For example, you can observe the anxiety level of family members and, if necessary, refer them to another member of the multidisciplinary team, such as a clinical social worker.

You can also help family members solve problems by assisting them to:
- verbalize the immediate problem
- identify support systems
- recall how they handled stress in the past.

Such assistance helps family members to focus on the present issue. It also allows them to solve problems and regain a sense of control over their lives.

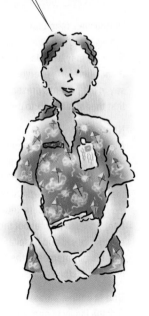

Stand by to answer whatever questions family members have. They may turn to you for guidance and support.

Lean on me

You can also help family members cope with their feelings during this stressful time. Two ways to do this are by encouraging expression of feelings (such as by crying or discussing the issue) and providing empathy.

Since you asked

During a patient's critical illness, family members come to rely on the opinions of professionals and commonly ask for their input. They need honest information given to them in terms they can understand. In many cases, you're the health care team member who provides this information. (See *Tips for helping the family cope.*)

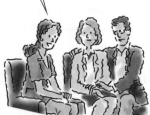

> Be prepared to orient the family to the critical care environment.

Tips for helping the family cope

A large role for the nurse is orienting a patient's family to the critical care unit. Here are some useful tips for dealing with family members of critically ill patients.

Please touch
Let family members know that it's okay to touch the patient. Many are afraid to touch a critically ill loved one for fear of interfering with monitoring equipment or invasive lines. Let them know if there are any special considerations when touching the patient.

Watch your language
Tell visitors that patients may not appear to respond but that they may be able to hear what's going on around them. Therefore, everyone should be careful of what they say in the patient's presence. Let family members know that they should talk to the patient as if he can hear.

How's the weather?
Many family members spend their visitation time looking at equipment in the room and asking the patient questions such as, "Are you in pain?" Encourage them to focus on the patient, not necessarily his pain or surroundings.

Let family members know how to be visitors. The patient wants to hear about the outside world—not reminders that he's ill and hospitalized. He wants to hear about other family members, the family pet, and who won the latest basketball game.

One at a time, please
Ask the family to appoint one spokesperson for the group. This is especially important when families are large.

The spokesperson is the person who should call the unit for updates on the patient's condition. The spokesperson can then spread the word to the rest of the family. It may also be helpful to identify a primary nursing contact for the family.

Should they stay or should they go?
Allow family members to stay at the patient's bedside when possible. For example, a patient may require constant monitoring to keep him from trying to climb out of bed. If a family member is available to stay with such a patient, the use of restraints could be avoided.

On the other hand, some patients appear to be agitated and have adverse changes in their vital signs when certain family members are present. Remember: Your first role is to be a patient advocate and to do what's best for the patient. Ask him whether he wants to have visitors and whom he wants to visit. If having a family member is best for the patient, then allow the visitor to stay. Many units have open visitation policies.

Ensure support
Ensure that support services are available to family members if they need them. If they belong to a particular church, offer to call someone if needed. Most facilities provide spiritual care for families if they request it.

A dose of reality

The best way to respond to concerned family members is to acknowledge their feelings and ambivalences and to lend reality to their statements.

Living with the decision

The nurse can use such phrases as "I know you would like me to decide what's best for your loved one, but I can't make that decision because you're the ones who will live with the consequences of your decision." The critical care nurse then needs to reinforce and acknowledge the family's decision and accept their feelings and decisions.

> As a patient advocate, make it a point to honor the cultural beliefs and values of patients and family members.

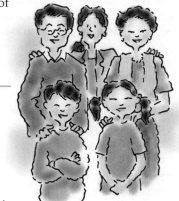

Cultural considerations

How a family copes with the hospitalization of a loved one can be influenced by cultural characteristics. A patient's cultural background can also affect many aspects of care, such as:

- patient and family roles during illness
- communication between health care providers and the patient and family members
- feelings of the patient and family members about end-of-life issues
- family views regarding health care practices
- pain management
- nutrition
- spiritual support.

Culture-clued for care

Because your knowledge about cultural characteristics affects care, you should perform a cultural assessment. (See *Assessing cultural considerations*, page 28.)

Conducting a cultural assessment enables you to:

- recognize a patient's cultural responses to illness and hospitalization
- determine how the patient and his family define health and illness
- determine the patient's and family's beliefs about the cause of the illness.

To provide effective holistic care, you must honor the patient's cultural beliefs and values.

> Although it's good to be aware of cultural considerations, make sure that you don't stereotype patients based on their cultural backgrounds.

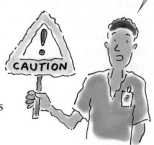

CAUTION

Assessing cultural considerations

A cultural assessment yields the information you need to administer high-quality nursing care to members of various cultural populations. The goal of the cultural assessment quest is to gain awareness and understanding of cultural variations and their effects on the care you provide. For each patient, you and other members of the multidisciplinary team use the findings of a cultural assessment to develop an individualized care plan.

When performing a cultural assessment, be sure to ask questions that yield information about the patient and his family, including information about:
- cultural health beliefs
- communication methods
- cultural restrictions
- social networks
- nutritional status
- religion
- values and beliefs.

Here are examples of the types of questions you should consider for each patient.

Cultural health beliefs
- What does the patient believe caused his illness? A patient may believe that his illness is the result of an imbalance in yin and yang, punishment for a past transgression, or the result of divine wrath.
- How does the patient express pain?
- What does the patient believe promotes health? Beliefs can range from eating certain foods to wearing amulets for good luck.
- In what types of healing practices (such as herbal remedies and healing rituals) does the patient engage?
- Who does the patient go to when he's ill? (Some patients may go to a doctor, a medicine man, or a holistic practitioner.)

Communication differences
- What language does the patient speak?
- Does the patient require an interpreter?
- How does the patient want to be addressed?
- What are the styles of nonverbal communication (eye contact, touching)?

Cultural restrictions
- How does the patient's cultural group express emotion?
- How are feelings about death, dying, and grief expressed?
- How is modesty expressed?
- Does the patient have restrictions related to exposure of any parts of the body?

Social networks
- What are the roles of each family member during health and illness?
- Who makes the decisions?

Nutrition
- What's the meaning of food and eating to the patient?
- What types of food does he eat?
- Does the patient's food need to be prepared a certain way?
- Are there dietary restrictions?

Religion
- What's the role of religious beliefs and practices during illness?
- Does the patient believe that special rites or blessings need to be performed?
- Are there healing rituals or practices that must be followed?

Cognitive issues

A patient on a critical care unit (CCU) may feel overwhelmed by all of the technology in the environment. Although this equipment is essential for patient care, it can create an environment that's foreign to the patient, which can result in disturbed cognition (thought-related function). In addition, the disease process can affect cognitive function in a critically ill patient. For example, patients with metabolic disturbances or hypoxia can experience confusion and changes in sensorium (mental clarity).

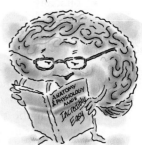

Uh-oh! It says here that the disease process can affect cognitive function.

The way things were

When assessing cognitive function, the first question you should ask is, "What activities were you able to perform by yourself?" If the patient can't answer this question, ask a family member. If the patient has been transferred to the CCU from another floor, ask the nurse who provided care before the transfer.

It's a factor

Many factors affect a patient's cognitive function while on the CCU, including:

- medications
- sensory input
- invasion of personal space
- emotional status
- medical diagnosis
- spiritual status.

Medications

Some medications that can cause adverse central nervous system reactions and affect cognitive function include:

- inotropics—such as digoxin (Lanoxin), which can cause agitation, hallucinations, malaise, dizziness, vertigo, and paresthesia
- corticosteroids—such as prednisone (Sterapred), which can cause euphoria, psychotic behavior, insomnia, vertigo, headache, paresthesia, and seizures
- benzodiazepines—such as lorazepam (Ativan), which can cause drowsiness, sedation, disorientation, amnesia, unsteadiness, and agitation
- opioid analgesics—such as oxycodone (Oxytocin), which can cause sedation, clouded sensorium, euphoria, dizziness, light-headedness, and somnolence.
  - antihypertensive drugs—such as lisinopril (Prinivil), which can increase the risk of falls due to dizziness or light-headedness as the body adjusts to the medication when first prescribed.

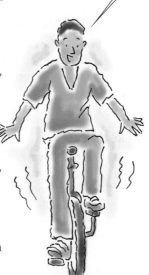

Benzodiazepine medications can cause a patient to become unsteady. Uh oh!

Sensory input

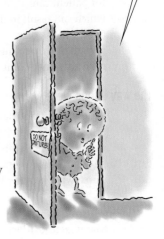

Shhh! Keep it down as much as possible because noise can result in delirium.

Sensory stimulation in any environment may be perceived as pleasant or unpleasant and comfortable or painful. The critical care environment tends to stimulate all five senses:

- auditory
- visual
- gustatory
- olfactory
- tactile.

Too much or too little

Patients on the CCU don't have control over the environmental stimulation around them. They may experience sensory deprivation, sensory overload, or both. Sensory deprivation can result from a reduction in the quantity and quality of normal and familiar sensory input, such as the normal sights and sounds encountered at home. Sensory overload results from an increase in the amount of unfamiliar sounds and sights in the critical care environment, such as beeping cardiac monitors, ringing telephones, overhead paging systems, and voices.

When environmental stimuli exceed the patient's ability to cope with the stimulation, the patient may experience anxiety, confusion, and panic as well as delusions.

A sensitive subject

Sensory deprivation or overload can lead to such problems as sleep disturbances, reality disturbances, and delirium.

Sleep disturbances

Because the critical care environment is typically noisy due to staff, other patients, and equipment alarms, patients on CCUs commonly experience sleep disturbances.

Other factors that interfere with sleep on the CCU include nursing interventions, pain, and fear.

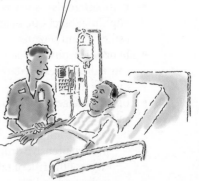

I know how hard it is when I don't get all my sleep. Imagine what it's like for a sleep-deprived patient on the CCU . . . pure torture!

Torture chamber

Sleep deprivation can cause anxiety, restlessness, disorientation, depression, irritability, confusion, combativeness, and hallucinations.

In addition, sleep deprivation can cause further medical problems, such as:

- immunosuppression
- decreased pain tolerance
- decreased muscle strength.

In other words, sleep deprivation can impede the recovery process and contribute to new problems. It has been shown to interfere with functional muscle recovery after an injury.

Quiet time

To promote rest, the critical care nurse can take steps to provide a quieter environment for patients.

For example, the nurse may reduce light and noise by not having loud conversations near the patient and by closing the door to the patient's room if it's safe to do so.

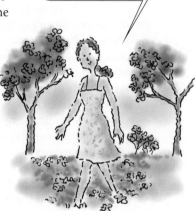

When your reality is altered, it isn't a pretty sight.

Reality disturbances

Integration of the senses is necessary for a person to process environmental information. Disturbances in reality occur when a patient's ability to interpret the environment is altered. Examples of reality disturbances are:

- disorientation to time
- inability to decipher whether it's night or day
- misinterpretation of environmental stimuli—for example, thoughts that alarms and noises from equipment are phones ringing for the patient.

The surreal world

Hearing or vision loss or loss of consciousness (caused, for example, by a head injury) can make a patient especially vulnerable to reality disturbances. Lack of one or more sensory mechanisms that are necessary to function make it hard for the patient to adapt to the critical care environment.

Delirium

Delirium (acute confusion) is an altered state of consciousness, consisting of confusion, distractibility, disorientation, delusional thinking, defective perception, and agitation. When it occurs in a critical care environment, it's commonly called *ICU psychosis*. It has a rapid onset and is generally reversible.

Common contributors

In addition to sensory deprivation or overload, contributing factors that affect most patients on the CCU include:

- infection
- immobility.

Anti-ICU psychosis

The nurse can assist the patient suffering from ICU psychosis by:

- promoting rest
- controlling pain

- monitoring the effects of new medications
- decreasing noise and light in the room
- encouraging mobility when possible
- providing orientation to the patient.

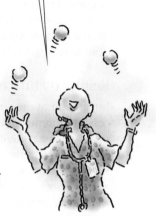

The critical care environment can be a circus. Try to show your patient common courtesies.

Invasion of personal space

Personal space is the unmarked boundary or territory around a person. Several factors—such as cultural background and social situation—influence a patient's interpretation of personal space. A patient's personal space is limited in many ways by the critical care environment—for example, due to the confines of bed rest, lack of privacy, and use of invasive equipment.

You can try to increase your patient's sense of personal space—even within the critical care environment—by simply remembering to show common courtesy, such as:

- asking permission to perform a procedure or look at a wound or dressing
- pulling the curtain or closing the door
- knocking before you enter the patient's room.

Pain control issues

Because fear of pain is a major concern for many critically ill patients, pain management is an important part of your care.

Critical care patients are exposed to many types of procedures—such as I.V. procedures, cardiac monitoring, and intubation—that cause discomfort and pain. Pain is classified as acute or chronic.

Acute pain can be managed effectively, and it generally subsides when the underlying problem is resolved. That's a relief!

Acute pain

Acute pain is caused by tissue damage due to injury or disease. It varies in intensity from mild to severe and lasts briefly (generally up to 6 months).

Acute pain is considered a protective mechanism because it warns of present or potential tissue damage or organ disease. It may result from a traumatic injury, surgical or diagnostic procedure, or medical disorder.

Examples of acute pain are:

- pain experienced during a dressing change
- pain related to surgery
- pain of acute myocardial infarction
- pain of immobility.

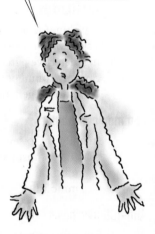

Help is at hand

Acute pain can be managed effectively with analgesics, such as opioids and nonsteroidal anti-inflammatory drugs (NSAIDs). It generally subsides when the underlying problem is resolved.

Chronic pain

Chronic pain is pain that has lasted 6 months or longer and is ongoing. It may be as intense as acute pain, but it isn't a warning of tissue damage. Some patients on the CCU experience chronic as well as acute pain.

Examples of chronic pain include:
- arthritis pain
- back pain
- pain from cancer.

Don't look for the signs

The nervous system adapts to chronic pain. This means that many typical manifestations of pain—such as abnormal vital signs and facial grimacing—cease to exist. Therefore, chronic pain should be assessed as often as acute pain (generally, at least every 2 hours or more often, depending on the patient's condition). Assess chronic pain by questioning the patient.

Pain assessment

When it comes to pain assessment for critical care patients, it's especially important for the nurse to have good assessment skills. The most valid pain assessment comes from the patient's own reports of pain.

A pain assessment includes questions about:
- *location*—Ask the patient to tell you where the pain is; there may be more than one area of pain.
- *intensity*—Ask the patient to rate the pain using a pain scale.
- *quality*—Ask how the pain feels: sharp, dull, aching, or burning.
- *onset, duration, and frequency*—Ask when the pain started, how long it lasts, and how often it occurs.
- *alleviating and aggravating factors*—Ask what makes the pain feel better and what makes it worse.
- *associated factors*—Ask whether other problems are associated with the pain, such as nausea and vomiting.
- *effects on lifestyle*—Ask whether appetite, sleep, relationships, emotions, and work are affected.

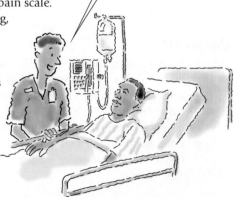

When it comes to pain, the best validation comes from the patient's own reports of pain.

Common pain-rating scales

These scales are examples of the rating systems you can use to help a patient quantify pain levels.

Visual analog scale

To use the visual analog scale, ask the patient to place a line across the scale to indicate the current level of pain. The scale is a 10-cm line with "No pain" at one end and "Pain as bad as it can be" at the other end. The pain rating is determined by using a ruler to measure the distance, in millimeters, from "No pain" to the patient's mark.

No pain _____ **Pain as bad as it can be**

Numeric rating scale

To use the numeric rating scale, ask the patient to choose a number from 0 (indicating no pain) to 10 (indicating the worst pain imaginable) to indicate the current pain level. The patient may circle the number on the scale or verbally state the number that best describes the pain.

No pain | 0   1   2   3   4   5   6   7   8   9   10 | **Pain as bad as it can be**

Faces scale

A pediatric or adult patient with language difficulty may not be able to describe the current pain level using the visual analog scale or the numeric rating scale. In that case, use a faces scale like the one below. Ask your patient to choose the face on a scale from 1 to 6 that best represents the severity of current pain.

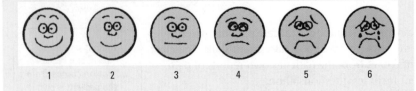

   1   2   3   4   5   6

Choose a tool

Many pain assessment tools are available. Whichever you choose, make sure it's used consistently so that everyone on the health care team is speaking the same language when addressing the patient's pain.

The three most common pain assessment tools used by clinicians are the visual analog scale, numeric rating scale, and faces scale. (See *Common pain-rating scales*.)

The sounds of silence

Many patients can't verbally express feelings of pain. For example, a patient may be unable to speak due to intubation or have an altered level of consciousness (LOC) ranging from confusion to unresponsiveness. In such cases, it's up to the nurse to ascertain the patient's pain level.

Body and mind

There are many physiologic and psychological responses to pain that the nurse should watch for during a pain assessment.

Some examples of the physiologic responses to pain are:
- tachycardia
- tachypnea
- dilated pupils
- increased or decreased blood pressure
- pallor
- nausea and vomiting
- loss of appetite.

Psychological responses to pain may manifest as:
- fear
- anxiety
- confusion
- depression
- sleep deprivation.

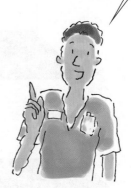

When a patient can't tell you about feelings of pain, it's up to you to see the unspoken signs.

Pain particulars

When communicating aspects of a patient's pain to his practitioner or other health care providers, make sure you:
- describe the pain by location, intensity, and duration
- indicate possible causes of the pain if known
- describe how the patient is responding to the pain or treatment interventions.

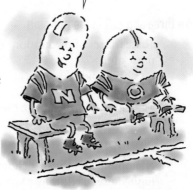

Enjoy the rest, pal. Once we're called up to the CCU, there's no break until the end of the first half.

Pain management

Achieving adequate pain control in critical care depends on effective pain assessment and the use of pharmacologic and nonpharmacologic treatments.

To provide the best holistic care possible, work with the practitioner and other members of the health care team to develop an individualized pain management program for each patient.

Pharmacologic pain management

Pharmacologic pain management is common on CCUs.

The WHO analgesic ladder

The World Health Organization (WHO) developed a three-step ladder (shown here) to guide pain-relief efforts for patients with cancer. Analgesics are selected based on the intensity of the patient's pain. The ladder includes three categories of drugs: nonopioids, opioids, and adjuvant drugs. Adjuvant drugs can be used on any step of the ladder.

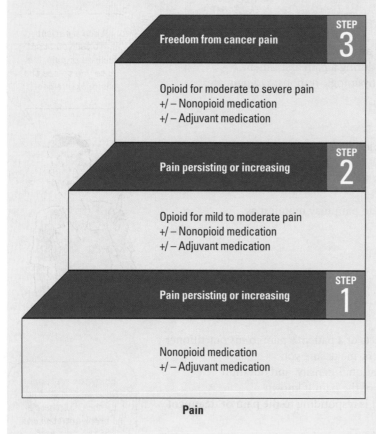

STEP 3
Freedom from cancer pain

Opioid for moderate to severe pain
+/ – Nonopioid medication
+/ – Adjuvant medication

STEP 2
Pain persisting or increasing

Opioid for mild to moderate pain
+/ – Nonopioid medication
+/ – Adjuvant medication

STEP 1
Pain persisting or increasing

Nonopioid medication
+/ – Adjuvant medication

Pain

When the patient's pain reaches the moderate to severe level, administer more potent opioid drugs, including morphine (Roxanol), oxycodone (Oxycontin), hydromorphone (Dilaudid), fentanyl (Sublimaze), and methadone (Dolophine). Nonopioid drugs may be continued.

Add opioid drugs, such as codeine or hydrocodone, for the patient with mild to moderate pain that isn't relieved by a nonopioid. If the patient is already taking NSAIDs, continue to use them, as they add to the analgesic effect.

Administer nonopioid analgesics, such as acetaminophen (Tylenol), aspirin (Ecotrin), and NSAIDs, to the patient just beginning to experience discomfort and mild pain. Although the patient's pain might not be adequately controlled with nonopioid drugs, their use may reduce the overall amount of opioids needed to achieve pain control.

Take three and call in the morning

Three classes of medications commonly used by the critical care nurse are:

- nonopioids
- opioids
- adjuvant medications. (See *The WHO analgesic ladder.*)

Nonopioids

Nonopioids are the first choice for managing mild pain but have a limited use in critically ill patients because of their adverse effects

A trio of opioids

Opioids block the release of neurotransmitters that send pain signals to the brain. The three categories of opioids are opioid agonists (narcotic analgesics), opioid antagonists (narcotic reversal agents), and mixed agonist–antagonists.

Opioid agonists
Opioid agonists relieve pain by binding to pain receptors, which, in effect, produces pain relief. Examples of opioid agonists are:
- morphine (Roxanol)
- fentanyl (Sublimaze)
- hydromorphone (Dilaudid)
- codeine
- oxycodone (Oxycontin).

Opioid antagonists
Opioid antagonists attach to opiate receptors without producing agonistic effects. They work by displacing the opioid at the receptor site and reversing the analgesic and respiratory depressant effects of the opioid.

Examples of opioid antagonists are:
- naloxone
- naltrexone (ReVia).

Mixed opioid agonist–antagonists
Mixed opioid agonist–antagonists relieve pain by binding to opiate receptors to effect varying degrees of agonistic and antagonistic activity.

They carry a lower risk of toxic effects and drug dependency than opioid agonists and opioid antagonists.

Examples of mixed opioid agonist–antagonists are:
- buprenorphine (Buprenex)
- butorphanol (Stadol)
- pentazocine.

and limited parenteral forms. They decrease pain by inhibiting inflammation at the injury site. Examples of nonopioids are:
- acetaminophen (Tylenol)
- NSAIDs, such as ibuprofen (Motrin) and naproxen (Naprosyn)
- salicylates such as aspirin
- tramadol (Ultram)
- lidocaine (Lidoderm)

Opioids

Opioids are narcotics that contain a derivative of the opium (poppy) plant and other synthetic drugs that imitate natural narcotics. Opioids work by blocking the release of neurotransmitters involved in transmitting pain signals to the brain. There are three categories of opioids. (See *A trio of opioids*.)

Adjuvant analgesics

Adjuvant analgesics are drugs that have other primary indications but are used as analgesics in some circumstances.

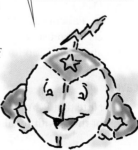

I'm ready to fight pain! Opioids work by blocking the release of neurotransmitters that send out pain signals.

Alone or together

Adjuvants may be given in combination with opioids or alone to treat patients with chronic pain. Drugs used as adjuvant analgesics include:

- anticonvulsants, such as carbamazepine (Tegretol), clonazepam (Klonopin), and gabapentin (Neurontin)
- tricyclic antidepressants, such as amitriptyline (Elavil) and nortriptyline (Aventyl)
- benzodiazepines, such as alprazolam (Xanax), diazepam (Valium), and lorazepam
- corticosteroids, such as dexamethasone (Decadron) and methyl-prednisolone (Medrol).

Drug administration

A common route of pain medication administration on the CCU is I.V. bolus on an as-needed basis. It's the preferred route for opioid therapy, especially when short-term pain relief is needed—for example, during procedures such as wound care. The benefit of this method is rapid pain control. On the downside, with I.V. bolus administration, the patient experiences alternating periods of pain control and pain.

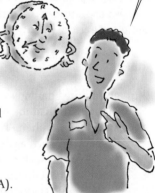

Round-the-clock dosing controls pain better than as-needed administration.

Round-the-clock control

Using around-the-clock dosing ensures that steady levels of drugs prevent exacerbations of pain. This type of dosing has many benefits for critically ill patients who have difficulty communicating their pain because of altered LOC or endotracheal intubation.

Patients overpower pain

Some patients are candidates for patient-controlled analgesia (PCA). PCA provides a constant level of pain medication while allowing the patient to self-administer more pain medication as needed. Controls are set to prevent excessive self-administration. (See *Understanding PCA.*)

Patients usually report that they have more control over pain levels when using PCA. Patients using PCA still require close assessment and evaluation for responses to treatment.

A caveat

Note that PCA may not be appropriate for patients with altered LOC or those with renal or hepatic abnormalities.

Understanding PCA

A PCA system provides an optimal opioid dose while maintaining a constant serum concentration of the drug.

Pump and port

A PCA system consists of a drug delivery injection pump that's piggybacked into an I.V. or subcutaneous infusion port.

By pressing a button, the patient receives a preset bolus dose of an opioid. The practitioner orders the bolus dose and the lockout time between boluses, thus preventing overdose. The device automatically records the number of times the patient presses the button, helping the doctor to adjust drug dosage.

Patient at the controls

Using a PCA system may reduce a patient's drug dosage need. This may be because the patient using PCA is more in control of pain and typically feels reassured knowing that an analgesic is quickly available.

Nonpharmacologic pain management

Pain control isn't achieved solely with medications. Nonpharmacologic means are useful adjuncts in managing pain.

Some common nonpharmacologic pain control methods are:

- distraction—such as television viewing and reading
- music therapy—a form of sound therapy using rhythmic sound to communicate, relax, and encourage healing (This method works for brief periods.)
- biofeedback—requires use of a biofeedback machine and allows the patient to recognize and control the relaxation process, thereby exerting conscious control over various autonomic functions.

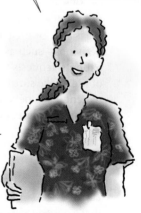

A biofeedback machine allows the patient to recognize and control the relaxation process, thereby controlling his pain.

You're getting sleepy

- hypnosis—used to achieve *symptom suppression*, to block awareness of pain, or *symptom substitution*, which allows a positive interpretation of pain
- imagery—in which the patient visualizes a soothing image while the nurse describes pleasant sensations (e.g., the patient may picture himself at the beach while you describe the sounds of the waves and birds and the feel of the warm sun and a breeze on the patient's skin)
- relaxation therapy—a form of meditation used to focus attention on a single sound or image or on the rhythm of breathing

- heat application (thermotherapy)—application of dry or moist heat to decrease pain (Heat enhances blood flow, increases tissue metabolism, and decreases vasomotor tone; it may also relieve pain due to muscle aches or spasms, itching, or joint pain.)
- cold application (cryotherapy)—constricts blood vessels at the injury site, reducing blood flow to the site (Cold slows edema development, prevents further tissue damage, and minimizes bruising; it may be more effective than heat in relieving such pain as muscle aches or spasms, itching, incision pain, headaches, and joint pain.)
- transcutaneous electrical nerve stimulator—in which electrodes transmit mild electrical impulses to the brain to block pain impulses
- massage therapy—used as an aid to relaxation
- reflexology—used as an aid to relaxation and to reduce pain.

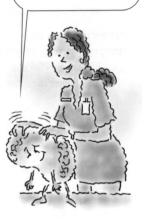

Massage therapy helps to control pain by inducing relaxation.

Ethical issues

Nurses who work on CCUs routinely deal with ethical dilemmas. You'll recognize a situation as an ethical dilemma in the following circumstances:

- More than one solution exists. That is, there's no clear "right" or "wrong" way to handle a situation.
- Each solution carries equal weight.
- Each solution is ethically defensible.

The value of values

Ethical dilemmas on CCUs commonly revolve around quality-of-life issues for the patient, especially as they relate to end-of-life decisions—such as do-not-resuscitate orders, life support, and patients' requests for no heroic measures. When considering quality of life, make sure others don't impose their own value system on the patient. Each person has a set of personal values that are influenced by environment and culture. Nurses also have a set of professional values.

Code of ethics

The American Nurses Association (ANA) has established a code of ethics. The ANA Code of Ethics for Nurses provides information that's necessary for the practicing nurse to use her professional skills in providing the most effective holistic care possible, such as serving as a patient advocate and striving to protect the health, safety, and rights of each patient.

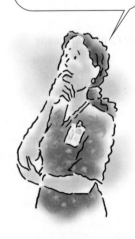

Ethical dilemmas are commonly faced by nurses on the CCU. Always remember to respect the patient's personal values.

End-of-life decisions

The threat of death is common on CCUs. Perhaps at no other time is the holistic care of patients and their families as important as it is during this time.

End-of-life decisions are almost always difficult for patients, families, and health care professionals to make. Nurses are in a unique position as advocates to assist patients and their families through this process.

Unsolvable mysteries

Your primary role as a patient advocate is to promote the patient's wishes. In many instances, however, a patient's wishes aren't known. That's when ethical decision making takes priority. Decisions aren't always easy to make, and the answers aren't usually clear-cut. At times, such ethical dilemmas may seem insolvable.

A question of quality

It's sometimes difficult to determine what can be done to achieve good quality of life and what can simply be achieved, technologically speaking.

Technological advances sometimes seem to exceed our ability to analyze the ethical dilemmas associated with them.

Years ago, death was considered a natural part of life, and most people died at home, surrounded by their families. Today, most people die in hospitals, and death is commonly regarded as a medical failure rather than a natural event. Sometimes it's hard for you to know whether you're assisting in extending the patient's life or delaying the patient's death.

Consulting the committee

Most hospitals have ethics committees that review ethical dilemmas. The nurse may consider consulting the ethics committee if:
- the practitioner disagrees with the patient or his family regarding treatment of the patient.
- health care providers disagree among themselves about treatment options.
- family members disagree about what should be done.

Determining medical futility

Medical futility refers to treatment that's hopeless or interventions that aren't likely to benefit the patient even though they may appear to be effective. For example, a patient with a terminal illness who's expected to die experiences cardiac arrest. Cardiopulmonary resuscitation may

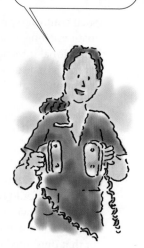

Futile treatment isn't a good use of health care resources and it doesn't change the patient's outcome.

Approaching ethical decisions

When faced with an ethical dilemma, consider these questions:
- What health issues are involved?
- What ethical issues are involved?
- What further information is necessary before a judgment can be made?
- Who will be affected by this decision? (Include the decision maker and other care-givers if they'll be affected emotionally or professionally.)
- What are the values and opinions of the people involved?
- What conflicts exist between the values and ethical standards of the people involved?
- Must a decision be made and, if so, who should make it?
- What alternatives are available?
- For each alternative, what are the ethical justifications?
- For each alternative, what are the possible outcomes?

be effective in restoring a heartbeat but may still be deemed futile because it doesn't change the patient's outcome.

Withholding or withdrawing treatment

The issue of withholding or withdrawing treatment on the CCU presents some ethical dilemmas. When withdrawing treatment from a patient—even at the patient's request—controversy over the principle of nonmaleficence (to prevent harm) may arise.

Harm alarm

Such controversy revolves around the definition of harm. Some feel that removing a patient from a ventilator and allowing death is an intentional infliction of harm. Others argue that keeping a person on a ventilator against the patient's will—thus prolonging death—is an intentional infliction of harm. (See *Approaching ethical decisions*.)

Dealing with cardiac arrest

In case of cardiac arrest (sudden stoppage of the heart), a critically ill patient may be described by a code status. This code status describes the orders written by the practitioner describing what resuscitation measures should be carried out by the nurse and should be based on the patient's wishes regarding resuscitation measures. When cardiac arrest occurs, you must ensure that resuscitative efforts are initiated or that unwanted resuscitation doesn't occur.

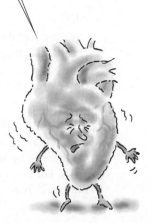

During cardiac arrest, it's typically up to you to ensure that resuscitation is initiated or that unwanted resuscitation doesn't occur.

Who decides?

The wishes of a competent, informed patient should always be honored. However, when a patient can't make decisions, the health care team—consisting of the patient's family, nursing staff, and doctors—may have to make end-of-life decisions for the patient.

Advance directives

Most people prefer to make their own decisions regarding end-of-life care. It's important that patients discuss their wishes with their loved ones; however, many don't. Instead, total strangers may be asked to make important health care decisions when a patient can't do so. That's why it's important for people to make choices ahead of time and to make these choices known by developing advance directives.

The Patient Self-Determination Act of 1990 requires hospitals and other institutions to make information available to patients on advance directives. However, it isn't mandatory for patients to have advance directives.

Where there's a will, there's a law

There are two types of advance directives:
- *a treatment directive*—sometimes known as a *living will*
- *an appointment directive*—sometimes called a *durable power of attorney for health care*.

A living will states which treatments a patient will accept and which the patient will refuse in case terminal illness renders the patient unable to make those decisions at the time. For example, a patient may be willing to accept artificial nutrition but not hemodialysis.

Durable power of attorney is the appointment of a person— chosen by the patient—to make decisions on the patient's behalf if the patient can no longer do so. Durable power of attorney for health care doesn't give the chosen individual authority to access business accounts; the power is strictly related to health care decisions.

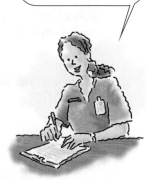

A living will states which treatments a patient will accept and which ones the patient will refuse in case of terminal illness.

It takes two

After an advance directive is written, two witnesses must sign it. This document can be altered or canceled at any time. For more information, check the laws regarding advance directives for the state in which you practice.

Organ donation

When asked, most people say that they support organ donation. However, only a small percentage of qualified organs are ever donated. Tens of thousands of names are on waiting lists for organs in the United States alone. Organ transplantation is successful for many patients, giving them additional, high-quality years of life.

The Uniform Anatomical Gift Act governs the donation of organs and tissues. In addition, most states have legislation governing the procurement of organs and tissues. Some require medical staff to ask about organ donation on every death. Other states require staff to notify a regional organ procurement agency that then approaches the family. Become familiar with the laws of your state and the policies of the facility in which you practice.

Crossing the line

Medical criteria for organ donation vary from state to state. Many organ procurement agencies want to be notified of all deaths and imminent deaths so that they, not the medical staff, can determine if the patient is a potential candidate for organ donation.

No, thank you

These conditions usually preclude any organ or tissue donation:
- metastatic cancer
- history of human immunodeficiency virus or acquired immunodeficiency syndrome
- sepsis.

Donations accepted

Any patient who donates organs must first be declared brain dead. The exceptions to this are living donors, who most commonly donate a kidney or a segment of the lung, liver, pancreas, or intestine. Death used to be defined as the cessation of respiratory and cardiac function. However, with developments in technology, this definition has become obsolete. We now rely on brain death criteria in determining death of an individual. (See *Assessing brain death*.)

Complex care

Care of a patient who's to be an organ donor is very complex. It's imperative that hemodynamic variables and electrolyte values be kept within very tight ranges for successful organ transplantation. You have a vital role in caring for the patient and in supporting the patient's family during this difficult time.

When caring for an organ donor, it's essential to:
- maintain hemodynamic stability so that vital organs are perfused adequately
- assess urine output hourly to detect diabetes insipidus
- monitor laboratory results—such as electrolyte levels, complete blood count, and liver and renal function tests—to assess organ function.

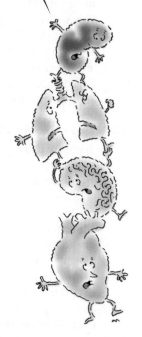

Despite the best intentions, only a small percentage of qualified organs are ever donated. Make sure you know your patient's wishes about organ donation before it's too late.

Assessing brain death

To determine brain death, a doctor must validate the presence of nonresponsive coma, the absence of brain stem reflexes, and the absence of respiratory drive after a carbon dioxide challenge. Methods for determining brain death vary, but several of these criteria are commonly used:
• The patient must be unresponsive to all stimuli.
• Pupillary responses are absent.
• All brain functions cease.
• No eye movements are noted when cold water is instilled into the ears (caloric test). Normally, the eyes move toward the ear irrigated with cold water.
• No corneal reflex is present.
• No gag reflex is present.
• Quick rotation of the patient's head from left to right (doll's eyes test) causes the eyes to remain fixed, suggesting brain death. Normally, the eyes move in the opposite direction of the head movement.
• No response to painful stimuli is present.
• An apnea test reveals no spontaneous breathing.
• EEG shows no brain activity or response.

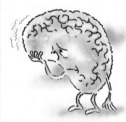

Although the methods for determining brain death vary, the most commonly used criteria are listed here.

Quick quiz

1. Which statement regarding a patient's culture and his hospitalization experience is true?
    A. Culture affects a patient's experience during hospitalization because the patient has to adapt to the hospital culture.
    B. Culture doesn't affect the patient's hospitalization.
    C. Cultural factors can affect patient and family roles during illness.
    D. Culture rarely affects decisions about health.

Answer: C. Cultural factors can have a major impact on patient and family roles during illness. Culture affects the patient's and family members' feelings about illness, pain, and end-of-life issues, among other things.

2. Factors that can affect a critically ill patient's cognitive function include:
    A. medications.
    B. health condition.
    C. sleep disturbances.
    D. all of the above.

Answer: D. All of these factors can affect the patient's cognitive function while on the CCU.

3.   When dealing with the family of a patient in critical care, the nurse should:
   A.   consider them an integral part of the team.
   B.   allow them to visit only during posted visiting times.
   C.   refer them to the patient's practitioner for all information.
   D.   tell them not to touch the patient.

Answer: A. Family members know the patient better than anyone else does and should be considered an important part of the team caring for the patient.

4.   Pain assessment in an unconscious patient:
   A.   isn't necessary because unconscious patients don't experience pain.
   B.   requires astute assessment skills by the nurse.
   C.   can be achieved through the use of visual analog scales.
   D.   is treated differently from pain in a conscious patient.

Answer: B. Nurses should be especially vigilant in assessing for nonverbal signs of pain in an unconscious patient.

5.   The Patient Self-Determination Act of 1990 states that:
   A.   all hospitalized patients must have advance directives.
   B.   hospitals must make information on advance directives available to all patients.
   C.   it's the practitioner's responsibility to obtain information about advance directives.
   D.   patients may have either a living will or a durable power of attorney for health care, but not both.

Answer: B. This act requires hospitals and other institutions to make information about advance directives available to patients, even though having an advance directive isn't mandatory.

Scoring

☆☆☆   If you answered all five questions correctly, jump for joy. You're wholly well versed in holistic care issues.

☆☆   If you answered four questions correctly, we won't issue a complaint. You're ready to join the team.

☆   If you answered fewer than four questions correctly, don't worry; it isn't an ethical dilemma. Just review the chapter and try again.

Suggested References

MedlinePlus. (n.d.). *Lisinopril.* Retrieved from http://www.nlm.nih.gov/medlineplus /druginfo/meds/a692051.html

Schwartz, P., Graham, W., Li, F., Locke, M., & Peever, J. (2013). Sleep deprivation impairs functional muscle recovery following injury. *Sleep Medicine, 14*(1), e262.

Chapter 3

Neurologic system

Just the facts

In this chapter, you'll learn:

♦ anatomy and physiology of the neurologic system

♦ assessment of the neurologic system

♦ diagnostic tests and procedures

♦ neurologic disorders and treatments.

Understanding the nervous system

The neurologic (or nervous) system is the organ system that coordinates all body functions. This complex system allows a person to adapt to changes within his body and in the environment.

Two systems in one

The nervous system consists of:

1. the central nervous system (CNS), which includes the brain and spinal cord
2. the peripheral nervous system, which includes the cranial nerves, spinal nerves, and autonomic system.

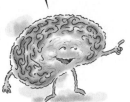

We're both central features of the central nervous system. I'm the smart one!

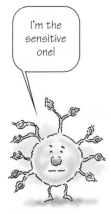

I'm the sensitive one!

Central nervous system

The organs of the CNS—the brain and spinal cord—collect and interpret motor and sensory stimuli. In the process, voluntary and involuntary sensory impulses travel along neural pathways to the brain. (See *A close look at the CNS*, page 48.)

A close look at the CNS

This illustration depicts a cross section of the brain and spinal cord, which together make up the CNS. The brain joins the spinal cord at the base of the skull and ends near the second lumbar vertebra. Note the H-shaped mass of gray matter in the spinal cord.

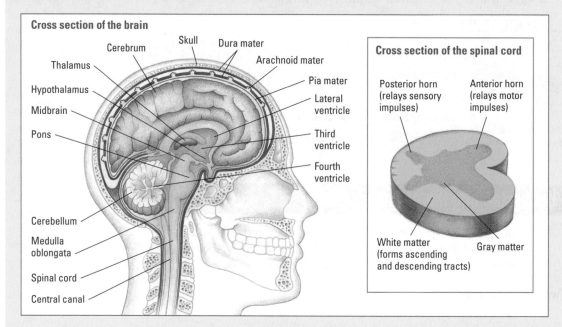

Cross section of the brain

Skull
Cerebrum
Dura mater
Thalamus
Arachnoid mater
Hypothalamus
Pia mater
Midbrain
Lateral ventricle
Pons
Third ventricle
Fourth ventricle
Cerebellum
Medulla oblongata
Spinal cord
Central canal

Cross section of the spinal cord

Posterior horn (relays sensory impulses)
Anterior horn (relays motor impulses)

White matter (forms ascending and descending tracts)
Gray matter

Brain

The brain consists of three parts:

- cerebrum
- cerebellum
- brain stem.

Brain work

The brain collects, integrates, and interprets all stimuli and initiates and regulates voluntary and involuntary motor activity. Four major arteries supply the brain with oxygen.

Cerebrum

The cerebrum, or cerebral cortex, is the largest part of the brain.

Nerve central station

Tissues of the cerebrum make up a nerve center that controls sensory and motor activities and intelligence. It's encased by the bones of the

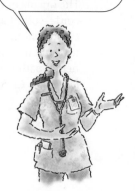

The cerebrum contains the nerve center that controls sensory and motor activities and intelligence.

skull and enclosed by three meninges (membrane layers): the dura mater, arachnoid mater, and pia mater.

Relay and regulate

The diencephalons, another part of the cerebrum, contain the thalamus and hypothalamus. The thalamus is a relay station for sensory and motor impulses.

The hypothalamus has many regulatory functions, such as:

- temperature control
- pituitary hormone production
- sleep and wake cycles
- water balance.

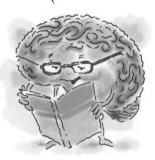

Two hemispheres . . . hmm . . . does that mean I have an equator somewhere down the middle?

Divided in two

The cerebrum is divided into two hemispheres, left and right. The right hemisphere controls the left side of the body. The left hemisphere controls the right side of the body.

The two hemispheres of the brain are composed of four lobes. Each of the four lobes controls different functions. (See *Basic brain functions*, page 50.)

Cerebellum

The cerebellum—the brain's second largest region—lies behind and below the cerebrum. Like the cerebrum, it has two hemispheres.

Smooth moves

The cerebellum contains the major motor and sensory pathways. It enables smooth, coordinated muscle movement and helps maintain equilibrium.

Brain stem

The brain stem lies below the diencephalons and includes the:

- midbrain
- pons
- medulla.

The brain stem is such a major pathway. How could I possibly be lost?

Pathway to the brain

The brain stem contains the nuclei, or cranial nerves III through XII. It's a major sensory and motor pathway for impulses running to and from the cerebral cortex. It also regulates automatic body functions, such as heart rate, breathing, swallowing, and coughing.

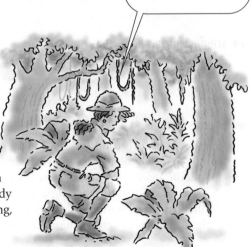

Basic brain functions

The basic structures and functions of the brain are depicted here. The cerebrum is divided into four lobes, based on location and function. The lobes—parietal, occipital, temporal, and frontal—are named for the cranial bones over them.

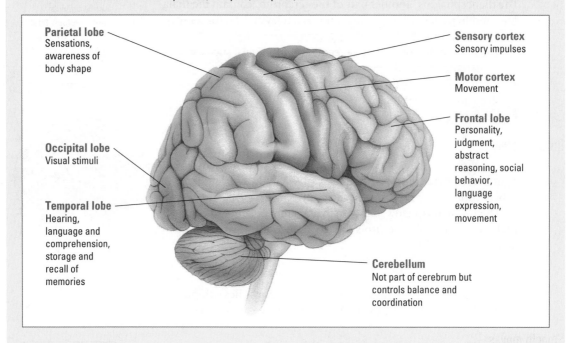

Parietal lobe
Sensations, awareness of body shape

Sensory cortex
Sensory impulses

Motor cortex
Movement

Frontal lobe
Personality, judgment, abstract reasoning, social behavior, language expression, movement

Occipital lobe
Visual stimuli

Temporal lobe
Hearing, language and comprehension, storage and recall of memories

Cerebellum
Not part of cerebrum but controls balance and coordination

Circulation to the brain

The four major blood vessels of the brain include two vertebral and two carotid arteries.

Two arteries converge

The two vertebral arteries converge to become the basilar artery. The basilar artery supplies oxygenated blood to the posterior parts of the brain.

Two arteries diverge

The common carotid arteries branch into the two internal carotids, which further divide to supply oxygenated blood to the anterior and middle areas of the brain. These vessels interconnect and form the circle of Willis at the base of the brain. The circle of Willis ensures that oxygen is continuously circulated to the brain even if any of the brain's major vessels is interrupted. (See *Arteries of the brain*.)

The circle of Willis ensures a constant supply of oxygen to the brain even if a major vessel is interrupted. Whew!

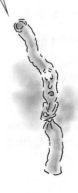

Arteries of the brain

Here's how the inferior surface of the brain appears. The anterior and posterior arteries join smaller arteries to form the circle of Willis.

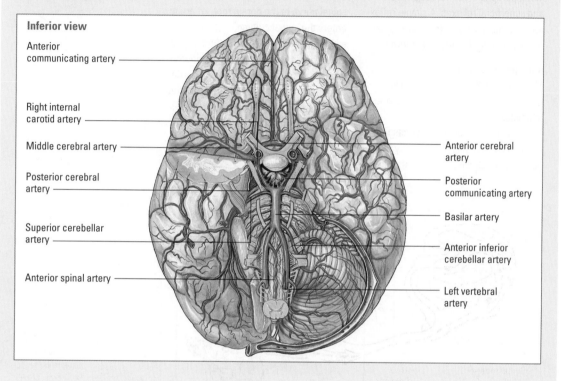

Inferior view

Anterior communicating artery

Right internal carotid artery

Middle cerebral artery

Posterior cerebral artery

Superior cerebellar artery

Anterior spinal artery

Anterior cerebral artery

Posterior communicating artery

Basilar artery

Anterior inferior cerebellar artery

Left vertebral artery

Spinal cord

The spinal cord extends from the upper border of the first cervical vertebra to the lower border of the first lumbar vertebra. It's encased by the same membrane structure as the brain and is protected by the bony vertebrae of the spine.

Long paths

The spinal cord is the primary pathway for messages traveling between the peripheral parts of the body and the brain.

Short paths

The spinal cord also mediates the sensory-to-motor transmission path known as the *reflex arc*. Because the reflex arc enters and exits the spinal cord at the same level, reflex pathways don't need to travel up and down the way other stimuli do. (See *Understanding the reflex arc*, page 52.)

Understanding the reflex arc

Spinal nerves—which have sensory and motor portions—control deep tendon and superficial reflexes. A simple reflex arc requires a sensory (or afferent) neuron and a motor (or efferent) neuron.

Knee jerk reaction

The knee jerk, or patellar, reflex illustrates the sequence of events in a normal reflex arc:

• First, a sensory receptor detects the mechanical stimulus produced by the reflex hammer striking the patellar tendon.

• Then the sensory neuron carries the impulse along its axon by way of the spinal nerve to the dorsal root, where it enters the spinal column.

• Next, in the anterior horn of the spinal cord, shown below, the sensory neuron joins with a motor neuron, which carries the impulse along its axon by way of the spinal nerve to the muscle. The motor neuron transmits the impulse to muscle fibers through stimulation of the motor end plate. This triggers the muscle to contract and the leg to extend.

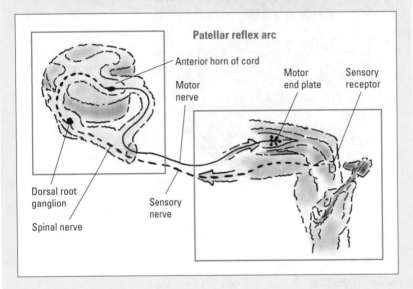

Patellar reflex arc

Anterior horn of cord

Motor nerve

Motor end plate

Sensory receptor

Dorsal root ganglion

Sensory nerve

Spinal nerve

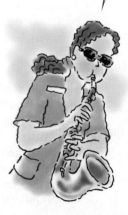

Even sax players have to practice their spinal chords to make it in the big league.

Neural horns

The H-shaped mass of gray matter in the spinal cord is divided into four horns, which consist mainly of neuron cell bodies.

Four horns

The main function of cells in the two dorsal (posterior) horns of the spinal cord is to relay sensations; those in the two ventral (anterior) horns play a part in voluntary and reflex motor activity.

White matter matters

White matter surrounds the four horns. This white matter consists of myelinated nerve fibers grouped in vertical columns, or tracts:

- The *dorsal* white matter contains the ascending tracts, which carry impulses up the spinal cord to higher sensory centers.
- The *ventral* white matter contains the descending tracts, which transmit motor impulses down from higher motor centers to the spinal cord.

Sensory impulse pathways

Sensory impulses travel along the afferent (sensory or ascending) neural pathways to the sensory cortex in the parietal lobe of the brain. There, the impulses are interpreted. The sensory impulses travel along two major pathways:

- dorsal horn
- ganglia.

"I admit it . . . I'm impulsive!"

Dorsal horn

Pain and temperature sensations enter the spinal cord through the dorsal horn. After immediately crossing to the opposite side of the cord, these impulses travel to the thalamus by way of the spinothalamic tract.

Ganglia

Sensations such as touch, pressure, and vibration enter the cord by way of relay stations, called *ganglia*, which are masses of nerve cell bodies on the dorsal roots of spinal nerves. Impulses travel up the dorsal column to the medulla, cross to the opposite side, and enter the thalamus. There, the sensory cortex interprets the impulses.

Motor impulse pathways

Motor impulses travel from the brain to muscles by way of the efferent (motor or descending) pathway. Motor impulses begin in the motor cortex of the frontal lobe and travel along the upper motor neurons to reach the lower motor neurons of the peripheral nervous system.

Upper motor neurons originate in the brain and form two major systems:

- the pyramidal system
- the extrapyramidal system.

Pyramidal system

The pyramidal system (corticospinal tract) is responsible for fine and skilled movements of skeletal muscle.

All the right moves

Impulses in this system travel from the motor cortex through the internal capsule to the medulla. At the medulla, they cross to the opposite side and continue down the spinal cord.

Extrapyramidal system

The extrapyramidal system (extracorticospinal tract) controls gross motor movements.

Extra, extra! Read all about it!

Impulses in this system originate in the premotor area of the frontal lobe. They then travel to the pons, where they cross to the opposite side and travel down the spinal cord to the anterior horns. They're then relayed to the lower motor neurons, which carry the impulses to muscles.

Peripheral nervous system

The peripheral nervous system includes the cranial nerves, spinal nerves, and autonomic nervous system.

Cranial nerves

The 12 pairs of cranial nerves are the primary motor and sensory pathways between the brain and the head and neck. All cranial nerves except the olfactory and optic nerves exit from the midbrain, pons, or medulla oblongata of the brain stem. (See *Identifying cranial nerves.*)

Spinal nerves

There are 31 pairs of spinal nerves, each named for the vertebra immediately below its exit point from the spinal cord.

The nerve of nerves

Each spinal nerve consists of afferent (sensory) and efferent (motor) neurons, which carry messages to and from specific body regions, called *dermatomes.*

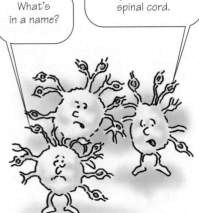

What's in a name?

Well, each pair of spinal nerves is named for the vertebra below its exit point from the spinal cord.

Identifying cranial nerves

The cranial nerves have either sensory or motor function or both. They're assigned Roman numerals and written this way: CN I, CN II, CN III, and so on. The locations of the cranial nerves as well as their functions are shown below.

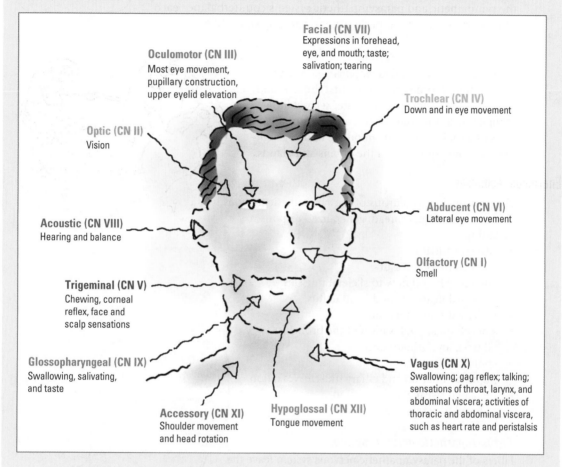

Facial (CN VII)
Expressions in forehead, eye, and mouth; taste; salivation; tearing

Oculomotor (CN III)
Most eye movement, pupillary construction, upper eyelid elevation

Trochlear (CN IV)
Down and in eye movement

Optic (CN II)
Vision

Abducent (CN VI)
Lateral eye movement

Acoustic (CN VIII)
Hearing and balance

Olfactory (CN I)
Smell

Trigeminal (CN V)
Chewing, corneal reflex, face and scalp sensations

Glossopharyngeal (CN IX)
Swallowing, salivating, and taste

Vagus (CN X)
Swallowing; gag reflex; talking; sensations of throat, larynx, and abdominal viscera; activities of thoracic and abdominal viscera, such as heart rate and peristalsis

Accessory (CN XI)
Shoulder movement and head rotation

Hypoglossal (CN XII)
Tongue movement

Autonomic nervous system

The large autonomic nervous system supplies nerves to all internal organs. These visceral efferent nerves carry messages to the viscera from the brain stem and neuroendocrine system.

Two sympathetic systems

The autonomic nervous system includes two major parts:
1. the sympathetic nervous system
2. the parasympathetic nervous system.

Balancing act

When one part of the autonomic nervous system stimulates smooth muscles to contract or a gland to secrete, the other part of the system inhibits that action. Through such dual innervation, the sympathetic and parasympathetic systems counterbalance each other's activities to keep body systems running smoothly.

Sympathetic nervous system

Sympathetic nerves, called *preganglionic neurons*, exit the spinal cord between the first thoracic and second lumbar vertebrae and enter relay stations (ganglia) near the cord. These ganglia form the links of a chain that sends impulses to postganglionic neurons, which reach the organs and glands.

Enormous responses

The postganglionic neurons of the sympathetic nervous system produce widespread, generalized responses, including:
- vasoconstriction
- elevated blood pressure
- enhanced blood flow to skeletal muscles
- increased heart rate and contractility
- increased respiratory rate
- smooth muscle relaxation of the bronchioles, GI tract, and urinary tract
- sphincter contraction
- pupillary dilation and ciliary muscle relaxation
- increased sweat gland secretion
- reduced pancreatic secretion.

Parasympathetic nervous system

Fibers of the parasympathetic nervous system leave the CNS by way of the cranial nerves from the midbrain and medulla and the spinal nerves between the second and fourth sacral vertebrae.

After leaving the CNS, the preganglionic fiber of each parasympathetic nerve travels to a ganglion near a specific organ or gland. The postganglionic fiber of the nerve enters that organ or gland.

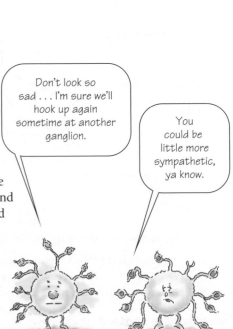

The autonomic nervous system supplies nerves to all internal organs.

Don't look so sad . . . I'm sure we'll hook up again sometime at another ganglion.

You could be little more sympathetic, ya know.

Subtle responses

The postganglionic fibers of the parasympathetic nervous system produce responses involving one specific organ or gland, such as:

- reductions in heart rate, contractility, and conduction velocity
- bronchial smooth muscle constriction
- increased GI tract tone and peristalsis, with sphincter relaxation
- increased bladder tone and urinary system sphincter relaxation
- vasodilatation of external genitalia, causing erection
- pupil constriction
- increased pancreatic, salivary, and lacrimal secretions.

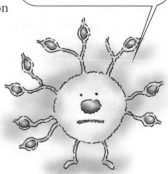

The postganglionic fibers of the parasympathetic nervous system produce responses that involve one specific organ or gland.

Neurologic assessment

Assessment of subtle and elusive changes in the complex nervous system can be difficult. When you assess a patient for possible neurologic impairment, be sure to collect a thorough health history and investigate physical signs of impairment.

Check the records

If you can't interview a critically ill patient due to impairment, you may gather history information from the patient's medical record. In some cases, you may need to ask his family members or the nurse transferring the patient to the critical care unit for information.

Health history

To collect a thorough health history, gather details about the patient's current state of health, previous health status, lifestyle, and family health.

With a little help from his friends (and family)

A patient with neurologic impairment may have trouble remembering. If members of the patient's family or close friends are available, include them in the assessment process. They may be able to corroborate or correct the details of the patient's health history.

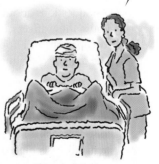

If the patient has a neurologic impairment, gather assessment data from his medical record and interview his family and close friends to get an accurate picture of his health history.

Current health

Discover the patient's chief complaint by asking such questions as, "Why did you come to the hospital?" or "What has been bothering you lately?" Use the patient's words when you document such chief complaints.

Common complaints

If your patient is suffering from a neurologic disorder, you may hear reports of headaches, motor disturbances (such as weakness, paresis, and paralysis), seizures, sensory deviations, and altered level of consciousness (LOC).

Details, please

Encourage the patient to describe details of the current condition by asking such questions as:

- Do you have headaches? How often do you have them? What precipitates them?
- Do you ever feel dizzy? How often do you feel this way? What seems to precipitate the episodes?
- Do you ever feel a tingling or prickling sensation or numbness? If so, where?
- Have you ever had seizures or tremors? Have you ever had weakness or paralysis in your arms or legs?
- Do you have trouble urinating, walking, speaking, understanding others, reading, or writing?
- How's your memory and ability to concentrate?

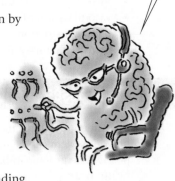

Yes ma'am . . . you seem to have a number of complaints. How may I direct your call?

Previous health

Many chronic diseases affect the neurologic system, so ask questions about the patient's past health and what medications he's taking. Specifically, ask whether the patient has had any:

- major illnesses
- recurrent minor illnesses
- accidents
- injuries
- surgical procedures
- allergies.

Lifestyle

Ask questions about the patient's cultural and social background because these affect care decisions. Note the patient's education level, occupation, and hobbies. As you gather this information, also assess the patient's self-image.

Family health

Information about the patient's family may reveal a hereditary disorder. Ask if anyone in the family has had diabetes, cardiac or renal disease, high blood pressure, cancer, a bleeding disorder, a mental disorder, or a stroke.

Physical examination

A complete neurologic examination can be long and detailed. It's unlikely that you would perform one in its entirety. However, if your initial screening suggests a neurologic problem, you may need to conduct a more detailed assessment.

Top-to-bottom examination

Examine the patient's neurologic system in an orderly way. Beginning with the highest levels of neurologic function and working down to the lowest, assess these five areas:
- mental status
- cranial nerve functions
- sensory function
- motor function
- reflexes.

Mental status

Mental status assessment begins when you talk to the patient during the health history. Responses to your questions reveal clues about the patient's orientation and memory. Use such clues as a guide during the physical assessment. Also observe expression, body language, and attentiveness, which provide clues to the patient overall status.

No easy answers

Make sure that you ask questions that require more than yes-or-no answers. Otherwise, confusion or disorientation might not be apparent. If you have doubts about a patient's mental status, perform a screening examination. (See *Quick check of mental status*, page 60.)

Three-part exam

Use the mental status examination to check these three parameters:
- LOC
- speech
- cognitive function.

Level of consciousness

Watch for any change in the patient's LOC. It's the earliest and most sensitive indicator that his neurologic status has changed.

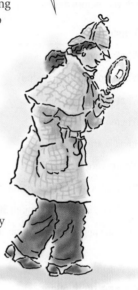

Mental status assessment begins with a health history. The patient's responses reveal clues about his mental status.

Quick check of mental status

To quickly screen your patient for disordered thought processes, ask the questions below. An incorrect answer to any question may indicate the need for a complete mental status examination. One quick tip: Make sure that you know the correct answers before asking the questions.

Question	Function screened
What's your name?	Orientation to person
What's your mother's name?	Orientation to other people
What year is it?	Orientation to time
Where are you now?	Orientation to place
How old are you?	Memory
Where were you born?	Remote memory
What did you have for breakfast?	Recent memory
Who's president of the United States now?	General knowledge
Can you count backward from 20 to 1?	Attention span and calculation skills

Let's be perfectly clear

Many terms are used to describe LOC, and definitions differ slightly among practitioners. To avoid confusion, clearly describe the patient's response to various stimuli using these definitions:

- *Alert*—Patient follows commands and responds completely and appropriately to stimuli.
- *Lethargic*—Patient is drowsy, has delayed but appropriate responses to verbal stimuli, and may drift off to sleep during the examination.
- *Stuporous*—Patient requires vigorous stimulation for a response. Responses vary in appropriateness.
- *Comatose*—Patient doesn't respond appropriately to verbal or painful stimuli and can't follow commands or communicate verbally.

> Watch for a change in the patient's LOC— the earliest and most sensitive indicator of neurologic status change.

Not too highly stimulating

Start by quietly observing the patient's behavior. If the patient is sleeping, try to rouse him by providing an appropriate stimulus, in this order:

1. auditory
2. tactile
3. painful.

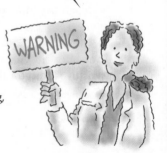

Always start with a minimal stimulus, increasing intensity as necessary. The Glasgow Coma Scale offers an objective way to assess the patient's LOC. (See *Using the Glasgow Coma Scale*, page 62.)

Speech
Listen to how well the patient expresses thoughts. Does he choose the correct words or seem to have problems finding or articulating words?

It's hard to say
To assess for dysarthria (difficulty forming words), ask the patient to repeat the phrase, "No ifs, ands, or buts." Assess speech comprehension by determining the patient's ability to follow instructions and cooperate with your examination.

Speaking of changes
Keep in mind that language performance tends to fluctuate with the time of day and changes in physical condition. A healthy person may have language difficulty when ill or fatigued. However, increasing speech difficulties may indicate deteriorating neurologic status, which warrants further evaluation.

Cognitive function
Assess cognitive function by testing the patient's:
- memory
- orientation
- attention span
- calculation ability
- thought content
- abstract thinking
- judgment
- insight
- emotional status.

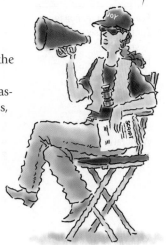

Listen up! Increasing speech difficulties may indicate deteriorating neurologic status.

Thanks for the memories
Short-term memory is commonly affected first in a patient with neurologic disease. A patient with intact short-term memory can generally remember and repeat five to seven nonconsecutive numbers right away and again 10 minutes later.

When then who
To quickly test your patient's orientation, memory, and attention span, use the mental status screening questions. Orientation to time is usually disrupted first; orientation to person, last.

Using the Glasgow Coma Scale

You can use the Glasgow Coma Scale to describe the patient's baseline mental status and detect and interpret changes in the LOC.

To use the scale, test the patient's ability to respond to verbal, motor, and sensory stimulation and base your findings on the scale. A patient who's alert, can follow simple commands, and is oriented to time, place, and person receives a score of 15 points. A lower score in one or more categories may signal an impending neurologic crisis. A total score of 7 or less indicates severe neurologic damage.

Test	Score	Patient's response
Eye-opening response		
Spontaneously	4	Opens eyes spontaneously
To speech	3	Opens eyes when told to
To pain	2	Opens eyes only on painful stimulus
None	1	Doesn't open eyes in response to stimulus
Motor response		
Obeys	6	Shows two fingers when asked
Localizes	5	Reaches toward painful stimulus and tries to remove it
Withdraws	4	Moves away from painful stimulus
Abnormal flexion	3	Assumes a decorticate posture (shown below)
Abnormal extension	2	Assumes a decerebrate posture (shown below)
None	1	No response, just lies flaccid—an ominous sign
Verbal response		
Oriented	5	Tells current date
Confused	4	Tells incorrect year
Inappropriate words	3	Replies randomly with incorrect word
Incomprehensible	2	Moans or screams
None	1	No response
Total score		

Always consider the patient's environment and physical condition when assessing orientation. For example, a patient admitted to the critical care unit for several days may not be oriented to time because of the constant activity and noise of the monitoring equipment.

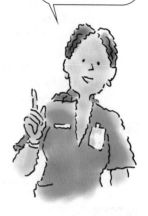

Orientation to time is usually disrupted first; orientation to person, last.

Attention and calculation

When testing attention span and calculation skills, keep in mind that lack of mathematical ability and anxiety can affect the patient's performance. If he has difficulty with numerical computation, ask him to spell the word "world" backwards. While he's performing these functions, note his ability to pay attention.

Thought content

Disordered thought patterns may indicate delirium or psychosis. Assess thought pattern by evaluating the clarity and cohesiveness of the patient's ideas. Is his conversation smooth, with logical transitions between ideas? Does he have hallucinations (sensory perceptions that lack appropriate stimuli) or delusions (beliefs not supported by reality)?

Hypothetically speaking . . .

Test the patient's judgment by asking him how he would respond to a hypothetical situation. For example, what would he do if he were in a public building and the fire alarm sounded? Evaluate the appropriateness of his answer.

Insight on insight

Test your patient's insight by finding out:
- whether the patient has a realistic view of himself
- whether he's aware of his illness and circumstances.

Assess insight by asking, for example, "What do you think caused your chest pain?" Expect different patients to have different degrees of insight. For instance, a patient may attribute chest discomfort to indigestion rather than acknowledge that he has had a heart attack.

Test the patient's judgment: Ask how he would respond to a hypothetical situation—like what he would do if he were in a public building and the fire alarm sounded—and then evaluate his answer.

Lost in emotion

Throughout the interview, assess your patient's emotional status. Note his mood, emotional lability or stability, and the appropriateness of his emotional responses. Also, assess the patient's mood by asking how he feels about himself and his future. Keep in mind that signs and symptoms of depression in an elderly patient may be atypical. (See *Depression and elderly patients*, page 64.)

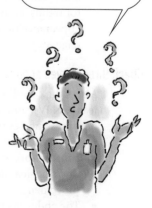

Cranial nerve function

Cranial nerve assessment reveals valuable information about the condition of the CNS, especially the brain stem.

Under pressure

Because of their location, some cranial nerves are more vulnerable to the effects of increasing intracranial pressure (ICP). Therefore, a neurologic screening assessment of the CNS focuses on these key nerves:
- optic (II)
- oculomotor (III)
- trochlear (IV)
- abducens (VI).

Go on

Also evaluate other nerves if the patient's history or symptoms indicate a potential CNS disorder or when performing a complete nervous system assessment. (See *Checking brain stem function*.)

Be nosey

Assess the olfactory nerve (cranial nerve [CN] I) first. Check the patency of each nostril. Then instruct the patient to close his eyes. Occlude one nostril and hold a familiar, pungent-smelling substance under the patient's nose and ask him to identify it. Repeat this with the other nostril.

See about sight

Next, assess the optic (CN II) and oculomotor (CN III) nerves:
- To assess the optic nerve, check visual acuity, visual fields, and retinal structures. Do this by asking the patient to read a newspaper, starting with large headlines and moving to small print.
- To assess the oculomotor nerve, check pupil size, pupil shape, and pupillary response to light. When assessing pupil size, look for trends, such as a gradual increase in the size of one pupil or appearance of unequal pupils. (See *Recognizing pupillary changes*, page 66.)

Check three nerves at once

Assess the coordinated function of the oculomotor (CN III), trochlear (CN IV), and abducens (CN VI) nerves simultaneously. Here's how these nerves normally work:
- The oculomotor nerve controls extraocular movement, pupillary constriction, and raising of the eyelid.
- The trochlear nerve controls downward and inward eye movement.
- The abducens nerve controls lateral eye movement.

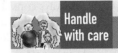

Handle with care

Depression and elderly patients

Symptoms of depression in elderly patients may be different from those found in other patients. For example, rather than the usual sad affect seen in patients with depression, your elderly patient may exhibit such atypical signs as decreased function and increased agitation.

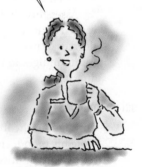

"Ah . . . the pungent aroma of hospital coffee—who could mistake it for anything else?"

Checking brain stem function

In an unconscious patient, assist the practitioner in assessing brain stem function by testing for the oculocephalic (doll's eye) reflex and the oculovestibular reflex. If the patient has a cervical spine injury, expect to use the oculovestibular reflex test as an alternative. The oculovestibular reflex test may also be used to determine the status of the vestibular portion of the acoustic nerve (CN VIII).

Oculocephalic reflex

Before beginning, examine the patient's cervical spine. Don't perform this procedure if you suspect the patient has a cervical spine injury. If the patient has no cervical spine injury, proceed as follows:
• Place both hands on either side of his head and use your thumbs to gently hold his eyelids open.
• While watching the patient's eyes, briskly rotate the head from side to side (as shown at right) or briskly flex and extend the patient's neck.
• Observe how the patient's eyes move in relation to head movement.

In a normal response, which indicates an intact brain stem, the eyes appear to move opposite to the movement of the head. For example, if the neck is flexed, the eyes appear to look upward. If the neck is extended, the eyes gaze downward.

Abnormal response

With an abnormal (doll's eye) response, the eyes appear to move passively in the same direction as the head, indicating the absence of oculocephalic reflex. Such a response suggests a severe brain stem damage at the level of the pons or midbrain.

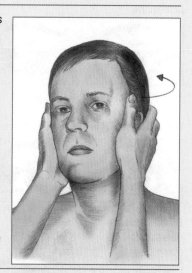

Oculovestibular reflex

To assess the oculovestibular reflex, the practitioner first determines that the patient has an intact tympanic membrane and a clear external ear canal. Then follow these steps:
• Elevate the head of the bed 30 degrees.
• Using a large syringe with a small catheter on the tip, slowly irrigate the external auditory canal with 20 to 200 ml of cold water or ice water (as shown at right).
• During irrigation, watch the patient's eye movements. In a patient with an intact oculovestibular reflex, the eyes deviate toward the side being irrigated with cold water.

Abnormal responses

If the patient is conscious to some degree, there may be nystagmus (involuntary, rapid movement of the eyeball) with rapid jerking of the eyes away from the side being irrigated. In an abnormal conscious individual, as little as 10 ml of ice water may produce such a response and may also cause nausea. In a comatose patient with an intact brain stem, the eyes tonically deviate toward the stimulated ear. Absence of eye movement suggests a brain stem lesion.

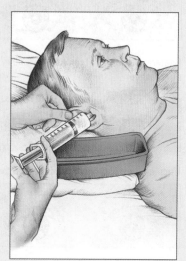

Recognizing pupillary changes

Use this table as a guide to recognize pupillary changes and identify possible causes.

Pupillary change	Possible causes
Unilateral, dilated (4 mm), fixed, and nonreactive 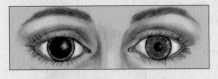	• Uncal herniation with oculomotor nerve damage • Brain stem compression • Increased ICP • Tentorial herniation • Head trauma with subdural or epidural hematoma • May be normal in some people
Bilateral, dilated (4 mm), fixed, and nonreactive 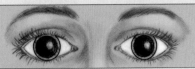	• Severe midbrain damage • Cardiopulmonary arrest (hypoxia) • Anticholinergic poisoning
Bilateral, midsize (2 mm), fixed, and nonreactive 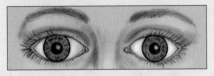	• Midbrain involvement caused by edema, hemorrhage, infarctions, lacerations, or contusions
Bilateral, pinpoint (<1 mm), and usually nonreactive 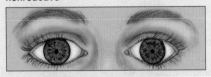	• Lesions of pons, usually after hemorrhage
Unilateral, small (1.5 mm), and nonreactive 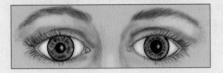	• Disruption of sympathetic nerve supply to the head caused by spinal cord lesion above the first thoracic vertebra

The cardinal rules

Make sure that the patient's pupils constrict when exposed to light and that his eyes adapt to seeing objects at various distances. Ask the patient to follow your finger through six cardinal positions of gaze:
1. left superior
2. left lateral
3. left inferior
4. right superior
5. right lateral
6. right inferior.

Pause slightly before moving from one position to the next, to assess the patient for nystagmus, or involuntary eye movement, and the ability to hold gaze in that particular position.

Focus on the face

To assess the sensory portion of the trigeminal nerve (CN V), gently touch the right and left sides of the patient's forehead with a cotton ball while his eyes are closed. Instruct him to tell you the moment the cotton touches each area. Compare the patient's responses on both sides.

Repeat the technique on the right and left cheek and on the right and left jaw. Next, repeat the entire procedure using a sharp object, such as the tip of a safety pin. Ask the patient to describe and compare both sensations.

To assess the motor function of the trigeminal nerve, ask the patient to clench his teeth while you palpate his temporal and masseter muscles.

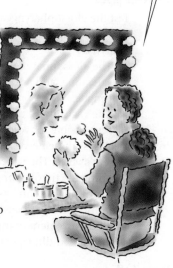

No need for safety pins. I can sense every line and wrinkle on my face. Pass the moisturizer, please!

Make someone smile

To test the motor portion of the facial nerve (CN VII), ask the patient to:
• wrinkle his forehead
• raise and lower his eyebrows
• smile to show his teeth
• puff out his cheeks.

Also, with the patient's eyes tightly closed, attempt to open his eyelids. As you conduct each part of this test, look for symmetry.

Keep it tasteful

The sensory portion of the facial nerve (CN VII) supplies taste sensation to the anterior two-thirds of the tongue. Test the taste sensation by placing items with various flavors on the patient's tongue. Use items such as sugar (sweet), salt, lemon juice (sour), and quinine (bitter). Between items, have the patient wash away each substance with a sip of water.

I'm still stuck on sweet. I'll get to salty, sour, and bitter after this cake. Could be a while, though.

Now hear this

To assess the acoustic nerve (CN VIII), first test the patient's hearing. Ask the patient to cover one ear. Then stand on the opposite side and whisper a few words. Find out whether the patient can repeat what you said. Test the other ear in the same way.

To test the vestibular portion of the acoustic nerve, observe the patient for nystagmus and disturbed balance. Note reports of the room spinning or dizziness.

Check the pipes

Test the glossopharyngeal nerve (CN IX) and vagus nerve (CN X) together because their innervation overlaps in the pharynx:

- The glossopharyngeal nerve is responsible for swallowing, salivating, and taste perception on the posterior one-third of the tongue.
- The vagus nerve controls swallowing and is responsible for voice quality.

Assess these nerves, first, by listening to the patient's voice. Then check the gag reflex by touching the tip of a tongue blade against the posterior pharynx and asking the patient to open wide and say "ah." Watch for the symmetrical upward movement of the soft palate and uvula and for the midline position of the uvula.

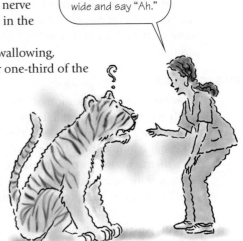

OK, let's try that again . . . open wide and say "Ah."

Shrug it off

To assess the spinal accessory nerve (CN XI), which controls the sternocleidomastoid muscles and the upper portion of the trapezius muscles, press down on the patient's shoulders while he attempts to shrug against this resistance. Note shoulder strength and symmetry while inspecting and palpating the trapezius muscles.

To further test the trapezius muscles, apply resistance from one side while the patient tries to return his head to midline position. Look for neck strength. Repeat on the other side.

Test tongue toughness

To assess the hypoglossal nerve (CN XII), follow these steps:

1. Ask the patient to stick out his tongue. Look for any deviation from the midline, atrophy, or fasciculations.
2. Test tongue strength by asking the patient to push his tongue against his cheek as you apply resistance. Observe the tongue for symmetry.
3. Test the patient's speech by asking him to repeat the sentence, "Round the rugged rock that ragged rascal ran."

Sensory function

Assess the sensory system to evaluate:
- ability of the sensory receptors to detect stimuli
- ability of the afferent nerves to carry sensory nerve impulses to the spinal cord
- ability of the sensory tracts in the spinal cord to carry sensory messages to the brain.

Five sensations

During your assessment, check five types of sensation, including pain, light touch, vibration, position, and discrimination.

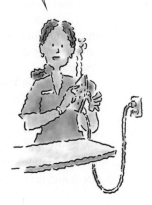

Ouch! To test for pain in a more sensible fashion, touch all the major dermatomes with the sharp end of a safety pin and then with the dull end.

This is gonna hurt

To test for pain sensation, have the patient close his eyes; then touch all the major dermatomes, first with the sharp end of a safety pin and then with the dull end. Proceed in this order:
- fingers
- shoulders
- toes
- thighs
- trunk.

While testing, occasionally alternate sharp and dull ends. Ask the patient to tell you when he feels the sharp stimulus. If the patient has known deficits, start in the area with the least sensation and move toward the area with the most sensation.

Use a light touch

To test for the sense of light touch, follow the instructions for pain sensation, using a wisp of cotton or tissue. Lightly touch the patient's skin; don't swab or sweep the skin. A patient with peripheral neuropathy might retain the sensation for light touch after losing pain sensation.

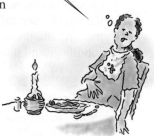

"All done with my fork, but I don't think it will help with testing sensory function. Check, please!"

Find the right vibe

To check for response to vibration, tap a low-pitched tuning fork on the heel of your hand and then place the base of the fork firmly over the distal interphalangeal joint of the index finger. Then move proximally until the patient feels the vibration; everything above that level is intact.

If the patient's vibratory sense is intact, further testing for position sense isn't necessary because they follow the same pathway.

Where the toes are

To experience position sense, the patient needs intact vestibular and cerebellar function. To assess for position sense, have the patient close his eyes. Then, grasp the sides of his big toe and move it up and down. Ask the patient what position the toe is in.

To perform the same test on the patient's upper extremities, grasp the sides of his index finger and move it back and forth. Ask the patient what position the finger is in.

Discrimination, integration, and extinction

Discrimination is the cortex's ability to integrate sensory input. Stereognosis is the ability to discriminate the shape, size, weight, texture, and form of an object by touching and manipulating it.

To test stereognosis, ask the patient to close both eyes and open one hand. Then place a common object, such as a key, in the hand and ask the patient to identify it. If the patient can't identify the object, test graphesthesia (ability to identify something by tactile sense). Here's how to do this: While the patient's eyes are closed, draw a large number on the palm of one hand and ask the patient to identify the number.

Extinction is the failure to perceive touch on one side. To test point localization, have the patient close his eyes, touch one of his limbs, and then ask where you touched him. To test two-point discrimination, touch the patient simultaneously in two contralateral areas and note whether he can identify touch on both sides.

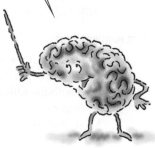

Discrimination is the ability to integrate sensory input to determine the shape, size, weight, texture, and form of an object.

Motor function

Assess motor function to aid evaluation of these structures and functions:
- the cerebral cortex and its initiation of motor activity by way of the pyramidal pathways
- the corticospinal tracts and their capacity to carry motor messages down the spinal cord
- the lower motor neurons and their ability to carry efferent impulses to the muscles
- the muscles and their capacity to carry out motor commands
- the cerebellum and basal ganglia and their capacity to coordinate and fine-tune movement.

A careful motor function assessment reveals a lot of information about neurologic structures and functions.

Tone test

Muscle tone represents muscular resistance to passive stretching. To test muscle tone of the arm, move the patient's shoulder through its passive range of motion (ROM); you should feel a slight resistance. When you let the patient's arm drop to his side, it should fall easily.

To test leg muscle tone, guide the patient's hip through its passive ROM and then let his leg fall to the bed. If it falls in an externally rotated position, note this abnormal finding.

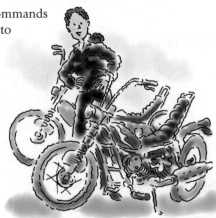

Feats of strength

To assess arm muscle strength, ask the patient to push you away as you apply resistance. To assess hand strength, ask the patient to grip your hand. Then ask the patient to extend both arms, palms up. Have him close his eyes and maintain this position for 20 to 30 seconds. Observe the arm for downward drifting and pronation.

Strength of feet

Assess leg movement by first asking the patient to move each leg and foot with and without applying resistance. If he fails to move the leg on command, watch for spontaneous movement.

Grace and gait

Assess the patient's coordination and balance through cerebellar testing. Note whether the patient can sit and stand without support. If appropriate, observe as the patient walks across the room, turns, and walks back.

While observing the patient, note imbalances and abnormalities. When cerebellar dysfunction is present, the patient has a wide-based, unsteady gait. Deviation to one side may indicate a cerebellar lesion on the side.

Synchronized standing

Perform Romberg's test to evaluate cerebellar synchronization of movement with balance. Have the patient stand with his feet together, arms at his sides, and without support. Note his ability to maintain balance with both eyes open and then closed. (Stand nearby in case the patient loses his balance.)

A small amount of swaying normally occurs when the eyes are closed. If the patient has trouble maintaining a steady position with eyes open or closed, cerebellar ataxia may be present.

Extreme coordination

Test the extremities for coordination by having the patient touch nose and then your outstretched finger as you move it. Have him do this faster and faster. His movements should be accurate and smooth.

Test cerebellar function further by assessing rapid alternating movements. Tell the patient to use the thumb of one hand to touch each finger of the same hand in rapid sequence. Repeat with the other hand.

To assess the legs, have the patient rapidly tap the floor with the ball of one foot. Test each leg separately. Note any slowness or awkwardness. Abnormalities can indicate cerebellar disease or motor weakness associated with extrapyramidal or pyramidal disease.

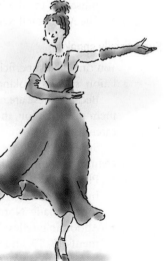

When assessing coordination and balance, note any imbalance or abnormality.

Present and absent actions

Motor responses in an unconscious patient may be appropriate, inappropriate, or absent. Appropriate responses, such as localization or withdrawal, mean that the sensory and corticospinal pathways are functioning. Inappropriate responses, such as decorticate or decerebrate posturing, indicate a dysfunction.

It can be challenging to assess motor responses in a patient who can't follow commands or is unresponsive. Make sure that you note whether any stimulus produces a response, what that response is, and the stimulus that was used.

Reflexes

Assess deep tendon and superficial reflexes to learn about the integrity of the sensory receptor organ. You can also evaluate how well afferent nerves relay sensory messages to the spinal cord or brain stem segment to mediate reflexes.

How deep is your reflex?

Test deep tendon reflexes by checking the responses of the biceps, triceps, brachioradialis, patellar, and Achilles tendons:
- The biceps reflex contracts the biceps muscle and forces flexion of the forearm.
- The triceps reflex contracts the triceps muscle and forces extension of the forearm.
- The brachioradialis reflex causes supination of the hand and flexion of the forearm at the elbow.
- The patellar reflex forces contraction of the quadriceps muscle in the thigh with extension of the leg.
- The Achilles reflex forces plantar flexion of the foot at the ankle.

Test deep tendon reflexes by checking responses of the biceps, triceps, brachioradialis, patellar, and Achilles tendons. Check superficial reflexes using light, tactile stimulation.

Superficially speaking

You can elicit superficial reflexes using light, tactile stimulation, such as stroking or scratching the skin.

Because these are cutaneous reflexes, the more you try to elicit them in succession, the less response you'll get. Therefore, observe carefully the first time you stimulate these reflexes.

Superficial reflexes include the pharyngeal, abdominal, and cremasteric reflexes. Here's how to test them:
- Pharyngeal reflex: To test CN IX and CN X, have the patient open his mouth wide. Then, touch the back of the pharynx with a tongue blade. Normally, this causes the patient to gag.
- Abdominal reflex: To test the intactness of thoracic spinal segments T8, T9, and T10, use the tip of the handle on the reflex hammer to stroke one side, and then the opposite side, of the patient's abdomen above the umbilicus. Repeat on the lower abdomen. Normally, the abdominal muscles contract and the umbilicus deviates toward the stimulated side.

- Cremasteric reflex: To test the intactness of lumbar spinal segments L1 and L2 in a male patient, use a tongue blade to scratch the inner aspects of each thigh gently. Normally, this action causes the testicles to lift.

Write it down

After you examine the patient, document your findings using a grading scale to rate each reflex. Document the rating for each reflex at the appropriate site on a stick figure. (See *Documenting reflex findings*.)

Documenting reflex findings

Use these grading scales to rate the strength of each reflex in a deep tendon and superficial reflex assessment.

Deep tendon reflex grades
0 absent
+ present but diminished
++ normal
+++ increased but not necessarily abnormal
++++ hyperactive or clonic (involuntary contraction and relaxation of skeletal muscle)

Superficial reflex grades
0 absent
+ present

Findings
Record the patient's reflex ratings on a drawing of a stick figure. The figures depict documentation of normal and abnormal reflex responses.

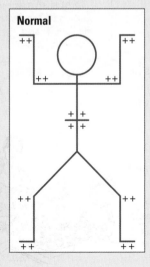

Normal

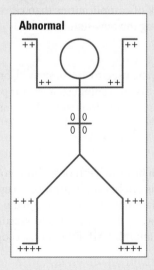

Abnormal

Diagnostic tests

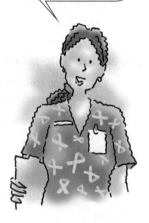

Diagnostic testing to evaluate the nervous system typically includes imaging studies, angiography, and electrophysiologic studies. Other tests, such as lumbar puncture and transcranial Doppler studies, may also be used.

Diagnostic testing can be frightening. Make sure that you prepare the patient and his family for each test.

Tell it like it is

Diagnostic testing may be routine for you, but it can be frightening for the patient. Make sure that you carefully prepare the patient and his family for each test and follow-up monitoring procedure. Some tests can be performed at the patient's bedside, but many require transportation to the imaging department.

Imaging studies

The most common imaging studies used to detect neurologic disorders include computed tomography (CT) scan, magnetic resonance imaging (MRI), positron emission tomography (PET) scan, and skull and spinal X-rays. Computed tomography angiography (CTA) and magnetic resonance angiography (MRA) are also available as diagnostic tools for cerebrovascular disease. (See *Understanding CTA and MRA*, page 76.)

Computed tomography scan

CT scanning of intracranial structures combines radiology and computer analysis of tissue density. CT angiography shows blood vessels, and it carries less risk of complications than cerebral angiography. CTA is becoming the new standard.

Before CT scanning of the brain, make sure that the patient isn't allergic to iodine or shellfish, which may foretell an adverse reaction to the contrast medium. Thankfully, we aren't allergic!

Spine scanning

CT scanning of the spine can be used to assess such disorders as herniated disk, spinal cord tumors, and spinal stenosis for patients that cannot have an MRI. It is best used to look at the bony architecture of the vertebral column.

Brain scanning

CT scanning of the brain can be done with or without contrast and is used to detect brain contusion, brain calcifications, cerebral atrophy, hydrocephalus, inflammation, space-occupying lesions (tumors, hematomas, edemas, and abscesses), and vascular anomalies (arteriovenous malformation [AVM], infarctions, blood clots, and hemorrhage).

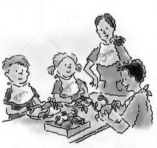

Nursing concerns

- If a contrast medium is ordered, confirm that the patient isn't allergic to iodine or shellfish to avoid an adverse reaction.
- If the test calls for a contrast medium, tell the patient that it's injected into an existing I.V. line or that a new line may be inserted.
- Preprocedure testing should include evaluation of renal function (serum creatinine and blood urea nitrogen [BUN] levels) because the contrast medium can cause acute renal failure.
- Warn the patient that he may feel flushed or notice a metallic taste in his mouth when the contrast medium is injected.
- Tell him that the CT scanner circles around him for 10 to 30 minutes, depending on the procedure and type of equipment.
- Explain that he must lie still during the test.
- Tell him that the contrast medium may discolor his urine for 24 hours. Suggest that he drink more fluids to flush the medium out of his body, unless this is contraindicated or he has oral intake restrictions; otherwise, the practitioner may write an order to increase the I.V. flow rate.

Magnetic resonance imaging

MRI generates detailed pictures of body structures. It is best for imaging soft tissue. The test may involve the use of a contrast medium such as gadolinium.

Sharper images

Compared with conventional X-rays and CT scans, MRI provides superior contrast of soft tissues, sharply differentiating healthy, benign, and cancerous tissue and clearly revealing blood vessels. In addition, MRI permits imaging in multiple planes, including sagittal and coronal views in regions where bones normally hamper visualization.

MRI is especially useful for studying the CNS because it can reveal structural and biochemical abnormalities associated with such conditions as transient ischemic attack (TIA), tumors, multiple sclerosis (MS), cerebral edema, and hydrocephalus.

Nursing concerns

- Confirm that the patient isn't allergic to the contrast medium (usually gadolinium).
- If the test calls for a contrast medium, tell the patient that it's injected into an existing I.V. line or that a new line may be inserted.
- Explain that the procedure can take up to 1½ hours; tell the patient that he must remain still for intervals of 5 to 20 minutes.
- Instruct the patient to remove all metallic items, such as hair clips, bobby pins, jewelry (including body-piercing jewelry), watches, eyeglasses, hearing aids, and dentures.

Understanding CTA and MRA

Because of the less invasive nature of CTA and MRA compared with conventional angiography, these two tests are becoming more readily available and being used more frequently. In addition, the lack of arterial access in CTA and MRA usually means fewer complications. Both scans typically take less time to perform than conventional angiography, which is especially helpful when your patient is critically ill.

CTA

CTA is a type of CT scan that uses a computer to produce images that are taken via X-ray. The type of CT scanner used must have a multidetector to be capable of performing a CTA. The multidetector functions by allowing the CT scanner to take high-quality pictures of the brain quickly. I.V. contrast media is used to help produce a clear picture of the cerebral arteries. With this type of scan, the doctor can see an aneurysm, even if it's ruptured.

Before a CTA

To prepare your patient for CTA, you'll need to establish vascular access for the contrast injection. Also, explain that it's important for the patient to lie still during the procedure to ensure good-quality images. Let the patient know that it will be possible to communicate with the technician and any other health care personnel that are present during the scan. Ask the patient about his history of adverse reactions to contrast medium and document what happened during that reaction. Be sure to communicate this information to the doctor and radiologist and follow your facility's policy on using contrast in these patients.

Intravascular contrast can make patients feel warm, so explain to the patient the difference between this type of expected reaction and unanticipated adverse reactions. Mild adverse reactions include nausea, vomiting, local urticaria, or pruritus; moderate adverse reactions include vasovagal reactions, bronchospasm, or mild laryngeal edema; and severe adverse reactions (rare) include seizures or cardiac arrest.

You may accompany a critically ill patient to the CTA scan; make sure that you use the necessary monitoring equipment and have resuscitation equipment available.

Because the patient must be supine for the duration of the scan, you may need to administer a diuretic before the procedure if the patient has ICP compromise.

After a CTA

Unless contraindicated, encourage oral fluid intake or administer I.V. fluids after the scan is complete to enhance urinary excretion of the contrast medium. Monitor the patient's renal function, assess for signs and symptoms of adverse reactions, and monitor ICP and neurologic status for signs of compromise.

MRA

MRA is a type of MRI. Magnetic resonance works by manipulating hydrogen, the most common element in human tissue. Hydrogen creates a radiofrequency signal when exposed to a magnetic field. A computer gathers the radiofrequency signals into a readable picture. In MRA, the radiofrequency signals created by hydrogen traveling in the arteries create an image. The computer removes the images of other structures and provides a clear image of the cerebral arteries and pathology. An I.V. contrast medium, gadolinium, is also injected to highlight the arteries in MRA. An MRA is valuable for evaluating intracranial or extracranial atherosclerosis, AVM, intact aneurysms, or other cerebrovascular disease.

Before an MRA

You should explain to your patient that it will be necessary for him to lie still during the procedure so that clear images can be obtained. Warn him that the scanner produces a loud jackhammer-like noise but that ear protection will be available. If not already present, you'll need to establish vascular access for the contrast medium injection.

Understanding CTA and MRA *(continued)*

Before the procedure, ask about any metal implants in his body and document your findings. Most facilities have an MRI/MRA screening form. You may want to also screen your patient for claustrophobia and obtain an order for anxiolytic if necessary. If you accompany a critically ill patient to the scan, make sure that you use the necessary monitoring equipment and have resuscitation equipment available. Assure the patient that he will be able to communicate with you and other health care personnel throughout the scan.

After an MRA

After the scan, monitor the patient's renal function. If you administered sedation, continue to monitor the patient's cardiopulmonary status. Encourage the patient to drink fluids or administer I.V. fluids for 24 to 48 hours after the MRA, unless contraindicated.

- Explain that the test is painless but that the machinery may seem loud and frightening and the tunnel confining. Tell the patient that he'll receive earplugs to reduce the noise.
- Provide sedation, as ordered, to promote relaxation during the test.
- After the procedure, increase the I.V. flow rate, as ordered, or encourage the patient to increase his fluid intake to flush the contrast medium from his system.

Positron emission tomography scan

PET scanning provides colorimetric information about the brain's metabolic activity. It works by detecting how quickly tissues consume radioactive isotopes.

PET scanning is used to reveal cerebral dysfunction associated with tumors, seizures, TIA, head trauma, Alzheimer's disease, Parkinson's disease, MS, and some mental illnesses. In addition, a PET scan can be used to evaluate the effect of treatment.

PET project

Here's how PET scanning works:
- A technician administers a radioactive gas or an I.V. injection of glucose or other biochemical substance tagged with isotopes, which act as tracers.
- The isotopes emit positrons that combine with negatively charged electrons in tissue cells to create gamma rays.
- The PET scanner registers the emitted gamma rays, and a computer translates the information into patterns that reflect cerebral blood flow, blood volume, and neuron and neurotransmitter metabolism.

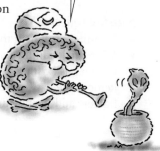

PET scanning is used to gather clues about cerebral blood flow, blood volume, and neuron and neurotransmitter metabolism. Don't worry, little buddy, it has nothing to do with you.

- Provide reassurance that PET scanning doesn't expose the patient to dangerous levels of radiation.
- Explain that insertion of an I.V. catheter may be required.
- Instruct the patient to lie still during the test.

Skull and spinal X-rays

Skull X-rays are typically taken from two angles: anteroposterior and lateral. The practitioner may order other angles, including Waters view, or occipitomental projection, to examine the frontal and maxillary sinuses, facial bones, and eye orbits.

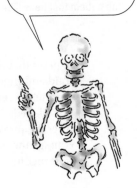

Skull X-rays are typically taken from the anteroposterior and lateral angles.

Having one's head examined

Skull X-rays are used to detect fractures; bony tumors or unusual calcifications; pineal displacement or skull or sella turcica erosion, which indicates a space-occupying lesion; and vascular abnormalities.

Spinal findings

The practitioner may order anteroposterior and lateral spinal X-rays when:
- spinal disease is suspected
- injury to the cervical, thoracic, lumbar, or sacral vertebral segments exists.

Depending on the patient's condition, other X-ray images may be taken from special angles, such as the open-mouth view (to confirm odontoid fracture).

Spinal X-rays are used to detect spinal fracture; displacement and subluxation due to partial dislocation; destructive lesions, such as primary and metastatic bone tumors; arthritic changes or spondylolisthesis; structural abnormalities, such as kyphosis, scoliosis, and lordosis; and congenital abnormalities.

Critical care nursing may seem like backbreaking work, but an X-ray is needed to confirm the diagnosis.

Nursing concerns
- Reassure the patient that X-rays are painless.
- As ordered, administer an analgesic before the procedure if the patient has existing pain, so he'll be more comfortable.
- Remove the patient's cervical collar if cervical X-rays reveal no fracture and the practitioner permits it.

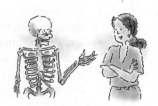

Angiography

Cerebral angiography

During cerebral angiography, the doctor injects a radiopaque contrast medium, usually into the brachial artery (through retrograde brachial injection) or femoral artery (through catheterization).

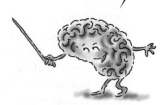

Cerebral angiography is used to detect and identify problems affecting the cerebral vessels.

Why it's done

This procedure highlights cerebral vessels, making it easier to:
- detect stenosis or occlusion associated with thrombus or spasm
- identify aneurysms and AVMs
- locate vessel displacement associated with tumors, abscesses, cerebral edema, hematoma, or herniation
- assess collateral circulation
- treat vasospasm.

Nursing concerns

- Explain the procedure to the patient and answer all questions honestly.
- Confirm that the patient isn't allergic to iodine or shellfish because a person with such allergies may have an adverse reaction to the contrast medium.
- Preprocedure testing should include evaluation of renal function (serum creatinine and BUN levels) and potential risk of bleeding (prothrombin time [PT], partial thromboplastin time [PTT], and platelet count). Notify the practitioner of abnormal results.
- Instruct the patient to lie still during the procedure.
- Explain that he'll probably feel a flushed sensation in his face as the dye is injected.
- Maintain bed rest, as ordered, and monitor the patient's vital signs.
- Monitor the catheter injection site for signs of bleeding.
- As ordered, keep a sandbag over the injection site.
- Monitor the patient's peripheral pulse in the arm or leg used for catheter insertion and mark the site of the pulse for reference.
- Unless contraindicated, encourage the patient to drink more fluids to flush the dye from the body; alternatively, increase the I.V. flow rate as ordered.
- Monitor the patient for neurologic changes and such complications as hemiparesis, hemiplegia, aphasia, and impaired LOC.
- Monitor for adverse reactions to the contrast medium, which may include restlessness, tachypnea and respiratory distress, tachycardia, facial flushing, urticaria, and nausea and vomiting.

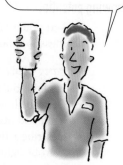

Encourage fluid consumption to flush out the contrast dye after testing, unless it's contraindicated.

Electrophysiologic studies

Common electrophysiologic studies include EEG and evoked potential studies.

Electroencephalography

During EEG, the brain's continuous electrical activity is recorded.

The results are used to identify seizure disorders; metabolic encephalopathy; other multifocal brain lesions, such as those caused by dementia or herpes; and brain death.

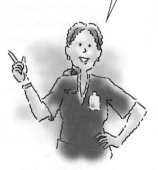

EEG is used to identify problems that affect the brain's electrical activity.

Nursing concerns

- Explain that a technician applies paste and attaches electrodes to areas of skin on the patient's head and neck after these areas have been lightly abraded to ensure good contact.
- Instruct the patient to remain still during the test.
- Discuss what the patient may be asked to do during the test, such as hyperventilating for 3 minutes or sleeping, depending on the purpose of the EEG.
- After the test, use acetone to remove any remaining paste from the patient's skin.

Evoked potential studies

Evoked potential studies are used to measure the nervous system's electrical response to a visual, auditory, or sensory stimulus. The results are used to detect subclinical lesions such as tumors of CN VIII and complicating lesions in a patient with MS.

Showing potential

Evoked potential studies are also useful in diagnosing blindness and deafness in infants.

Nursing concerns

- Explain to the patient that he must remain still during the test.
- Describe how a technician applies paste and electrodes to the head and neck before testing.
- Describe activities—such as gazing at a checkerboard pattern or a strobe light or listening with headphones to a series of clicks—performed during testing. The patient may have electrodes placed on an arm and leg and be asked to respond to a tapping sensation.
- Explain that the test equipment may emit noises.

Other tests

Other neurologic tests include lumbar puncture and transcranial Doppler studies.

Lumbar puncture

During lumbar puncture, a sterile needle is inserted into the subarachnoid space of the spinal canal, usually between the third and fourth lumbar vertebrae. A doctor does the lumbar puncture, with a nurse assisting. It requires sterile technique and careful patient positioning.

Why do it?

Lumbar puncture is used to:
- detect blood in cerebrospinal fluid (CSF)
- obtain CSF specimens for laboratory analysis
- inject dyes or gases for contrast in radiologic studies.
  It's also used to administer drugs or anesthetics.

Contraindications and cautions

Lumbar puncture is contraindicated in patients with lumbar deformity or infection at the puncture site. It's not performed in patients with increased ICP because the rapid decrease of pressure that follows withdrawal of CSF can cause tonsillar herniation and medullary compression.

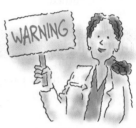

Be careful! If the patient has increased ICP, the rapid drop in ICP after CSF is withdrawn can lead to serious problems.

Nursing concerns
- Calmly describe lumbar puncture to the patient, explaining that the procedure may cause some discomfort.
- Reassure the patient that a local anesthetic is administered before the test. Tell him to report any tingling or sharp pain he feels as the anesthetic is injected.
- To prevent headache after the test, instruct the patient to lie flat for 4 to 6 hours after the procedure.
- Monitor the patient for neurologic deficits and complications, such as headache, fever, back spasms, or seizures, according to facility policy.
- Administer analgesics as needed.
- Monitor the puncture site for signs of infection.

Transcranial Doppler studies

In transcranial Doppler studies, the velocity of blood flow through cerebral arteries is measured. The results provide information about the presence, quality, and changing nature of blood flow to an area of the brain.

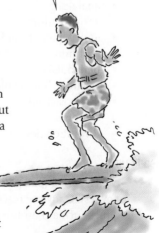

In transcranial Doppler studies, waveforms and velocities of blood flow are measured. High velocities are typically abnormal.

What blood flow tells you

The types of waveforms and velocities obtained by testing indicate whether disease exists. Test results commonly aren't definitive, but this is a noninvasive way to obtain diagnostic information.

High velocities are typically abnormal, suggesting that blood flow is too turbulent or the vessel is too narrow. They may also indicate stenosis or vasospasm. High velocities may also indicate AVM due to the extra blood flow associated with stenosis or vasospasm.

Nursing concerns
- Tell the patient that the study usually takes less than 1 hour, depending on the number of vessels examined and on any interfering factors.
- Explain that a small amount of gel is applied to the skin and that a probe is then used to transmit a signal to the artery being studied.

Treatments

Treatments for patients with neurologic dysfunction may include medication therapy, surgery, and other forms of treatment.

Medication therapy

For many of your patients with neurologic disorders, medication or drug therapy is essential. For example:
- thrombolytics are used to treat patients with acute ischemic stroke
- anticonvulsants are used to control seizures
- corticosteroids are used to reduce inflammation.

Typical types

Types of drugs commonly used to treat patients with neurologic disorders include:
- analgesics
- anticonvulsants
- anticoagulants and antiplatelets
- barbiturates
- benzodiazepines
- calcium channel blockers
- corticosteroids
- diuretics
- thrombolytics.

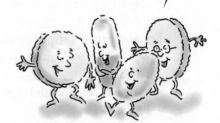

Watch for severe adverse reactions and interactions with other drugs.

Heads up!

When caring for a patient undergoing medication therapy, stay alert for severe adverse reactions and interactions with other drugs. Some drugs such as barbiturates also carry a high risk of toxicity.

Stay the course

Successful therapy hinges on strict adherence to the medication schedule. Compliance is especially critical for drugs that require steady blood levels for therapeutic effectiveness such as anticonvulsants. (See *Common neurologic drugs*, pages 84 to 87.)

Surgery

Life-threatening neurologic disorders usually call for emergency surgery.
Surgery commonly involves craniotomy, a procedure to open the skull and expose the brain.

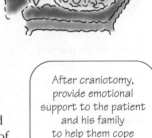

I feel so exposed. Life-threatening neurologic disorders may call for emergency surgery, beginning with craniotomy.

Be ready before and after

You may be responsible for the patient's care before and after surgery.
Here are some general preoperative and postoperative pointers:
- The prospect of surgery usually causes fear and anxiety, so give ongoing emotional support to the patient and his family. Make sure that you're ready to answer their questions.
- Postoperative care may include teaching about diverse topics, such as ventricular shunt care and tips about cosmetic care after craniotomy. Be ready to give good advice after surgery.

Craniotomy

During craniotomy, a surgical opening into the skull exposes the brain. This procedure allows various treatments, such as ventricular shunting, excision of a tumor or abscess, hematoma aspiration, and aneurysm clipping (placing one or more surgical clips on the neck of an aneurysm to destroy it).

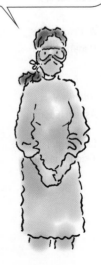

After craniotomy, provide emotional support to the patient and his family to help them cope with any remaining deficits.

Condition and complexity count

The degree of risk depends on your patient's condition and the complexity of the surgery. Craniotomy raises the risk of having various complications, such as:
- infection
- hemorrhage
- respiratory compromise
- increased ICP.

Nursing concerns
- Encourage the patient and his family to ask questions about the procedure. Provide clear, honest answers to reduce their confusion and anxiety and to enhance effective coping.
- Explain that the patient's head will be shaved before surgery in the area where the incision will be made.

(Text continues on page 86.)

Common neurologic drugs

Use this table to find out about common neurologic drugs, their indications and adverse effects, and related monitoring measures.

Drugs	Indications	Adverse effects
Nonopioid analgesics Acetaminophen (Tylenol)	• Mild pain, headache	• Severe liver damage, neutropenia, thrombocytopenia
Opioid analgesics Morphine (MS Contin) Codeine	• Severe pain • Mild to moderate pain	• Respiratory depression, apnea, bradycardia, seizures, sedation • Respiratory depression, bradycardia, sedation, constipation
Anticonvulsants Carbamazepine (Tegretol) Fosphenytoin (Cerebyx) Levetiracetam (Keppra) Phenytoin (Dilantin) Primidone (Mysoline) Valproic acid, valproate (Depakene)	• Generalized tonic-clonic seizures, complex partial seizures, mixed seizures • Status epilepticus, seizures during neurosurgery • Generalized tonic-clonic seizures, partial-onset seizures, juvenile myoclonic epilepsy • Generalized tonic-clonic seizures, status epilepticus, nonepileptic seizures after head trauma • Generalized tonic-clonic seizures, focal seizures, and complex partial seizures • Complex partial seizures, simple and complex absence seizures	• Heart failure, hepatitis, Stevens-Johnson syndrome, aplastic anemia • Increased ICP, cerebral edema, somnolence, ventricular fibrillation, hepatotoxicity • Leukopenia, neutropenia, somnolence, asthenia, dizziness • Agranulocytosis, thrombocytopenia, toxic hepatitis, slurred speech, Stevens-Johnson syndrome, ataxia • Thrombocytopenia, drowsiness, ataxia • Thrombocytopenia, pancreatitis, toxic hepatitis, sedation, Stevens-Johnson syndrome
Anticoagulants Heparin	• Embolism prophylaxis	• Hemorrhage, thrombocytopenia, prolonged clotting time
Antiplatelets Aspirin (Ecotrin) Clopidogrel (Plavix) Ticlopidine (Ticlid)	• TIAs, prophylaxis for TIAs • Thrombotic stroke prophylaxis • Thrombotic stroke prophylaxis	• GI bleeding, acute renal insufficiency, thrombocytopenia, liver dysfunction, angioedema • Purpura, dizziness, rash, epistaxis • Thrombocytopenia, agranulocytosis, intracranial bleeding, hepatitis

Practice pointers

• Monitor total daily intake of acetaminophen because of risk of liver toxicity. Use with caution in elderly patients and those with liver disease.

• Monitor for respiratory depression. Use with caution in elderly patients and those with head injury, seizures, or increased ICP. Contraindicated in patients with acute bronchial asthma.
• Monitor for respiratory depression. Use with caution in elderly patients and those with head injury, seizures, or increased ICP.

• Use cautiously in patients with mixed seizure disorders because it can increase the risk of seizure. Use cautiously in patients with hepatic dysfunction. Obtain baseline liver function studies, complete blood count (CBC), and BUN level. Monitor blood levels of the drug; therapeutic level is 4 to 12 mcg/ml.
• Stop drug with acute hepatotoxicity. May cause hyperglycemia; monitor blood glucose in diabetic patients. Fosphenytoin should be prescribed and dispensed in phenytoin sodium equivalent units. Monitor for cardiac arrhythmias and QT prolongation.
• Use cautiously in immunocompromised patients and patients with a history of psychotic symptoms and behaviors. Use only with other anticonvulsants. Monitor renal function.
• Abrupt withdrawal can trigger status epilepticus. Contraindicated in patients with heart block. Use cautiously in patients with hepatic disease and myocardial insufficiency. Monitor blood levels of the drug; therapeutic range is 10 to 20 mcg/ml. If rash appears, stop the drug.
• Abrupt withdrawal can cause status epilepticus. Reduce dosage in elderly patients.

• Obtain baseline liver function tests. Avoid use in patients at high risk for hepatotoxicity. Abrupt withdrawal may worsen seizures. Monitor blood levels of the drug; therapeutic range is 50 to 100 mcg/ml.

• Monitor for bleeding. Obtain baseline prothrombin time/International Normalized Ratio (PT/INR) and PTT. Monitor PTT at regular intervals. Protamine sulfate reverses the effects of heparin.

• Monitor for bleeding. Avoid use in patients with active peptic ulcer and GI inflammation.

• Monitor for signs of thrombotic thrombocytopenia purpura.
• Monitor for bleeding. Avoid use in patients with hepatic impairment and peptic ulcer disease.

(continued)

Common neurologic drugs *(continued)*

Drugs	Indications	Adverse effects
Barbiturates Phenobarbital (Solfoton)	• All types of seizures except absence seizures, febrile seizures in children; also used for status epilepticus, sedation, and drug withdrawal	• Respiratory depression, apnea, bradycardia, angioedema, Stevens-Johnson syndrome
Benzodiazepines Clonazepam (Klonopin) Diazepam (Valium) Lorazepam (Ativan)	• Absence and atypical seizures, status epilepticus, panic disorders • Status epilepticus, anxiety, acute alcohol withdrawal, muscle spasm, repetitive seizure activity • Status epilepticus, anxiety, agitation	• Respiratory depression, thrombocytopenia, leukopenia, drowsiness, ataxia • Bradycardia, cardiovascular collapse, drowsiness, acute withdrawal syndrome, ataxia • Drowsiness, acute withdrawal syndrome
Corticosteroids Dexamethasone, methylprednisolone (Medrol)	• Cerebral edema associated with brain tumors, severe inflammation	• Heart failure, cardiac arrhythmias, circulatory collapse, thromboembolism, pancreatitis, peptic ulceration
Diuretics Furosemide (Lasix) (loop) Mannitol (Osmitrol)	• Edema, hypertension • Cerebral edema, increased ICP	• Renal failure, thrombocytopenia, agranulocytosis, volume depletion, dehydration, hypokalemia • Seizures, fluid and electrolyte imbalance, diarrhea
Thrombolytics Alteplase (Activase) (recombinant tissue plasminogen activator)	• Acute ischemic stroke	• Cerebral hemorrhage, spontaneous bleeding, allergic reaction

- Discuss the recovery period so the patient understands what to expect. Explain that he'll awaken with a dressing on his head to protect the incision and may have a surgical drain.
- Tell him to expect a headache and facial swelling for 2 to 3 days after surgery and reassure him that he'll receive pain medication.
- Monitor the patient's neurologic status and vital signs and report any acute change immediately. Watch for signs of increased ICP, such as pupil changes, weakness in extremities, headache, and change in LOC.

Practice pointers

• Monitor for respiratory depression and bradycardia. Keep resuscitation equipment on hand when administering I.V. dose; monitor respirations.

• Abrupt withdrawal may precipitate status epilepticus. Withdrawal of drug may cause insomnia, tremors, and hallucinations.
• Monitor for respiratory depression and cardiac arrhythmia. Don't stop suddenly; can cause acute withdrawal in physically dependent persons.

• Don't stop abruptly; can cause withdrawal. Monitor for CNS depressant effects in elderly patients.

• Use cautiously in patients with recent myocardial infarction, hypertension, renal disease, and GI ulcer. Monitor blood pressure and blood glucose levels. Monitor the patient's potassium level (can cause hypokalemia).

• Monitor blood pressure, pulse, and intake and output. Monitor serum electrolyte levels, especially potassium levels. Monitor for cardiac arrhythmias.

• Contraindicated in severe pulmonary congestion and heart failure. Monitor blood pressure, heart rate, and intake and output. Monitor serum electrolyte levels. Use with caution in patients with renal dysfunction.

• Contraindicated in patients with intracranial or subarachnoid hemorrhage. The patient must meet criteria for thrombolytic therapy before initiation of therapy. Monitor baseline laboratory values: hemoglobin (Hb) level, hematocrit (HCT), PTT, PT/INR. Monitor vital signs. Monitor for signs of bleeding. Monitor puncture sites for bleeding.

- Monitor the incision site for signs of infection or drainage.
- Provide emotional support to the patient and his family as they cope with remaining neurologic deficits.

Cerebral aneurysm repair

Surgical intervention is the only sure way to prevent rupture or rebleeding of a cerebral aneurysm.

Endovascular aneurysm repair

An alternative to craniotomy and clipping for intracranial aneurysm repair, an endovascular treatment method called *embolization*, may be used. Embolization is most successful in aneurysms with small necks and those without significant intrafundal thrombus.

Embolization

Here's what happens in embolization:
• A microcatheter with a coil attached is introduced through the initial catheter.
• After the coil is positioned within the fundus of the aneurysm, it is detached from the catheter using an electrical current.
• The delivery catheter is removed, leaving the platinum coil in place, and another coil is introduced into the fundus.

• The process is continued until the aneurysm is densely packed with platinum and no longer opacifies during diagnostic contrast injections.

How it works

The positively charged platinum left in the aneurysm theoretically attracts negatively charged blood elements, such as white and red blood cells, platelets, and fibrinogen. This induces intra-aneurysmal thrombosis.

The coils provide immediate protection against further hemorrhage by reducing blood pulsations in the fundus and sealing the hole or weak portion of the artery wall. Eventually, clots form, and the aneurysm is separated from the parent vessel by the formation of new connective tissue.

Northern exposure

In cerebral aneurysm repair, a craniotomy is performed to expose the aneurysm. Depending on the shape and location of the aneurysm, the surgeon then uses one of several corrective techniques, such as:
• clamping the affected artery
• wrapping the aneurysm wall with a biologic or synthetic material
• clipping or ligating the aneurysm.

New and improved

Other techniques for surgery include *interventional radiology* in conjunction with endovascular balloon therapy. This technique occludes the aneurysm or vessel and uses cerebral angiography to treat arterial vasospasm.

In some cases, a type of nonsurgical repair called *embolization* is used. (See *Endovascular aneurysm repair*.)

Nursing concerns
• Tell the patient and his family that monitoring is done in the critical care unit before and after surgery. Explain that several I.V. lines, intubation, and mechanical ventilation may be needed.
• Monitor the incision site for signs of infection or drainage.
• Monitor the patient's neurologic status and vital signs and report acute changes immediately. Watch for signs of increased ICP, such as pupil changes, weakness in extremities, headache, and a change in LOC.
• Give emotional support to the patient and his family to help them cope with remaining neurologic deficits.

Other treatments

Other treatments include barbiturate coma, CSF drainage, ICP monitoring, and plasmapheresis.

Barbiturate coma

The practitioner may order barbiturate coma when conventional treatments, such as fluid restriction, diuretic or corticosteroid therapy, or ventricular shunting, don't correct sustained or acute episodes of increased ICP.

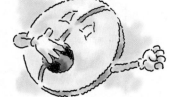

A barbiturate coma produces a drug-induced state that reduces the patient's metabolic rate and cerebral blood flow. I suddenly feel very sleepy . . .

High I.V.

During barbiturate coma, the patient receives high I.V. doses of a short-acting barbiturate (such as pentobarbital [Nembutal]) to produce a comatose state. The drug reduces the patient's metabolic rate and cerebral blood flow.

Last resort

The goal of barbiturate coma is to relieve increased ICP and protect cerebral tissue. It's a last resort for patients with:
- acute ICP elevation (over 40 mm Hg)
- persistent ICP elevation (over 20 mm Hg)
- rapidly deteriorating neurologic status that's unresponsive to other treatments.

If barbiturate coma doesn't reduce ICP, the patient's prognosis for recovery is poor.

Nursing concerns
- Focus your attention on the patient's family. The patient's condition and apprehension about the treatment is likely to frighten them. Provide clear explanations of the procedure and its effects and encourage them to ask questions. Convey a sense of optimism but provide no guarantees of the treatment's success.
- Prepare the family for expected changes in the patient during therapy, such as decreased respirations, hypotension, and loss of muscle tone and reflexes.
- Closely monitor the patient's ICP, electrocardiogram (ECG), bispectral index, and vital signs. Notify the practitioner of increased ICP, arrhythmias, or hypotension.
- Because the patient is in a drug-induced coma, devote special care to safety measures to prevent injury.

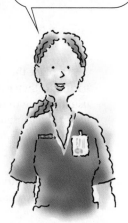

Devote special care to pressure ulcer prevention when the patient is in a drug-induced coma.

Cerebrospinal fluid drainage

The goal of CSF drainage is to reduce ICP to the desired level and keep it at that level. Fluid is withdrawn from the lateral ventricle through an external ventricular catheter (EVD).

CSF closed drainage system

The goal of CSF drainage is to control ICP during treatment for traumatic injury or other conditions that cause increased ICP. Here's one common procedure.

External ventricular drain

For a ventricular drain, the neurosurgeon makes a burr hole in the patient's skull and inserts the catheter into the ventricle. The distal end of the catheter is connected to a closed drainage system.

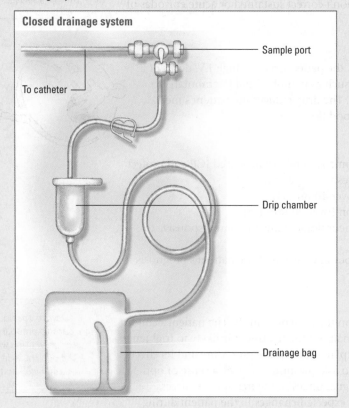

Closed drainage system

Sample port

To catheter

Drip chamber

Drainage bag

> Observe for complications such as rapid or excessive CSF drainage—an emergency! Signs and symptoms include headache, tachycardia, diaphoresis, and nausea.

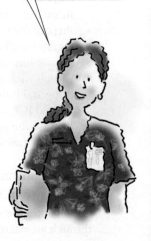

To place the ventricular drain, a neurosurgeon inserts a ventricular catheter through a burr hole in the patient's skull. This is usually done in the operating room but can be done in the emergency department (ED) or at the bedside in the intensive care unit. (See *CSF closed drainage system.*)

Nursing concerns

- For continuous drainage of CSF by maintaining the drainage system, drip chamber at the desired level.

- To intermittently drain the CSF, put on gloves and turn the main stopcock on to drainage and allow the CSF to collect in the drip chamber according to ordered parameters.
- To stop drainage, turn off the stopcock to drainage. Record the time and the amount of collected CSF as well as its color.
- Check the patient's dressing frequently for drainage or bleeding.
- Check the tubing for patency by watching the CSF drops in the drip chamber.
- Observe the CSF for color, clarity, amount, blood, and sediment.
- Maintain the patient on bed rest with the head of the bed at 30 degrees to promote venous drainage that will also help control ICP.
- Observe for complications, such as excessive CSF drainage, characterized by headache, tachycardia, diaphoresis, and nausea. Overly rapid accumulation of drainage can be a neurosurgical emergency by causing a subdural hematoma. Cessation of drainage may indicate clot formation or collapse of ventricles.

Intracranial pressure monitoring

In ICP monitoring, pressure exerted by the brain, blood, and CSF against the inside of the skull is measured. ICP monitoring enables prompt intervention, which can avert damage caused by cerebral hypoxia and shifts of brain mass.

Indications for ICP monitoring include:
- closed head injury with severe neurologic deficit
- overproduction or insufficient absorption of CSF (hydrocephalus)
- cerebral hemorrhage
- space-occupying lesions.

Four similar systems

There are four basic types of ICP monitoring systems. (See *Monitoring ICP*, page 92.) Regardless of which system is used, the insertion procedure is always performed by a neurosurgeon in the operating room, ED, or critical care unit. Insertion of an ICP monitoring device requires sterile technique to reduce the risk of CNS infection.

Doctors do this

The neurosurgeon inserts a ventricular catheter or subarachnoid screw through a twist-drill hole created in the skull. The device is attached to a transducer that converts ICP to electrical impulses displayed as waveforms, allowing constant monitoring.

Nursing concerns
- Observe digital ICP readings and waveforms. (See *Interpreting ICP waveforms*, page 93.)

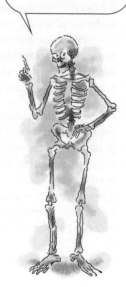

Pressure exerted by the brain, blood, and CSF against the inside of my skull can cause cerebral hypoxia and shifts in brain mass. That can hurt!

Monitoring ICP

ICP can be monitored using one of four systems.

1 Intraventricular catheter monitoring

In intraventricular catheter monitoring, used to monitor ICP directly, the doctor inserts a small polyethylene or silicone rubber catheter into the lateral ventricles through a burr hole.

Although this method is most accurate for measuring ICP, it carries the greatest risk of infection. This is the only type of ICP monitoring that allows evaluation of brain compliance and significant drainage of CSF.

Contraindications usually include stenotic cerebral ventricles, cerebral aneurysms in the path of catheter placement, and suspected vascular lesions.

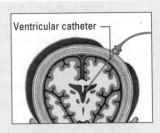

Ventricular catheter

2 Subarachnoid bolt monitoring

Subarachnoid bolt monitoring involves insertion of a special bolt into the subarachnoid space through a twist-drill burr hole in the front of the skull, behind the hairline.

Placing the bolt is easier than placing an intraventricular catheter, especially if a CT scan reveals that the cerebrum has shifted or the ventricles have collapsed. This type of ICP monitoring carries less risk of infection and parenchymal damage because the bolt doesn't penetrate the cerebrum.

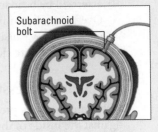

Subarachnoid bolt

3 Epidural or subdural sensor monitoring

ICP can also be monitored from the epidural or subdural space. For epidural monitoring, a fiber-optic sensor is inserted into the epidural space through a burr hole. This system's main drawback is its questionable accuracy because ICP isn't being measured directly from a CSF-filled space.

For subdural monitoring, a fiber-optic transducer-tipped catheter is tunneled through a burr hole and is placed on brain tissue under the dura mater. The main drawback to this method is its inability to drain CSF.

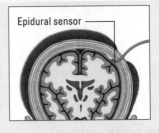

Epidural sensor

4 Intraparenchymal monitoring

In intraparenchymal monitoring, the doctor inserts a catheter through a small subarachnoid bolt and, after punctuating the dura mater, advances the catheter a few centimeters into the brain's white matter. There's no need to balance or calibrate the equipment after insertion.

This method doesn't provide direct access to CSF, but measurements are accurate because brain tissue pressure correlates well with ventricular pressures. Intraparenchymal monitoring may be used to obtain ICP measurements in patients with compressed or dislocated ventricles.

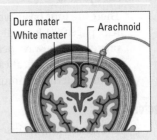

Dura mater
White matter
Arachnoid

Interpreting ICP waveforms

Three waveforms—A, B, and C—are used to monitor ICP. A waves are an ominous sign of intracranial decompensation and poor compliance, B waves correlate with changes in respiration, and C waves correlate with changes in arterial pressure.

Normal waveform

A normal ICP waveform typically shows a steep upward systolic slope followed by a downward diastolic slope with a dicrotic notch. In most cases, this waveform is continuous and indicates an ICP between 0 and 15 mm Hg (normal blood pressure).

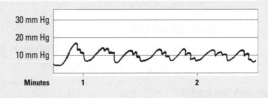

A waves

The most clinically significant ICP waveforms are A waves, which may reach elevations of 50 to 200 mm Hg, persist for 5 to 20 minutes, then drop sharply, signaling exhaustion of the brain's compliance mechanisms.

A waves may come and go, spiking from temporary increases in thoracic pressure or from any condition that increases ICP beyond the brain's compliance limits. A waves are commonly associated with a temporary decrease in neurologic status.

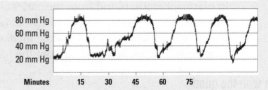

B waves

B waves, which appear sharp and rhythmic with a sawtooth pattern, occur every 30 seconds to 2 minutes and may reach an elevation of 50 mm Hg. The clinical significance of B waves isn't clear; however, the waves correlate with respiratory changes and may occur more frequently with decreasing compensation.

Because B waves sometimes precede A waves, notify the practitioner if B waves occur frequently.

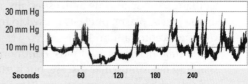

C waves

Like B waves, C waves are rapid and rhythmic, but they aren't as sharp. They may reach an elevation of 20 mm Hg and occur up to six times per minute. They're clinically insignificant and may fluctuate with respirations or systemic blood pressure changes.

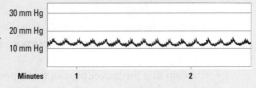

Waveform showing equipment problem

A waveform like the one shown at right signals a problem with the transducer or monitor. Check for line obstruction and determine whether the transducer needs rebalancing.

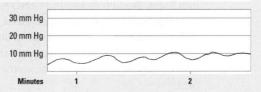

- Assess the patient's clinical status and monitor routine and neurologic vital signs every hour or as ordered.
- Calculate cerebral perfusion pressure (CPP) hourly. To calculate CPP, subtract ICP from mean arterial pressure (MAP).
- Inspect the insertion site at least every 24 hours for redness, swelling, and drainage.

Plasmapheresis

Symptoms of several neurologic disorders are reduced through plasma exchange or plasmapheresis.

Out with the bad

In plasmapheresis, blood from the patient flows into a cell separator, which separates plasma from formed elements. The plasma is then filtered to remove toxins and disease mediators, such as immune complexes and autoantibodies, from the patient's blood.

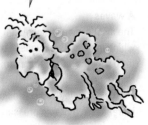

Looks like I'm movin' out! In plasmapheresis, plasma is filtered to remove toxins and disease mediators from the patient's blood.

In with the good

The cellular components are then transfused back into the patient using fresh frozen plasma or albumin in place of the plasma removed.

Who benefits?

Plasmapheresis benefits patients with neurologic disorders such as Guillain-Barré syndrome and, especially, myasthenia gravis. In myasthenia gravis, plasmapheresis is used to remove circulating antiacetylcholine receptor antibodies.

Plasmapheresis is used most commonly for patients with long-standing neuromuscular disease, but it can also be used to treat patients with acute exacerbations. Some acutely ill patients require treatment up to four times per week; others about once every 2 weeks. When it's successful, treatment may relieve symptoms for months, but results vary.

Administer prescribed medications after plasmapheresis; otherwise, they're removed from the blood during treatment.

Nursing concerns

- Discuss the treatment and its purpose with the patient and his family.
- Explain that the procedure can take up to 5 hours. During that time, blood samples are taken frequently to monitor calcium and potassium levels. Blood pressure and heart rate are checked regularly. Tell the patient to report any paresthesia (numbness, burning, tingling, prickling, or increased sensitivity) during treatment.
- If possible, give the patient prescribed medications after treatment because they're removed from the blood during treatment.
- Monitor the patient's vital signs according to your facility's policy.
- Check puncture sites for signs of bleeding or extravasation.

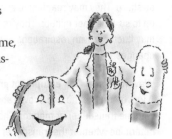

Neurologic system disorders

In the critical care unit, you're likely to encounter patients with common neurologic disorders, especially acute spinal cord injury, AVM, cerebral aneurysm, encephalitis, Guillain-Barré syndrome, head injury, meningitis, seizure disorders, and stroke.

Acute spinal cord injury

Spinal injuries include fractures, contusions, and compressions of the vertebral column. They usually result from trauma to the head or neck. Fractures of the 5th, 6th, or 7th cervical; 12th thoracic; and 1st lumbar vertebrae are most common.

Dangerous damage

The real danger with spinal injury is spinal cord damage due to cutting, pulling, twisting, and compression. Spinal cord injury can occur at any level, and the damage it causes may be partial or involve the entire cord.

Complications of spinal cord injury include neurogenic shock and spinal shock. (See *Complications of spinal cord injury*, page 96.)

> "Diving injuries can cause the most serious spinal cord trauma."

What causes it

The most serious spinal cord trauma typically results from motor vehicle accidents, falls, sports injuries, diving into shallow water, and gunshot or stab wounds. Less serious injuries commonly occur from lifting heavy objects and minor falls.

Spinal dysfunction may also result from hyperparathyroidism and neoplastic lesions.

How it happens

Spinal cord trauma results from acceleration, deceleration, or other deforming forces. Types of trauma include:
- hyperextension due to acceleration–deceleration forces
- hyperflexion from sudden and excessive force
- vertebral compression from downward force from the top of the cranium, along the vertical axis, and through the vertebra
- rotational twisting, which adds shearing forces.

Trauma trail

Here's what happens during spinal cord trauma:
- An injury causes microscopic hemorrhages in the gray matter and pia–arachnoid.
- The hemorrhages gradually increase in size until all of the gray matter is filled with blood, which causes necrosis.

Take charge!

Complications of spinal cord injury

When you assess your patient, watch for these two complications related to spinal cord injuries.

Neurogenic shock

Neurogenic shock is an abnormal vasomotor response that occurs secondary to disruption of sympathetic impulses from the brain stem to the thoracolumbar area. It's most common in patients with cervical cord injury. It causes temporary loss of autonomic function below the level of injury and leads to cardiovascular changes.

Signs of neurogenic shock include:
- orthostatic hypotension
- bradycardia
- inability to sweat below the level of the injury.

Spinal shock

Spinal shock is the loss of autonomic, reflex, motor, and sensory activity below the level of the cord lesion. It occurs secondary to damage of the spinal cord.

Signs of spinal shock include:
- flaccid paralysis
- loss of deep tendon and perianal reflexes
- loss of motor and sensory function.

- From the gray matter, the blood enters the white matter, where it impedes circulation within the spinal cord.
- Resulting edema causes compression and decreases the blood supply.
- The spinal cord loses perfusion and becomes ischemic. The edema and hemorrhage are usually greatest in the two segments above and below the injury.
- The edema temporarily adds to the patient's dysfunction by increasing pressure and compressing the nerves. For example, edema near the 3rd to 5th cervical vertebrae may interfere with respiration.

After acute injury

Here's what happens following acute trauma:
- In the white matter, circulation usually returns to normal within 24 hours after injury.
- In the gray matter, an inflammatory reaction prevents restoration of circulation.
- Phagocytes appear at the site within 35 to 48 hours after injury.
- Macrophages engulf degenerating axons, and collagen replaces the normal tissue.

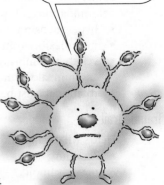

After acute spinal injury, scarring and meningeal thickening leave the nerves in the area blocked or tangled.

- Scarring and meningeal thickening leave the nerves in the area blocked or tangled.

What to look for

In your assessment, look for:
- history of trauma, a neoplastic lesion, an infection that could produce a spinal abscess, or an endocrine disorder
- muscle spasm and back or neck pain that worsens with movement; in cervical fractures, pain that causes point tenderness; in dorsal and lumbar fractures, pain that may radiate to other areas, such as the legs
- mild paresthesia to quadriplegia and shock, if the injury damages the spinal cord.

Speaking specifically

Specific signs and symptoms depend on the type and degree of injury. (See *Types of spinal cord injury*, page 98.)

What tests tell you

Diagnoses of acute spinal cord injuries are based on the results of these tests:
- Spinal X-rays reveal fracture.
- CT scan and MRI show the location of fracture and the site of compression and reveal spinal cord edema and a possible spinal cord mass.
- Neurologic assessment is essential to determine the level of injury and detect cord damage.

I think the correct treatment option is sandbags on both sides of the head. Can anyone reach that shovel?

How it's treated

The primary treatment after spinal injury is immediate immobilization to stabilize the spine and prevent further damage. Other treatment is supportive.

Cervical injuries require immobilization, using sandbags on both sides of the patient's head, a hard cervical collar, or skeletal traction with skull tongs or a halo device.

What to do

Here's what you should do for patients with spinal cord injuries:
- Immediately stabilize the patient's spine. As with all spinal injuries, suspect cord damage until proven otherwise.
- Perform a neurologic assessment to establish a baseline and continually reassess neurologic status for changes.
- Assess respiratory status closely at least every hour, initially. Obtain baseline tidal volume, vital capacity, negative inspiratory forces, and minute volume.
- Auscultate breath sounds and check secretions as necessary.

Types of spinal cord injury

A patient with an acute spinal cord injury (SCI) typically has pain at the site of the spinal fracture. However, it's important to remember that these patients also often have associated brain and systemic injuries that may limit the patient's ability to report localized pain.

Immediately after an SCI, there may be a physiologic loss of all spinal cord function caudal to the level of the injury, with flaccid paralysis, anesthesia, absent bowel and bladder control, and loss of reflex activity. In males, especially those with a cervical cord injury, priapism may develop. This altered physiologic state may last several hours to several weeks and is sometimes referred to as *spinal shock*.

SCI may be complete or incomplete.

Complete injury

Description

- All tracts below the level of the injury are disrupted.
- Loss of motor and sensory function below the level of the injury
  - Cervical cord level—quadriplegia
  - Thoracic level—paraplegia
- Loss is complete and permanent.

Signs and symptoms

- Muscle flaccidity
- Loss of all reflexes and sensory function
- Bowel and bladder atony
- Spinal shock—loss of vasomotor tone
- May have respiratory impairment if the level is at or above C4

Incomplete injury

There are varying degrees of preserved neurologic function depending on the spinal tracts involved.

Description: central cord syndrome

- Injury involves the more centrally located motor fibers.
- Common in elderly after a fall—related to the degenerative changes
- Often a hyperextension/flexion injury

Signs and symptoms

- Motor weakness greater in the upper extremities than the lower extremities

- Often accompanied by a burning dysesthesia in the hands

Description: anterior cord syndrome

- Injury involves the more anterior fibers both motor and sensory.
- Can be the result of a vascular compromise

Signs and symptoms

- Loss of motor function below the level of the injury
- Loss of pain and temperature below the level of the injury
- Maintenance of light touch, pressure, position, and vibratory sensation

Description: Brown-Séquard syndrome

- Damage to only one side of the cord
- Common with gunshot wounds or stabbing

Signs and symptoms

- Ipsilateral loss of motor function below the level of the injury
- Ipsilateral loss of light touch, pressure, position, and vibratory sensation below the level of the injury
- Contralateral loss of pain and temperature below the level of the injury

- Monitor oxygen saturation levels as ordered. Administer supplemental oxygen as indicated.
- Assess cardiac status frequently, at least every hour initially. Begin cardiac monitoring. Monitor blood pressure and hemodynamic status frequently. If a pulmonary artery catheter is in place, inform the practitioner if there's a decrease in right atrial pressure, pulmonary artery pressure, pulmonary wedge pressure, and systemic vascular resistance that indicates neurogenic shock.

- If your patient becomes hypotensive, prepare to administer vasopressors.
- Prepare the patient for surgical stabilization, if necessary.
- Assess GI status closely for signs of ulceration or bleeding. Anticipate nasogastric (NG) tube insertion and low intermittent suctioning. Assess the abdomen for distention, auscultate bowel sounds, and report any decrease or absence. Be alert for paralytic ileus, which usually occurs 72 hours after injury.
- Monitor intake and output for fluid imbalance.
- Insert an indwelling urinary catheter as ordered.
- Begin measures to prevent skin breakdown due to immobilization, including repositioning, padding, and care of equipment such as halo or traction devices.
- Monitor laboratory and diagnostic test results, including BUN and creatinine levels, CBC, and urine culture (if indicated).
- Monitor the patient for deep vein thrombosis and pulmonary embolism. Apply antiembolism stockings or intermittent sequential compression devices as ordered.
- Provide emotional support to the patient and his family.
- Begin rehabilitation as soon as possible. An obese patient with spinal cord injury may have additional needs. (See *Obesity and acute spinal cord injury.*)

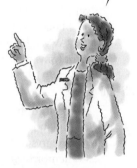

Whew! This is quite a list. Spinal injuries are very serious and require careful assessment and monitoring.

Weighing the evidence

Obesity and acute spinal cord injury

In people with SCI, obesity is commonly cited as one of the major risk factors for the higher prevalence of cardiovascular disease (CVD). Studies on SCI have shown relationships between measures of adiposity and CVD risk factors, such as abnormalities in carbohydrate metabolism and serum lipid levels and hypertension. For example, body mass index (BMI) or upper body obesity is positively correlated with serum triglycerides, insulin, glucose, and C-reactive protein levels.

A recent study using a combination of self-reported and measured heights and weights to determine BMI and a blood pressure level of <120/80 mm Hg as the reference showed that borderline and high blood pressure levels were positively related to being overweight or obese in veterans with SCI. However, data on smoking, a variable related to BMI and blood pressure, were lacking in this study. Findings from these studies on obesity and health outcomes must be interpreted cautiously, keeping in mind that cross-sectional associations don't prove causality.

Source: Rajan, S., McNeely, M. J., Warms, C., & Goldstein, B. (2008). Clinical assessment and management of obesity in individuals with spinal cord injury: A review. *Journal of Spinal Cord Medicine, 31*(4), 361–372.

Arteriovenous malformation

AVMs are tangled masses of thin-walled, dilated blood vessels between arteries and veins that aren't connected by capillaries. Abnormal channels between the arterial and venous system mix oxygenated and unoxygenated blood. This prevents adequate perfusion of brain tissue.

Looking for AVMs

AVMs are common in the brain, especially in the posterior parts of the cerebral hemispheres. They range in size from a few millimeters to large malformations extending from the cerebral cortex to the ventricles. More than one AVM is commonly found.

Males and females are affected equally, and some evidence exists that AVMs occur in families. Most AVMs are present at birth, but symptoms typically occur later, when the person is 10 to 20 years old.

Uh-oh

Complications depend on the severity (location and size) of the AVM and include:
- aneurysm development and subsequent rupture
- hemorrhage (intracerebral, subarachnoid, or subdural, depending on the location of the AVM)
- hydrocephalus.

What causes it

Causes of AVMs may be either:
- congenital—due to a hereditary defect
- acquired—due to penetrating injuries such as trauma.

How it happens

AVMs lack the typical structural characteristics of the blood vessels; the vessels of an AVM are very thin.

Blood pressure, aneurysm, and hemorrhage

One or more arteries feed into the AVM; the typically high-pressured arterial blood flow moves into the venous system through connecting channels. This increases venous pressure, engorging and dilating the venous structures, which may result in the development of an aneurysm.

If the AVM is large enough, the shunting can deprive the surrounding tissue of adequate blood flow. Additionally, the thin-walled vessels may ooze small amounts of blood or rupture, causing hemorrhage into the brain or subarachnoid space.

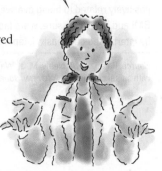

Most patients with AVM exhibit few, if any, signs or symptoms—unless the AVM is large or it leaks or ruptures.

What to look for

Typically, patients exhibit few, if any, signs and symptoms unless the AVM is large or it leaks or ruptures.

Some signs and symptoms

In some patients, signs and symptoms include:
- chronic mild headache and confusion from AVM dilation, vessel engorgement, and increased pressure
- seizures secondary to compression of the surrounding tissues by the engorged vessels
- systolic bruit over the carotid artery, mastoid process, or orbit, indicating turbulent blood flow
- focal neurologic deficits (depending on the location of the AVM) resulting from compression and diminished perfusion
- symptoms of intracranial (intracerebral, subarachnoid, or subdural) hemorrhage, including sudden severe headache, seizures, confusion, lethargy, and meningeal irritation from bleeding into the brain tissue or subarachnoid space
- hydrocephalus from AVM extension into the ventricular lining.

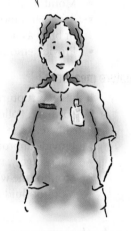

Loss of blood through thin-walled vessels can lead to rupture and hemorrhage.

What tests tell you

The following tests are used to diagnose AVM:
- Cerebral angiography yields the most definitive diagnostic information. It's used to localize the AVM and allow visualization of large feeding arteries and drainage veins.
- MRI/MRA is used to determine the location and size of AVM.

How it's treated

The choice of treatment depends on the:
- size and location of the AVM
- feeder vessels supplying it
- age and condition of the patient.

Supportive, corrective, or both

Treatment can be supportive, corrective, or both, including:
- support measures, such as aneurysm precautions to prevent possible rupture
- surgery—block dissection, laser, or ligation—to repair the communicating channels and remove the feeding vessels
- embolization or stereotactic radiosurgery if surgery isn't possible, to close the communicating channels and feeder vessels and thus reduce blood flow to the AVM.

What to do

If hemorrhage hasn't occurred in your patient with AVM, focus your efforts on bleeding prevention.

Steps to take

To prevent bleeding, follow these steps to control hypertension and seizure activity:
- Maintain a quiet therapeutic environment.
- Monitor and control associated hypertension with drug therapy as ordered.
- Conduct ongoing neurologic assessments.
- Monitor vital signs frequently.
- Assess and monitor characteristics of headache, seizure activity, or bruit as needed.
- Provide emotional support.

Rupture measures

If the AVM ruptures, work to control elevated ICP and intracranial hemorrhage. Follow the previously described steps as well as those listed here:
- Provide appropriate preoperative teaching.
- After surgery, monitor neurologic status and vital signs frequently.
- Monitor the wound for signs of infection.
- Monitor fluid balance and electrolyte levels.

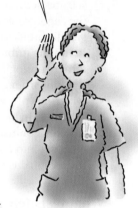

Listen up! To prevent bleeding, maintain a quiet, therapeutic environment and take the necessary steps to control hypertension and seizure activity.

Cerebral aneurysm

In intracranial or cerebral aneurysm, a weakness in the wall of a cerebral artery causes that area of the artery to dilate or bulge. The most common form is the berry aneurysm, a saclike outpouching in a cerebral artery.

The usual place

Cerebral aneurysms usually arise at an arterial junction in the circle of Willis, the circular anastomosis forming the major cerebral arteries at the base of the brain. Cerebral aneurysms commonly rupture and cause subarachnoid hemorrhage.

The usual patient

The incidence of cerebral aneurysm is slightly higher in women than in men, especially those in their late 40s or early to mid-50s, but a cerebral aneurysm can occur at any age in either sex.

The usual prognosis

The prognosis for any patient with cerebral aneurysm is guarded. About 50% of all patients who suffer a subarachnoid hemorrhage die immediately.

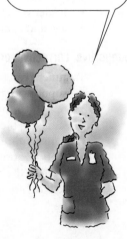

In cerebral aneurysm, blood pressure against a weak arterial wall stretches the vessel like a balloon, making it likely to rupture.

Signs of increased ICP

The earlier you spot signs of increased ICP, the quicker you can intervene and the better your patient's chance of recovery. By the time late signs appear, interventions may be useless.

Assessment area	Early signs	Late signs
LOC	• Requires increased stimulation • Subtle orientation loss • Restlessness and anxiety • Sudden quietness	• Unarousable
Pupils	• Pupil changes on side of lesion • One pupil constricts but then dilates (unilateral hippus). • Sluggish reaction of both pupils • Unequal pupils	• Pupils fixed and dilated or "blown"
Motor response	• Sudden weakness • Motor changes on side opposite the lesion • Positive pronator drift: With palms up, one hand pronates.	• Profound weakness • Decorticate or decerebrate posturing
Vital signs	• Intermittent increases in blood pressure	• Increased systolic blood pressure with widening pulse pressure, bradycardia, and abnormal respirations (Cushing's triad)

Of those who survive untreated, 40% die from the effects of hemorrhage and another 20% die later from recurring hemorrhage. New treatments are improving the prognosis.

The major complications of cerebral aneurysm include death from increased ICP and brain herniation, rebleeding, and vasospasm. (See *Signs of increased ICP*.)

What causes it

Causes of cerebral aneurysm include:
• congenital defect
• degenerative process
• combination of congenital defect and degenerative process
• trauma.

How it happens

Blood flow exerts pressure against a weak arterial wall, stretching it like an overblown balloon and making it likely to rupture.

Right after rupture

Rupture causes a subarachnoid hemorrhage, in which blood spills into the space normally occupied by CSF. Sometimes, blood also spills into brain tissue, where a clot can cause potentially fatal increased ICP and brain tissue damage.

What to look for

Occasionally, your patient may exhibit signs and symptoms due to blood oozing into the subarachnoid space. The symptoms, which may persist for several days, include:
- headache
- intermittent nausea
- nuchal rigidity
- stiff back and legs.

Rupture without warning

Aneurysm rupture usually occurs abruptly and without warning, causing:
- sudden severe headache caused by increased pressure from bleeding into a closed space
- nausea and projectile vomiting related to increased ICP
- altered LOC, possibly including deep coma, depending on the severity and location of bleeding, due to increased pressure caused by increased cerebral blood volume
- meningeal irritation due to bleeding into the meninges and resulting in nuchal rigidity, back and leg pain, fever, restlessness, irritability, occasional seizures, photophobia, and blurred vision
- hemiparesis, hemisensory defects, dysphagia, and visual defects due to bleeding into the brain tissues
- diplopia, ptosis, dilated pupil, and inability to rotate the eye caused by compression on the oculomotor nerve if the aneurysm is near the internal carotid artery.

Grading severity

Typically, the severity of a ruptured cerebral aneurysm is graded according to the patient's signs and symptoms. (See *Grading cerebral aneurysm rupture.*)

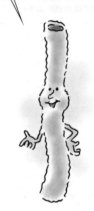

Reports of headache, nausea, and back and leg stiffness lasting several days may signal an impending aneurysm rupture.

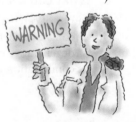

A cerebral aneurysm typically ruptures before symptoms are seen. Signs after rupture are sudden and severe.

WARNING

Grading cerebral aneurysm rupture

The severity of symptoms varies from patient to patient, depending on the site and amount of bleeding. Five grades characterize ruptured cerebral aneurysm:

• *Grade I: minimal bleeding*—The patient is alert, with no neurologic deficit; he may have a slight headache and nuchal rigidity.

• *Grade II: mild bleeding*—The patient is alert, with a mild to severe headache and nuchal rigidity; he may have third nerve palsy.

• *Grade III: moderate bleeding*—The patient is confused or drowsy, with nuchal rigidity and, possibly, a mild focal deficit.

• *Grade IV: severe bleeding*—The patient is stuporous, with nuchal rigidity and, possibly, mild to severe hemiparesis.

• *Grade V: moribund (usually fatal)*—If the rupture is nonfatal, the patient is in a deep coma or decerebrate.

What tests tell you

The following tests help diagnose cerebral aneurysm:

• Cerebral angiography confirms a cerebral aneurysm that isn't ruptured and reveals altered cerebral blood flow, vessel lumen dilation, and differences in arterial filling.

• CT scan, CTA, or MRA reveals evidence of aneurysm and possible hemorrhage.

• Transcranial Doppler sonography is used to detect vasospasm.

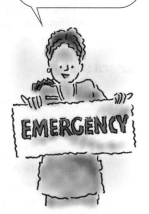

Think fast! Emergency treatment begins with oxygenation and ventilation before the doctor attempts aneurysm repair.

How it's treated

Emergency treatment begins with oxygenation and ventilation. Then, to reduce the risk of rebleeding, the doctor may attempt to repair the aneurysm. Surgical repair usually includes clipping, ligating, or wrapping the aneurysm neck with muscle, or embolization.

Conservative whys

The patient may receive conservative treatment when surgical correction poses too much risk, such as when:

• the patient is elderly

• the patient has heart, lung, or other serious disease

• the aneurysm is in a dangerous location

• the vasospasm necessitates a delay in surgery.

Conservative ways

Conservative treatment methods include:

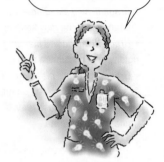

- bed rest in a quiet, darkened room with the head of bed flat or raised less than 30 degrees, which may continue for 4 to 6 weeks
- avoidance of coffee, other stimulants, and aspirin to reduce the risk of rupture and elevation of blood pressure
- possible administration of codeine or another analgesic
- administration of hydralazine (Apresoline) or another antihypertensive, if the patient is hypertensive
- administration of corticosteroids to reduce inflammation
- administration of phenobarbital (Solfoton) or another sedative
- administration of a vasoconstrictor to maintain an optimum blood pressure level (20 to 40 mm Hg above normal), if necessary
- administration of nimodipine to reduce vasospasm.

What to do

When caring for a patient with an intact cerebral aneurysm, an accurate neurologic assessment, good patient care, patient and family teaching, and psychological support can speed recovery and reduce complications.

Your next step

During the initial treatment after hemorrhage, follow these steps:

- Establish and maintain a patent airway and anticipate the need for supplementary oxygen or mechanical ventilatory support. Monitor arterial blood gas (ABG) levels.
- Position the patient to promote pulmonary drainage and prevent upper airway obstruction. If intubated, preoxygenate with 100% oxygen before suctioning.
- Impose aneurysm precautions (such as bed rest, limited visitors, and avoidance of coffee and physical activity) to minimize the risk of rebleeding and avoid increased ICP.
- Administer a stool softener, as ordered, to prevent straining.
- Monitor LOC and vital signs frequently. Avoid rectal temperatures.
- Determine the CPP. Institute cerebral blood flow monitoring as ordered to determine CPP. If not available, calculate CPP by subtracting the patient's ICP from the MAP (systolic blood pressure plus twice the diastolic blood pressure divided by 3).
- Accurately measure intake and output.

- Be alert for danger signs that may indicate an enlarging aneurysm, rebleeding, intracranial clot, increased ICP, or vasospasm, including decreased LOC, unilateral enlarged pupil, onset or worsening of hemiparesis or motor deficit, increased blood pressure, slowed pulse rate, worsening of headache or sudden onset of a headache, renewed or worsened nuchal rigidity, and renewed or persistent vomiting.
- If the patient develops vasospasm—evidenced by focal motor deficits, increasing confusion, and worsening headache—initiate hypervolemic-hemodilution therapy, as ordered, such as the administration of normal saline, whole blood, packed red blood cells, albumin plasma protein fraction, and crystalloid solution. A calcium channel blocker may reduce smooth muscle spasm and maximize perfusion during spasm. During therapy, assess the patient for fluid overload.
- Turn the patient often, apply antiembolism stockings or intermittent sequential compression devices to the patient's legs, and begin measures to prevent skin breakdown.
- If the patient has facial weakness, assist during meals. If he can't swallow, insert an NG tube, as ordered. Give all tube feedings slowly.
- Prepare the patient for surgery, as appropriate, and provide preoperative teaching if the patient's condition permits.
- Teach the patient and his family about the condition and how to recognize and report signs of rebleeding.

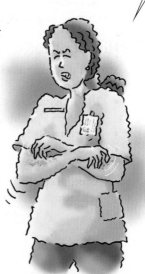

Encephalitis is usually caused by a mosquito-borne virus, but it can be acquired in other ways, too. Think I'll stock up on some new netting as a precaution, though.

Encephalitis

Encephalitis is severe inflammation of the brain, usually caused by a mosquito-borne or, in some areas, a tick-borne virus. Other means of transmission include ingestion of infected goat's milk and accidental injection or inhalation of the virus.

What causes it

Encephalitis results from infection with arboviruses specific to rural areas. In urban areas, it's most commonly caused by enteroviruses (coxsackievirus, poliovirus, and echovirus).

Other causes include herpesvirus, mumps virus, human immunodeficiency virus, adenoviruses, and demyelinating diseases following measles, varicella, rubella, or vaccination.

How it happens

With encephalitis, intense lymphocytic infiltration of brain tissues and the leptomeninges causes cerebral edema, degeneration of the brain's ganglion cells, and diffuse nerve cell destruction.

What to look for

Watch for the signs and symptoms that signal the beginning of acute illness, including:
- fever (102° to 105° F [38.9° to 40.6° C])
- headache
- vomiting.

Negative progression

The illness can progress to include signs and symptoms of meningeal irritation, such as stiff neck and back. Be alert for signs of neuron damage, such as:
- drowsiness
- coma
- paralysis
- seizures
- ataxia
- organic psychoses.

What tests tell you

These tests help diagnose encephalitis:
- CSF or blood analysis used to identify the causative virus confirms the diagnosis.
- Technetium-99 scan results may show localized abnormalities.
- CT scan may disclose localized abnormalities.

How it's treated

Most of the treatments for patients with encephalitis are entirely supportive:
- The antiviral agent acyclovir (Zovirax) is effective in treatment herpes encephalitis.
- Anticonvulsants to prevent or control seizures
- Furosemide (Lasix) or mannitol reduces cerebral swelling.
- Sedatives are given to alleviate restlessness.
- Aspirin (Ecotrin) or acetaminophen (Tylenol) relieves headache and reduces fever.

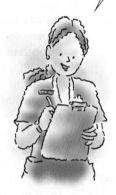

When a patient presents with fever, headache, vomiting, and stiff neck and back, suspect encephalitis.

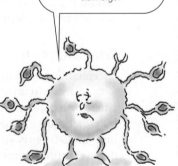

Stay alert for changes! Symptoms can escalate to include drowsiness, coma, paralysis, and other signs of neuron damage.

- Fluids and electrolytes prevent dehydration and electrolyte imbalance.
- Antibiotics are used to fight an associated infection such as pneumonia.

What to do

During the acute phase of the illness, follow these guidelines:

- Assess neurologic function frequently. Check for changes in LOC and signs of increased ICP. Watch for signs and symptoms of cranial nerve involvement, such as ptosis, strabismus, diplopia, abnormal sleep patterns, and behavior changes.
- Monitor intake and output carefully to maintain fluid balance. Be aware that fluid overload can increase cerebral edema.
- Position the patient carefully and turn him often to prevent joint stiffness and neck pain.
- Perform ROM exercises to prevent contractures.
- Provide a quiet, darkened room to ease headache and photophobia.
- Maintain adequate nutrition by giving small, frequent meals and NG tube or parenteral feedings, as ordered.
- Reassure the patient and his family that behavior changes caused by encephalitis usually disappear.
- If the patient is disoriented or confused, attempt to reorient him frequently. Place a calendar or clock in the patient's room to aid in orientation.

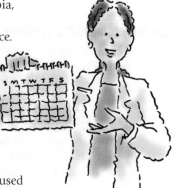

If the patient with encephalitis is disoriented, place a calendar or clock in the room.

Guillain-Barré syndrome

Guillain-Barré syndrome, or acute idiopathic polyneuritis, is also known as *infectious polyneuritis*. It's an acute, rapidly progressive, and potentially fatal form of polyneuritis that causes muscle weakness and mild distal sensory loss.

Equal opportunity syndrome

This syndrome can occur at any age but is most common in people between ages 30 and 50. It affects both sexes equally.

Recovery is spontaneous and complete in about 95% of patients; however, mild motor or reflex deficits may persist in the feet and legs. The prognosis is best when symptoms resolve sooner than 15 to 20 days after onset.

Three-phase syndrome

Guillain-Barré syndrome occurs in three phases:
1. The acute phase begins with the onset of the first definitive symptom and ends 1 to 3 weeks later. Further deterioration doesn't occur after the acute phase.
2. The plateau phase lasts several days to 2 weeks.
3. The recovery phase coincides with remyelinization and regrowth of axonal processes. Recovery commonly takes 4 to 6 months but may take as long as 2 to 3 years in severe cases.

Commonly complicated syndrome

Common complications include thrombophlebitis, pressure ulcers, muscle wasting, sepsis, joint contractures, respiratory tract infections, respiratory failure, and loss of bladder and bowel control.

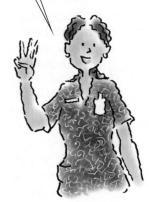

In a severe case, the patient with Guillain-Barré syndrome may take up to 3 years to recover.

What causes it

The precise cause of Guillain-Barré syndrome isn't known, but it may be a cell-mediated immune response to a virus. About 50% of patients with Guillain-Barré syndrome have a recent history of minor febrile illness, usually an upper respiratory tract infection or, less commonly, gastroenteritis. When infection precedes the onset of Guillain-Barré syndrome, signs of infection subside before neurologic features appear.

Possible precipitators

Other possible precipitating factors include:
- surgery
- rabies or swine influenza vaccination
- Hodgkin's or other malignant disease
- systemic lupus erythematosus.

How it happens

The major pathologic feature of Guillain-Barré syndrome is segmental demyelination of the peripheral nerves, which prevents the normal transmission of electrical impulses along the sensorimotor nerve roots.

Double trouble

Guillain-Barré syndrome causes inflammation and degenerative changes in both posterior (sensory) and the anterior (motor) nerve roots. That's why

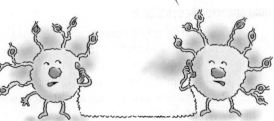

My sensorimotor nerve roots are fried . . . nothing's getting through! Hello . . . ?

signs of sensory and motor losses occur simultaneously. Additionally, autonomic nerve transmission may be impaired.

What to look for

During your assessment, look for symptoms that are progressive and include:
- symmetrical muscle weakness (the major neurologic sign), appearing first in the legs (in the ascending type of the syndrome, which is the most common form) and then extending to the arms and facial nerves within 24 to 72 hours, due to impaired anterior nerve root transmission
- muscle weakness developing in the brain stem, in the cranial nerves, and progressing downward in the arms first (in the descending type of the syndrome) or in the arms and legs simultaneously, due to impaired anterior nerve root transmission
- normal muscle strength (in mild forms of the syndrome) or weakness affecting only the cranial nerves
- paresthesia, sometimes preceding muscle weakness but vanishing quickly, due to impairment of the dorsal nerve root transmission
- diplegia, possibly with ophthalmoplegia (ocular paralysis), from impaired motor nerve root transmission and involvement of cranial nerves III, IV, and VI
- dysphagia or dysarthria and, less commonly, weakness of the muscles supplied by CN XI (the spinal accessory nerve)
- hypotonia and areflexia from interruption of the reflex arc.

What tests tell you

These tests help diagnose Guillain-Barré syndrome:
- CSF analysis reveals protein levels that begin to increase several days after the onset of symptoms and peak in 4 to 6 weeks.
- CBC early in illness shows leukocytosis and immature forms of white blood cells (WBCs; immature neutrophils, called *bands*).
- Electromyography may show repeated firing of the same motor unit instead of widespread sectional stimulation.
- Nerve conduction velocities slow soon after paralysis develops.
- Serum immunoglobulin levels are elevated due to an inflammatory response.

How it's treated

- Treatments are primarily supportive and include endotracheal (ET) intubation or tracheotomy if respiratory muscle involvement causes difficulty in clearing secretions.
- A trial dose (7 days) of prednisone (Deltasone) is given to reduce inflammatory response if the disease is relentlessly progressive; if prednisone produces no noticeable improvement, the drug is discontinued.
- Plasmapheresis is useful during the initial phase but of no benefit if started 2 weeks after onset.
- Continuous ECG is used to monitor for possible arrhythmias due to autonomic dysfunction. Propranolol (Inderal) is used to reduce tachycardia and hypertension. Atropine is given for bradycardia. Volume replacement is used in treating patients with severe hypotension.

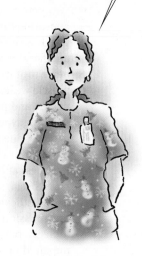

Stand by to provide supportive treatments, such as ET intubation or tracheotomy.

What to do

When caring for a patient with Guillain-Barré syndrome:
- Watch for ascending sensory loss, which precedes motor loss.
- Monitor vital signs and LOC.
- Assess and treat patients with respiratory dysfunction.
- Auscultate breath sounds, turn and position the patient, and encourage coughing and deep breathing. Begin respiratory support at the first sign of respiratory failure, which may include ET intubation and mechanical ventilation.
- Provide meticulous skin care to prevent skin breakdown.
- Perform passive ROM exercises within the patient's pain limits.
- To prevent aspiration, test the gag reflex and elevate the head of the bed before the patient eats. If the gag reflex is absent, give NG tube feedings until the gag reflex returns.
- As the patient regains strength and can tolerate a vertical position, be alert for hypotension. Change the patient's position slowly.
- Apply antiembolism stockings and a sequential compression device to the legs.
- If the patient has facial paralysis, provide eye and mouth care every 4 hours.
- Watch for urine retention. Use an indwelling urinary catheter if necessary.
- To prevent constipation, provide a high-fiber diet and offer prune juice. Administer a suppository or bisacodyl (Fleet enema), as ordered.
- Refer the patient to physical therapy.

Head injury

Head injury is any traumatic insult to the brain that causes physical, intellectual, emotional, social, or vocational changes. Children ages 6 months to 2 years, adults ages 15 to 24, and elderly adults are most at risk for head injury.

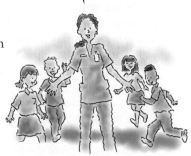

It's no surprise that children are particularly at-risk for head injury.

To put it bluntly

Head injury is generally categorized as closed trauma or open trauma. Closed (or blunt) trauma is more common. It typically occurs when the head strikes a hard surface or a rapidly moving object strikes the head. The dura mater is intact, and no brain tissue is exposed to the external environment.

In open trauma, as the name suggests, an opening in the scalp, skull, meninges, or brain tissue (the dura mater) exposes the cranial contents to the environment. The risk of infection is high.

Complications are possible

Possible complications include:
- increased ICP
- infection (in open trauma)
- respiratory depression and failure
- brain herniation.

On the decline

Mortality from head injury has declined as a result of:
- advances in preventive measures, such as air bags, seat belts, and helmets
- quicker emergency response and transport times
- improved treatment measures.

Think safety. Always wear your helmet on the field.

What causes it

Head injury commonly results from:
- motor vehicle collisions (the number one cause)
- falls
- sports-related accidents
- assaults and other crimes.

How it happens

The patient's brain is shielded by the cranial vault (composed of skin, bone, meninges, and CSF), which intercepts the force of a physical blow. Below a certain level of force, the cranial vault prevents energy from affecting the brain.

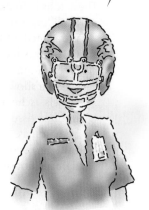

The degree of traumatic head injury is usually proportional to the amount of force reaching the cranial tissues. In addition, unless it's ruled out, you may presume that neck injuries are present in patients with traumatic head injuries.

Case closed

Closed trauma is typically a sudden acceleration–deceleration or coup–contrecoup injury. In coup–contrecoup injury, the head hits a more stationary object, injuring cranial tissues near the point of impact (coup); the remaining force then pushes the brain against the opposite side of the skull, causing a second impact and injury (contrecoup).

Contusions and lacerations may also occur during contrecoup as the brain's soft tissues slide over the rough bone of the cranial cavity. The cerebrum may endure rotational shear, damaging the upper midbrain and areas of the frontal, temporal, and occipital lobes.

What to look for

Types of head trauma include:
- concussion
- contusion
- epidural hematoma
- subdural hematoma
- intracerebral hematoma
- skull fractures.

Each type is associated with specific signs and symptoms. (See *Types of head injury*, pages 116 to 119.) Signs and symptoms of head trauma in elderly patients may not be readily apparent. (See *Hidden hematoma*.)

What tests tell you

These tests help diagnose head injury:
- Skull X-rays show the location of the fracture, unless the cranial vault is fractured. (A CT scan will show a fracture of the cranial vault.)
- CTA shows the location of vascular disruption due to internal pressure or injuries that result from cerebral contusion or skull fracture.
- CT scan shows intracranial hemorrhage from ruptured blood vessels; ischemic or necrotic tissue; cerebral edema; a shift in brain tissue; and subdural, epidural, and intracerebral hematomas.
- MRI may show intracranial hemorrhage, edema, or neuronal damage not seen on CT such as diffuse axonal injury.

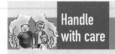

Handle with care

Hidden hematoma

An older person with cerebral atrophy can tolerate a larger subdural hematoma for a longer time than a younger person can before the hematoma causes neurologic changes. That's why a hematoma in an older patient can become rather large before you see any symptoms, even in an acute condition.

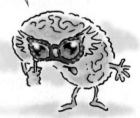

Remember, signs and symptoms of head trauma in elderly patients may not be obvious at first. They often take longer to develop than in a younger person.

How it's treated

Treatment may be surgical or supportive.

It's surgical

Surgical treatment includes:
* evacuation of a hematoma
* elevation of a depressed skull fracture
* decompressive craniotomy.
   The goal of surgery is reduce pressure on the brain, debride damaged tissue, and restore the cranial vault.

It's supportive

Provide supportive treatment, which includes:
* close observation to detect changes in neurologic status suggesting further damage or expanding hematoma
* cleaning and debridement of any wounds associated with skull fractures
* diuretics such as mannitol to reduce cerebral edema
* analgesics such as acetaminophen to relieve complaints of headache
* anticonvulsants such as phenytoin (Dilantin) or fosphenytoin (Cerebyx) to prevent seizures
* respiratory support, including mechanical ventilation and ET intubation for patients with respiratory failure from brain stem involvement
* only contaminated open fractures require antibiotics.

What to do

* Initially monitor vital signs continuously and check for additional injuries.
* Continue to check vital signs and neurologic status, including LOC and pupil size, every 15 minutes.
* Maintain a patent airway. Monitor oxygen saturation levels through pulse oximetry and ABG analysis as ordered.
* Assess hemodynamic parameters to aid in evaluating CPP.
* Administer medications as ordered. If necessary, use continuous infusions of such agents as midazolam (Versed), fentanyl (Sublimaze), morphine, or propofol (Diprivan) to reduce metabolic demand and the risk for increased ICP.
* Observe the patient closely for signs of hypoxia or increased ICP, such as headache, dizziness, irritability, anxiety, and changes in behavior such as agitation.

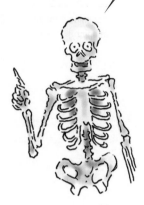

Check skull X-rays for the location of a fracture.

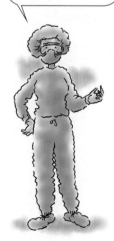

Surgical intervention may be needed to reduce a patient's risk for infection and further brain damage due to fractures.

(Text continues on page 120.)

Types of head injury

Here's a summary of the signs and symptoms and diagnostic test findings for different types of head injury.

Type	Description
Concussion (closed head injury)	• Characterized as a blow to the head hard enough to make the brain hit the skull but not hard enough to cause a cerebral contusion; causes temporary neural dysfunction • Recovery is usually complete within 24 to 48 hours. • Repeated injuries have a cumulative effect on the brain.
Epidural hematoma (bleeding above the dura mater)	• It's most common in 20- to 40-year-olds. • Most result from arterial bleeding. • Blood commonly accumulates between skull and dura mater. Injury to middle meningeal artery in parietotemporal area is most common and is typically accompanied by linear skull fractures in temporal region over middle meningeal artery. • It less commonly arises from dural venous sinuses.
Contusion	• Acceleration–deceleration or coup–contrecoup injuries disrupt normal nerve functions in bruised area. • Injury is directly beneath the site of impact when the brain rebounds against the skull from the force of a blow (e.g., a beating with a blunt instrument), when the force of the blow drives the brain against the opposite side of the skull, or when the head is hurled forward and stopped abruptly (as in an automobile crash when a driver's head strikes the windshield). • Brain continues moving and slaps against the skull (acceleration), then rebounds (deceleration). Brain may strike bony prominences inside the skull (especially the sphenoidal ridges), causing intracranial hemorrhage or hematoma that may result in tentorial herniation.

Signs and symptoms	Diagnostic test findings
• May occur without loss of consciousness. A short-term loss of consciousness is secondary to disruption of reticular activating system, possibly due to abrupt pressure changes in the areas responsible for consciousness, changes in polarity of the neurons, ischemia, or structural distortion of neurons. • Anterograde and retrograde amnesia (patient can't recall events immediately after the injury or events that led up to the traumatic incident) correlating with severity of injury; all related to disruption of reticular activating system • Irritability or lethargy • Behavior out of character • Complaints of dizziness, nausea, or severe headache	• CT scan or MRI reveals no sign of fracture, bleeding, or other nervous system lesion.
• Severe scalp wounds from direct injury • Brief period of unconsciousness after injury reflecting the concussive effects of head trauma, followed by a lucid interval varying from 10 to 15 minutes to hours or, rarely, days • Labored respiration and loss of consciousness secondary to increased pressure from bruising • Hemiparesis related to interrupted blood flow to the site of injury • Decorticate or decerebrate posturing from cortical damage or hemispheric dysfunction r/t increased ICP • Unequal pupillary response from brain stem involvement—third cranial nerve	• CT scan shows changes in tissue density, possible displacement of the surrounding structures, and evidence of ischemic tissue, hematomas, and fractures. • EEG recordings directly over the area of contusion reveal progressive abnormalities by appearance of high-amplitude theta and delta waves.
• Drowsiness, confusion, disorientation, agitation, or violence from increased ICP associated with trauma • Severe headache • Edema forms around the contusion increasing the ICP, which can lead to decreased LOC, worsening of neurologic deficit—depending on the location of the contusion—may include. • Respirations, initially deep and labored, becoming shallow and irregular as brain stem is impacted • Contralateral motor deficits reflecting compression of corticospinal tracts that pass through the brain stem • Ipsilateral (same-side) pupillary dilation due to compression of third cranial nerve • Seizures possibly from high ICP • Continued bleeding leading to progressive neurologic degeneration (evidenced by bilateral pupillary dilation, bilateral decerebrate response, increased systemic blood pressure, decreased pulse, and profound coma with irregular respiratory patterns)	• CT scan or MRI identifies abnormal masses or structural shifts within the cranium.

(continued)

Types of head injury *(continued)*

Type	Description
Subdural hematoma	• Meningeal hemorrhage results from accumulation of blood in subdural space (between dura mater and arachnoid mater). • It may be acute, subacute, and chronic: unilateral or bilateral. • It's usually associated with torn connecting veins in cerebral cortex; rarely from arteries. • Large acute hematomas are a surgical emergency. • Subacute hematomas have better prognosis because they occur over a longer period of time.
Intracerebral hematoma	• Traumatic or spontaneous disruption of cerebral vessels in brain parenchyma cause neurologic deficits, depending on site and amount of bleeding. • Shear forces from brain movement frequently cause vessel laceration and hemorrhage into the parenchyma. • Frontal and temporal lobes are common sites. Trauma is associated with few intracerebral hematomas; most are caused by hypertension.
Skull fracture	• There are four types: linear, comminuted, depressed, and basilar. • Fractures of anterior and middle fossae are associated with severe head trauma and are more common than those of posterior fossa. • A blow to the head causes one or more of the types. It may not be problematic unless the brain is exposed or bone fragments are driven into neural tissue.

Signs and symptoms	Diagnostic test findings
• Similar to epidural hematoma but significantly slower in onset because bleeding is typically of venous origin	• CT scan, confirming a hematoma • CT scan or MRI reveals evidence of masses and tissue shifting. • CT scan or MRI /MRA Identify the hemorrhage
• Headache • May have loss of consciousness—depends on size of hematoma • Possible motor deficits and decorticate or decerebrate responses from compression of corticospinal tracts and brain stem	
• May not produce symptoms, depending on underlying brain trauma • Discontinuity and displacement of bone structure with severe fracture • Motor sensory and cranial nerve dysfunction with associated facial fractures • May cause periorbital ecchymosis (raccoon eyes), anosmia (loss of smell due to first cranial nerve involvement), and pupil abnormalities (second and third cranial nerve involvement) in those with anterior fossa basilar skull fractures • CSF rhinorrhea (leakage through nose), CSF otorrhea (leakage from the ear), hemotympanum (blood accumulation at the tympanic membrane), ecchymosis over the mastoid bone (Battle's sign), and facial paralysis (seventh cranial nerve injury) in those with middle fossa basilar skull fractures • Signs of medullary dysfunction such as cardiovascular and respiratory failure in those with posterior fossa basilar skull fractures	• CT scan and MRI reveal swelling and intracranial hemorrhage from ruptured blood vessels. • Skull X-ray may reveal a fracture.

- Monitor elderly patients especially closely because they may have brain atrophy and, therefore, more space for cerebral edema. This means ICP may increase without showing signs.
- If an ICP monitoring system is inserted, continuously monitor ICP waveforms and pressure.
- Carefully observe the patient for CSF leakage. Check the bed sheets for a blood-tinged spot surrounded by a lighter ring (halo sign). If the patient has CSF leakage or is unconscious, elevate the head of the bed 30 degrees.
- Position the patient so that secretions drain properly. If you detect CSF leakage from the nose, place a gauze pad under the nostrils. Don't suction through the nose but use the mouth. If CSF leaks from the ear, position the patient so his ear drains naturally.
- Monitor intake and output frequently to maintain fluid balance.
- Institute seizure precautions as necessary. Use safety precautions to minimize the risk of injury.
- Cluster nursing activities to provide rest periods, thus reducing metabolic demands and reducing the risk of sustained increases in ICP.
- Prepare the patient for craniotomy as indicated.
- After the patient is stabilized, clean and dress superficial scalp wounds using strict sterile technique. Monitor wounds for signs and symptoms of infection.
- Explain all procedures and treatments to the patient and his family.

Meningitis

In meningitis, the brain and the spinal cord meninges become inflamed, usually because of bacterial infection. Such inflammation may involve all three meningeal membranes—the dura mater, arachnoid mater, and pia mater.

Promptness improves prognosis

If meningitis is recognized early and the infecting organism responds to treatment, the prognosis is good. Complications are rare and may include increased ICP, hydrocephalus, cerebral infarction, cranial nerve deficits causing optic neuritis and deafness, brain abscess, seizures, or coma.

Time matters. Prompt recognition and treatment improves the meningitis patient's prognosis.

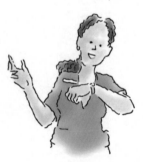

What causes it

Meningitis is usually a complication of bacteremia, especially from pneumonia, empyema, osteomyelitis, or endocarditis. Aseptic meningitis may result from a virus or other organism. Sometimes no causative organism can be found.

Uh–oh, other infections

Other infections associated with meningitis include:
- sinusitis
- otitis media
- encephalitis
- myelitis
- brain abscess, usually caused by *Neisseria meningitidis*, *Haemophilus influenzae*, *Streptococcus pneumoniae*, and *Escherichia coli*.

Any opening

Meningitis may follow trauma or invasive procedures, including skull fracture, penetrating head wound, lumbar puncture, and ventricular shunting.

How it happens

Meningitis commonly begins as inflammation of the pia–arachnoid tissue. It may progress to congestion of adjacent tissues and destroy some nerve cells.

It enters here . . .

The causative organism typically enters the CNS by one of four routes:
1. the blood (most common)
2. a direct opening between the CSF and the environment as a result of trauma
3. along the cranial and peripheral nerves
4. through the mouth or nose.

. . . and triggers a response . . .

The invading organism triggers an inflammatory response in the meninges. To ward off the invasion, neutrophils gather in the area and produce an exudate in the subarachnoid space, causing the CSF to thicken. The thickened CSF flows less readily around the brain and spinal cord. This can block the arachnoid villi, further obstructing CSF flow and causing hydrocephalus.

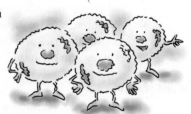

"Hey neutrophils, let's gather with our friends for an inflammatory response!"

... and yet more responses

The exudate also:

- exacerbates the inflammatory response, increasing the pressure in the brain
- can extend to the cranial and peripheral nerves, triggering additional inflammation
- irritates the meninges, disrupting their cell membranes, and causing edema.

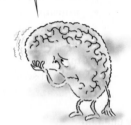

Thickened CSF flows slowly around the brain and spinal cord, sometimes causing hydrocephalus.

Truth or consequences

The consequences of meningitis are:

- elevated ICP
- engorged blood vessels
- disrupted cerebral blood supply
- possible thrombosis or rupture
- cerebral infarction if ICP isn't reduced
- possible encephalitis (a secondary infection of the brain tissue).
  In aseptic meningitis, lymphocytes infiltrate the pia–arachnoid layers but usually not as severely as in bacterial meningitis; no exudate is formed. Thus, this type of meningitis is self-limiting.

What to look for

Look for the signs of meningitis, which typically include:

- fever, chills, and malaise resulting from infection and inflammation
- headache, vomiting and, rarely, papilledema (inflammation and edema of the optic nerve) from increased ICP.
  Bacterial meningitis (meningococcal) has a characteristic petechial rash.

Fever is one of the classic signs of meningitis. Others include chills, malaise, headache, and, in some cases, papilledema.

Signs of irritation

Signs of meningeal irritation include:

- nuchal rigidity
- positive Brudzinski's and Kernig's signs
- exaggerated and symmetrical deep tendon reflexes
- opisthotonos (a spasm more common in infants and children in which the back and extremities arch backward so that the body rests on the head and heels).

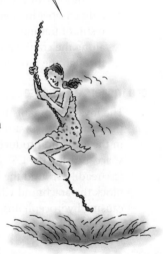

Further features

Other features of meningitis may include:

- sinus arrhythmias due to irritation of autonomic nerves
- irritability due to increasing ICP
- photophobia, diplopia, and other visual problems due to cranial nerve irritation

- delirium, deep stupor, and coma due to increased ICP and cerebral edema.

What tests tell you

- Lumbar puncture shows elevated CSF pressure (from obstructed CSF outflow at the arachnoid villi), cloudy or milky-white CSF, high protein levels, positive Gram stain and culture (unless a virus is responsible), presence of enterovirus by Xpert EV test, and decreased glucose concentration.
- Positive Brudzinski's and Kernig's signs indicate meningeal irritation.
- Cultures of blood, urine, and nose and throat secretions reveal the offending organism.
- Chest X-ray may reveal pneumonitis or lung abscess, tubercular lesions, or granulomas secondary to a fungal infection.
- Sinus and skull X-rays may identify paranasal sinusitis as the underlying infectious process or a skull fracture as the mechanism for entrance of microorganisms.
- WBC count reveals leukocytosis.

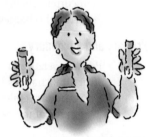

Various specimens will be collected and tests ordered to confirm the diagnosis and identify a causative organism.

How it's treated

Treatment includes administration of:
- antibiotic therapy, usually for 2 weeks
- digoxin (Lanoxin) to control arrhythmia
- mannitol to decrease cerebral edema
- anticonvulsant to prevent seizures
- sedative to reduce restlessness
- acetaminophen to relieve headache and fever.

Supportive measures

Supportive measures include bed rest; fever reduction, which may include tepid baths or cooling the patient with a hyperthermia-hypothermia blanket; and isolation, if necessary.

What to do

Take the following steps when caring for a patient with meningitis:
- Assess neurologic function often.
- Watch for deterioration, especially temperature increase, deteriorating LOC, onset of seizures, and altered respirations.
- Monitor fluid balance. Maintain adequate fluid intake to avoid dehydration but avoid fluid overload because of the danger of cerebral edema.
- Position the patient to prevent joint stiffness and neck pain. Assist with ROM exercises.
- Maintain adequate nutrition and elimination.
- Maintain a quiet environment.

- Follow strict sterile technique when treating patients with head wounds or skull fractures.
- Provide emotional support.
- Administer medications as ordered.

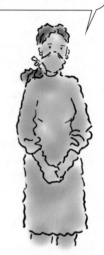

Remember: Meningitis is usually due to infection, so use sterile technique for patients with a head or skull injury.

Seizure disorder

Seizure disorder, or epilepsy, is a condition of the brain characterized by recurrent seizures (paroxysmal events associated with abnormal electrical discharges of neurons in the brain).

Primary and secondary

Primary seizure disorder or epilepsy is idiopathic without apparent structural changes in the brain.

Secondary epilepsy, characterized by structural changes or metabolic alterations of the neuronal membranes, causes increased automaticity.

Who's affected . . .

Epilepsy affects 1% to 2% of the population; approximately 2 million people live with epilepsy. The incidence is highest in childhood and old age. The prognosis is good if the patient adheres strictly to the prescribed treatment.

. . . and how

Complications of epilepsy may include hypoxia or anoxia due to airway occlusion, traumatic injury, brain damage, and depression and anxiety.

What causes it

In about one-half of seizure disorder cases, the cause is unknown. Some possible causes are:
- birth trauma (such as inadequate oxygen supply to the brain, blood incompatibility, or hemorrhage)
- perinatal infection
- anoxia
- infectious diseases (meningitis, encephalitis, or brain abscess)
- head injury or trauma.

How it happens

Some neurons in the brain may depolarize easily or be hyperexcitable, firing more readily than normal when stimulated. On stimulation, the electrical current spreads to surrounding cells, which fire in turn. The impulse thus cascades to:
- one side of the brain (a partial seizure)
- both sides of the brain (a generalized seizure)
- cortical, subcortical, and brain stem areas.

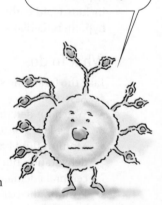

Don't be fooled . . . without the right treatment, I'm prone to recurrent seizures and possible hypoxia, traumatic injury, and even brain damage.

Increase O$_2$, or else

The brain's metabolic demand for oxygen increases dramatically during a seizure. If this demand isn't met, hypoxia and brain damage result.

Firing of inhibitory neurons causes the excited neurons to slow their firing and eventually stop. Without this inhibitory action, the result is status epilepticus (seizures occurring one right after another). Without treatment, resulting anoxia is fatal.

What to look for

The hallmarks of seizure disorders are recurring seizures, which can be classified as partial or generalized. Some patients are affected by more than one type. (See *Types of seizures*, page 126.)

What tests tell you

The results of primary diagnostic tests for seizure disorders may include the following:
- CT scan to show density readings of the brain may indicate abnormalities in internal structures.
- MRI may indicate abnormalities in internal brain structures.
- EEG is used to confirm the diagnosis of epilepsy by documenting changes in the brain's electrical conduction.
- Long-term or continuous EEG monitoring can be used to confirm seizure spikes.
- PET scan can help locate the focus of the seizures.

How it's treated

Generally, treatment consists of drug therapy specific to the type of seizures. The goal is to reduce seizures using a combination of the fewest drugs.

For tonic–clonic seizures

The most commonly prescribed drugs for generalized tonic-clonic seizures (alternating episodes of muscle spasm and relaxation) include phenytoin, carbamazepine (Tegretol), phenobarbital, and primidone (Mysoline).

For absence seizures

Drugs commonly prescribed for absence seizures (brief changes in LOC) include valproic acid (Depakene), clonazepam (Klonopin), and ethosuximide (Zarontin).

"The fewer the better. The goal is to reduce seizures using the fewest of us as possible!"

Types of seizures

Use the guidelines below to understand different seizure types. Keep in mind that some patients may be affected by more than one type.

Partial seizures

Partial seizure activity arising from a localized area in the brain may spread to the entire brain, causing a generalized seizure. There are several types and subtypes of partial seizures:
- simple partial seizures, which include jacksonian and sensory seizures
- complex partial seizures
- secondarily generalized partial seizures (partial onset leading to generalized tonic-clonic seizure).

Jacksonian seizures

A jacksonian seizure begins as a localized motor seizure, characterized by a spread of abnormal activity to adjacent areas of the brain.

The patient experiences stiffening or jerking in one extremity, with a tingling sensation in the same area. The patient seldom loses consciousness, but the seizure may progress to a generalized tonic-clonic seizure.

Sensory seizure

Symptoms of a sensory seizure include hallucinations, flashing lights, tingling sensations, vertigo, déjà vu, and smelling a foul odor.

Complex partial seizure

Signs and symptoms of a complex partial seizure are variable but usually include purposeless behavior, including a glassy stare, picking at clothes, aimless wandering, lip-smacking or chewing motions, and unintelligible speech.

An aura may occur first, and seizures may last a few seconds to 20 minutes. Afterward, mental confusion may last for several minutes and may be mistaken for alcohol or drug intoxication or psychosis. The patient has no memory of his actions during the seizure.

Secondarily generalized partial seizure

A secondarily generalized partial seizure can be simple or complex and can progress to a generalized seizure. An aura may occur first, with loss of concentration immediately or 1 to 2 minutes later.

Generalized seizure

Generalized seizures cause a generalized electrical abnormality in the brain. Types include absence, myoclonic, clonic, tonic, generalized tonic-clonic, and atonic.

Absence seizure

Absence seizure, also known as *petit mal seizure*, is most common in children. It usually begins with a brief change in the LOC, signaled by blinking or rolling of the eyes, a blank stare, and slight mouth movements. The patient retains his posture and continues preseizure activity without difficulty.

Such seizures last 1 to 10 seconds, and impairment is so brief that the patient may be unaware of it. If not properly treated, seizures can recur up to 100 times a day and progress to a generalized tonic-clonic seizure.

Myoclonic seizure

Myoclonic seizure is marked by brief, involuntary muscle jerks of the body or extremities and typically occurs in early morning.

Clonic seizure

Clonic seizure is characterized by bilateral rhythmic movements.

Tonic seizure

Tonic seizure is characterized by a sudden stiffening of muscle tone, usually of the arms but may also include the legs.

Generalized tonic-clonic seizure

Typically, a generalized tonic-clonic seizure begins with a loud cry, caused by air rushing from the lungs and through the vocal cords. The patient falls to the ground, losing consciousness. The body stiffens (tonic phase) and then alternates between episodes of muscle spasm and relaxation (clonic phase). Tongue biting, incontinence, labored breathing, apnea, and cyanosis may also occur.

The seizure stops in 2 to 5 minutes, when abnormal electrical conduction of the neurons is completed. Afterward, the patient regains consciousness but is somewhat confused. He may have difficulty talking and may have drowsiness, fatigue, headache, muscle soreness, and arm or leg weakness. He may fall into a deep sleep afterward.

Atonic seizure

Atonic seizure is characterized by a general loss of postural tone and temporary loss of consciousness. It occurs in children and is sometimes called a *drop attack* because the child falls.

Understanding status epilepticus

Status epilepticus is a continuous seizure state that must be interrupted by emergency measures. It can occur during all types of seizures. For example, generalized tonic-clonic status epilepticus is a continuous generalized tonic-clonic seizure without an intervening return of consciousness.

Always an emergency
Status epilepticus is accompanied by respiratory distress. It can result from withdrawal of antiepileptic medications, hypoxic or metabolic encephalopathy, acute head trauma, or septicemia secondary to encephalitis or meningitis.

Act fast
Emergency treatment usually consists of diazepam, phenytoin, or phenobarbital; I.V. dextrose 50% when seizures are secondary to hypoglycemia; and I.V. thiamine in patients with chronic alcoholism or those who are undergoing withdrawal.

Surgery and emergencies

Emergency treatment for patients with status epilepticus usually includes:
- administration of diazepam (Valium), lorazepam (Ativan), fosphenytoin (Cerebyx), or phenobarbital
- 50% dextrose I.V. (when seizures are secondary to hypoglycemia)
- thiamine I.V. (in chronic alcoholism or withdrawal). (See *Understanding status epilepticus*.)

A nonpharmacologic approach for managing seizures is vagus nerve stimulation. The vagus nerve stimulation device acts on the brain the way a pacemaker acts on the heart. It sends electrical signals to the brain to inhibit seizure activity.

Because the device is implanted in the chest and neck, adverse effects include voice changes, throat discomfort, and shortness of breath, all of which usually occur when the device is turned on.

What to do

- Monitor a patient taking anticonvulsants constantly for signs of toxicity, such as nystagmus, ataxia, lethargy, dizziness, drowsiness, slurred speech, irritability, nausea, and vomiting.
- When administering fosphenytoin I.V., use a large vein, administer according to guidelines (not more than 150 mg/minute), and monitor vital signs often.

Did you know that the vagus nerve stimulation device is like a pacemaker for the brain? It sends electrical signals to me to inhibit seizure activity.

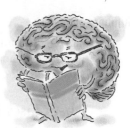

- Encourage the patient and his family to express their feelings about the patient's condition.
- Stress the need for compliance with the prescribed drug schedule.
- Emphasize the importance of having blood levels of anticonvulsants checked at regular intervals.

Tonic-clonic interventions

Generalized tonic-clonic seizures may necessitate the following interventions:

- Avoid restraining the patient during a seizure.
- Help the patient to a lying position, loosen any tight clothing, and place something flat and soft, such as a pillow, under his head.
- Clear the area of hard objects.
- Don't force anything into the patient's mouth if his teeth are clenched.
- Turn the patient's head or turn him on his side to provide an open airway.
- After the seizure, reassure the patient that he's all right, orient him to time and place, and tell him that he had a seizure.

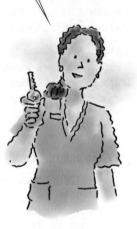

The key during a generalized tonic-clonic seizure is to take necessary precautions to prevent injury and maintain a patent airway.

Stroke

Stroke, also known as a *cerebrovascular accident* or *brain attack*, is a sudden impairment of cerebral circulation in one or more blood vessels. A stroke interrupts or diminishes oxygen supply and commonly causes serious damage or necrosis in the brain tissues.

The sooner, the better

The sooner circulation returns to normal after a stroke, the better your patient's chances are for a complete recovery. However, about one-half of the patients who survive a stroke remain permanently disabled and experience a recurrence within weeks, months, or years. It's the leading cause of admission to long-term care.

Numbers and odds

Stroke is the third most common cause of death in the United States and the most common cause of neurologic disability. It affects more than 700,000 people each year and is fatal in about one-half of these cases.

What causes it

Stroke typically results from one of three causes:

1. thrombosis of the cerebral arteries supplying the brain or of the intracranial vessels occluding blood flow

2. embolism from a thrombus outside the brain, such as in the heart, aorta, or common carotid artery

3. hemorrhage from an intracranial artery or vein, such as from hypertension, ruptured aneurysm, AVM, trauma, hemorrhagic disorder, or septic embolism.

Risk factor facts

Risk factors that predispose patients to stroke include:

* hypertension
* family history of stroke
* history of TIA (See *TIA and elderly patients.*)
* cardiac disease, including arrhythmias, coronary artery disease, acute myocardial infarction, dilated cardiomyopathy, and valvular disease
* diabetes
* familial hyperlipidemia
* cigarette smoking
* increased alcohol intake
* obesity, sedentary lifestyle (See *Obesity and stroke.*)
* use of hormonal contraceptives.

How it happens

Regardless of the cause, the underlying event leading to stroke is oxygen and nutrient deprivation. Here's what happens:

* Normally, if the arteries become blocked, autoregulatory mechanisms maintain cerebral circulation until collateral circulation develops to deliver blood to the affected area.
* If the compensatory mechanisms become overworked or cerebral blood flow remains impaired for more than a few minutes, oxygen deprivation leads to infarction of brain tissue.

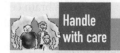

TIA and elderly patients

During your assessment, ask an elderly patient about recent falls—especially frequently occurring falls. This is important because an older patient is less likely to forget about or minimize frequent falls than he is to report other signs of a TIA.

Handle with care

Obesity and stroke

The degree of obesity—defined by BMI, waist circumference, or waist-to-hip ratio—has been found to be a significant risk factor for ischemic stroke incidence, regardless of gender or race. It's important to encourage your obese patients to lose weight, eat a healthy diet, and exercise as potential measures to reduce the incidence of ischemic stroke.

- The brain cells cease to function because they can't engage in anaerobic metabolism or store glucose or glycogen for later use.

Ischemic stroke

Here's what happens when a thrombotic or embolic stroke causes ischemia:
- Some of the neurons served by the occluded vessel die from lack of oxygen and nutrients.
- The result is cerebral infarction, in which tissue injury triggers an inflammatory response that in turn increases ICP.
- Injury to the surrounding cells disrupts metabolism and leads to changes in ionic transport, localized acidosis, and free radical formation.
- Calcium, sodium, and water accumulate in the injured cells, and excitatory neurotransmitters are released.
- Consequent continued cellular injury and swelling set up a vicious cycle of further damage.

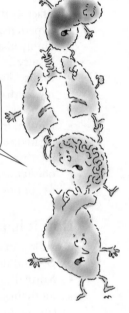

Uh-oh!

What's that old saying? "United we stand, divided we fall."

Hemorrhagic stroke

Here's what happens when a hemorrhage causes a stroke:
- Impaired cerebral perfusion causes infarction, and the blood acts as a space-occupying mass, exerting pressure on the brain tissues.
- The brain's regulatory mechanisms attempt to maintain equilibrium by increasing blood pressure to maintain CPP. The increased ICP forces CSF out, thus restoring equilibrium.
- If the hemorrhage is small, the patient may have minimal neurologic deficits. If the bleeding is heavy, ICP increases rapidly and perfusion stops. Even if the pressure returns to normal, many brain cells die.
- Initially, the ruptured cerebral blood vessels may constrict to limit the blood loss. This vasospasm further compromises blood flow, leading to more ischemia and cellular damage.
- If a clot forms in the vessel, decreased blood flow also promotes ischemia. If the blood enters the subarachnoid space, meningeal irritation occurs.
- Blood cells that pass through the vessel wall into the surrounding tissue may break down and block the arachnoid villi, causing hydrocephalus.

What to look for

Clinical features of stroke vary, depending on the artery affected (and, consequently, the portion of the brain it supplies), the severity of the damage, and the extent of collateral circulation that develops to help the brain compensate for decreased blood supply. (See *Stroke signs and symptoms*, page 132.)

Left is right and right is left

A stroke in the left hemisphere produces symptoms on the right side of the body; in the right hemisphere, symptoms on the left side.

Common signs and symptoms of stroke include sudden onset of:

- hemiparesis on the affected side (may be more severe in the face and arm than in the leg)
- unilateral sensory defect (such as numbness, or tingling) generally on the same side as the hemiparesis
- slurred or indistinct speech or the inability to understand speech
- blurred or indistinct vision, double vision, or vision loss in one eye (usually described as a curtain coming down or gray-out of vision)
- mental status changes or loss of consciousness (particularly if associated with one of the above symptoms)
- very severe headache (with hemorrhagic stroke).

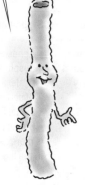

"The features of stroke vary, depending on the artery affected."

What tests tell you

Here are some test findings that can help diagnose a stroke:

- CT scan discloses structural abnormalities, edema, hemorrhage, and lesions, such as nonhemorrhagic infarction and aneurysms. Results are used to differentiate a stroke from other disorders, such as a tumor or hematoma. Patients with TIA generally have a normal CT scan. CT scan shows evidence of hemorrhagic stroke immediately and of ischemic (thrombotic or embolic) stroke within 72 hours after onset of symptoms. CT scan should be obtained within 25 minutes after the patient arrives in the ED, and results should be available within 45 minutes of arrival to determine whether hemorrhage is present. If hemorrhagic stroke is present, thrombolytic therapy is contraindicated.
- MRI is used to identify areas of ischemia and infarction and cerebral swelling. MRA/CTA can be used to evaluate the cerebral vessels.
- Cerebral angiography shows details of disruption or displacement of the cerebral circulation by occlusion or hemorrhage and can be used to treat occlusion or vasospasm.
- Carotid duplex scan is a high-frequency ultrasound that shows blood flow through the carotid arteries and reveals stenosis due to atherosclerotic plaque and blood clots.
- Transcranial Doppler studies are used to evaluate the velocity of blood flow through major intracranial vessels, which can indicate vessel diameter.

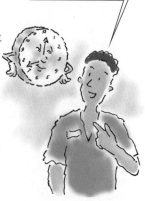

A CT scan should be taken within 25 minutes after the patient arrives in the emergency department. This will determine within minutes whether hemorrhage is present.

Stroke signs and symptoms

With stroke, functional loss reflects damage to the area of the brain that's normally perfused by the occluded or ruptured artery. Although one patient may experience only mild hand weakness, another may develop unilateral paralysis.

Hypoxia and ischemia may produce edema that affects distal parts of the brain, causing further neurologic deficits. Here are the signs and symptoms that accompany stroke at different sites.

Site	Signs and symptoms	Site	Signs and symptoms
Middle cerebral artery	• Aphasia • Dysphasia • Dyslexia (reading problems) • Dysgraphia (inability to write) • Visual field cuts • Hemiparesis on the affected side, which is more severe in the face and arm than in the leg	Anterior cerebral artery	• Confusion • Weakness • Numbness on the affected side (especially in the arm) • Paralysis of the contralateral foot and leg • Incontinence • Poor coordination • Impaired motor and sensory functions • Personality changes, such as flat affect and distractibility
Internal carotid artery	• Headaches • Weakness • Paralysis • Numbness • Sensory changes • Visual disturbances such as blurring on the affected side • Altered LOC • Bruits over the carotid artery • Aphasia • Dysphagia • Ptosis	Vertebral or basilar artery	• Mouth and lip numbness • Dizziness • Weakness on the affected side • Visual deficits, such as color blindness, lack of depth perception, and diplopia • Poor coordination • Dysphagia • Slurred speech • Amnesia • Ataxia
		Posterior cerebral artery	• Visual field cuts • Sensory impairment • Dyslexia • Coma • Blindness from ischemia in the occipital area

- Brain scan shows ischemic areas but may not be conclusive for up to 2 weeks after stroke.
- Single photon emission CT scanning and PET scan show areas of altered metabolism surrounding lesions that aren't revealed by other diagnostic tests.
- No laboratory tests confirm the diagnosis of stroke, but some tests aid diagnosis and some are used to establish a baseline for thrombolytic treatment. A blood glucose test shows whether the patient's symptoms are related to hypoglycemia. Hb level and HCT may be elevated in severe occlusion. Baselines obtained before thrombolytic therapy begins include CBC, platelet count, PTT, PT, fibrinogen level, and chemistry panel.

After a definitive diagnosis has been made, treatment with thrombolytics begins—if the patient meets the criteria—within 60 minutes after arrival in the emergency department.

How it's treated

The goal is to begin treatment within 3 hours of symptom onset.

Drugs of choice

Thrombolytics (also called *fibrinolytics*) are the drugs of choice in treating a stroke patient. The patient must first meet certain criteria to be considered for this type of treatment. (See *Who's suited for thrombolytic therapy?*, page 134.)

Drugs of choice for management

Drug therapy for the management of stroke includes:
- thrombolytics for emergency treatment of ischemic stroke (See *Adult suspected stroke algorithm*, page 135.)
- aspirin or clopidogrel (Plavix) as an antiplatelet agent to prevent recurrent stroke
- benzodiazepines to treat patients with seizure activity
- anticonvulsants to treat seizures or to prevent them after the patient's condition has stabilized
- stool softeners to avoid straining, which increases ICP
- antihypertensives and antiarrhythmics to treat patients with risk factors for recurrent stroke
- analgesics to relieve the headaches that may follow a hemorrhagic stroke.

Antihypertensives and antiarrhythmics are given to patients with risk factors for recurrent stroke.

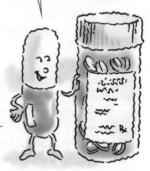

Medical management

Medical management of stroke commonly includes physical rehabilitation, dietary and drug regimens to reduce risk factors, surgery, and care measures to help the patient adapt to deficits, such as motor impairment and paralysis.

Who's suited for thrombolytic therapy?

Not every stroke patient is a candidate for thrombolytic therapy. Each is evaluated to see whether established criteria are met.

Criteria that must be present

Criteria that must be present for a patient to be considered for thrombolytic therapy include:
- acute ischemic stroke associated with significant neurologic deficit
- onset of symptoms less than 3 hours before treatment begins
- age 18 or older.

Criteria that must not be present

In addition to meeting the above criteria, the patient must not:
- have a history of head trauma or prior stroke in the past 3 months
- exhibit evidence of subarachnoid hemorrhage during pretreatment evaluation
- have a history of arterial puncture at a noncompressible site in the past 7 days
- have a history of previous intracranial hemorrhage
- have an elevated blood pressure (systolic blood pressure greater than 185 mm Hg or diastolic blood pressure less than 110 mm Hg) at the time of treatment
- have evidence of active bleeding on examination
- have a blood glucose concentration less than 50 mg/dl (2.7 mmol/L)
- have a CT scan that demonstrates multilobar infarction (hypodensity greater than 1/3 cerebral hemisphere)
- have a known bleeding diathesis, involving but not limited to:
  - platelet count less than 100,000/mm^3
  - receipt of heparin within 48 hours before the onset of stroke and having an elevated activated PTT (greater than the upper limit of normal)
  - current use of oral anticoagulants such as warfarin, international normalized ratio greater than 1.7, or PT greater than 15 seconds.

Criteria that must be evaluated individually

Recent experience suggests that under some circumstances and with careful evaluation, a patient may receive fibrinolytic therapy despite the presence of one or more of the following criteria. The doctor must weigh the risk to benefit for each patient.

The criteria include:
- evidence of only minor or rapidly improving stroke symptoms that clear spontaneously
- seizure at onset with postictal residual neurologic impairments
- major surgery or serious trauma within previous 14 days
- GI or urinary tract hemorrhage within the previous 21 days
- acute myocardial infarction within the previous 3 months.

Adult suspected stroke algorithm

Identify signs of possible stroke

Critical EMS assessments and actions

- Support airway, breathing, and circulation (ABCs); give **oxygen** if needed
- Perform prehospital stroke assessment
- Establish time when patient last known normal (Note: therapies may be available beyond 3 hours from onset)
- Transport; consider triage to a center with a stroke unit if appropriate; consider bringing a witness, family member, or caregiver
- Alert hospital
- Check glucose if possible

Immediate general assessment and stabilization

- Assess ABCs, vital signs
- Provide **oxygen** if hypoxemic
- Obtain I.V. access and blood samples
- Check glucose; treat if indicated
- Perform neurologic screening assessment
- Activate stroke team
- Order emergency computed tomography (CT) scanning of brain
- Obtain 12-lead electrocardiogram

Immediate neurologic assessment by stroke team or designee

- Review patient history
- Establish symptom onset
- Perform neurologic examination (NIH Stroke Scale or Canadian Neurologic Scale)

Does CT scan show any hemorrhage?

No hemorrhage

Probable acute ischemic stroke; consider fibrinolytic therapy

- Check for fibrinolytic exclusions
- Repeat neurologic examination: Are deficits rapidly improving to normal?

Hemorrhage

Consult neurologist or neurosurgeon; consider transfer if not available

Patient remains candidate for fibrinolytic therapy?

Not a candidate

Administer **aspirin**

Candidate

Review risks/benefits with patient and family: If acceptable

- Give **rtPA**
- No anticoagulants or antiplatelet treatment for 24 hours

- Begin stroke or hemor-rhage pathway
- Admit to stroke unit or intensive care unit if available

- Begin post-rtPA stroke pathway
- Aggressively monitors
  – BP per protocol
  – for neurologic deterioration
- Emergent admission to stroke unit or intensive care unit

Under the knife

Depending on the cause and extent of the stroke, the patient may undergo:
- a craniotomy to remove a hematoma
- a carotid endarterectomy to remove atherosclerotic plaques from the inner arterial wall
- an extracranial bypass to circumvent an artery that's blocked by occlusion or stenosis.

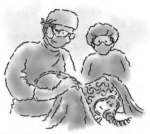

Surgical intervention after stroke is called for in some cases.

Call the "S" team

Your facility may have a stroke protocol and stroke team composed of specially trained nurses who respond to potential stroke patients. When a patient shows signs and symptoms of a stroke, first assess the patient using a stroke assessment tool such as the Cincinnati Stroke Scale. (See *Cincinnati prehospital stroke scale*.)

After your initial assessment, call the stroke team nurse, who will evaluate the patient; complete a neurologic assessment; report findings to the practitioner; and facilitate rapid and appropriate care of the patient, including emergency interventions, diagnostic tests, and transfer to the critical care unit.

Cincinnati prehospital stroke scale

The Cincinnati Prehospital Stroke Scale is a simplified scale for evaluating stroke patients that was derived from the National Institutes of Health Stroke Scale. It's used to evaluate facial palsy, arm weakness, and speech abnormalities. An abnormality in any one of the categories below is highly suggestive of stroke.

Facial droop (The patient shows teeth or smiles.)
- Normal—Both sides of the face move equally.
- Abnormal—One side of the face doesn't move as well as the other.

Arm drift (The patient closes eyes and extends both arms straight out for 10 seconds.)
- Normal—Both arms move the same or both arms don't move at all.
- Abnormal—One arm either doesn't move or one arm drifts downward as compared with the other.

Speech (The patient repeats, "The sky is blue in Cincinnati.")
- Normal—The patient says the correct words with no slurring of words.
- Abnormal—The patient slurs words, says the wrong words, or can't speak.

From Kothari, R. U., Pancioli, A., Liu, T., Brott, T., & Broderick, J. (1999). Cincinnati Prehospital Stroke Scale: Reproducibility and validity. *Annals of Emergency Medicine, 33*, 373–378. Adapted with permission from the American College of Emergency Physicians.

What to do

- If the patient has an altered LOC, secure and maintain the patient's airway and anticipate the need for ET intubation and mechanical ventilation.
- Monitor oxygen saturation levels via pulse oximetry and ABG levels as ordered. Administer supplemental oxygen as ordered to maintain oxygen saturation greater than 90%.
- Place the patient on a cardiac monitor and monitor for cardiac arrhythmias. Monitor blood pressure carefully. The current guideline for patients with ischemic stroke that have not received tissue plasminogen activator (tPa) is for permissive hypertension—not treating unless the blood pressure is greater than 220 mm Hg systolic. For patients who have received tPa, blood pressure of greater than 180/105 mm Hg is treated to reduce the risk of posttreatment hemorrhage.
- Assess the patient's neurologic status frequently, at least every 15 to 30 minutes, initially, then hourly as indicated. Observe for signs of increased ICP.
- If cerebral edema is suspected, maintain ICP sufficient for adequate cerebral perfusion but low enough to avoid brain herniation. Elevate the head of the bed 25 to 30 degrees. (See *Positioning the head of the bed*.)

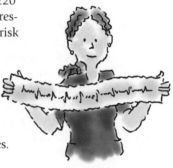

As you can see, nursing care of a stroke patient is pretty intensive. It demands careful monitoring and measures to prevent further progression of neurologic and other body system problems.

Weighing the evidence

Positioning the head of the bed

Positioning of the head of the bed must be individualized for each patient. The traditional positioning at 25 to 30 degrees is commonly used for potentially increased ICP. Stroke patients with increased ICP and chronic respiratory conditions may need head elevation for maximum oxygenation. The head of the bed should be elevated at least 30 degrees if the patient is at risk for aspiration or airway obstruction due to dysphagia.

Researchers haven't identified the optimal position of the head of the bed, but it seems that positioning depends on the individual patient's condition. Recent studies have suggested that positioning the head of the bed can facilitate an increase in cerebral blood flow and maximize oxygenation to cerebral tissue. A study using transcranial Doppler technology found that the head-flat position maximized blood flow to the brain. Further studies on head positioning of acute ischemic stroke patients need to be completed; if a patient has a lower risk for increased ICP and isn't at risk for aspiration, the head-down position has been shown to be beneficial.

Source: Summers, D., Leonard, A., Wentworth, D., Saver, J. L., Simpson, J., Spilker, J. A., . . . Mitchelle, P. H. (2009). Comprehensive overview of nursing and interdisciplinary care of the acute ischemic stroke patient: A scientific statement from the American Heart Association. *Stroke, 40*(8), 2911–2944.

- Assess hemodynamic status frequently. Give fluids as ordered and monitor I.V. infusions to avoid overhydration, which may increase ICP.
- For a patient receiving thrombolytic therapy, assess the patient for signs and symptoms of bleeding every 15 to 30 minutes and institute bleeding precautions. Monitor results of coagulation studies.
- Monitor the patient for seizures and administer anticonvulsants as ordered. Institute safety precautions to prevent injury.
- If the patient had a TIA, administer antiplatelet agents.
- Turn the patient often and position him using careful body alignment. Apply antiembolism stockings or intermittent sequential compression devices.
- Take steps to prevent skin breakdown.
- Begin exercises as soon as possible. Perform passive ROM exercises for both the affected and unaffected sides. Teach and encourage the patient to use his unaffected side to exercise his affected side.
- Manage GI problems. Be alert for signs of straining at stool as it increases ICP. If the patient is receiving steroids, monitor for signs of GI irritation.
- Modify the patient's diet, as appropriate, such as by increasing fiber.
- Provide meticulous eye and mouth care.
- Maintain communication with the patient. If he's aphasic, set up a simple method of communicating.
- Provide psychological support.

Quick quiz

1. The most sensitive indicator of neurologic status change is:
    A. LOC.
    B. speech.
    C. behavior.
    D. cognitive function.

Answer: A. Change in LOC is the earliest and most sensitive indicator of neurologic status change.

2. Signs of an adverse reaction to contrast medium include all of the following except:
    A. restlessness.
    B. bradycardia.
    C. urticaria.
    D. facial flushing.

Answer: B. A sign of adverse reaction to the contrast medium is tachycardia.

3. The major neurologic symptom of Guillain-Barré syndrome is:
    A. headache.
    B. nuchal rigidity.
    C. muscle weakness.
    D. altered LOC.

Answer: C. Muscle weakness usually appears in the legs first, then extends to the arms and face within 2 weeks or less.

4. Which type of seizure is characterized by brief, involuntary muscle movements?
    A. Jacksonian
    B. Myoclonic
    C. Generalized tonic-clonic
    D. Akinetic

Answer: B. During myoclonic seizures, the patient has brief, involuntary muscle movements.

5. Which condition may have delayed symptoms in an older person?
    A. stroke
    B. cerebral aneurysm
    C. seizure disorder
    D. subdural hematoma

Answer: D. An older person with cerebral atrophy can tolerate a larger subdural hematoma for a longer time than a younger person can before the hematoma causes neurologic changes.

6. In order for a patient experiencing an ischemic stroke to receive thrombolytic therapy, which criteria must be present?
    A. onset of symptoms less than 3 hours before treatment begins
    B. evidence of only minor or rapidly improving stroke symptoms that clear spontaneously
    C. seizure at onset with postictal residual neurologic impairments
    D. evidence of active bleeding on examination

Answer: A. Criteria that must be present for a patient to be considered for thrombolytic therapy include acute ischemic stroke associated with significant neurologic deficit, onset of symptoms less than 3 hours before treatment begins, and age 18 or older.

Scoring

☆☆☆   If you answered all six questions correctly, you may already know this: You're a brainiac!

☆☆   If you answered six questions correctly, cheer up. You have all the brainpower you need to succeed.

☆   If you answered fewer than six questions correctly, don't become irritable. Review the chapter and then take the test again.

Suggested References

Barrett, K. M., & Meschia, J. F. (2010). Acute ischemic stroke management: Medical management. *Seminars in Neurology, 30*(5), 461–468.

Blissitt, P. (Ed.). (2011). *Care of the patient undergoing intracranial pressure monitoring/external ventricular drainage or lumbar drainage.* Glenview, IL: American Association of Neuroscience Nurses.

Carney, N., Ghajar, J., Jagoda, A., Bedrick, S., Davis-O'Reilly, C., du Coudray, H., . . . Riggio, S. (2014). Concussion guidelines step 1: Systematic review of prevalent indicators. *Neurosurgery, 75*(3), 53–64.

Herzig, R., Burval, S., Krupka, B., Vlachova, I., Urbanek, K., & Mares, J. (2004). Comparison of ultrasonography, CT angiography, and digital subtraction angiography in severe carotid stenoses. *European Journal of Neurology, 11*(11), 774–775.

Hickey, J. (2014). *Clinical practice of neurological and neurosurgical nursing* (7th ed.). Philadelphia, PA: Lippincott Williams & Wilkins.

Saver, J., & Lutsep, H. (2014). *Thrombolytic therapy in stroke.* Retrieved from http://emedicine.medscape.com/article/1160840-overview

Steiner, I., Budka, H., Chaudhuri, A., Koskiniemi, M., Sainio, K., Salonen, O., & Kennedy, P. G. (2005). Viral encephalitis: A review of diagnostic methods and guidelines for management. *European Journal of Neurology, 12*(5), 331–343.

Thompson, H. J. (Ed.). (2008). *AANN clinical practice guidelines for the management of adults with severe traumatic brain injury.* Glenview, IL: American Association of Neuroscience Nurses.

Chapter 4

Cardiovascular system

Just the facts

In this chapter, you'll learn:

- ◆ structures and functions of the cardiovascular system
- ◆ assessment of the cardiovascular system
- ◆ diagnostic tests and procedures for the cardiovascular system
- ◆ cardiovascular disorders and treatments.

Understanding the cardiovascular system

The cardiovascular system consists of the heart and the blood vessels.

Bring it on . . . and take it away

This complex system functions to:
- carry life-sustaining oxygen and nutrients in the blood to all cells of the body
- remove metabolic waste products from the cells
- move hormones from one part of the body to another.

Heart

The heart is about the size of a closed fist. It lies beneath the sternum in the mediastinum (the cavity between the lungs), between the second and sixth ribs.

The right border of the heart aligns with the right border of the sternum. The left border aligns with the midclavicular line. The exact position of the heart varies slightly in each patient.

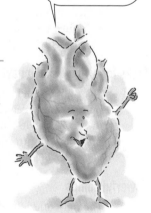

You might say the cardiovascular system is a mover and remover!

Pericardium

The pericardium is a sac that surrounds the heart. It's composed of an outer (fibrous) layer and an inner (serous) layer. The serous layer of the pericardium is composed of a visceral (inner) layer and a parietal (outer) layer.

Liquid cushion

The pericardial space separates the visceral and parietal layers of the serous pericardium. This space contains 10 to 30 ml of thin, clear pericardial fluid, which lubricates the two surfaces of the serous pericardium and cushions the heart.

Heart wall

The heart's wall is composed of three layers:
1. *Epicardium* includes the outer layer of the heart wall and the visceral layer of the serous pericardium. It's made up of squamous epithelial cells overlying connective tissue.
2. *Myocardium* is the middle and largest portion of the heart wall. This layer of muscle tissue contracts with each heartbeat.
3. *Endocardium* is the innermost layer of the heart wall. It contains endothelial tissue made up of small blood vessels and bundles of smooth muscle.

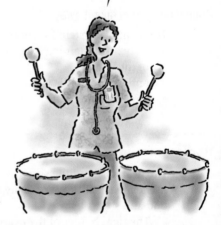

The myocardium is composed of muscle tissue that contracts with each heartbeat.

Four chambers

The heart has four chambers:
- right atrium
- left atrium
- right ventricle
- left ventricle. (See *A close look at the heart.*)

Tanks for giving blood today!

The right and left atria serve as reservoirs for blood. The right atrium receives deoxygenated blood returning from the body. The left atrium receives oxygenated blood from the lungs. Contraction of the atria forces blood into the ventricles below.

Powerful pumps

The right and left ventricles are the pumping chambers of the heart. The ventricles—which have thicker walls and are larger than the atria—are composed of highly developed muscles.

A close look at the heart

This illustration provides a detailed look at the internal structures of the heart.

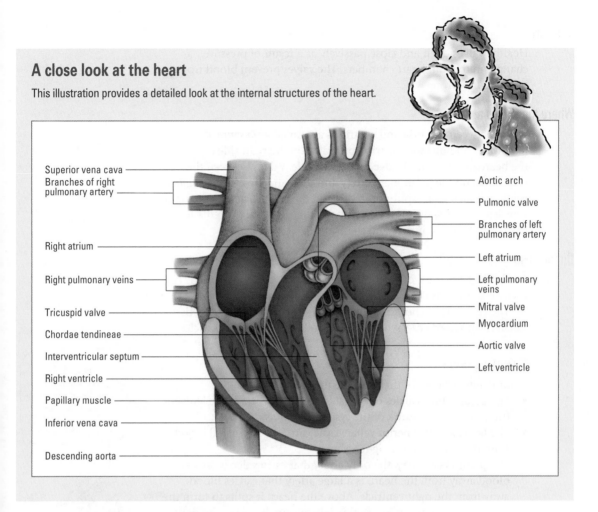

Superior vena cava

Branches of right pulmonary artery

Right atrium

Right pulmonary veins

Tricuspid valve

Chordae tendineae

Interventricular septum

Right ventricle

Papillary muscle

Inferior vena cava

Descending aorta

Aortic arch

Pulmonic valve

Branches of left pulmonary artery

Left atrium

Left pulmonary veins

Mitral valve

Myocardium

Aortic valve

Left ventricle

The right ventricle receives blood from the right atrium and pumps it through the pulmonary arteries to the lungs, where it picks up oxygen and drops off carbon dioxide. The left ventricle receives oxygenated blood from the left atrium and pumps it through the aorta and then out to the rest of the body. The interventricular septum separates the ventricles and helps them to pump.

Heart valves

Valves in the heart keep blood flowing in one direction.

One way

Healthy valves open and close passively as a result of pressure changes in the four heart chambers. The valves prevent blood from traveling the wrong way.

Where the valves are

Valves between the atria and ventricles are called *atrioventricular* (*AV*) *valves* and include the tricuspid valve on the right side of the heart and the mitral valve on the left side. Valves between the ventricles and the pulmonary artery and the aorta are called *semilunar valves* and include the pulmonic valve on the right (between the right ventricle and the pulmonary artery) and the aortic valve on the left (between the left ventricle and the aorta).

On the cusp

The leaflets, or cusps, of each valve keep the valves tightly closed. The tricuspid valve has three cusps. The mitral valve has two.

The cusps are anchored to the heart wall by cords of fibrous tissue called *chordae tendineae*, which are controlled by papillary muscles.

Great vessels

Leading into and out of the heart are the great vessels:

- The aorta, which carries oxygenated blood away from the left ventricle, is the main trunk of the systemic artery system.
- The inferior and superior venae cavae carry deoxygenated blood from the body into the right atrium.
- The pulmonary artery, the only artery that carries deoxygenated blood away from the heart, is a large artery that carries blood away from the right ventricle. Above the heart, it splits to form the right and left pulmonary arteries, which carry blood to the right and left lungs.
- The four pulmonary veins—two on the left and two on the right—carry oxygenated blood from the left and right lungs to the left atrium.

Coronary arteries

Like all other organs, the heart needs an adequate blood supply to survive. The coronary arteries, which lie on the surface of the heart, supply the heart muscle with blood and oxygen. (See *Heart vessels*.)

Coronary ostium

The coronary ostium is an opening in the aorta above the aortic valve. It feeds blood to the coronary arteries.

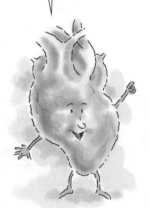

The vessels carry blood into and out of the heart. Aren't they great?

Heart vessels

These two views of the heart depict the great vessels and some of the major coronary vessels.

Anterior view

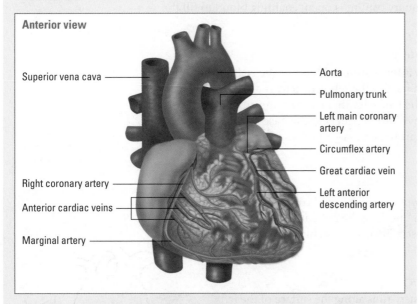

Superior vena cava

Aorta

Pulmonary trunk

Left main coronary artery

Circumflex artery

Great cardiac vein

Right coronary artery

Left anterior descending artery

Anterior cardiac veins

Marginal artery

Posterior view

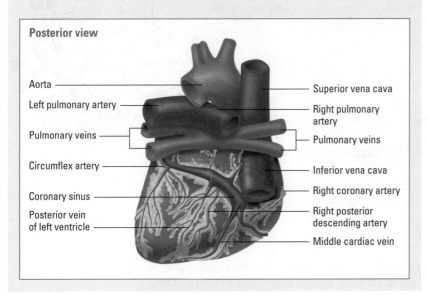

Aorta

Left pulmonary artery

Pulmonary veins

Circumflex artery

Coronary sinus

Posterior vein of left ventricle

Superior vena cava

Right pulmonary artery

Pulmonary veins

Inferior vena cava

Right coronary artery

Right posterior descending artery

Middle cardiac vein

Ostium action

When the left ventricle is pumping blood through the aorta, the aortic valve is open and the coronary ostium is partly covered. When the left ventricle is filling with blood, the aortic valve is closed and the coronary ostium is open, enabling blood to fill the coronary arteries.

Right coronary artery

The right coronary artery supplies blood to the right atrium, the right ventricle, and part of the left ventricle. It also supplies blood to the bundle of His (muscles that connect the atria with the ventricles) and the AV node (fibers at the base of the interatrial septum that transmit the cardiac impulses from the sinoatrial [SA] node).

What do you SA about that?

In about half the population, the right coronary artery also supplies blood to the SA node of the right atrium. The SA node consists of atypical muscle fibers that establish the rhythm of cardiac contractions.

Left coronary artery

The left coronary artery runs along the surface of the left atrium, where it splits into two major branches: the left anterior descending artery and the left circumflex artery.

Left out

The left anterior descending artery supplies blood to the:
- anterior wall of the left ventricle
- interventricular septum
- right bundle branch (a branch of the bundle of His)
- left anterior fasciculus (small cluster) of the left bundle branch.

The branches of the left anterior descending artery—the septal perforators and the diagonal arteries—supply blood to the walls of both ventricles.

Circumflex-ability

The circumflex artery supplies oxygenated blood to the lateral walls of the left ventricle, the left atrium, and, in about 50% of the population, the SA node.

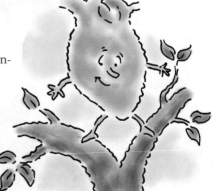

The left coronary artery splits into two major branches that supply blood to the rest of the heart.

Circle left

In addition, the circumflex artery supplies blood to the left posterior fasciculus of the left bundle branch. This artery circles around the left ventricle and provides blood to the ventricle's posterior portion.

Veins

Like other parts of the body, the heart has veins, called *cardiac veins*, that collect deoxygenated blood from the capillaries of the myocardium. These cardiac veins join together to form an enlarged vessel called the *coronary sinus*. The right atrium receives deoxygenated blood from the heart through the coronary sinus.

Pulmonary circulation

During pulmonary circulation, blood travels to the lungs to pick up oxygen in exchange for carbon dioxide.

Heart to lungs to heart

Here's what happens during pulmonary circulation:
- Deoxygenated blood travels from the right ventricle through the pulmonary semilunar valve into the pulmonary arteries.
- Blood passes through smaller arteries and arterioles into the capillaries of the lungs.
- Blood reaches the alveoli and exchanges carbon dioxide for oxygen.
- Oxygenated blood returns through the venules and veins to the pulmonary veins.
- The pulmonary veins carry the oxygenated blood back to the left atrium of the heart.

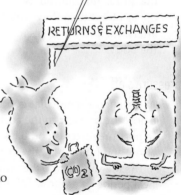

Cardiac rhythm

Contractions of the heart occur in a rhythm that's regulated by impulses initiated at the SA node.

Nature's pacemaker

The SA node is the heart's pacemaker. Impulses initiated at the SA node are conducted from there throughout the heart. Impulses from the autonomic nervous system affect the SA node and alter its firing rate to meet the body's needs.

The cardiac cycle

The cardiac cycle consists of two phases: systole and diastole.

Out with systole, in with diastole

During systole, the ventricles contract and send blood on its outward journey. During diastole, the ventricles relax and fill with blood; the mitral and tricuspid valves are open, and the aortic and pulmonic valves are closed.

Filling and more filling

Diastole consists of ventricular filling and atrial contraction. During ventricular filling, 70% of the blood in the atria drains into the ventricles passively, by gravity. The active period of diastole, atrial contraction (also called *atrial kick*), accounts for the remaining 30% of blood that passes into the ventricles.

The pressure's on

When the pressure in the ventricles is greater than the pressure in the aorta and pulmonary artery, the aortic and pulmonic valves open. Blood then flows from the ventricles into the pulmonary artery, then to the lungs and into the aorta, and then to the rest of the body.

The pressure's off

At the end of ventricular contraction, pressure in the ventricles drops below the pressure in the aorta and pulmonary artery. The difference in pressure forces blood back up toward the ventricles and causes the aortic and pulmonic valves to snap shut.

As the valves shut, the atria fill with blood in preparation for the next period of diastolic filling, and the cycle begins again.

Out in a minute

Cardiac output is the amount of blood the heart pumps in 1 minute. It's equal to the heart rate multiplied by the stroke volume (the amount of blood ejected with each heartbeat).

Stroke volume depends on three major factors:
1. preload, the amount of blood volume the heart has to work with
2. afterload, the resistance the heart is working against
3. contractility. (See *Understanding preload, afterload, and contractility.*)

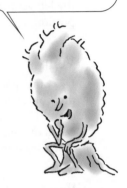

During diastole, the ventricles relax and fill with blood.

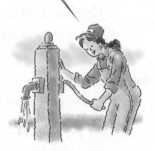

Cardiac output is the amount of blood the heart pumps in 1 minute.

Understanding preload, afterload, and contractility

If you think of the heart as a balloon, it will help you understand preload, afterload, and contractility.

Blowing up the balloon

Preload is the stretching of muscle fibers in the ventricles. This stretching results from blood volume in the ventricles at end diastole. According to Starling's law, the more the heart muscles stretch during diastole, the more forcefully they contract during systole. Think of preload as the balloon stretching as air is blown into it. The more air, the greater the stretch.

The balloon's stretch

Contractility refers to the inherent ability of the myocardium to contract normally. Contractility is influenced by preload. The greater the stretch, the more forceful the contraction—or, the more air in the balloon, the greater the stretch, and the farther the balloon will fly when air is allowed to expel.

The knot that ties the balloon

Afterload refers to the pressure that the ventricular muscles must generate to overcome the higher pressure in the aorta to get the blood out of the heart. *Resistance* is the knot on the end of the balloon, which the balloon has to work against to get the air out.

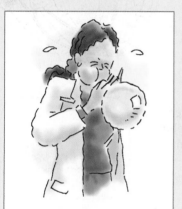 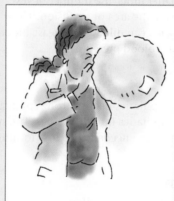 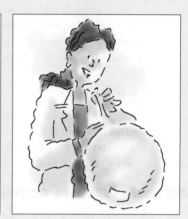

Blood vessels

The vascular system is the complex network of blood vessels throughout the body that conducts systemic circulation. Blood carries oxygen and other nutrients to body cells and transports waste products for excretion.

Arteries

The major artery—the aorta—branches into vessels that supply blood to specific organs and areas of the body.

Upper blood suppliers

Three arteries arise from the arch of the aorta and supply blood to the brain, arms, and upper chest. These are the:
- left common carotid artery
- left subclavian artery
- brachiocephalic artery (also called the *innominate artery*).

Descending distribution

As the aorta descends through the thorax and abdomen, its branches supply blood to the GI and genitourinary organs, spinal column, and lower chest and abdominal muscles. Then the aorta divides into the iliac arteries, which further divide into the femoral arteries.

Arterioles

As the arteries divide into smaller units, the number of vessels increases, thereby increasing the area of perfusion. These smaller units, known as *arterioles*, can dilate to decrease blood pressure or constrict to increase blood pressure.

Capillaries

Where the arterioles end, the capillaries begin. Strong sphincters control blood flow from the capillaries into the tissues. The sphincters open to permit more flow when needed and close to shunt blood to other areas.

Small vessels, large area of distribution

Although the capillary bed contains the smallest vessels, it supplies blood to the largest area. Capillary pressure is extremely low to allow for exchange of nutrients, oxygen, and carbon dioxide with body cells.

Venules and veins

From the capillaries, returning blood flows into venules and, eventually, into veins. Valves in the veins prevent blood backflow, and the pumping action of skeletal muscles assists venous return.

Branching back to the right atrium

The veins merge until they form branches that return blood to the right atrium. The two main branches include the superior vena cava and the inferior vena cava.

> Dilated arterioles decrease blood pressure. Constricted arterioles increase blood pressure.

> Low capillary pressure allows for the exchange of nutrients, oxygen, and carbon dioxide with body cells. Looks yummy . . . can't wait to dig in!

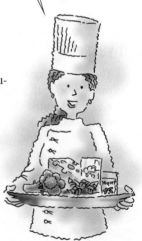

Cardiovascular assessment

Assessment of a patient's cardiovascular system includes a health history and physical examination.

Health history

To obtain a health history of a patient's cardiovascular system, begin by introducing yourself and explaining what happens during the health history and physical examination. Then obtain the following information.

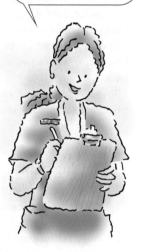

During your assessment, collect a health history and perform a physical examination.

Chief complaint

Ask for details about the patient's chief complaint. Patients with cardiovascular problems typically cite specific complaints, including:
- chest pain
- irregular heartbeat or palpitations
- shortness of breath on exertion, when lying down, or at night
- cough
- weakness or fatigue
- unexplained weight change
- swelling of the extremities
- dizziness
- headache
- peripheral skin changes, such as decreased hair distribution, skin color changes, a thin shiny appearance to the skin, or an ulcer on the lower leg that fails to heal
- pain in the extremities, such as leg pain or cramps.

Personal and family health

Ask the patient for details about his family history and past medical history. Also ask about:
- stressors in the patient's life and coping strategies he uses to deal with them
- current health habits, such as smoking, alcohol intake, caffeine intake, exercise, and dietary intake of fat and sodium
- drugs the patient is taking, including prescription drugs, over-the-counter drugs, and herbal preparations
- previous surgeries
- environmental or occupational considerations
- activities of daily living (ADLs)
- menopause (if applicable).

Cardiac questions

To thoroughly assess your patient's cardiac function, be sure to ask these questions:
- Are you in pain?
- Where is the pain located?
- Does the pain feel like a burning, tight, or squeezing sensation?
- Does the pain radiate to your arm, neck, back, or jaw?
- When did the pain begin?
- What relieves or aggravates it?
- Are you experiencing nausea, dizziness, or sweating?
- Do you feel short of breath? Has breathing trouble ever awakened you from sleep?
- Does your heart ever pound or skip a beat? When?
- Do you ever get dizzy or faint? When?
- Do you experience swelling in your ankles or feet? When? Does anything relieve the swelling?
- Do you urinate frequently at night?
- Have you had to limit your activities?

Rating pain

Many patients with cardiovascular problems complain of chest pain. If the patient is experiencing chest pain, ask him to rate the pain on a scale of 0 to 10, in which 0 indicates no pain and 10 indicates the worst chest pain imaginable. It's vital to thoroughly assess pain.

Where, what, and why

If the patient isn't in distress, ask questions that require more than a yes-or-no response. Use familiar expressions rather than medical terms whenever possible. (See *Cardiac questions.*) The nurse can also utilize the PQRST method to help focus the cardiac pain assessment. The P stands for precipitating factors: what brings on the pain? The Q represents quality of pain: have the patient use descriptive words including tight or burning? The R stands for radiation: does the pain radiate, and where does it radiate? The S is the severity of the pain on the 0 to 10 scale as described above. Finally, the T is for treatments: what treatments has the patient tried to relieve the chest pain and are they effective?

In his own words

Let the patient describe his condition in his own words. Ask him to describe the location, radiation, intensity, and duration of pain and any precipitating, exacerbating, or relieving factors to obtain an accurate description of chest pain. (See *Understanding chest pain.*)

"Just give me a second . . . I'm trying to think of the exact word to describe the pain."

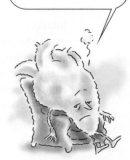

Understanding chest pain

Use this table to help you more accurately assess chest pain.

What it feels like	Where it's located	What makes it worse	What causes it	What makes it better
Aching, squeezing, pressure, heaviness, burning pain; usually subsides within 10 minutes	Substernal; may radiate to jaw, neck, arms, and back	Eating, physical effort, smoking, cold weather, stress, anger, hunger, lying down	Angina pectoris	Rest, nitroglycerin (*Note:* Unstable angina appears even at rest.)
Tightness or pressure; burning, aching pain, possibly accompanied by shortness of breath, diaphoresis, weakness, anxiety, or nausea; sudden onset; ½ hour to 2 hours	Typically across chest but may radiate to jaw, neck, arms, or back	Exertion, anxiety	Acute myocardial infarction (MI)	Opioid analgesics such as morphine, nitroglycerin
Sharp and continuous; may be accompanied by friction rub; sudden onset	Substernal; may radiate to neck, left arm, or back	Deep breathing (inspiration), supine position	Pericarditis	Sitting up, leaning forward, anti-inflammatory drugs
Excruciating, tearing pain; may be accompanied by blood pressure difference between right and left arm; sudden onset	Retrosternal, upper abdominal, or epigastric; may radiate to back, neck, or shoulders	Not applicable	Dissecting aortic aneurysm	Analgesics, surgery
Sudden, stabbing pain; may be accompanied by cyanosis, dyspnea, or cough with hemoptysis	Over lung area	Inspiration	Pulmonary embolus	Analgesics
Sudden and severe pain; sometimes accompanied by dyspnea, increased pulse rate, decreased breath sounds, or deviated trachea	Lateral thorax	Normal respiration	Pneumothorax	Analgesics, chest tube insertion

Physical examination

Cardiovascular disease affects people of all ages and can take many forms. To best identify abnormalities, use a consistent, methodical approach to the physical examination.

First things first

Before you begin the physical examination, wash your hands thoroughly. Obtain a stethoscope with a bell and a diaphragm, an appropriate-sized blood pressure cuff, and a penlight. Also, make sure the room is quiet.

Ask the patient to remove all clothing except his underwear and to put on an examination gown. Have the patient lie on his back, with the head of the bed at a 30- to 45-degree angle.

The heart of it

When performing an assessment of a patient's heart health, proceed in this order:
1. inspection
2. palpation
3. percussion
4. auscultation.

Inspection

First, take a moment to assess the patient's general appearance.

First impressions

Is the patient too thin or obese? Is he alert? Does he appear anxious? Note the patient's skin color. Are his fingers clubbed? (Clubbing is a sign of chronic hypoxia caused by a lengthy cardiovascular or respiratory disorder.) If the patient is dark-skinned, inspect his mucous membranes for pallor. The nurse can also inspect the skin noting if it is warm or dry or if the patient appears diaphoretic.

Check the chest

Next, inspect the chest. Note landmarks you can use to describe your findings as well as structures underlying the chest wall. (See *Cardiovascular landmarks*.)

Look for pulsations, symmetry of movement, retractions, or heaves (strong outward thrusts of the chest wall that occur during systole).

Inspecting the impulse

Then position a light source, such as a penlight, so that it casts a shadow on the patient's chest. Note the location of the apical impulse. This is also usually the point of maximal impulse (PMI) and should be located in the fifth intercostal space medial to the left midclavicular line.

The apical impulse gives an indication of how well the left ventricle is working because it corresponds to the apex of the heart. To

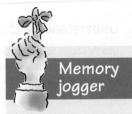

Memory jogger

To remember the order in which you should perform assessment of the cardiovascular system, just think, "I'll **P**roperly **P**erform **A**ssessment."

Inspection

Palpation

Percussion

Auscultation

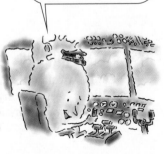

"Let's see, I should be looking for pulsations, symmetry of movement, retractions, and heaves, but all I see are clouds."

Cardiovascular landmarks

Here's a guide to finding the critical landmarks used in cardiovascular assessment.

Anterior thorax

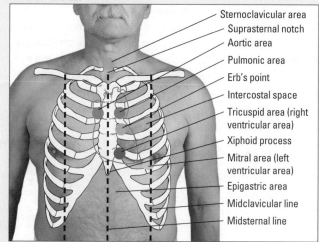

- Sternoclavicular area
- Suprasternal notch
- Aortic area
- Pulmonic area
- Erb's point
- Intercostal space
- Tricuspid area (right ventricular area)
- Xiphoid process
- Mitral area (left ventricular area)
- Epigastric area
- Midclavicular line
- Midsternal line

Lateral thorax

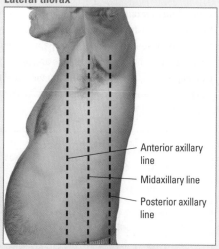

- Anterior axillary line
- Midaxillary line
- Posterior axillary line

find the apical impulse in a woman with large breasts, displace the breasts during the examination.

Abnormal findings on inspection

Here are some of the abnormal findings you may note on inspection and what such findings tell you:

- Inspection may reveal cyanosis, pallor, or cool or cold skin, which may indicate poor cardiac output and tissue perfusion.
- Skin may be flushed if the patient has a fever.
- Absence of body hair on the arms or legs may indicate diminished arterial blood flow to those areas. (See *Assessing arterial and venous insufficiency*, page 156.)
- Swelling, or edema, may indicate heart failure or venous insufficiency. It may also be caused by varicosities or thrombophlebitis.
- Chronic right-sided heart failure may cause ascites and generalized edema.

A chest of clues

- Inspection may reveal barrel chest (rounded thoracic cage caused by chronic obstructive pulmonary disease), scoliosis (lateral curvature of the spine), or kyphosis (convex curvature of the thoracic

Edema is a telltale sign of possible heart failure, venous insufficiency, varicosities, or thrombophlebitis.

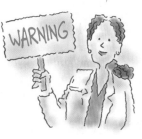

WARNING

Assessing arterial and venous insufficiency

You should be aware of how assessment findings differ between healthy patients and those with arterial insufficiency or chronic venous insufficiency.

Arterial insufficiency

In a patient with arterial insufficiency, pulses may be decreased or absent. The skin is cool, pale, and shiny, and the patient may have pain in his legs and feet. Ulcerations typically occur in the area around the toes, and the foot usually turns deep red when dependent. Nails may be thick and ridged.

Chronic venous insufficiency

In a patient with chronic venous insufficiency, check for ulcerations around his ankle. Pulses are present but may be difficult to find because of pitting edema. The foot may become cyanotic when dependent, and you may see a brown pigmentation and thickening of the skin around the ankle.

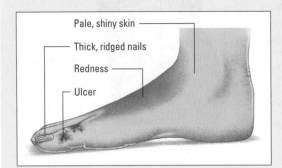

Pale, shiny skin
Thick, ridged nails
Redness
Ulcer

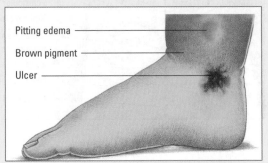

Pitting edema
Brown pigment
Ulcer

spine). If severe enough, these conditions can impair cardiac output by preventing chest expansion and inhibiting heart muscle movement.

- Retractions (visible indentations of the soft tissue covering the chest wall) and the use of accessory muscles to breathe typically result from a respiratory disorder but may also occur with a congenital heart defect or heart failure.

Palpation

Note skin temperature, turgor, and texture. Using the ball of your hand and then your fingertips, gently palpate over the precordium to find the apical impulse. Note heaves or thrills (fine vibrations that feel like the purring of a cat). (See *Assessing apical impulse.*)

Elusive impulse

The apical impulse may be difficult to palpate in patients who are obese or pregnant and in patients with thick chest walls. If it's difficult to palpate with the patient lying on his back, have him lie on his left side or sit upright.

> If the apical impulse is unpalpable with the patient on his back, have him lie on his left side or sit upright.

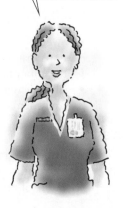

Plus, palpate

Also palpate the sternoclavicular, aortic, pulmonic, tricuspid, and epigastric areas for abnormal pulsations. Pulsations aren't usually felt in those areas. However, an aortic arch pulsation in the sternoclavicular area or an abdominal aorta pulsation in the epigastric area may be a normal finding in a thin patient.

Percussion

Percussion is less useful than other assessment methods, but it may help you locate the cardiac borders.

Border patrol

Begin percussing at the anterior axillary line and continue toward the sternum along the fifth intercostal space. The sound changes from resonance to dullness over the left border of the heart, normally at the midclavicular line. The right border of the heart is usually aligned with the sternum and can't be percussed.

Auscultation

You can learn a great deal about the heart by auscultating for heart sounds. Cardiac auscultation requires a methodical approach and lots of practice.

Here's the plan

First, identify the auscultation sites, which include the sites over the four cardiac valves, at Erb's point, and at the third intercostal space at the left sternal border. Use the bell to hear low-pitched sounds and the diaphragm to hear high-pitched sounds. (See *Heart sound sites*, page 158.)

Auscultate for heart sounds with the patient in three positions:
1. lying on his back with the head of the bed raised 30 to 45 degrees
2. sitting up
3. lying on his left side.

Upward, downward, zigward, zagward

Use a zigzag pattern over the precordium. Start at the apex and work upward or at the base and work downward. Whichever approach you use, be consistent.

Use the diaphragm to listen as you go in one direction; use the bell as you come back in the other direction. Be sure to listen over the entire precordium, not just over the valves. Note the patient's heart rate and rhythm.

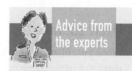

Advice from the experts

Assessing apical impulse

The apical impulse is associated with the first heart sound and carotid pulsation. To ensure that you're feeling the apical impulse and not a muscle spasm or some other pulsation, use one hand to palpate the patient's carotid artery and the other to palpate the apical impulse. Then compare the timing and regularity of the impulses. The apical impulse should roughly coincide with the carotid pulsation.

Note the amplitude, size, intensity, location, and duration of the apical impulse. You should feel a gentle pulsation in an area about ½" to ¾" (1.5 to 2 cm) in diameter.

Heart sound sites

When auscultating for heart sounds, place the stethoscope over the four different sites illustrated below.

Normal heart sounds indicate events in the cardiac cycle, such as the closing of heart valves, and are reflected to specific areas of the chest wall. Auscultation sites are identified by the names of heart valves but aren't located directly over the valves. Rather, these sites are located along the pathway blood takes as it flows through the heart's chambers and valves.

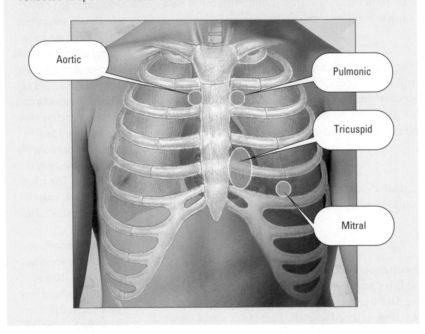

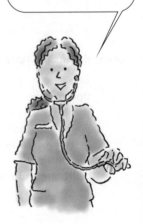

Rubs and dub-lubs, three heart sounds in a tub, and which will sound the loudest?

1, 2, 3, 4, and more

Systole is the period of ventricular contraction. As pressure in the ventricles increases, the mitral and tricuspid valves snap close. The closure produces the first heart sound, S_1.

At the end of ventricular contraction, the aortic and pulmonic valves snap shut. This produces the second heart sound, S_2.

Always identify S_1 and S_2 and then listen for adventitious sounds, such as third and fourth heart sounds (S_3 and S_4). (See *Extra heart sounds in the cardiac cycle*.)

Also listen for murmurs (vibrating, blowing, or rumbling sounds) and rubs (harsh, scratchy, scraping, or squeaking sounds).

Extra heart sounds in the cardiac cycle

To understand where extra heart sounds fall in relation to systole, diastole, and normal heart sounds, compare the illustrations of normal and extra heart sounds below.

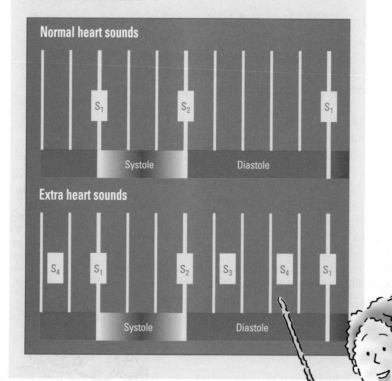

Those sounds don't belong there!

Listen for the "dub"

Start auscultating at the aortic area where the S_2 is loudest.

An S_2 is best heard at the base of the heart at the end of ventricular systole. It occurs when the pulmonic and aortic valves close and is generally described as sounding like "dub." It's a shorter, higher pitched, and louder sound than S_1.

When the pulmonic valve closes later than the aortic valve during inspiration, you hear a split S_2.

Listen for the "lub"

From the base of the heart, move to the pulmonic area and then down to the tricuspid area. Then move to the mitral area, where S_1 is the loudest.

An S_1 is best heard at the apex of the heart. It occurs with closure of the mitral and tricuspid valves and is generally described as sounding like "lub." It's low-pitched and dull.

An S_1 occurs at the beginning of ventricular systole. It may be split if the mitral valve closes just before the tricuspid valve.

Abnormal findings on heart auscultation

On auscultation, you may detect S_1 and S_2 heart sounds that are accentuated, diminished, or inaudible. Other abnormal heart sounds—such as S_3, S_4, and murmurs—may result from pressure changes, valvular dysfunctions, and conduction defects.

Third heart sound

The third heart sound—known as S_3 or *ventricular gallop*—is a low-pitched noise best heard by placing the bell of the stethoscope at the apex of the heart.

Kentucky galloper

Its rhythm resembles a horse galloping, and its cadence resembles the word "Ken-tuc-ky" (lub-dub-by). Listen for S_3 with the patient in a supine or left lateral decubitus position.

An S_3 usually occurs during early diastole to middiastole, at the end of the passive-filling phase of either ventricle. Listen for this sound immediately after S_2. It may signify that the ventricle isn't compliant enough to accept the filling volume without additional force.

Age-related adversity

An S_3 may occur normally in a child or young adult. In a patient older than age 30, however, it usually indicates a disorder, such as:
- right-sided heart failure
- left-sided heart failure
- pulmonary congestion
- intracardiac shunting of blood
- MI
- anemia
- thyrotoxicosis
- mitral insufficiency
- tricuspid insufficiency.

Fourth heart sound

The fourth heart sound, or S_4, is an abnormal, low-frequency sound that occurs late in diastole, just before the pulse upstroke. It imme-

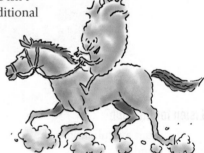

A ventricular gallop in a young person—even a 3-year-old filly—may be normal. But in someone older than age 30, it usually indicates a disorder.

diately precedes the S_1 of the next cycle. It's known as the *atrial* or *presystolic gallop*, and it occurs during atrial contraction.

Tennessee walker

An S_4 shares the same cadence as the word "Ten-nes-see" (le-lub-dub). It's heard best on expiration with the bell of the stethoscope and with the patient in the supine position.

What S_4 says

An S_4 may indicate cardiovascular disease, such as:
- acute MI
- hypertension
- coronary artery disease (CAD)
- cardiomyopathy
- angina
- anemia
- elevated left ventricular pressure
- aortic stenosis
- left ventricular hypertrophy
- pulmonary hypertension
- pulmonary embolism.

If the S_4 sound persists, it may indicate impaired ventricular compliance or volume overload. S_4 commonly appears in elderly patients with age-related systolic hypertension and aortic stenosis.

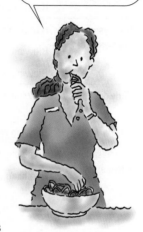

"I finally figured out that the turbulence I kept hearing between breakfast and lunch wasn't a murmur after all . . . just my stomach telling me it needed a little snack."

Murmurs

A murmur, which is longer than a heart sound, makes a vibrating, blowing, or rumbling noise. Just as turbulent water in a stream babbles as it passes through a narrow point, turbulent blood flow produces a murmur.

If you detect a murmur, identify where it's loudest, pinpoint the time it occurs during the cardiac cycle, and describe its pitch, pattern, quality, and intensity. (See *Identifying heart murmurs*, page 162.)

Location and timing

Murmurs can occur in any cardiac auscultatory site and may radiate from one site to another.

Marking murmurs

To identify the radiation area, auscultate from the site where the murmur seems loudest to the farthest site it's still heard. Note the anatomic landmark of this farthest site.

Identifying heart murmurs

To identify a heart murmur, first listen closely to determine its timing in the cardiac cycle. Then determine its other characteristics, including quality, pitch, and location as well as possible causes.

Timing	Quality and pitch	Location	Possible causes
Midsystolic (systolic ejection)	Harsh, rough with medium to high pitch	Pulmonic	Pulmonic stenosis
	Harsh, rough with medium to high pitch	Aortic and suprasternal notch	Aortic stenosis
Holosystolic (pansystolic)	Harsh with high pitch	Tricuspid	Ventricular septal defect
	Blowing with high pitch	Mitral, lower left sternal border	Mitral insufficiency
	Blowing with high pitch	Tricuspid	Tricuspid insufficiency
Early diastolic	Blowing with high pitch	Midleft sternal edge (not aortic area)	Aortic insufficiency
	Blowing with high pitch	Pulmonic	Pulmonic insufficiency
Middiastolic to late diastolic	Rumbling with low pitch	Apex	Mitral stenosis
	Rumbling with low pitch	Tricuspid, lower right sternal border	Tricuspid stenosis

Pinpoint its presence

Determine if the murmur occurs during systole (between S_1 and S_2) or diastole (between S_2 and the next S_1). Then pinpoint when in the cardiac cycle the murmur occurs—for example, during middiastole or late systole. A murmur heard throughout systole is called a *holosystolic* or *pansystolic* murmur, and a murmur heard throughout diastole is called a *pandiastolic* murmur. Occasionally, murmurs occur during both portions of the cycle (continuous murmur).

Describe the quality of a patient's murmur using terms like musical, blowing, harsh, rasping, rumbling, or machinelike.

Pitch

Depending on the rate and pressure of blood flow, pitch may be high, medium, or low. A low-pitched murmur can be best heard with the bell of the stethoscope, a high-pitched murmur with the diaphragm, and a medium-pitched murmur with both.

Pattern

Crescendo occurs when the velocity of blood flow increases and the murmur becomes louder. Decrescendo occurs when velocity decreases and the murmur becomes quieter.

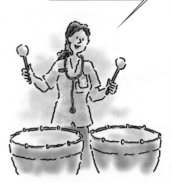

Up and down

A crescendo–decrescendo pattern describes a murmur with increasing loudness followed by increasing softness.

Quality

The volume of blood flow, the force of the contraction, and the degree of valve compromise all contribute to murmur quality. Terms used to describe quality include *musical, blowing, harsh, rasping, rumbling,* or *machinelike.*

Intensity

Use a standard, six-level grading scale to describe the intensity of the murmur:
1. grade I—extremely faint; barely audible even to the trained ear
2. grade II—soft and low; easily audible to the trained ear
3. grade III—moderately loud; about equal to the intensity of normal heart sounds
4. grade IV—loud with a palpable thrill at the murmur site
5. grade V—very loud with a palpable thrill; audible with the stethoscope in partial contact with the chest
6. grade VI—extremely loud, with a palpable thrill; audible with the stethoscope over, but not in contact with, the chest.

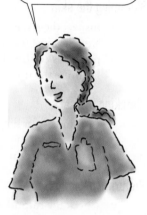

Grade the patient's murmur using a standard, 6-grade scale. This ensures consistency among all health care providers evaluating the murmur.

Rubs

To detect a pericardial friction rub, use the diaphragm of the stethoscope to auscultate in the third left intercostal space along the lower left sternal border.

Rubs the wrong way

Listen for a harsh, scratchy, scraping, or squeaking sound that occurs throughout systole, diastole, or both. To enhance the sound, have the patient sit upright and lean forward or exhale. A rub usually indicates pericarditis, but it may also occur in infections or neoplasms or after cardiac surgery.

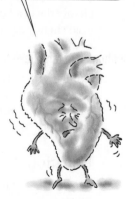

A rub often indicates pericarditis. That really rubs me the wrong way!

Assessing the vascular system

Assessment of the vascular system is an important part of a full cardiovascular assessment.

Inspection

Start your assessment of the vascular system the same way you start an assessment of the cardiac system—by making general observations.

To arms! ... and legs!

Examination of the patient's arms and legs can reveal arterial or venous disorders. Examine the patient's arms when you take his vital signs. Are the arms equal in size? Evaluate the legs when the patient is standing. Are the legs symmetrical? Check the legs later during the physical examination as well, with the patient lying on his back.

Skimming the skin

Inspect the patient's skin color. Note how body hair is distributed. Note lesions, scars, clubbing, and edema of the extremities. If the patient is confined to bed, be sure to check the sacrum for swelling. Examine the fingernails and toenails for abnormalities.

Checking the neck

Continue your inspection by observing vessels in the neck. Inspection of these vessels can provide information about blood volume and pressure in the right side of the heart.

Picturing pulsations

Check the carotid artery pulsations. The carotid artery should have a brisk, localized pulsation—not weak or bounding. The carotid pulsation doesn't decrease when the patient is upright, when he inhales, or when you palpate the carotid artery.

Inspect the jugular veins. The internal jugular vein has a softer, undulating pulsation. The internal jugular pulsation changes in response to position, breathing, and palpation.

Going for the jugular

To check the jugular venous pulse, have the patient lie on his back. Elevate the head of the bed 30 to 45 degrees and turn the patient's head slightly away from you.

Pulsations a notch above the notch

Normally, the highest pulsation occurs no more than ½" (4 cm) above the sternal notch. If pulsations appear higher, it indicates elevation in central venous pressure (CVP) and jugular vein distention.

Palpation

The first step in palpation is to assess skin temperature, texture, and turgor.

If you detect pulsations too far above the sternal notch, it's due to elevated CVP and jugular vein distention.

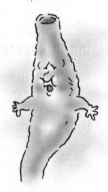

Note nail beds

Next, check capillary refill by assessing the nail beds on the fingers and toes. Refill time should be no more than 3 seconds or long enough to say "capillary refill."

Palpate pulses

Palpate for the pulse on each side of the neck, comparing pulse volume and symmetry. Don't palpate both carotid arteries at the same time or press too firmly. If you do, the patient may faint or become bradycardic.

Making the grade

All pulses should be regular in rhythm and equal in strength. Pulses are graded on a scale from 0 to 4+:

- 4+ is bounding.
- 3+ is increased.
- 2+ is normal.
- 1+ is weak.
- 0 is absent.

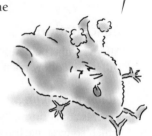

Don't palpate both carotid arteries at once or press too firmly. If you do, the patient may faint or become bradycardic.

Abnormal findings

Abnormal findings on palpation may reveal:

- weak pulse, indicating low cardiac output or increased peripheral vascular resistance such as in arterial atherosclerotic disease (Note that elderly patients commonly have weak pedal pulses.)
- strong bounding pulse, which occurs in hypertension and in high cardiac output states, such as exercise, pregnancy, anemia, and thyrotoxicosis
- apical impulse that exerts unusual force and lasts longer than one-third of the cardiac cycle—a possible indication of increased cardiac output
- displaced or diffuse impulse, which is a possible indication of left ventricular hypertrophy
- pulsation in the aortic, pulmonic, or right ventricular area, which is a sign of chamber enlargement or valvular disease
- pulsation in the sternoclavicular or epigastric area, which is a sign of an aortic aneurysm
- palpable thrill, which is an indication of blood flow turbulence and is usually related to valvular dysfunction; determine how far the thrill radiates and make a mental note to listen for a murmur at this site during auscultation
- heave along the left sternal border, which is an indication of right ventricular hypertrophy
- heave over the left ventricular area, which is a sign of a ventricular aneurysm; a thin patient may experience a heave with exercise,

fever, or anxiety because of increased cardiac output and more forceful contraction
- displaced PMI, which is a possible indication of left ventricular hypertrophy caused by volume overload from mitral or aortic stenosis, septal defect, acute MI, or other disorder.

Percussion

Percussion isn't used when assessing the vascular system.

Auscultation

After vascular palpation, use the bell of the stethoscope to begin auscultation. Follow the palpation sequence and listen over each artery.

Abnormal findings

Sounds aren't normally heard over the carotid arteries. A bruit, which sounds like buzzing or blowing, could indicate arteriosclerotic plaque formation.

> Uh-oh! A bruit over the abdominal aorta usually indicates an aneurysm or a dissection.

Brutish bruits

When you auscultate for the femoral and popliteal pulses, check for a bruit or other abnormal sounds. A bruit over the femoral or popliteal artery usually indicates narrowed vessels.

During auscultation of the central and peripheral arteries, you may notice a continuous bruit, caused by turbulent blood flow. A bruit over the abdominal aorta usually indicates an aneurysm (weakness in the arterial wall that allows a sac to form) or a dissection (a tear in the layers of the arterial wall).

Diagnostic tests

Advances in diagnostic testing allow for earlier and easier diagnosis and treatment of cardiovascular disorders. For example, in some patients, echocardiography—a noninvasive and risk-free test—can provide as much diagnostic information on valvular heart disease as can cardiac catheterization—an invasive and high-risk test.

12-Lead electrocardiogram

The 12-lead electrocardiogram (ECG) measures the heart's electrical activity and records it as waveforms. It's one of the most valuable and commonly used diagnostic tools.

A test with 12 views

The standard 12-lead ECG uses a series of electrodes placed on the patient's extremities and chest wall to assess the heart from 12 different views (leads). The 12 leads include three bipolar limb leads (I, II, and III), three unipolar augmented limb leads (aV_R, aV_L, and aV_F), and six unipolar precordial limb leads (V_1 to V_6). The limb leads and augmented leads show the heart from the frontal plane. The precordial leads show the heart from the horizontal plane. If the patient presents to the emergency department with chest pain, the ECG needs to be done right away!

ECG can be used to identify myocardial ischemia and infarction, rhythm and conduction disturbances, chamber enlargement, electrolyte imbalances, and drug toxicity.

In addition to the 12-lead ECG, two other ECGs may be used for diagnostic purposes, the right chest-lead ECG and posterior-lead ECG. (See *Understanding right chest-lead and posterior-lead ECGs.*)

Nursing considerations

* Use a systematic approach to interpret the ECG recording. (See *Normal ECG waveforms*, page 168.) Compare the patient's previous ECG with the current one, if available. This will help you identify changes.

Understanding right chest-lead and posterior-lead ECGs

The right chest-lead ECG and posterior-lead ECG use chest leads to assess areas that standard 12-lead ECGs can't.

Checking out the right chest

The usual 12-lead ECG evaluates only the left ventricle. If the right ventricle needs to be assessed for damage or dysfunction, the doctor may order a right chest-lead ECG. For example, a patient with an inferior wall MI might have a right chest-lead ECG to rule out right ventricular involvement.

With this type of ECG, the six chest leads are placed on the right side of the chest in a mirror image of the standard precordial lead placement. Electrodes start at the left sternal border and swing down the right side of the breast area.

Seeing behind your back

Because of lung and muscle barriers, the usual chest leads can't "see" the heart's posterior surface to record myocardial damage there. Some doctors add three posterior leads to the 12-lead ECG: leads V_7, V_8, and V_9. These leads are placed opposite the anterior leads V_4, V_5, and V_6 on the left side of the patient's back following the same horizontal line. V_7 is placed at the posterior axillary line, lead V_9 at the paraspinal line, and lead V_8 halfway between leads V_7 and V_9.

Normal ECG waveforms

Each of the 12 standard leads of an ECG takes a different view of heart activity, and each generates its own characteristic tracing. The tracings shown here represent a normal heart rhythm viewed from each of the 12 leads. Keep these facts in mind:

• An upward (positive) deflection indicates that the wave of depolarization flows toward the positive electrode.

• A downward (negative) deflection indicates that the wave of depolarization flows away from the positive electrode.

• An equally positive and negative (biphasic) deflection indicates that the wave of depolarization flows perpendicularly to the positive electrode.

Each lead represents a picture of a different anatomic area; when you find abnormal tracings, compare information from the different leads to pinpoint areas of cardiac damage.

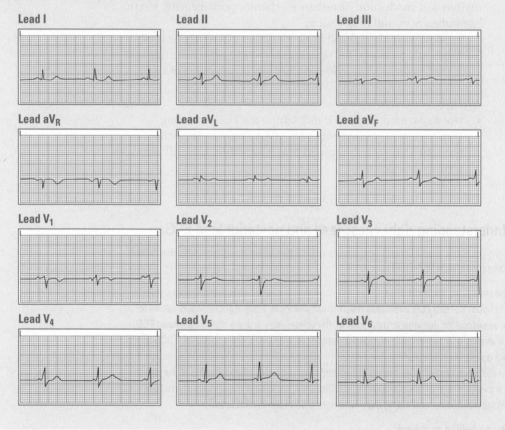

Lead I   Lead II   Lead III

Lead aV$_R$ Lead aV$_L$ Lead aV$_F$

Lead V$_1$ Lead V$_2$ Lead V$_3$

Lead V$_4$ Lead V$_5$ Lead V$_6$

Waves of waves

- P waves should be upright; however, they may be inverted in lead aV_R or biphasic or inverted in leads III, aV_L, and V_1.
- A P wave should be present and look the same before each QRS complex.
- PR intervals should always be constant, just like QRS-complex durations.
- QRS-complex deflections vary in different leads. Observe for pathologic Q waves.
- ST segments should be isoelectric or have minimal deviation.
- ST-segment elevation greater than 1 mm above the baseline and ST-segment depression greater than 0.5 mm below the baseline are considered abnormal. Leads facing an injured area have ST-segment elevations, and leads facing away show ST-segment depressions.
- The T wave normally deflects upward in leads I, II, and V_3 through V_6. It's inverted in lead aV_R and variable in the other leads. T-wave changes have many causes and aren't always a reason for alarm. Excessively tall, flat, or inverted T waves occurring with symptoms, such as chest pain, may indicate ischemia.
- A normal Q wave generally has a duration less than 0.04 second. An abnormal Q wave has either a duration of 0.04 second or more, a depth greater than 4 mm, or a height one-fourth of the R wave. Abnormal Q waves indicate myocardial necrosis, developing when depolarization can't follow its normal path because of damaged tissue in the area.
- Remember that aV_R normally has a large Q wave, so disregard this lead when searching for abnormal Q waves.

Holter monitor

This test is used to detect suspected dysrhythmias. The patient is connected to a small portable recorder with 3 to 5 electrodes. The recorder is worn for 24 to 48 hours, and the patient will engage in normal activities keeping a log of anytime symptoms are felt. The recordings are then analyzed for abnormalities with the documented activities and symptoms.

Cardiac marker studies

Analysis of cardiac markers (proteins) aids diagnosis of acute MI.

Release the enzymes!

After infarction, damaged cardiac tissue releases significant amounts of enzymes into the blood. Serial measurement of enzyme levels reveals the extent of damage and helps to monitor the progress of healing.

Heart-zymes

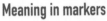

The cardiac enzymes include creatine kinase (CK) and its isoenzyme MB (found specifically in heart muscle).

Tests for troponin T and I and myoglobin are more specific to cardiac muscle and can be used to detect damage more quickly, allowing faster and more effective treatment.
- Ischemia modified albumin (IMA) measures changes in serum albumin when it comes in contact with ischemic tissue. IMA rises faster than any other cardiac enzyme.

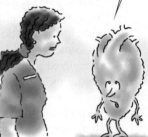

Did you know that troponin levels stay elevated for a long time and can indicate an infarction that occurred several days earlier?

Meaning in markers

Here's what the results of cardiac marker studies mean:
- CK-MB levels increase 4 to 8 hours after the onset of acute MI, peak after 20 hours, and may remain elevated for up to 72 hours.
- Troponin levels increase within 3 to 6 hours after myocardial damage. Troponin I peaks in 14 to 20 hours, with a return to baseline in 5 to 7 days. Troponin T peaks in 12 to 24 hours, with a return to baseline in 10 to 15 days. Because troponin levels stay elevated for a long time, they can be used to detect an infarction that occurred several days earlier.
- Myoglobin levels may increase within 30 minutes to 4 hours after myocardial damage, peak within 6 to 7 hours, and return to baseline after 24 hours. However, because skeletal muscle damage may cause myoglobin levels to increase, it isn't specific to myocardial injury.
- IMA levels rise within minutes of myocardial ischemia. Levels peak in 6 hours and return to baseline within 12 hours. IMA levels are best interpreted when used in conjunction with troponin, myoglobin, and CK-MB levels.

Nursing considerations
- Before CK measurement, withhold alcohol, aminocaproic acid (Amicar), and lithium (Eskalith) as ordered. If the patient must continue taking these substances, note this on the laboratory request. Inform your patient that serial blood tests are necessary.
- Avoid administering I.M. injections because they can cause muscle damage and elevate some cardiac markers.
- After any cardiac enzyme test, handle the collection tube gently to prevent hemolysis and send the sample to the laboratory immediately. A delay can affect test results.

Echocardiography

Echocardiography is used to examine the size, shape, and motion of cardiac structures. It's done using a transducer placed at an acoustic window (an area where bone and lung tissue are absent) on the patient's chest. The transducer directs sound waves toward cardiac structures, which reflect these waves.

Echo, echo

The transducer picks up the echoes, converts them to electrical impulses, and relays them to an echocardiography machine for display on a screen and for recording on a strip chart or videotape. The most commonly used echocardiographic techniques are M-mode and two-dimensional.

Motion mode

In M-mode (motion mode) echocardiography, a single, pencil-like ultrasound beam strikes the heart, producing an "ice pick," or vertical, view of cardiac structures. This mode is especially useful for precisely viewing cardiac structures.

Echo in 2-D

In two-dimensional echocardiography, the ultrasound beam rapidly sweeps through an arc, producing a cross-sectional, or fan-shaped, view of cardiac structures; this technique is useful for recording lateral motion and providing the correct spatial relationship between cardiac structures. In many cases, both techniques are performed to complement each other.

TEE combination

In TEE, ultrasonography is combined with endoscopy to provide a better view of the heart's structures. (See *A closer look at TEE*.)

Echo abnormalities

The echocardiogram may detect mitral stenosis, mitral valve prolapse, aortic insufficiency, wall motion abnormalities, and pericardial effusion (excess pericardial fluid).

Nursing considerations
- Explain the procedure to the patient and advise him to remain still during the test because movement can distort results. Tell him that conductive gel is applied to the chest, and a quarter-sized transducer is placed directly over it. Because pressure is exerted to

---

A closer look at TEE

In transesophageal echocardiography (TEE), ultrasonography is combined with endoscopy to provide a better view of the heart's structures. Similar to other endoscopic procedures, a TEE will require the patient to have conscious sedation.

How it's done
A small transducer is attached to the end of a gastroscope and inserted into the esophagus so that images of the heart's structure can be taken from the posterior of the heart. This test causes less tissue penetration and interference from chest wall structures and produces high-quality images of the thoracic aorta (except for the superior ascending aorta, which is shadowed by the trachea).

And why
TEE is used to diagnose:
- thoracic and aortic disorders
- endocarditis
- congenital heart disease
- intracardiac thrombi
- tumors.
  It's also used to evaluate valvular disease or repairs.

keep the transducer in contact with the skin, warn the patient that he may feel minor discomfort.

- After the procedure, remove the conductive gel from the skin.

Stress Testing

Exercise stress testing

This is a noninvasive test in which the patient is connected to an ECG while exercising. As physical stress causes an increase in myocardial oxygen consumption, ischemia may result showing changes to the ECG. If ischemia is noted during the test, the provider should stop the test.

Pharmacologic stress testing

If a patient is physically unable to perform an exercise stress test, a pharmacologic stress test can be done. This is done with radionuclide echocardiography. Medications are used because they cause vasodilation of normal coronary arteries, which will show ischemia if stenosis is occurring.

Cardiac magnetic resonance imaging

Magnetic resonance imaging (MRI) is a noninvasive test that evaluates tissues, structures, and blood flow. The images from the MRI are fed into a computer that reconstructs the image that will differentiate between healthy and ischemic tissue. It can be used to diagnose CAD, aortic aneurysm, congenital heart disease, left ventricular function, cardiac tumors, thrombus, valvular disease, and pericardial disorders. MRI is contraindicated in patients with pacemakers, defibrillators, brain clips, and cochlear implants.

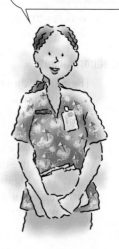

Cardiac catheterization is used to confirm CAD and other common abnormalities.

Cardiac catheterization

Cardiac catheterization involves passing a catheter into the right, left, or both sides of the heart.

A multipurpose procedure

Cardiac catheterization permits measurement of blood pressure and blood flow in the chambers of the heart. It also allows the doctor to visualize the coronary arteries and determine the presence of any narrowing or occlusions. It's used to determine valve competence and cardiac wall contractility and to detect intracardiac shunts.

Left sided catheterization is completed to visualize the coronary arteries and note extent of lesions within native vessels as well as bypass grafts. Balloon catheter treatments, such as angioplasty or placement of a coronary stent, may be done with cardiac catheterization.

Right-sided catheterization is performed by placing a pulmonary artery (PA) catheter in the femoral or brachial vein and then advancing it into the right atrium, ventricle, and pulmonary artery. This enables the health care provider to measure pressures in the right atrium, pulmonary artery, and also the pulmonary artery occlusion pressure.

The procedure also enables collection of blood samples and taking of diagnostic films of the ventricles (contrast ventriculography) and arteries (coronary arteriography or angiography).

Cardiac calculations

Use of thermodilution catheters allows calculation of cardiac output. Such calculations are used to evaluate valvular insufficiency or stenosis, septal defects, congenital anomalies, myocardial function and blood supply, and heart wall motion.

Confirming common problems

Common abnormalities and defects that can be confirmed by cardiac catheterization include CAD, myocardial incompetence, valvular heart disease, and septal defects.

Nursing considerations
When caring for a patient undergoing a cardiac catheterization, describe the procedure and events after it and take steps to prevent postoperative complications.

Before the procedure
- Explain that this test is used to evaluate the function of the heart and its vessels. Instruct the patient to restrict food and fluids for at least 6 hours before the test. Tell him the procedure takes 1 to 2 hours and that he may receive a mild sedative during the procedure.
- Tell the patient that the catheter is inserted into an artery or vein in the arm or leg. Tell him he'll experience a transient stinging sensation when a

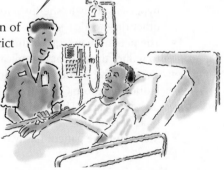

Reassure the patient that a local anesthetic is used to numb the incision site before catheter insertion.

Cardiac catheterization complications

Cardiac catheterization carries more patient risk than most other diagnostic tests. Although infrequent, complications can become life-threatening. Observe the patient carefully during the procedure. Notify the practitioner promptly and carefully document complications such as those listed here.

Left- or right-sided catheterization
- Cardiac tamponade
- Arrhythmias
- Hematoma or blood loss at insertion site
- Hypovolemia
- Infection (systemic or local)

- MI
- Pulmonary edema
- Reaction to contrast medium

Left-sided catheterization
- Arterial embolus or thrombus in limb
- Stroke or transient ischemic attack

Right-sided catheterization
- Pulmonary embolism
- Thrombophlebitis
- Vagal response
- Vagus nerve endings irritated in SA node, atrial muscle tissue, or atrioventricular junction

local anesthetic is injected to numb the incision site for catheter insertion.
- Inform the patient that injection of the contrast medium through the catheter may produce a hot, flushing sensation or nausea that quickly passes; instruct him to follow directions to cough or breathe deeply. Explain that medication will be given if he experiences chest pain during the procedure and that he may also be given nitroglycerin (Nitrostat) periodically to dilate coronary vessels and aid visualization. Reassure him that complications, such as MI and thromboembolism, are rare. (See *Cardiac catheterization complications*, page 174.)
- Make sure that the patient or a responsible family member has signed a consent form. Check for and tell the practitioner about hypersensitivity to shellfish, iodine, or contrast media used in other diagnostic tests.
- The patient may require anticoagulant therapy to be discontinued to reduce the risk for complications from bleeding.
- Contrast dye needed for the procedure can result in a decline in kidney function. Check the patient's renal function tests (blood urea nitrogen [BUN] and creatinine) and notify the practitioner of abnormalities.
- Make sure the patient has two patent I.V. access sites.

- Review activity restrictions that may be required of the patient after the procedure, such as lying flat with the limb extended for 4 to 6 hours and use of sandbags, if a femoral sheath is used.
- Document the presence of peripheral pulses, noting their intensity. Mark the pulses so they may be easily located after the procedure.

After the procedure

- Determine if a hemostatic device, such as a collagen plug or suture closure system, was used to close the vessel puncture site. A hemostatic bandage may also be used, and there are other commercial devices, including the FemoStop, which can help with pressure for the first 15 to 30 minutes. With any method, inspect the site for bleeding or oozing, redness, swelling, or hematoma formation. Maintain the patient on bed rest for 1 to 2 hours.
- Enforce bed rest for 8 hours if no hemostatic device was used. If the femoral route was used for catheter insertion, keep the patient's leg extended for 6 to 8 hours; if the antecubital fossa route was used, keep the arm extended for at least 3 hours.
- Monitor vital signs every 15 minutes for 2 hours, then every 30 minutes for the next 2 hours, and then every hour for 4 hours. If no hematoma or other problems arise, check every 4 hours. If signs are unstable, check every 5 minutes and notify the practitioner.
- Continually assess the insertion site for a hematoma or blood loss and reinforce the pressure dressing as needed.
- Check the patient's color, skin temperature, and peripheral pulse below the puncture site.
- Administer I.V. fluids as ordered (usually 100 ml/hour) to promote excretion of the contrast medium. Monitor for signs of fluid overload.
- Watch for signs of chest pain, shortness of breath, abnormal heart rate, dizziness, confusion, diaphoresis, nausea or vomiting, or extreme fatigue. Notify the practitioner immediately if these complications occur.

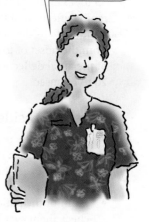

After catheter insertion, continually assess the site for a hematoma or blood loss.

Electrophysiology studies

Electrophysiology studies (EPS) are used to diagnose and treat abnormal heart rhythms. The procedure involves passing two to four temporary electrode catheters into multiple heart chambers. The electrodes are usually positioned in the right atrium, the AV node, the bundle of His region, and the apex of the right ventricle. The electrodes stimulate (pace) the heart and record the heart's electrical conduction.

Normal conduction intervals in adults are as follows: HV interval (measured from the earliest onset of the bundle of His deflection to the earliest registered surface or intracardiac ventricular activation), 35 to 55 msec; AH interval (represents the interval from the earliest rapid deflection of the atrial recording to the earliest onset of the bundle of His deflection), 45 to 150 msec; and PA interval (measured from the onset of the earliest registered surface P wave to the onset of the atrial deflection on the bundle of His catheter recording), 20 to 60 msec.

Nursing considerations

- Explain to the patient that EPS evaluate the heart's conduction system. Instruct him to restrict food and fluids for at least 6 hours before the test. Inform him that the studies take 1 to 3 hours.
- Have the patient void before the test.
- Monitor the patient's vital signs, as ordered. If they're unstable, check them every 15 minutes and alert the doctor. Observe for shortness of breath, chest pain, pallor, or changes in pulse rate, cardiac rhythm, or blood pressure. Enforce bed rest for 4 to 6 hours.
- Check the catheter insertion site for bleeding; apply a pressure bandage and sandbag to the site until bleeding stops.

Hemodynamic monitoring

Hemodynamic monitoring is used to assess cardiac function and determine the effectiveness of therapy by measuring:
- cardiac output
- mixed venous blood
- oxygen saturation
- intracardiac pressures
- blood pressure. (See *Putting hemodynamic monitoring to use.*)

The methods behind the monitoring

Follow your facility's procedure for setting up, zero referencing, calibrating, maintaining, and troubleshooting equipment. Common uses of hemodynamic monitoring include arterial blood pressure

Putting hemodynamic monitoring to use

Hemodynamic monitoring provides information on intracardiac pressures, arterial pressure, and cardiac output. To understand intracardiac pressures, picture the heart and vascular system as a continuous loop with constantly changing pressure gradients that keep the blood moving. Hemodynamic monitoring records the gradients within the vessels and heart chambers. Cardiac output indicates the amount of blood ejected by the heart each minute.

Pressure and description	Normal values	Causes of increased pressure	Causes of decreased pressure
Central venous pressure or right atrial pressure The CVP or right atrial pressure shows right ventricular function and end-diastolic pressure.	Normal mean pressure ranges from 1 to 6 mm Hg (1.34 to 8 cm H_2O).	• Right-sided heart failure • Volume overload • Tricuspid valve stenosis or insufficiency • Constrictive pericarditis • Pulmonary hypertension • Cardiac tamponade • Right ventricular infarction	• Reduced circulating blood volume • Vasodilation
Right ventricular pressure Typically, the doctor measures right ventricular pressure only when initially inserting a PA catheter. Right ventricular systolic pressure normally equals pulmonary artery systolic pressure; right ventricular end-diastolic pressure, which reflects right ventricular function, equals right atrial pressure.	Normal systolic pressure ranges from 20 to 30 mm Hg; normal diastolic pressure, from 0 to 5 mm Hg.	• Mitral stenosis or insufficiency • Pulmonary disease • Hypoxemia • Constrictive pericarditis • Chronic heart failure • Atrial and ventricular septal defects • Patent ductus arteriosus	• Reduced circulating blood volume • Vasodilation
Pulmonary artery pressure Pulmonary artery systolic pressure shows right ventricular function and pulmonary circulation pressures. Pulmonary artery diastolic pressure reflects left ventricular pressures, specifically left ventricular end-diastolic pressure, in a patient without significant pulmonary disease.	Systolic pressure normally ranges from 20 to 30 mm Hg. The mean pressure usually ranges from 10 to 15 mm Hg.	• Left-sided heart failure • Increased pulmonary blood flow (left or right shunting, as in atrial or ventricular septal defects) • Any condition causing increased pulmonary arteriolar resistance (such as pulmonary hypertension, volume overload, mitral stenosis, or hypoxia)	• Reduced circulating blood volume • Vasodilation
Pulmonary artery wedge pressure Pulmonary artery wedge pressure (PAWP) reflects left atrial and left ventricular pressures, unless the patient has mitral stenosis. Changes in PAWP reflect changes in left ventricular filling pressure.	The mean pressure normally ranges from 6 to 12 mm Hg.	• Left-sided heart failure • Mitral stenosis or insufficiency • Pericardial tamponade	Reduced circulating blood volume

Understanding minimally and noninvasive hemodynamic monitoring

Minimally and noninvasive hemodynamic monitoring techniques are easier to use and have been shown to provide reproducible, valid results. Minimally invasive techniques include esophageal Doppler hemodynamic monitoring and arterial pressure-based cardiac output (APCO) monitoring. Impedance cardiography is a noninvasive alternative for tracking hemodynamic status.

Esophageal Doppler hemodynamic monitoring

Esophageal Doppler hemodynamic monitoring uses ultrasound to measure heart function. It involves placement of a probe into the esophagus. By measuring blood flow through the heart valves or ventricular outflow tracks, this monitoring system can monitor:

- cardiac output (CO)
- stroke volume (SV)
- cardiac index (CI)
- systemic vascular resistance (SVR)
- SVR index.

This type of monitoring is appropriate for sedated critically ill patients with difficult fluid management or for use during and after cardiac surgery.

Transducer probe placement for esophageal Doppler hemodynamic monitoring is similar to inserting a nasogastric (NG) or orogastric tube and typically can be performed at the bedside. When the probe is positioned properly, it's ready to measure blood flow in the descending thoracic arch. The normal waveform should show good capture of blood flow. The monitor automatically measures such values as heart rate, peak velocity (PV), and flow time corrected (FTc). Other hemodynamic monitoring parameters are then derived from these measurements including CO, CI, SV, SV index, and SVR.

Arterial pressure-based cardiac output monitoring

In APCO, a patient's existing arterial catheter is used to continuously calculate and display CO. The arterial catheter and line are connected to a sensor, transducer, and specialized monitor preprogrammed with a clinically validated algorithm for determining CO.

Three devices are currently available. One system requires that the patient's age, gender, height, and weight be entered into the computer but no external calibration. Two others require an external calibration method. APCO is very useful in helping to determine a patient's fluid status and his potential response to a fluid challenge before he has significant changes in blood pressure.

Factors that may interfere with APCO include:

- incorrect leveling of transducer and sensor
- incorrect zeroing
- intra-aortic balloon pump (IABP)
- arrhythmias
- artificial heart or ventricular assist device (VAD)
- dampened pressure waveforms
- air bubbles in the fluid line.

Impedance cardiography

Impedance cardiography provides a noninvasive alternative for tracking hemodynamic status. This technique provides information about a patient's CI, preload, afterload, contractility, CO, and blood flow by measuring low-level electricity that flows harmlessly through the body from electrodes placed on the patient's thorax. These electrodes detect signals elicited from the changing volume and velocity of blood flow through the aorta. The signals are interpreted by the impedance monitor as a waveform. CO is computed from this waveform and the ECG.

Impedance cardiography monitoring eliminates the patient's risk for infection, bleeding, pneumothorax, emboli, and arrhythmias associated with traditional invasive hemodynamic monitoring. The accuracy of results obtained by this method is comparable to that obtained by thermodilution. In addition, the impedance cardiography monitor automatically updates information every 2nd to 10th heartbeat, providing real-time data.

monitoring, CVP monitoring, and pulmonary artery pressure (PAP) monitoring.

Minimally and noninvasive hemodynamic monitoring techniques are also proving to be reliable, safe options that are easier to use and can be applied in many clinical settings. (See *Understanding minimally and noninvasive hemodynamic monitoring.*)

Arterial blood pressure monitoring

In arterial blood pressure monitoring, the practitioner inserts a catheter into the radial or femoral artery to measure blood pressure or obtain samples of arterial blood for diagnostic tests such as arterial blood gas (ABG) studies.

A transducer transforms the flow of blood during systole and diastole into a waveform, which appears on an oscilloscope. The waveform has five distinct components. (See *Normal arterial waveform.*)

Normal arterial waveform

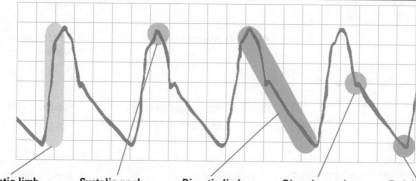

Anacrotic limb
The *anacrotic limb* marks the waveform's initial upstroke, which occurs as blood is rapidly ejected from the ventricle through the open aortic valve into the aorta.

Systolic peak
Arterial pressure then rises sharply, resulting in the *systolic peak*—the waveform's highest point.

Dicrotic limb
As blood continues into the peripheral vessels, arterial pressure falls and the waveform begins a downward trend, called the *dicrotic limb*. Arterial pressure usually keeps falling until pressure in the ventricle is less than the pressure in the aortic root.

Dicrotic notch
When ventricular pressure is lower than aortic root pressure, the aortic valve closes. This event appears as a small notch on the waveform's downside, called the *dicrotic notch*.

End diastole
When the aortic valve closes, diastole begins, progressing until aortic root pressure gradually falls to its lowest point. On the waveform, this is known as *end diastole*.

Nursing considerations
- Explain the procedure to the patient and his family, including the purpose of arterial pressure monitoring.
- After catheter insertion, observe the pressure waveform to assess arterial pressure. (See *Recognizing abnormal arterial waveforms.*)
- The four major components of validating the accuracy of the hemodynamic arterial line are patient positioning, zeroing the transducer, leveling the air–fluid interface to the phlebostatic axis, and assessing dynamic responsiveness with the square wave test.

Recognizing abnormal arterial waveforms

Use this chart to help you recognize and resolve waveform abnormalities.

Waveform	Abnormality	Possible causes
	Alternating high and low waves in a regular pattern	Ventricular bigeminy
	Flattened waveform	Overdamped waveform or hypotensive patient
	Slightly rounded waveform with consistent variations in systolic height	Patient on ventilator with positive end-expiratory pressure
	Slow upstroke	Aortic stenosis
	Diminished amplitude on inspiration	Pulsus paradoxus, possibly from cardiac tamponade, constrictive pericarditis, or lung disease
	Alteration in beat-to-beat amplitude (in otherwise normal rhythm)	Pulsus alternans, which may indicate left ventricular failure

- Assess the insertion site for signs of infection, such as redness and swelling. Notify the practitioner immediately if you note such signs.
- Ensure all connections are tightly closed and stopcock is in the correct position to prevent arterial bleeding
- Maintain 300 mm Hg pressure in the pressure bag to allow a flush flow of 3 to 6 ml per hour.
- Document the date and time of catheter insertion, catheter insertion site, type of flush solution used, type of dressing applied, and patient's tolerance of the procedure.

Nursing interventions

- Check the patient's ECG to confirm ventricular bigeminy. The tracing should reflect premature ventricular contractions (PVCs) every second beat.

- Check the patient's blood pressure with a sphygmomanometer. If you obtain a higher reading, suspect overdamping. Correct the problem by trying to aspirate the arterial line. If you succeed, flush the line. If the reading is very low or absent, suspect hypotension.

- Check the patient's systolic blood pressure regularly. The difference between the highest and lowest systolic pressure reading should be less than 10 mm Hg. If the difference exceeds that amount, suspect pulsus paradoxus, possibly from cardiac tamponade.

- Check the patient's heart sounds for signs of aortic stenosis. Also notify the practitioner, who will document suspected aortic stenosis in his notes.

- Note systolic pressure during inspiration and expiration. If inspiratory pressure is at least 10 mm Hg less than expiratory pressure, call the practitioner.
- If you're also monitoring PAP, observe for a diastolic plateau. This abnormality occurs when the mean CVP (right atrial pressure), mean PAP, and mean PAWP (pulmonary artery obstructive pressure) are within 5 mm Hg of one another.

- Observe the patient's ECG, noting any deviation in the waveform.
- Notify the practitioner if this is a new and sudden abnormality.

Central venous pressure

In CVP monitoring, the doctor inserts a catheter through a vein and advances it until its tip lies in or near the right atrium. Because no major valves lie at the junction of the vena cava and right atrium, pressure at end diastole reflects back to the catheter. In critically ill patients, when connected to the transducer or manometer, the catheter measures CVP, an index of right ventricular function, and central venous blood volume.

Nursing considerations

- Explain the procedure, including the purpose of CVP monitoring, to the patient and his family.
- After catheter insertion, observe the waveform to assess CVP. (See *Recognizing abnormal CVP waveforms.*)

Recognizing abnormal CVP waveforms

These illustrations show a normal CVP waveform and abnormal CVP waveforms, along with possible causes of abnormal waveforms.

Normal CVP waveform	Elevated *a* wave	Elevated *v* wave
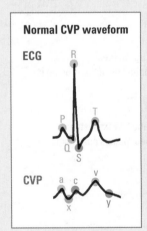	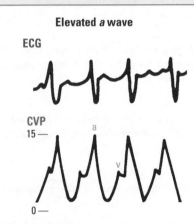	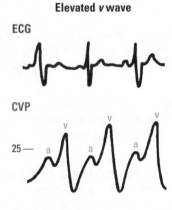

Elevated *a* wave

Physiologic causes
- Increased resistance to ventricular filling
- Increased atrial contraction

Associated conditions
- Heart failure
- Tricuspid stenosis
- Pulmonary hypertension

Elevated *v* wave

Physiologic cause
- Regurgitant flow

Associated conditions
- Tricuspid insufficiency
- Inadequate closure of the tricuspid valve due to heart failure

- Monitor the patient for infection. The U.S. Centers for Disease Control and Prevention estimates that 250,000 catheter-related bloodstream infections occur annually within the United States.
- Monitor for complications including pneumothorax, air embolism, and thrombosis. Notify the practitioner immediately if you notice such complications.
- Adhere to your facility's policy for dressing, tubing, catheter, and flush changes; use caution to prevent infection when changing dressing, tubing, and catheters.
- Document the date and time of catheter insertion, catheter insertion site, type of flush solution used, type of dressing applied, and patient's tolerance of the procedure.
- Document the CVP per your facility's policy or as ordered.

Elevated *a* and *v* waves

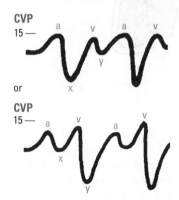

Physiologic causes
- Increased resistance to ventricular filling, which causes an elevated *a* wave
- Functional regurgitation, which causes an elevated *v* wave

Associated conditions
- Cardiac tamponade (smaller *y* descent than *x* descent)
- Constrictive pericardial disease (*y* descent exceeds *x* descent)
- Heart failure
- Hypervolemia
- Atrial hypertrophy

Absent *a* wave

ECG

CVP
10 —

Physiologic cause
- Decreased or absent atrial contraction

Associated conditions
- Atrial fibrillation
- Junctional arrhythmias
- Ventricular pacing

Understanding pulmonary artery pressures

PA systolic pressure

PA systolic pressure measures right ventricular systolic ejection or, simply put, the amount of pressure needed to open the pulmonic valve and eject blood into the pulmonary circulation. When the pulmonic valve is open, PA systolic pressure should be the same as right ventricular pressure.

PA diastolic pressure

PA diastolic pressure represents the resistance of the pulmonary vascular bed as measured when the pulmonic valve is closed and the tricuspid valve is open. To a limited degree (under absolutely normal conditions), PA diastolic pressure also reflects left ventricular end-diastolic pressure.

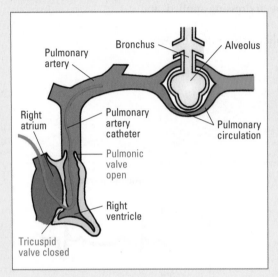

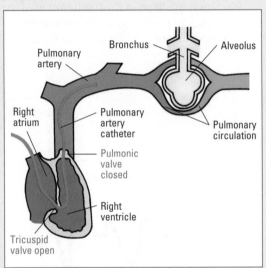

Pulmonary artery pressure monitoring

Continuous PAP and intermittent PAWP measurements provide important information about left ventricular function and preload. (See *Understanding pulmonary artery pressures*.) Use this information for monitoring and for aiding diagnosis, refining assessment, guiding interventions, and projecting patient outcomes.

PAP purposes

PAP monitoring is indicated for patients who:
- are hemodynamically unstable
- need fluid management or continuous cardiopulmonary assessment
- are receiving multiple or frequently administered cardioactive drugs.
  PAP monitoring is also crucial for patients experiencing shock, trauma, pulmonary or cardiac disease, or multiple organ dysfunction syndrome.

PAP's parts

A PA catheter has up to six lumens that gather hemodynamic information. In addition to distal and proximal lumens used to measure pressures, a PA catheter has a balloon inflation lumen that inflates the balloon for PAWP measurement and a thermistor connector lumen that allows cardiac output measurement.

Some catheters also have a pacemaker wire lumen that provides a port for pacemaker electrodes and measures continuous mixed venous oxygen saturation. (See *PA catheter ports*.)

PAP and PAWP procedures

The doctor inserts the balloon-tipped, multilumen catheter into the patient's internal jugular or subclavian vein. When the catheter reaches the right atrium, the balloon is inflated to float the catheter through the right ventricle into the pulmonary artery. This permits PAWP measurement through an opening at the catheter's tip. Thermodilution PA catheters that have the ability to obtain PAPs and cardiac output measurements are now considered the gold standard to hemodynamic monitoring.

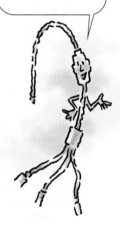

PA catheters have up to six lumens, so various hemodynamic information can be gathered.

PA catheter ports

A PA catheter contains several lumen ports to allow various catheter functions:
• The balloon inflation lumen inflates the balloon at the distal tip of the catheter for PAWP measurement.
• A distal lumen measures PAP when connected to a transducer and measures PAWP during balloon inflation. It also permits drawing of mixed venous blood samples.
• A proximal lumen measures right atrial pressure (CVP).
• The thermistor connector lumen contains temperature-sensitive wires, which feed information into a computer for CO calculation.
• Another lumen may provide a port for pacemaker electrodes or measurement of mixed venous oxygen saturation (SvO_2).

Five-lumen PA catheter

Balloon inflation lumen

Distal lumen

Proximal lumen

Thermistor connector lumen

Lumen for pacemaker electrodes or measuring SvO_2

The deflated catheter rests in the pulmonary artery, allowing diastolic and systolic PAP readings. The balloon should be totally deflated except when taking a PAWP reading because prolonged wedging can cause pulmonary infarction. (See *Normal PA waveforms.*)

Nursing considerations

- Inform the patient he'll be conscious during catheterization and he may feel temporary local discomfort from the administration of the local anesthetic. Catheter insertion takes about 15 to 30 minutes.
- After catheter insertion, you may inflate the balloon with a syringe to take PAWP readings. Be careful not to inflate the balloon with more than 1.5 cc of air. Overinflation could distend the pulmonary artery causing vessel rupture. Don't leave the balloon wedged for a prolonged period because this could lead to a pulmonary infarction.
- After each PAWP reading, flush the line; if you encounter difficulty, notify the practitioner.
- Maintain 300 mm Hg pressure in the pressure bag to allow a flush flow of 3 to 6 ml per hour.
- If fever develops when the catheter is in place, inform the practitioner; he may remove the catheter and send its tip to the laboratory for culture.
- Make sure stopcocks are properly positioned and connections are secure. Loose connections may introduce air into the system or cause blood backup, leakage of deoxygenated blood, or inaccurate pressure readings. Also make sure the lumen hubs are properly identified to serve the appropriate catheter ports.
- Because the catheter can slip back into the right ventricle and irritate it, check the monitor for a right ventricular waveform to detect this problem promptly. Be aware that running a continuous infusion through the distal lumen will interfere with your ability to monitor this waveform for changes.
- To minimize valvular trauma, make sure the balloon is deflated whenever the catheter is withdrawn from the pulmonary artery to the right ventricle or from the right ventricle to the right atrium.
- Adhere to your facility's policy for dressing, tubing, catheter, and flush changes.
- Document the date and time of catheter insertion, the doctor who performed the procedure, the catheter insertion site, pressure waveforms and values for the various heart chambers, balloon inflation volume required to obtain a wedge tracing, arrhythmias that occurred during or after the procedure, type of flush solution used and its heparin concentration (if any), type of dressing applied, and the patient's tolerance of the procedure.

Remember, don't leave the balloon wedged for a prolonged period because this could lead to a pulmonary infarction.

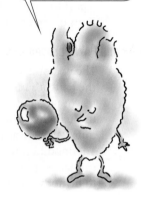

Normal PA waveforms

During PA catheter insertion, the waveforms on the monitor change as the catheter advances through the heart.

Right atrium

When the catheter tip enters the right atrium, the first heart chamber on its route, a waveform like the one shown below appears on the monitor. Note the two small upright waves. The *a* waves represent the right ventricular end-diastolic pressure; the *v* waves, right atrial filling.

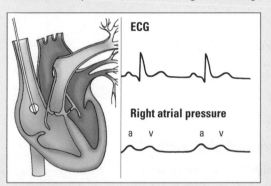

Pulmonary artery

The catheter then floats into the pulmonary artery, causing a PAP waveform such as the one shown below. Note that the upstroke is smoother than on the right ventricle waveform. The dicrotic notch indicates pulmonic valve closure.

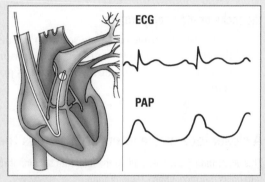

Right ventricle

As the catheter tip reaches the right ventricle, you'll see a waveform with sharp systolic upstrokes and lower diastolic dips, as shown below.

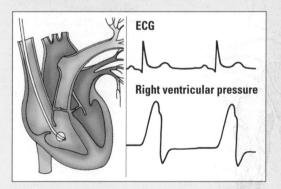

PAWP

Floating into a distal branch of the pulmonary artery, the balloon wedges where the vessel becomes too narrow for it to pass. The monitor now shows a PAWP waveform, with two small upright waves, as shown below. The *a* wave represents left ventricular end-diastolic pressure, the *v* wave, left atrial filling. The balloon is then deflated, and the catheter is left in the pulmonary artery.

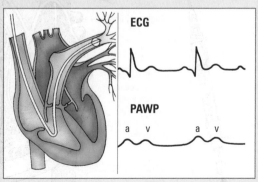

Cardiac output monitoring

Cardiac output—the amount of blood ejected by the heart in 1 minute—is monitored to evaluate cardiac function. The normal range for cardiac output is 4 to 8 L per minute.

The most widely used method for monitoring cardiac output is the intermittent bolus thermodilution technique. (See *A closer look at the intermittent bolus thermodilution method*.) The ability to continuously monitor cardiac output is also available. (See *A closer look at the continuous cardiac output method*.)

On the rocks or room temperature

To measure cardiac output, a solution is injected into the right atrium through a port on a PA catheter. Iced or room-temperature injectant may be used depending on your facility's policy and on the patient's status.

A closer look at the intermittent bolus thermodilution method

This illustration shows the path of the injectate solution through the heart during intermittent bolus thermodilution CO monitoring.

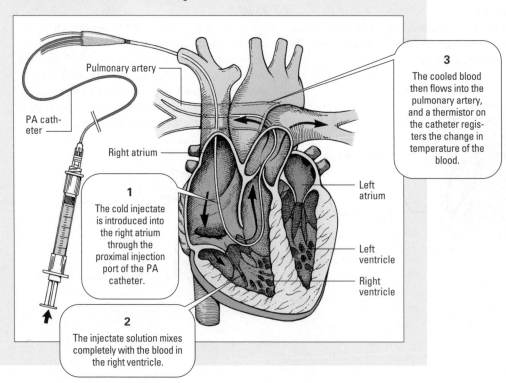

Pulmonary artery

PA catheter

Right atrium

1
The cold injectate is introduced into the right atrium through the proximal injection port of the PA catheter.

2
The injectate solution mixes completely with the blood in the right ventricle.

3
The cooled blood then flows into the pulmonary artery, and a thermistor on the catheter registers the change in temperature of the blood.

Left atrium

Left ventricle

Right ventricle

A closer look at the continuous cardiac output method

Measuring CO using a continuous cardiac output (CCO) system requires a modified PA catheter and CO computer. Rather than using a cooler-than-blood injectant as the input signal, the CCO system relies on a thermal filament on the catheter's outer surface. The thermal filament creates an input signal by emitting pulses of low heat energy, warming blood as it flows by; a thermistor then measures the temperature downstream. A computer algorithm identifies when the pulmonary artery temperature change matches the temperature of the input signal and produces a thermodilution washout curve and the CO value.

The monitor measures CO about every 30 to 60 seconds and displays a continuously updated CO value, averaged from the previous 3 to 6 minutes of data collected.

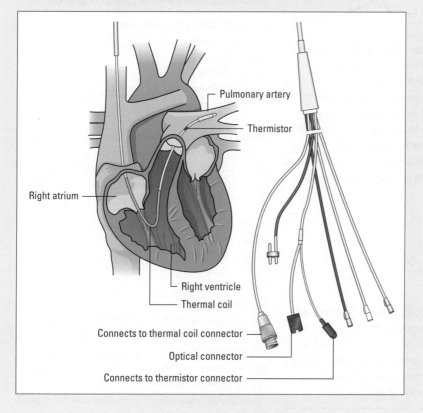

This indicator solution mixes with the blood as it travels through the right ventricle into the pulmonary artery, and a thermistor on the catheter registers the change in temperature of the flowing blood. A computer then plots the temperature change over time as a curve and calculates flow based on the area under the curve. (See *Analyzing thermodilution curves*, page 190.)

Analyzing thermodilution curves

The thermodilution curve provides valuable information about CO, injection technique, and equipment problems. When studying the curve, keep in mind that the area under the curve is inversely proportionate to CO: The smaller the area under the curve, the higher the CO; the larger the area under the curve, the lower the CO.

Besides providing a record of CO, the curve may indicate problems related to technique, such as erratic or slow injectate instillations, or other problems, such as respiratory variations or electrical interference. The curves below correspond to those typically seen in clinical practice.

Normal thermodilution curve

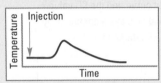

With an accurate monitoring system and a patient who has adequate CO, the thermodilution curve begins with a smooth, rapid upstroke and is followed by a smooth, gradual downslope. The curve shown below indicates that the injectate instillation time was within the recommended 4 seconds and that the temperature curve returned to baseline blood temperature.

The height of the curve will vary, depending on whether you use a room temperature or an iced injectate. Room-temperature injectate produces an upstroke of lower amplitude.

Low CO curve

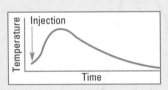

A thermodilution curve representing low CO shows a rapid, smooth upstroke (from proper injection technique). However, because the heart is ejecting blood less efficiently from the ventricles, the injectate warms slowly and takes longer to be ejected from the ventricle. Consequently, the curve takes longer to return to baseline. This slow return produces a larger area under the curve, corresponding to low CO.

High CO curve

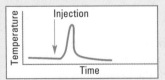

Again, the curve has a rapid, smooth upstroke from proper injection technique. But because the ventricles are ejecting blood too forcefully, the injectate moves through the heart quickly, and the curve returns to baseline more rapidly. The smaller area under the curve suggests higher CO.

Curve reflecting poor technique

This curve results from an uneven and too slow (taking more than 4 seconds) administration of injectate. The

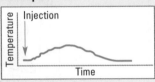

uneven and slower than normal upstroke and the larger area under the curve erroneously indicate low CO. A kinked catheter, unsteady hands during the injection, or improper placement of the injectate lumen in the introducer sheath may also cause this type of curve.

Curve associated with respiratory variations

To obtain a reliable CO measurement, you need a steady baseline pulmonary artery blood temperature. If the patient has rapid or labored respirations or if he's receiving mechanical ventilation, the thermodilution curve may reflect inaccurate CO values. The curve shown below from a patient receiving mechanical ventilation reflects fluctuating pulmonary artery blood temperatures. The thermistor interprets the unsteady temperature as a return to baseline. The result is a curve erroneously showing a high CO (small area under the curve). (*Note:* In some cases, the equipment senses no return to baseline at all and produces a sine-like curve recorded by the computer as 0.00.)

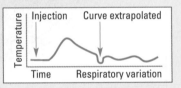

To be continued

Some PA catheters contain a filament that permits continuous cardiac output monitoring. Using such a device, an average cardiac output value is determined over a 3-minute span; the value is updated every 30 to 60 seconds. This type of monitoring allows close scrutiny of the patient's hemodynamic status and prompt intervention in case problems arise.

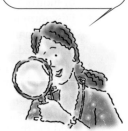

> Continuous cardiac output monitoring allows close scrutiny of the patient's hemodynamic status.

Better assessor

Cardiac output is better assessed by calculating cardiac index, which takes body size into account. To calculate the patient's cardiac index, divide his cardiac output by his body surface area, a function of height and weight. The normal cardiac index for adults ranges from 2.5 to 4.2 L per minute per m^2; for pregnant women, 3.5 to 6.5 L per minute per m^2. There are several other measurements of cardiac function that combine cardiac output values with other values obtained from a PA catheter and an arterial line. (See *Measuring cardiac function*.)

Measuring cardiac function

Listed here are several common measures of cardiac function that are based on information obtained from a PA catheter. Most CO systems will compute these values automatically.

	Normal values	Formula for calculation	Causes of increased values	Causes of decreased values
Stroke volume Volume of blood pumped by the ventricle in one contraction	60 to 130 ml per beat	SV = CO × 1,000/HR	• Sepsis • Hypervolemia • Inotrope administration	• Arrhythmias • Hypovolemia • Decreased contractility • Increased afterload
Stroke volume index Determines if the SV is adequate for patient's body size	30 to 65 ml/beat/m^2	SVI = SV/BSA or SVI = CI/HR	• Same as SV	• Same as SV
Systemic vascular resistance Degree of left ventricular resistance, or afterload	800 to 1,400 dynes/sec/cm^{-5}	SVR = MAP − CVP/CO × 80	• Hypothermia • Hypovolemia • Vasoconstriction	• Vasodilation • Vasodilators • Shock (anaphylactic, neurogenic, or septic)
Pulmonary vascular resistance	20 to 200 dynes/sec/cm^{-5}	PVR = MPAP − PAWP/CO × 80	• Hypoxemia • Pulmonary embolism • Pulmonary hypertension	• Pulmonary vasodilating drugs (morphine)

Nursing considerations

- Make sure your patient doesn't move during the procedure because movement can cause an error in measurement.
- Perform cardiac output measurements and monitoring at least every 2 to 4 hours, especially if the patient is receiving vasoactive or inotropic agents or if fluids are being added or restricted.
- Discontinue cardiac output measurements when the patient is hemodynamically stable and weaned from his vasoactive and inotropic medications.
- Monitor the patient for signs and symptoms of inadequate perfusion, including restlessness, fatigue, changes in level of consciousness (LOC), decreased capillary refill time, diminished peripheral pulses, oliguria, and pale, cool skin.
- Add the fluid volume injected for cardiac output determinations to the patient's total intake.
- Record the patient's cardiac output, cardiac index, and other hemodynamic values and vital signs at the time of measurement. Note the patient's position during measurement.

Treatments

Many treatments are available for patients with cardiovascular disease; the dramatic ones, such as heart transplantation and the artificial heart, have received a lot of publicity. Commonly used treatment measures include drug therapy; surgery; balloon catheter treatments; and other treatments, such as defibrillation, synchronized cardioversion, and pacemaker insertion.

Drug therapy

Types of drugs used to improve cardiovascular function include cardiac glycosides and phosphodiesterase (PDE) inhibitors, antiarrhythmic drugs, antianginal drugs, antihypertensive drugs, diuretic drugs, adrenergic drugs, and beta-adrenergic blockers.

Cardiac glycosides and PDE inhibitors

Cardiac glycosides and PDE inhibitors increase the force of the heart's contractions.

More force

Increasing the force of contractions is known as a *positive inotropic effect*, so these drugs are also called *inotropic agents* (affecting the force or energy of muscular contractions). (See *Understanding cardiac glycosides and PDE inhibitors.*)

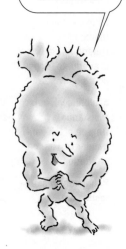

Cardiac glycosides and PDE inhibitors increase the force of the heart's contractions.

Understanding cardiac glycosides and PDE inhibitors

Cardiac glycosides and PDE inhibitors have a positive inotropic effect on the heart, meaning they increase the force of contraction. Use this table to learn about the indications, adverse reactions, and practice pointers associated with these drugs.

Drugs	Indications	Adverse reactions	Practice pointers
Cardiac glycoside			
Digoxin (Lanoxin)	Heart failure, supraventricular arrhythmias	• Digoxin toxicity (nausea, abdominal pain, headache, irritability, depression, insomnia, vision disturbances, arrhythmias) • Arrhythmias • Anorexia	• If immediate effects are required (as with a supraventricular arrhythmia), a loading dose of digoxin is required. • Check apical pulse for 1 minute before administration; report pulse less than 60 beats/minute. • Therapeutic serum levels are 0.5 to 2 ng per ml.
PDE inhibitors			
Inamrinone, milrinone	Heart failure refractory to digoxin, diuretics, and vasodilators	• Arrhythmias • Nausea • Vomiting • Headache • Fever • Chest pain • Hypokalemia • Thrombocytopenia	• These drugs are contraindicated in patients in the acute phase of MI and after an MI. • Serum potassium levels should be within normal limits before and during therapy.

Slower rate

Cardiac glycosides, such as digoxin (Lanoxin), also slow the heart rate (called a *negative chronotropic effect*) and slow electrical impulse conduction through the AV node (called a *negative dromotropic effect*).

The short and long of it

PDE inhibitors, such as inamrinone and milrinone, are typically used for short-term management of heart failure or long-term management in patients awaiting heart transplant surgery.

Boosting output

PDE inhibitors improve cardiac output by strengthening contractions. These drugs are thought to help move calcium into the cardiac cell or to increase calcium storage in the sarcoplasmic reticulum.

Understanding antiarrhythmics

Antiarrhythmics are used to restore normal heart rhythm in patients with arrhythmias. Check this table for information about the indications, adverse reactions, and practice pointers associated with these drugs.

Drugs	Indications	Adverse reactions	Practice pointers
Class IA antiarrhythmics			
Disopyramide (Norpace), procainamide, quinidine sulfate, quinidine gluconate	• Ventricular tachycardia • Atrial fibrillation • Atrial flutter • Paroxysmal atrial tachycardia	• Diarrhea • Nausea • Vomiting • Arrhythmias • ECG changes • Hepatotoxicity • Respiratory arrest	• Check apical pulse rate before therapy. If you note extremes in pulse rate, hold the dose and notify the practitioner. • Use cautiously in patients with asthma.
Class IB antiarrhythmics			
Lidocaine (Xylocaine), mexiletine	• Ventricular tachycardia, ventricular fibrillation	• Drowsiness • Hypotension • Bradycardia • Arrhythmias • Widened QRS complex	• IB antiarrhythmics may potentiate the effects of other antiarrhythmics. • Administer I.V. infusions using an infusion pump.
Class IC antiarrhythmics			
Flecainide (Tambocor), propafenone (Rythmol)	• Ventricular tachycardia, ventricular fibrillation, supraventricular arrhythmias	• New arrhythmias • Heart failure • Cardiac death	• Correct electrolyte imbalances before administration. • Monitor the patient's ECG before and after dosage adjustments.
Class II antiarrhythmics			
Acebutolol (Sectral), esmolol (Brevibloc), propranolol (Inderal)	• Atrial flutter, atrial fibrillation, paroxysmal atrial tachycardia • Ventricular arrhythmias	• Arrhythmias • Bradycardia • Heart failure • Hypotension • Nausea and vomiting • Bronchospasm	• Monitor apical heart rate and blood pressure. • Abruptly stopping these drugs can exacerbate angina and precipitate MI.

Understanding antiarrhythmics

Drugs	Indications	Adverse reactions	Practice pointers
Class III antiarrhythmics			
Amiodarone (Cordarone), ibutilide fumarate (Corvert)	• Life-threatening arrhythmias resistant to other antiarrhythmics	• Aggravation of arrhythmias • Hypotension • Anorexia • Severe pulmonary toxicity (amiodarone) • Hepatic dysfunction	• Amiodarone increases the risk of digoxin toxicity in patients also taking digoxin. • Monitor blood pressure, heart rate, and rhythm for changes. • Monitor for signs of pulmonary toxicity (dyspnea, nonproductive cough, and pleuritic chest pain).
Class IV antiarrhythmics			
Diltiazem (Cardizem), verapamil (Calan)	• Supraventricular arrhythmias	• Peripheral edema • Hypotension • Bradycardia • AV block • Flushing (with diltiazem) • Heart failure • Pulmonary edema	• Monitor heart rate and rhythm and blood pressure carefully when initiating therapy or increasing dose. • Calcium supplements may reduce effectiveness.
Miscellaneous			
Adenosine (Adenocard)	• Paroxysmal supraventricular tachycardia	• Facial flushing • Shortness of breath • Dyspnea • Chest discomfort	• Adenosine must be administered over 1 to 2 seconds, followed by a 20 ml flush of normal saline solution. • Record rhythm strip during administration.

By directly relaxing vascular smooth muscle, they also decrease peripheral vascular resistance (afterload) and the amount of blood returning to the heart (preload).

Antiarrhythmics

Antiarrhythmic drugs are used to treat arrhythmias, which are disturbances of the normal heart rhythm. (See *Understanding antiarrhythmics.*)

Benefits vs. risks

Unfortunately, many antiarrhythmic drugs can worsen or cause arrhythmias, too. In any case, the benefits of antiarrhythmic therapy need to be weighed against its risks.

Four classes plus . . .

Antiarrhythmics are categorized into four major classes: I (which includes IA, IB, and IC), II, III, and IV. The mechanisms of action of antiarrhythmic drugs vary widely, and a few drugs exhibit properties common to more than one class. One drug, adenosine, doesn't fall into any of these classes.

Class I antiarrhythmics

Class I antiarrhythmics are sodium channel blockers. This is the largest group of antiarrhythmic drugs. Class I agents are commonly subdivided into classes IA, IB, and IC. With the development of newer drugs, the use of this class of antiarrhythmics is decreasing.

Class IA antiarrhythmics

Class IA antiarrhythmics control arrhythmias by altering the myocardial cell membrane and interfering with autonomic nervous system control of pacemaker cells. Class IA antiarrhythmics include:
- disopyramide (Norpace)
- procainamide
- quinidine sulfate
- quinidine gluconate.

No (para)sympathy

Class IA antiarrhythmics also block parasympathetic stimulation of the SA and AV nodes. Because stimulation of the parasympathetic nervous system causes the heart rate to slow down, drugs that block the parasympathetic nervous system increase the conduction rate of the AV node.

Rhythmic risks

This increase in the conduction rate can produce dangerous increases in the ventricular heart rate if rapid atrial activity is present, as in a patient with atrial fibrillation. In turn, the increased ventricular heart rate can offset the ability of the antiarrhythmics to convert atrial arrhythmias to a regular rhythm.

Class IB antiarrhythmics

Lidocaine (Xylocaine), a class IB antiarrhythmic, is one of the antiarrhythmics commonly used in treating patients with acute ventricular arrhythmias. Mexiletine is another drug in this class.

Class IB drugs work by blocking the rapid influx of sodium ions during the depolarization phase of the heart's depolarization–repolarization cycle, resulting in a decreased refractory period, which reduces the risk of arrhythmia.

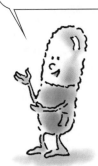

Class IA antiarrhythmics block parasympathetic stimulation and increase the conduction rate of the AV node.

Make an IB-line for the ventricle

Because class IB antiarrhythmics especially affect the Purkinje fibers (fibers in the conducting system of the heart) and myocardial cells in the ventricles, they're used only in treating patients with ventricular arrhythmias.

Class IC antiarrhythmics

Class IC antiarrhythmics are used to treat patients with certain severe, refractory (resistant) ventricular arrhythmias. Class IC antiarrhythmics include flecainide (Tambocor) and propafenone (Rythmol).

Slowing the seeds of conduction

Class IC antiarrhythmics primarily slow conduction along the heart's conduction system. Moricizine decreases the fast inward current of sodium ions of the action potential. This depresses the depolarization rate and effective refractory period.

Class II antiarrhythmics

Class II antiarrhythmics include the beta-adrenergic antagonists, also known as *beta-adrenergic blockers*. Beta-adrenergic blockers used as antiarrhythmics include:
- acebutolol (Sectral)
- esmolol (Brevibloc)
- propranolol (Inderal).

Don't be so impulsive

Class II antiarrhythmics block beta-adrenergic receptor sites in the conduction system of the heart. As a result, the ability of the SA node to fire spontaneously (automaticity) is slowed. The ability of the AV node and other cells to receive and conduct an electrical impulse to nearby cells (conductivity) is also reduced.

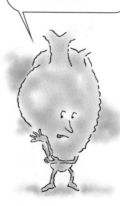

Maybe being less impulsive and spontaneous isn't such a bad thing after all.

Sometimes weaker is better

Class II antiarrhythmics also reduce the strength of the heart's contractions. When the heart beats less forcefully, it doesn't require as much oxygen to do its work.

Class III antiarrhythmics

Class III antiarrhythmics are used to treat patients with ventricular arrhythmias. Amiodarone (Cordarone) is the most widely used class III antiarrhythmic.

One-way to two-way

Although the exact mechanism of action isn't known, class III antiarrhythmics are thought to suppress arrhythmias by converting a unidirectional block to a bidirectional block. They have little or no effect on depolarization.

Class IV antiarrhythmics

The class IV antiarrhythmics include the calcium channel blockers. These drugs block the movement of calcium during phase 2 of the action potential and slow conduction and the refractory period of calcium-dependent tissues, including the AV node. The calcium channel blockers used to treat patients with arrhythmias are verapamil (Calan) and diltiazem (Cardizem).

Adenosine

Adenosine (Adenocard) is an injectable antiarrhythmic drug indicated for acute treatment for paroxysmal supraventricular tachycardia.

Depressing the pacemaker

Adenosine depresses the pacemaker activity of the SA node, reducing the heart rate and the ability of the AV node to conduct impulses from the atria to the ventricles.

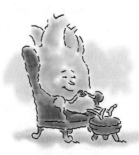

Antianginal drugs take away the pain of angina by reducing myocardial oxygen demand or increasing the supply of oxygen to the heart. Either way, I have more time to relax and just feel good!

Antianginal drugs

When the oxygen demands of the heart exceed the amount of oxygen being supplied, areas of heart muscle become ischemic (not receiving enough oxygen). When the heart muscle is ischemic, a person experiences chest pain. This condition is known as *angina* or *angina pectoris*.

Reduce demand, increase supply

Although angina's cardinal symptom is chest pain, the drugs used to treat angina aren't typically analgesics. Instead, antianginal drugs correct angina by reducing myocardial oxygen demand (the amount of oxygen the heart needs to do its work), increasing the supply of oxygen to the heart, or both.

The top three

The three classes of commonly used antianginal drugs include:
- nitrates (for acute angina)
- beta-adrenergic blockers (for long-term prevention of angina)
- calcium channel blockers (used when other drugs fail to prevent angina). (See *Understanding antianginal drugs*.)

Nitrates

Nitrates are the drug of choice for relieving acute angina. Nitrates commonly prescribed to correct angina include:
- isosorbide dinitrate (Isordil)

Understanding antianginal drugs

Antianginal drugs are effective in treating patients with angina because they reduce myocardial oxygen demand, increase the supply of oxygen to the heart, or both. Use this table to learn about the indications, adverse reactions, and practice pointers associated with these drugs.

Drugs	Indications	Adverse reactions	Practice pointers
Nitrates			
Isosorbide dinitrate (Isordil), isosorbide mononitrate (Imdur), nitroglycerin (Nitro-Bid)	• Relief and prevention of angina	• Headache • Hypotension • Dizziness • Increased heart rate	• Only sublingual and translingual forms should be used to treat an acute angina attack. • Monitor the patient's blood pressure before and after administration. • Avoid administering nitrates to patients taking erectile dysfunction drugs due to the risk for severe hypotension.
Beta-adrenergic blockers			
Atenolol (Tenormin), carvedilol (Coreg), metoprolol (Lopressor), propranolol (Inderal)	• Long-term prevention of angina • First-line therapy for hypertension • Stable heart failure due to decreased left ventricle ejection fraction	• Bradycardia • Fainting • Fluid retention • Heart failure • Arrhythmias • Nausea • Diarrhea • AV blocks • Bronchospasm • Hypoglycemia	• Monitor apical pulse rate before administration. Monitor blood pressure, ECG, and heart rate and rhythm frequently. • Signs of hypoglycemic shock may be masked; watch diabetic patients for sweating, fatigue, and hunger. • Monitor patients with a history of respiratory problems for breathing difficulty if using a nonselective beta-adrenergic blocker.
Calcium channel blockers			
Amlodipine (Norvasc), diltiazem (Cardizem), nifedipine (Adalat), verapamil (Calan)	• Long-term prevention of angina (especially Prinzmetal's angina) • Hypertension	• Orthostatic hypotension • Heart failure • Hypotension • Arrhythmias • Dizziness • Headache • Persistent peripheral edema • Pulmonary edema	• Monitor cardiac rate and rhythm and blood pressure carefully when initiating therapy or increasing the dose. • Calcium supplementation may decrease the effects of calcium channel blockers.

- isosorbide mononitrate (Imdur)
- nitroglycerin.

Anti-angina effect

Nitrates cause the smooth muscle of the veins and, to a lesser extent, the arteries to relax and dilate. This is what happens:
- When the veins dilate, less blood returns to the heart.
- This, in turn, reduces the amount of blood in the ventricles at the end of diastole, when the ventricles are full. (This blood volume in the ventricles just before contraction is called *preload*.)
- By reducing preload, nitrates reduce ventricular size and ventricular wall tension so the left ventricle doesn't have to stretch much to pump blood. This, in turn, reduces the oxygen requirements of the heart.
- As the coronary arteries dilate, more blood is delivered to the myocardium, improving oxygenation of the ischemic tissue.

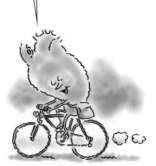

Nitrates cause veins and arteries to relax and dilate, so more blood is delivered to the myocardium. Gotta go . . . I'm on a tight schedule!

Reducing resistance

The arterioles provide the most resistance to the blood pumped by the left ventricle (called *peripheral vascular resistance*). Nitrates decrease afterload by dilating the arterioles, reducing resistance, easing the heart's workload, and easing oxygen demand.

Beta-adrenergic blockers

Beta-adrenergic blockers are used for long-term prevention of angina and are one of the main types of drugs used to treat hypertension. Beta-adrenergic blockers include:
- atenolol (Tenormin)
- carvedilol (Coreg)
- metoprolol (Lopressor)
- propranolol (Inderal).

Down with everything

Beta-adrenergic blockers decrease blood pressure and block beta-adrenergic receptor sites in the heart muscle and conduction system, decreasing heart rate and reducing the force of the heart's contractions, resulting in lower demand for oxygen.

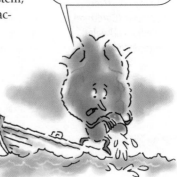

I should have listened to those calcium channel blocker border guards . . . milk overboard!

Calcium channel blockers

Calcium channel blockers are commonly used to prevent angina that doesn't respond to drugs in either of the other antianginal classes. Some calcium channel blockers are also used as antiarrhythmics.

Calcium channel blockers include:
- amlodipine (Norvasc)
- diltiazem (Cardizem)

- nifedipine (Adalat)
- verapamil (Calan).

Preventing passage

Calcium channel blockers prevent the passage of calcium ions across the myocardial cell membrane and vascular smooth muscle cells. This causes dilation of the coronary and peripheral arteries, which decreases the force of the heart's contractions and reduces the workload of the heart.

Rate reduction

By preventing arterioles from constricting, calcium channel blockers also reduce afterload. In addition, decreasing afterload decreases oxygen demands of the heart.

Calcium channel blockers also reduce the heart rate by slowing conduction through the SA and AV nodes. A slower heart rate reduces the heart's need for oxygen.

Antihypertensive drugs

Antihypertensive drugs, which act to reduce blood pressure, are used to treat patients with hypertension, a disorder characterized by high systolic blood pressure, diastolic blood pressure, or both.

Know the program

Treatment for hypertension begins with beta-adrenergic blockers and diuretics. If those drugs aren't effective, treatment continues with sympatholytic drugs (other than beta-adrenergic blockers), vasodilators, angiotensin-converting enzyme (ACE) inhibitors, angiotensin receptor blockers, or a combination of drugs. (See *Understanding antihypertensives*, page 202.)

Sympatholytic drugs

The sympatholytic drugs include several different types of drugs but work by inhibiting or blocking the sympathetic nervous system, which causes dilation of the peripheral blood vessels or decreases cardiac output, thereby reducing blood pressure.

The sympatholytic drugs are classified by their site or mechanism of action and include:

- central-acting sympathetic nervous system inhibitors, such as clonidine (Catapres), guanabenz, guanfacine (Tenex), and methyldopa
- alpha blockers, such as doxazosin (Cardura), phentolamine, prazosin (Minipress), and terazosin (Hytrin)
- mixed alpha- and beta-adrenergic blockers such as labetalol (Trandate)
- norepinephrine depletors, such as guanadrel (Hylorel).

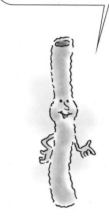

Antihypertensives act to reduce blood pressure. Treatment for hypertension begins with beta-adrenergic blockers and diuretics and may require the use of additional drugs if these treatments are ineffective.

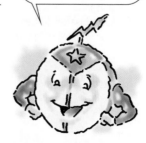

We sympatholytic drugs reduce blood pressure by blocking the sympathetic nervous system. Just try to get by me!

Understanding antihypertensives

Antihypertensives are prescribed to reduce blood pressure in patients with hypertension. Use this table to learn about the indications, adverse reactions, and practice pointers associated with these drugs.

Drugs	Indications	Adverse reactions	Practice pointers
Sympatholytic drugs			
• *Central-acting sympathetic nervous system inhibitors* (such as clonidine [Catapres], guanabenz, guanfacine [Tenex], and methyldopa) • *Alpha blockers* (such as doxazosin [Cardura], phentolamine, prazosin [Minipress], and terazosin [Hytrin]) • *Mixed alpha- and beta-adrenergic blockers* (such as labetalol [Trandate]) • *Norepinephrine depletors* (such as guanadrel [Hylorel])	• Hypertension	• Hypotension (alpha blockers) • Depression • Drowsiness • Edema • Vertigo (central-acting drugs) • Bradycardia • Hepatic necrosis • Arrhythmias	• Monitor blood pressure and pulse before and after administration.
Vasodilators			
• Hydralazine, minoxidil, nitroprus-side (Nipride)	• Used in combination with other drugs to treat moderate to severe hypertension • Hypertensive crisis	• Tachycardia • Palpitations • Angina • Fatigue • Headache • Severe pericardial effusion • Hepatotoxicity • Nausea • Stevens-Johnson syndrome	• Monitor blood pressure and pulse before and after administration. • Monitor patient receiving nitroprusside for signs of cyanide toxicity.
Angiotensin-converting enzyme inhibitors			
• Benazepril (Lotensin), captopril (Capoten), enalapril (Vasotec), lisino-pril (Prinivil), quinapril (Accupril), ramipril (Altace)	• Hypertension • Heart failure	• Angioedema • Persistent cough • Rash • Renal insufficiency	• Monitor blood pressure and pulse before and after administration.
Angiotensin-converting enzyme inhibitors			
• Candesartan (Atacand), irbesartan (Avapro), losartan (Cozaar), olmesar-tan (Benicar), valsartan (Diovan)	• Hypertension • Heart failure resis-tant to ACE inhibitors	• Fatigue • Abdominal pain • Rash • Hypotension	• Monitor blood pressure and pulse before and after administration.

Vasodilating drugs

The two types of vasodilating drugs include calcium channel blockers and direct vasodilators. These drugs decrease systolic and diastolic blood pressure.

Calcium stoppers

Calcium channel blockers produce arteriolar relaxation by preventing the entry of calcium into the cells. This prevents the contraction of vascular smooth muscle.

Direct dilators

Direct vasodilators act on arteries, veins, or both. They work by relaxing peripheral vascular smooth muscles, causing the blood vessels to dilate. This decreases blood pressure by increasing the diameter of the blood vessels, reducing total peripheral resistance.

The direct vasodilators include:
- hydralazine
- minoxidil
- nitroprusside (Nitropress).

Hydralazine and minoxidil are usually used to treat patients with resistant or refractory hypertension. Nitroprusside is reserved for use in hypertensive crisis.

ACE inhibitors

ACE inhibitors reduce blood pressure by interrupting the renin-angiotensin-aldosterone system. These drugs are the prime choice in preventing heart failure in a patient with a recent MI.

Commonly prescribed ACE inhibitors include:
- benazepril (Lotensin)
- captopril (Capoten)
- enalapril (Vasotec)
- lisinopril (Prinivil)
- quinapril (Accupril)
- ramipril (Altace).

Without ACE interference

Here's how the renin-angiotensin-aldosterone system works:
- Normally, the kidneys maintain blood pressure by releasing the hormone renin.
- Renin acts on the plasma protein angiotensinogen to form angiotensin I.
- Angiotensin I is then converted to angiotensin II.
- Angiotensin II, a potent vasoconstrictor, increases peripheral resistance and promotes the excretion of aldosterone.
- Aldosterone, in turn, promotes the retention of sodium and water, increasing the volume of blood the heart needs to pump.

> Vasodilators cause the blood vessels to dilate, which decreases blood pressure.

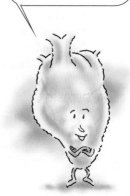

> ACE inhibitors reduce blood pressure by interrupting the renin-angiotensin-aldosterone system.

With ACE interference

ACE inhibitors work by preventing the conversion of angiotensin I to angiotensin II. As angiotensin II is reduced, arterioles dilate, reducing peripheral vascular resistance.

Less water, less work

By reducing aldosterone secretion, ACE inhibitors promote the excretion of sodium and water, reducing the amount of blood the heart needs to pump, resulting in a lowered blood pressure.

Angiotensin II receptor blockers

Unlike ACE inhibitors, which prevent production of angiotensin, angiotensin II receptor blockers (ARBs) inhibit the action of angiotensin II by attaching to tissue-binding receptor sites.

Commonly prescribed ARBs include:

- candesartan (Atacand)
- irbesartan (Avapro)
- losartan (Cozaar)
- olmesartan (Benicar)
- valsartan (Diovan).

Diuretics

Diuretics are used to promote the excretion of water and electrolytes by the kidneys. By doing so, diuretics play a major role in treating hypertension and other cardiovascular conditions. (See *Understanding diuretics.*)

The major diuretics used as cardiovascular drugs include:

- thiazide and thiazide-like diuretics
- loop diuretics
- potassium-sparing diuretics.

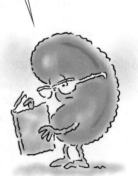

Thiazide and thiazide-like diuretics work by preventing sodium reabsorption in the kidney.

Thiazide and thiazide-like diuretics

Thiazide and thiazide-like diuretics are sulfonamide derivatives. Thiazide diuretics include hydrochlorothiazide, hydroflumethiazide (Saluron), and methyclothiazide (Enduron). Thiazide-like diuretics include indapamide.

Sodium stoppers

Thiazide and thiazide-like diuretics work by preventing sodium from being reabsorbed in the kidney. As sodium is excreted, it pulls water along with it. Thiazide and thiazide-like diuretics also increase the

Understanding diuretics

Diuretics are used to treat patients with various cardiovascular conditions. They work by promoting the excretion of water and electrolytes by the kidneys. Use this table to learn about the indications, adverse reactions, and practice pointers associated with these drugs.

Drugs	Indications	Adverse reactions	Practice pointers
Thiazide and thiazide-like diuretics			
Hydrochlorothiazide hydroflumethiazide (Saluron), indapamide, methyclothiazide (Enduron)	• Hypertension • Edema	• Hypokalemia • Orthostatic hypotension • Hyponatremia • Dizziness • Nausea	• Monitor serum potassium levels. • Monitor intake and output. • Monitor blood glucose values in diabetic patients. Thiazide diuretics can cause hyperglycemia.
Loop diuretics			
Bumetanide (Bumex), ethacrynic acid (Edecrin), furosemide (Lasix)	• Hypertension • Heart failure • Edema	• Dehydration • Orthostatic hypotension • Hyperuricemia • Hypokalemia • Hyponatremia • Dizziness • Muscle cramps • Rash	• Monitor for signs of excess diuresis (hypotension, tachycardia, poor skin turgor, and excessive thirst). • Monitor blood pressure, heart rate, and intake and output. • Monitor serum electrolyte levels.
Potassium-sparing diuretics			
Amiloride (Midamor), spironolactone (Aldactone), triamterene (Dyrenium)	• Edema • Diuretic-induced hypokalemia in patients with heart failure • Cirrhosis • Nephrotic syndrome • Hypertension	• Hyperkalemia • Headache • Nausea • Rash	• Monitor ECG for arrhythmias. • Monitor serum potassium levels. • Monitor intake and output.

excretion of chloride, potassium, and bicarbonate, which can result in electrolyte imbalances.

Stability with time

Initially, these drugs decrease circulating blood volume, leading to a reduced cardiac output. However, if the therapy is maintained, cardiac output stabilizes, but plasma fluid volume decreases.

Loop diuretics

Loop (high-ceiling) diuretics are highly potent drugs. They include:
- bumetanide (Bumex)
- ethacrynic acid (Edecrin)
- furosemide (Lasix).

High potency, big risk

The loop diuretics are the most potent diuretics available, producing the greatest volume of diuresis (urine production). They also have a high potential for causing severe adverse reactions.

Bumetanide is the shortest acting diuretic. It's even 40 times more potent than another loop diuretic, furosemide.

Locating the loop

Loop diuretics receive their name because they act primarily on the thick ascending loop of Henle (the part of the nephron responsible for concentrating urine) to increase the secretion of sodium, chloride, and water. These drugs may also inhibit sodium, chloride, and water reabsorption.

Potassium-sparing diuretics

Potassium-sparing diuretics have weaker diuretic and antihypertensive effects than other diuretics, but they have the advantage of conserving potassium.

The potassium-sparing diuretics include:
- amiloride (Midamor)
- spironolactone (Aldactone)
- triamterene (Dyrenium).

Potassium-sparing effects

The direct action of the potassium-sparing diuretics on the distal tubule of the kidneys produces:
- increased urinary excretion of sodium and water
- increased excretion of chloride and calcium ions
- decreased excretion of potassium and hydrogen ions.

These effects lead to reduced blood pressure and increased serum potassium levels.

Aping aldosterone

Spironolactone, one of the main potassium-sparing diuretics, is structurally similar to aldosterone and acts as an aldosterone antagonist.

Aldosterone promotes the retention of sodium and water and loss of potassium; spironolactone counteracts these effects by competing with aldosterone for receptor sites. As a result, sodium, chloride, and water are excreted, and potassium is retained.

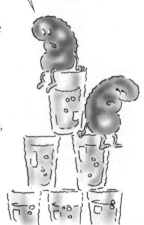

Loop diuretics are the most potent diuretics, producing the most amount of urine. But they also carry the highest risk for severe adverse reactions.

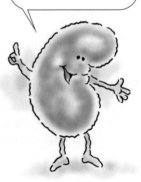

Potassium-sparing diuretics have weaker diuretic and antihypertensive effects than other diuretics, but they conserve potassium.

Understanding anticoagulants

Anticoagulants reduce the blood's ability to clot and are included in the treatment plans for many patients with cardiovascular disorders. Use this table to learn about the indications, adverse reactions, and practice pointers associated with these drugs.

Drugs	Indications	Adverse reactions	Practice pointers
Heparins			
Heparin and low-molecular-weight heparins, such as dalteparin (Fragmin) and enoxaparin (Lovenox)	• Deep vein thrombosis (treatment and prevention) • Embolism prophylaxis • Disseminated intravascular coagulation (heparin) • Prevention of complications after MI	• Bleeding • Hemorrhage • Thrombocytopenia	• Monitor thromboplastin time; the therapeutic range is 1½ to 2½ times the control. • Monitor the patient for signs of bleeding. • Concomitant administration with nonsteroidal anti-inflammatory drugs (NSAIDs), iron dextran, or an antiplatelet drug increases the risk of bleeding. • Protamine sulfate reverses the effects of heparin.
Factor Xa inhibitor			
Fondaparinux (Arixtra)	• Deep vein thrombosis (treatment and prevention) • Acute pulmonary embolism	• Hemorrhage • Thrombocytopenia • Nausea • Fever	• This drug is not interchangeable with heparin or low-dose heparins. • Monitor the patient for signs of bleeding. • Monitor complete blood count (CBC) and platelet count. • Monitor anti-Xa results; the goal for prophylaxis is 0.2 to 0.4 anti-Xa units/ml; the goal for therapy is 0.5 to 1.0 anti-Xa units/ml.
Oral anticoagulants			
Warfarin (Coumadin)	• Deep vein thrombosis prophylaxis • Prevention of complications of prosthetic heart valves or diseased mitral valves • Atrial arrhythmias	• Bleeding (may be severe) • Hepatitis • Diarrhea	• Monitor prothrombin time and International Normalized Ratio. • Monitor the patient for signs of bleeding. • The effects of oral anticoagulants can be reversed with phytonadione (vitamin K_1).
Antiplatelet drugs			
Aspirin (Ecotrin), dipyridamole (Persantine), ticlopidine (Ticlid), clopidogrel (Plavix)	• Decreases the risk of death post MI • Prevention of complications of prosthetic heart valves • Reduction of risk of MI • Prevention of reocclusion in coronary revascularization procedures	• GI distress • Bleeding • Thrombocytopenia • Angioedema	• Monitor the patient for signs of bleeding. • Aspirin and ticlopidine should be taken with meals to prevent GI irritation. • Dipyridamole should be taken with a full glass of fluid at least 1 hour before meals.

Anticoagulants

Anticoagulants are used to reduce the ability of the blood to clot. (See *Understanding anticoagulants*, page 207.) Major categories of anticoagulants include heparin, oral anticoagulants, and antiplatelet drugs.

Heparin

Heparin, prepared commercially from animal tissue, is used to prevent clot formation. Low-molecular-weight heparin, such as dalteparin (Fragmin) and enoxaparin (Lovenox), prevents deep vein thrombosis (a blood clot in the deep veins, usually of the legs) in surgical patients.

No new clots

Because it doesn't affect the synthesis of clotting factors, heparin can't dissolve already formed clots. It does prevent the formation of new thrombi, though. Here's how it works:

- Heparin inhibits the formation of thrombin and fibrin by activating antithrombin III.
- Antithrombin III then inactivates factors IXa, Xa, XIa, and XIIa in the intrinsic and common pathways. The end result is prevention of a stable fibrin clot.
- In low doses, heparin increases the activity of antithrombin III against factor Xa and thrombin and inhibits clot formation. Much larger doses are necessary to inhibit fibrin formation after a clot has formed. This relationship between dose and effect is the rationale for using low-dose heparin to prevent clotting.
- Whole blood clotting time, thrombin time, and partial thromboplastin time are prolonged during heparin therapy. However, these times may be only slightly prolonged with low or ultra-low preventive doses.

Circulate freely

Heparin can be used to prevent clotting when a patient's blood must circulate outside the body through a machine, such as a cardiopulmonary bypass machine or hemodialysis machine.

Factor Xa inhibitors

Factor Xa inhibitors are new class of anticoagulants. At this time, the only drug in this class is fondaparinux (Arixtra). Fondaparinux works by inhibiting only factor Xa—the common point in the intrinsic and extrinsic clotting pathways. Inhibition of factor Xa prevents the formation of thrombin and the formation of a clot.

Oral anticoagulants

Oral anticoagulants alter the ability of the liver to synthesize vitamin K–dependent clotting factors, including prothrombin and factors VII, IX, and X. Clotting factors already in the bloodstream continue to coagulate blood until they become depleted, so anticoagulation doesn't begin immediately.

Warfarin vs. coagulation

The major oral anticoagulant used in the United States is warfarin (Coumadin).

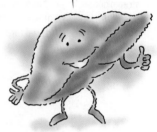

Oral anticoagulants alter my ability to synthesize vitamin K–dependent clotting factors.

Antiplatelet drugs

Examples of antiplatelet drugs are:
- aspirin (Ecotrin)
- dipyridamole (Persantine)
- ticlopidine (Ticlid)
- clopidogrel (Plavix).

Thromboembolism prevention

Antiplatelet drugs are used to prevent arterial thromboembolism, especially in patients at risk for MI, stroke, and arteriosclerosis (hardening of the arteries). They interfere with platelet activity in different drug-specific and dose-related ways.

Not just for "babies"

Low dosages of aspirin (81 mg/day) appear to inhibit clot formation by blocking the synthesis of prostaglandin, which in turn prevents formation of the platelet-aggregating substance thromboxane A_2. Dipyridamole and clopidogrel may inhibit platelet aggregation.

Broken bindings

Ticlopidine inhibits the binding of fibrinogen to platelets during the first stage of the clotting cascade.

Thrombolytic drugs

Thrombolytic drugs are used to dissolve a preexisting clot or thrombus and are commonly used in an acute or emergency situation. They work by converting plasminogen to plasmin, which lyse (dissolve) thrombi, fibrinogen, and other plasma proteins. (See *Understanding thrombolytics*, page 210.)

Some commonly used thrombolytic drugs include:
- alteplase (Activase)
- reteplase (Retavase)
- streptokinase (Streptase).

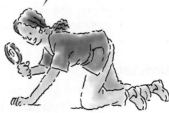

Low doses of aspirin help inhibit clot formation by blocking the synthesis of prostaglandin and formation of thromboxane A_2.

Understanding thrombolytics

Sometimes called *clot busters*, thrombolytic drugs are prescribed to dissolve a preexisting clot or thrombus. These drugs are typically used in acute or emergency situations. Use this table to learn about the indications, adverse reactions, and practice pointers associated with these drugs.

Drugs	Indications	Adverse reactions	Practice pointers
Thrombolytics			
Alteplase, reteplase, streptokinase	• Acute MI • Acute ischemic stroke • Pulmonary embolus • Catheter occlusion • Arterial thrombosis	• Bleeding • Allergic reaction	• Monitor partial thromboplastin time, prothrombin time, International Normalized Ratio, hemoglobin, and hematocrit before, during, and after administration. • Monitor vital signs frequently during and immediately after administration. Don't use an automatic blood pressure cuff to monitor blood pressure. • Monitor puncture sites for bleeding. Don't use a tourniquet when obtaining blood specimens. • Monitor for signs of bleeding.

Adrenergic drugs

Adrenergic drugs are also called *sympathomimetic drugs* because they produce effects similar to those produced by the sympathetic nervous system.

Classified by chemical

Adrenergic drugs are classified into two groups based on their chemical structure—catecholamines (both naturally occurring and synthetic) and noncatecholamines. (See *Understanding adrenergics*.)

Which receptor?

Therapeutic use of adrenergic drugs depends on which receptors they stimulate and to what degree. Adrenergic drugs can affect:
• alpha-adrenergic receptors
• beta-adrenergic receptors
• dopamine receptors.

Mimicking

Most of the adrenergic drugs produce their effects by stimulating alpha- and beta-adrenergic receptors. These drugs mimic the action of norepinephrine or epinephrine.

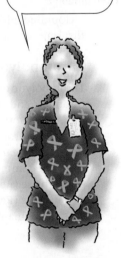

Most adrenergic drugs mimic the action of norepinephrine or epinephrine.

Understanding adrenergics

Adrenergic drugs produce effects similar to those produced by the sympathetic nervous system. Adrenergic drugs can affect alpha-adrenergic receptors, beta-adrenergic receptors, or dopamine receptors. However, most of the drugs stimulate the alpha- and beta-receptors, mimicking the effects of norepinephrine and epinephrine. Dopaminergic drugs act on receptors typically stimulated by dopamine.

Use this table to learn about the indications, adverse reactions, and practice pointers associated with these drugs.

Drugs	Indications	Adverse reactions	Practice pointers
Catecholamines			
Dobutamine	• Increase CO in short-term treatment of cardiac decompensation from depressed contractility.	Headache, tingling sensation, bronchospasm, palpitations, tachycardia, cardiac arrhythmias (PVCs), hypotension, hypertension and hypertensive crisis, angina, nausea, vomiting, tissue necrosis and sloughing (if catecholamine given I.V. leaks into surrounding tissue)	• Correct hypovolemia before administering drug. • Incompatible with alkaline solution (sodium bicarbonate); don't mix or give through same line; don't mix with other drugs. • Administer continuous drip on infusion pump. • Give drug into a large vein to prevent irritation or extravasation at site. • Monitor cardiac rate and rhythm and blood pressure carefully when initiating therapy or increasing the dose.
Dopamine	• Shock and correct hemodynamic imbalances. • Increase CO. • Hypotension	Headache, bradycardia, palpitations, tachycardia, conduction disturbance, cardiac arrhythmias (ventricular), hypotension, hypertension and hypertensive crisis, azotemia, angina, nausea, vomiting, gangrene of extremities in high dose, tissue necrosis and sloughing (if catecholamine given I.V. leaks into surrounding tissue), bronchospasm	• Correct hypovolemia before administering drug. • Administer continuous drip on infusion pump. • Give drug into a large vein to prevent extravasation; if extravasation occurs, stop infusion and treat site with phentolamine (Regitine) infiltrate to prevent tissue necrosis. • Monitor cardiac rate and rhythm and blood pressure carefully when initiating therapy or increasing the dose. • Monitor urine output during treatment, especially at high doses.
Epinephrine (Adrenalin)	• Bronchospasm • Hypersensitivity reactions • Anaphylaxis • Restoration of cardiac rhythm in cardiac arrest	Restlessness, anxiety, dizziness, headache, tachycardia, palpitations, cardiac arrhythmias (ventricular fibrillation), hypertension, stroke, cerebral hemorrhage, angina, increased blood glucose levels, tissue necrosis and sloughing (if catecholamine given I.V. leaks into surrounding tissue)	• Correct hypovolemia before administering drug. • Administer continuous drip on infusion pump. • Give drug into a large vein to prevent irritation or extravasation at site. • Monitor cardiac rate and rhythm and blood pressure carefully when initiating therapy or increasing the dose.

(continued)

Understanding adrenergics *(continued)*

Drugs	Indications	Adverse reactions	Practice pointers
Catecholamines *(continued)*			
Norepinephrine (Levophed)	• Maintain blood pressure in acute hypotensive states.	Anxiety, dizziness, headache, bradycardia, cardiac arrhythmias, hypotension, hypertension, tissue necrosis and sloughing (if catecholamine given I.V. leaks into surrounding tissue), fever, metabolic acidosis, increased blood glucose levels, dyspnea	• Correct hypovolemia before administering drug. • Administer continuous drip on infusion pump. • Give drug into a large vein to prevent extravasation; if extravasation occurs, stop infusion and treat site with phentolamine infiltrate to prevent tissue necrosis. • Monitor cardiac rate and rhythm and blood pressure carefully when initiating therapy or increasing the dose.
Noncatecholamines			
Ephedrine	• Maintain blood pressure in acute hypotensive states, especially with spinal anesthesia. • Treatment of orthostatic hypotension and bronchospasm	Anxiety, dizziness, headache, palpitations, hypotension, hypertension, nausea, vomiting, tachycardia	• Correct hypovolemia before administering drug. • Give drug into a large vein to prevent irritation or extravasation at site. • Monitor cardiac rate and rhythm and blood pressure carefully when initiating therapy or increasing the dose.
Phenylephrine (Neo-Synephrine)	• Maintain blood pressure in hypotensive states, especially hypotensive emergencies with spinal anesthesia.	Restlessness, anxiety, dizziness, headache, palpitations, cardiac arrhythmias, hypertension, tissue necrosis and sloughing (if noncatecholamine given I.V. leaks into surrounding tissue)	• Correct hypovolemia before administering drug. • Administer continuous drip on infusion pump. • Give drug into a large vein to prevent extravasation; if extravasation occurs, stop infusion and treat site with phentolamine infiltrate to prevent tissue necrosis. • Monitor cardiac rate and rhythm and blood pressure carefully when initiating therapy or increasing the dose.

Doing it like dopamine

Dopaminergic drugs act primarily on receptors in the sympathetic nervous system that are stimulated by dopamine.

Catecholamines

Because of their common basic chemical structure, catecholamines share certain properties. They stimulate the nervous system, constrict

peripheral blood vessels, increase the heart rate, and dilate the bronchi. They can be manufactured in the body or in a laboratory. Common catecholamines include:
- dobutamine
- dopamine
- epinephrine (Adrenalin)
- norepinephrine (Levophed).

Direct-acting and excitatory or inhibitory

Catecholamines are primarily direct-acting. When catecholamines combine with alpha- or beta-receptors, they cause either an excitatory or inhibitory effect. Typically, activation of alpha-receptors generates an excitatory response except for intestinal relaxation. Activation of the beta-receptors mostly produces an inhibitory response except in the cells of the heart, where norepinephrine produces excitatory effects.

How heartening

The clinical effects of catecholamines depend on the dosage and the route of administration. Catecholamines are potent inotropes, meaning they make the heart contract more forcefully. As a result, the ventricles empty more completely with each heartbeat, increasing the workload of the heart and the amount of oxygen it needs to do this harder work.

Rapid rates

Catecholamines also produce a positive chronotropic effect, which means they cause the heart to beat faster. That's because the pacemaker cells in the SA node of the heart depolarize at a faster rate. As catecholamines cause blood vessels to constrict and blood pressure to increase, the heart rate decreases as the body tries to prevent an excessive increase in blood pressure.

Fascinating rhythm

Catecholamines can cause the Purkinje fibers (an intricate web of fibers that carry electrical impulses into the ventricles of the heart) to fire spontaneously, possibly producing abnormal heart rhythms, such as PVCs and fibrillation. Epinephrine is likelier than norepinephrine to produce this spontaneous firing.

Noncatecholamines

Noncatecholamine adrenergic drugs have a variety of therapeutic uses because of the many effects these drugs can have on the body, such as the local or systemic constriction of blood vessels by phenylephrine.

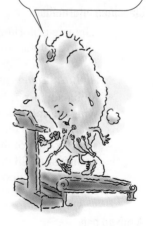

Catecholamines make the heart contract more forcefully so the ventricles empty more completely with each heartbeat, allowing me to do more work.

Alpha active . . .

Direct-acting noncatecholamines that stimulate alpha activity include methoxamine and phenylephrine.

Beta active . . .

Those that selectively exert beta$_2$ activity include:
- albuterol (Proventil)
- isoetharine
- metaproterenol.

. . . or both

Dual-acting noncatecholamines combine both actions such as ephedrine.

Adrenergic blocking drugs

Adrenergic blocking drugs, also called *sympatholytic drugs*, are used to disrupt sympathetic nervous system function. (See *Understanding adrenergic blockers*.)

Impeding impulses

These drugs work by blocking impulse transmission (and thus sympathetic nervous system stimulation) at adrenergic neurons or adrenergic receptor sites. The action of the drugs at these sites can be exerted by:
- interrupting the action of sympathomimetic (adrenergic) drugs
- reducing available norepinephrine
- preventing the action of cholinergic drugs.

Classified information

Adrenergic blocking drugs are classified according to their site of action as alpha-adrenergic blockers or beta-adrenergic blockers.

Alpha-adrenergic blocking drugs

Alpha-adrenergic blocking drugs work by interrupting the actions of sympathomimetic drugs at alpha-adrenergic receptors.
This results in:
- relaxation of the smooth muscle in the blood vessels
- increased dilation of blood vessels
- decreased blood pressure.
Drugs in this class include phentolamine and prazosin.

A mixed bag

Ergotamine is a mixed alpha agonist and antagonist. At high doses, it acts as an alpha-adrenergic blocker.
Alpha-adrenergic blockers work in one of two ways:
1. They interfere with or block the synthesis, storage, release, and reuptake of norepinephrine by neurons.

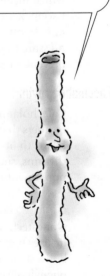

Alpha-adrenergic blocking drugs help to relax smooth muscle in blood vessels, increase dilation of blood vessels, and decrease blood pressure. I tell you, I'm so relaxed, I feel like a wet noodle!

Understanding adrenergic blockers

Adrenergic blockers block impulse transmission at adrenergic receptor sites by interrupting the action of adrenergic drugs, reducing the amount of norepinephrine available, and blocking the action of cholinergics.

Use this table to learn the indications, adverse reactions, and practice pointers needed to safely administer these drugs.

Drugs	Indications	Adverse reactions	Practice pointers
Alpha-adrenergic blockers			
Phentolamine, prazosin (Minipress)	• Hypertension • Pheochromocytoma	Orthostatic hypotension, bradycardia, tachycardia, edema, difficulty breathing, flushing, weakness, palpitations, nausea	• Monitor vital signs and heart rhythm before, during, and after administration. • Instruct the patient to rise slowly to a standing position to avoid orthostatic hypotension.
Beta-adrenergic blockers			
Nonselective Carvedilol (Coreg), labetalol (Trandate), propranolol (Inderal), sotalol (Betapace), timolol *Selective* Acebutolol (Sectral), atenolol (Tenormin), esmolol (Brevibloc), metoprolol (Lopressor)	• Prevention of complications after MI, angina, hypertension, supraventricular arrhythmias, anxiety, essential tremor, cardiovascular symptoms associated with thyrotoxicosis, migraine headaches, pheochromocytoma	Hypotension, bradycardia, peripheral vascular insufficiency, bronchospasm (nonselective), sore throat, atrioventricular block, thrombocytopenia, hypoglycemia	• Monitor vital signs and heart rhythm frequently. • Beta-adrenergic blockers can alter the requirements for insulin and oral antidiabetic agents.

2. They antagonize epinephrine, norepinephrine, or adrenergic (sympathomimetic) drugs at alpha-receptor sites.

Not very discriminating

Alpha-receptor sites are either alpha₁ or alpha₂ receptors. Alpha-adrenergic blockers include drugs that block stimulation of alpha₁ receptors and that may block alpha₂ stimulation.

Reducing resistance

Alpha-adrenergic blockers occupy alpha-receptor sites on the smooth muscle of blood vessels.

This prevents catecholamines from occupying and stimulating the receptor sites. As a result, blood vessels dilate, increasing local blood flow to the skin and other organs. The decreased peripheral vascular resistance (resistance to blood flow) helps to decrease blood pressure.

Beta-adrenergic blockers

Beta-adrenergic blockers, the most widely used adrenergic blockers, prevent stimulation of the sympathetic nervous system by inhibiting the action of catecholamines and other sympathomimetic drugs at beta-adrenergic receptors.

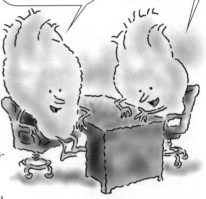

Nonselective beta-adrenergic drugs affect the heart and other sites.

Selective beta-adrenergic drugs primarily affect the heart only.

Selective (or not)

Beta-adrenergic drugs are selective or nonselective. Nonselective beta-adrenergic drugs affect:

- $beta_1$-receptor sites (located mainly in the heart)
- $beta_2$-receptor sites (located in the bronchi, blood vessels, and the uterus).

Nonselective beta-adrenergic drugs include carvedilol, labetalol, propranolol, sotalol (Betapace), and timolol.

Highly discriminating

Selective beta-adrenergic drugs primarily affect the $beta_1$-adrenergic sites. They include acebutolol, atenolol, esmolol, and metoprolol tartrate.

Intrinsically sympathetic

Some beta-adrenergic blockers, such as acebutolol, have intrinsic sympathetic activity. This means that instead of attaching to beta-receptors and blocking them, these beta-adrenergic blockers attach to beta-receptors and stimulate them. These drugs are sometimes classified as partial agonists.

Nonselective beta-adrenergic blockers reduce heart stimulation, but they can cause bronchospasm in a patient with a chronic obstructive lung disorder.

Widely effective

Beta-adrenergic blockers have widespread effects in the body because they produce their blocking action not only at the adrenergic nerve endings but also in the adrenal medulla. Effects on the heart include:

- increased peripheral vascular resistance
- decreased blood pressure
- decreased force of contractions of the heart
- decreased oxygen consumption by the heart
- slowed conduction of impulses between the atria and ventricles
- decreased cardiac output.

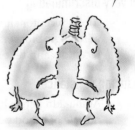

Selective or nonselective

Some of the effects of beta-adrenergic blocking drugs depend on whether the drug is classified as selective or nonselective. Selective beta-adrenergic blockers, which preferentially block beta$_1$ receptor sites, reduce stimulation of the heart. They're commonly called *cardioselective beta-adrenergic blockers*.

Nonselective beta-adrenergic blockers, which block both beta$_1$ and beta$_2$ receptor sites, reduce stimulation of the heart and cause the bronchioles of the lungs to constrict. This can cause bronchospasm in patients with chronic obstructive lung disorders.

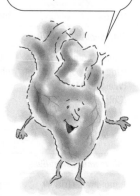

Weight loss, a proper diet, exercise, and the right antilipemic drug may be just the ticket I need to lower my lipid level.

Antilipemics

Antilipemic drugs are used to lower abnormally high blood levels of lipids, including cholesterol, triglycerides, and phospholipids.

Lipid-busting combo

Antilipemics can be used in combination with lifestyle changes (proper diet, weight loss, and exercise) to lower a patient's lipid level.

A class act

Major classes of antilipemic drugs include:
- bile-sequestering drugs
- fibric acid derivatives
- HMG-CoA reductase inhibitors
- cholesterol absorption inhibitors. (See *Understanding antilipemics*, page 218.)

I do what I can to get rid of the bad cholesterol.

Bile-sequestering drugs

Bile-sequestering drugs help lower blood levels of low-density lipoproteins (LDLs, or bad cholesterol) by combining with bile acids in the intestines to form an insoluble compound that's then excreted in the feces.

Follow the exit signs, please

The decreasing level of bile acid in the gallbladder triggers the liver to synthesize more bile acids from their precursor, cholesterol. As cholesterol leaves the bloodstream and other storage areas to replace the lost bile acids, blood cholesterol levels decrease.

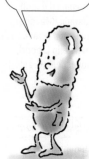

It's all in the family

Bile-sequestering drugs are the drugs of choice for treating familial hypercholesterolemia when the patient isn't able to reduce his LDL levels through dietary changes. Examples of bile-sequestering drugs include:
- cholestyramine (Questran)
- colesevelam (Welchol)
- colestipol hydrochloride (Colestid).

Understanding antilipemics

Antilipemics are used to lower high blood levels of lipids by combining with bile acids, reducing cholesterol formation, inhibiting enzymes, and inhibiting cholesterol absorption.

Use this table to learn the indications, adverse reactions, and practice pointers needed to safely administer these drugs.

Drugs	Indications	Adverse reactions	Practice pointers
Bile-sequestering drugs			
Cholestyramine (Questran), colesevelam (Welchol), colestipol (Colestid)	• Elevated serum cholesterol	• Constipation • Increased bleeding tendencies • Muscle and joint pain • Nausea, heartburn • Headache	• Tell the patient he'll need periodic blood tests. • Administer the drug before meals. • Don't administer the powder in dry form; mix with fluid. • Administer other medications 1 hour before or 4 to 6 hours after these drugs.
Fibric acid derivatives			
Fenofibrate (TriCor), gemfibrozil (Lopid)	• Hypercholesterolemia • Hypertriglyceridemia	• Rash, nausea, vomiting, diarrhea • Myalgia, flulike syndromes • Impotence • Dizziness, blurred vision • Abdominal pain, epigastric pain	• Tell the patient he'll need periodic blood tests. • Educate the patient on dietary and lifestyle changes to help lower cholesterol and triglyceride levels. • Administer these drugs with meals.
HMG-CoA reductase inhibitors			
Atorvastatin (Lipitor), fluvastatin (Lescol), lovastatin (Mevacor), pravastatin (Pravachol), simvastatin (Zocor), rosuvastatin (Crestor)	• Elevated cholesterol, triglyceride, and LDL levels • Prevention of cardiovascular disease in adults without clinically evident coronary disease but with multiple risk factors	• Rhabdomyolysis with acute renal failure • Headache • Flatulence, abdominal pain, constipation, nausea	• Tell the patient he'll need periodic blood tests. • Monitor periodic liver function tests. • Administer the drug at the same time each day; doesn't need to be administered with food. • Educate the patient on dietary and lifestyle changes to help lower cholesterol and triglyceride levels.
Cholesterol absorption inhibitors			
Ezetimibe (Zetia)	• Elevated cholesterol, triglyceride, and LDL levels • May be administered as adjunctive treatment with simvastatin	• Cough • Myalgia, arthralgia • Headache, dizziness	• Tell the patient he'll need periodic blood tests. • Educate the patient on dietary and lifestyle changes to help lower cholesterol and triglyceride levels. • If administering with an HMG-CoA reductase inhibitor, administer both drugs together.

Fibric acid derivatives

Fibric acid derivatives reduce high triglyceride levels and, to a lesser extent, high LDL levels.

Keeping the highs low

It isn't known exactly how these drugs work, although it's thought that they:
- reduce cholesterol production early in its formation
- mobilize cholesterol from the tissues
- increase cholesterol excretion
- decrease synthesis and secretion of lipoproteins
- decrease synthesis of triglycerides.

A common answer

Fenofibrate (TriCor) and gemfibrozil (Lopid), two commonly used fibric acid derivatives, both reduce triglyceride levels and blood cholesterol levels. Gemfibrozil also increases the high-density lipoprotein (HDL) levels in the blood and increases the serum's capacity to dissolve additional cholesterol.

HMG-CoA reductase inhibitors

Also known as *statins*, HMG-CoA reductase inhibitors lower lipid levels by interfering with cholesterol synthesis. More specifically, they inhibit the enzyme that's responsible for converting HMG-CoA to mevalonate, an early rate-limiting step in the biosynthesis of cholesterol.

Statins with status

Commonly prescribed HMG-CoA reductase inhibitors include:
- atorvastatin (Lipitor)
- fluvastatin (Lescol)
- lovastatin (Mevacor)
- pravastatin (Pravachol)
- simvastatin (Zocor)
- rosuvastatin (Crestor).

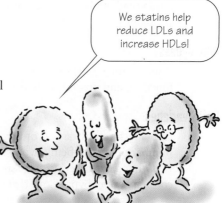

We statins help reduce LDLs and increase HDLs!

Highs, lows, and a bonus or two

Statin drugs are used primarily to reduce LDLs and total blood cholesterol levels. They also produce a mild increase in HDLs (or good cholesterol). Because of their effect on LDL and total cholesterol, these drugs are used not only to treat hypercholesterolemia but also for primary and secondary prevention of cardiovascular events.

Cholesterol absorption inhibitors

As their name implies, cholesterol absorption inhibitors inhibit the absorption of cholesterol and related phytosterols from the intestine.

In a class by itself

At this time, ezetimibe (Zetia) is the only drug in the class. Ezetimibe reduces blood cholesterol levels by inhibiting the absorption of cholesterol by the small intestine. This leads to a decrease in delivery of intestinal cholesterol to the liver, causing a reduction in hepatic cholesterol stores and an increase in clearance from the blood.

A two-drug punch

Ezetimibe may be used alone or with statins to help lower cholesterol. There is currently one drug on the market that combines the statin simvastatin and ezetimibe (Vytorin) to help decrease total cholesterol and LDLs and increase HDLs.

Surgery

Surgeries for treatment of cardiovascular system disorders include coronary artery bypass graft (CABG), heart transplantation, valve surgery, vascular repair, and insertion of a VAD.

Coronary artery bypass graft

CABG circumvents an occluded coronary artery with an autogenous graft (usually a segment of the saphenous vein from the leg or internal mammary artery), thereby restoring blood flow to the myocardium.

CABG is one of the most commonly performed surgeries because it's done to prevent MI in a patient with acute or chronic myocardial ischemia. The need for CABG is determined from the results of cardiac catheterization and patient symptoms. (See *Bypassing coronary occlusions*.)

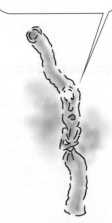

CABG surgery—circumventing an occluded artery with an autogenous graft—may be a viable option for your patient with acute or chronic myocardial ischemia.

Why bypass?

If successful, CABG can relieve anginal pain, improve cardiac function, and possibly enhance the patient's quality of life.

CABG varieties

CABG techniques vary according to the patient's condition and the number of arteries being bypassed.

Other surgical techniques, such as the mini-CABG and direct coronary artery bypass, can reduce the risk for cerebral complications

Bypassing coronary occlusions

After the patient receives general anesthesia, surgery begins with graft harvesting. The surgeon makes a series of incisions in the patient's thigh or calf and removes a saphenous vein segment for grafting. Most surgeons prefer to use a segment of the internal mammary artery.

Exposing the heart

After the autografts are obtained, the surgeon performs a medial sternotomy to expose the heart and then initiates cardiopulmonary bypass.

To reduce myocardial oxygen demands during surgery and to protect the heart, the surgeon induces cardiac hypothermia and standstill by injecting a cold cardioplegic solution (potassium-enriched saline solution) into the aortic root.

One fine sewing lesson

After the patient is prepared, the surgeon sutures one end of the venous graft to the ascending aorta and the other end to a patent coronary artery that's distal to the occlusion. The graft is sutured in a reversed position to promote proper blood flow. The surgeon repeats this procedure for each occlusion to be bypassed.

In the example depicted below, saphenous vein segments bypass occlusions in three sections of the coronary arteries.

Finishing up

After the grafts are in place, the surgeon flushes the cardioplegic solution from the heart and discontinues cardiopulmonary bypass. He then implants epicardial pacing electrodes, inserts a chest tube, closes the incision, and applies a sterile dressing.

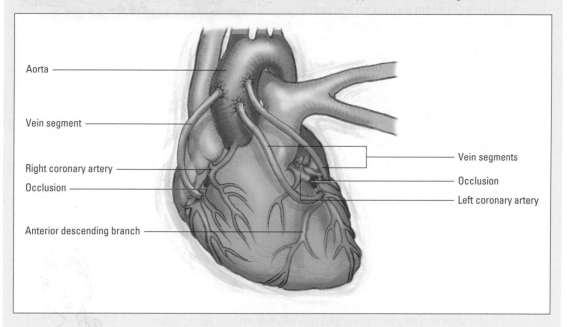

Aorta

Vein segment

Right coronary artery

Occlusion

Anterior descending branch

Vein segments

Occlusion

Left coronary artery

and accelerate recovery for patients requiring grafts of only one or two arteries.

In some patients, it's possible to perform the CABG procedure without using a cardiopulmonary bypass machine. This decreases recovery time and complications.

Short and sweet

Minimally invasive coronary artery surgery is also called *limited-access coronary surgery*. It has two standard methods including port-access coronary bypass (PACB) and minimally invasive direct coronary artery bypass (MIDCAB). A MIDCAB is also performed on a beating heart, but instead of the traditional midsternal incision, the surgeon uses a small thoracotomy incision. MIDCAB procedures usually result in shorter hospital stays and fewer complications than traditional CABG.

> A MIDCAB procedure will have your patient back home much quicker. It usually results in a shorter hospital stay and fewer complications than traditional CABG surgery.

Nursing considerations

When caring for a CABG patient, your major roles include patient instruction and caring for the patient's changing cardiovascular needs.

Before surgery
- Reinforce the doctor's explanation of the surgery.
- Explain the complex equipment and procedures used in the critical care unit (CCU) or postanesthesia care unit (PACU).
- Explain that the patient awakens from surgery with an endotracheal (ET) tube in place and connected to a mechanical ventilator. He'll also be connected to a cardiac monitor and may have in place an NG tube, a chest tube, an indwelling urinary catheter, arterial lines, epicardial pacing wires, and a PA catheter. Tell him that discomfort is minimal and that the equipment is removed as soon as possible.
- Review incentive spirometry techniques and range-of-motion (ROM) exercises with the patient.
- Make sure that the patient or a responsible family member has signed a consent form.
- Before surgery, prepare the patient's skin as ordered.
- Immediately before surgery, begin cardiac monitoring and then assist with PA catheterization and insertion of arterial lines. Some facilities insert PA catheters and arterial lines in the operating room before surgery.

> After CABG, look for signs of hemodynamic compromise and be ready to assist with epicardial pacing, cardioversion, or defibrillation.

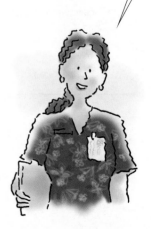

After surgery
- After CABG, look for signs of hemodynamic compromise, such as severe hypotension, decreased cardiac output, and shock.
- Begin warming procedures according to your facility's policy.

- Check and record vital signs and hemodynamic parameters every 5 to 15 minutes until the patient's condition stabilizes. Administer medications and titrate according to the patient's response, as ordered.
- Monitor ECGs continuously for disturbances in heart rate and rhythm. If you detect serious abnormalities, notify the practitioner and be prepared to assist with epicardial pacing or, if necessary, cardioversion or defibrillation.
- To ensure adequate myocardial perfusion, keep arterial pressure within the limits set by the doctor. Usually, mean arterial pressure (MAP) less than 70 mm Hg results in inadequate tissue perfusion; pressure greater than 110 mm Hg can cause hemorrhage and graft rupture. Monitor PAP, CVP, left atrial pressure, and cardiac output as ordered.
- Frequently evaluate the patient's peripheral pulses, capillary refill time, and skin temperature and color and auscultate for heart sounds; report abnormalities.
- Evaluate tissue oxygenation by assessing breath sounds, chest excursion, and symmetry of chest expansion. Check ABG results every 2 to 4 hours and adjust ventilator settings to keep ABG values within ordered limits.
- Maintain chest tube drainage at the ordered negative pressure (usually -10 to -40 cm H_2O) and assess regularly for hemorrhage, excessive drainage (greater than 200 ml/hour), and sudden decrease or cessation of drainage.
- Monitor the patient's intake and output. Assess urine output at least hourly during the immediate postoperative period and then less frequently as the patient's condition stabilizes.
- Assess for electrolyte imbalances, especially hypokalemia and hypomagnesemia, and replace electrolytes as ordered.
- As the patient's incisional pain increases, give an analgesic as ordered. Give other drugs as ordered.
- Throughout the recovery period, assess for symptoms of stroke, pulmonary embolism, and impaired renal perfusion.
- After weaning the patient from the ventilator and removing the ET tube, provide chest physiotherapy. Start with incentive spirometry and encourage the patient to cough, turn frequently, and deep breathe. Assist with ROM exercises, as ordered, to enhance peripheral circulation and prevent thrombus formation.
- Explain that postpericardiotomy syndrome commonly develops after open heart surgery. Instruct the patient about signs and symptoms, such as fever, muscle and joint pain, weakness, and chest discomfort.
- Prepare the patient for the possibility of postoperative depression, which may not develop until weeks after discharge. Reassure him that this depression is normal and should pass quickly.

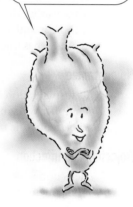

Don't be fooled by the fact that CABG is a fairly common procedure. Remember, my heart is in your hands—right up to the time I'm discharged home.

- Maintain nothing by mouth status until bowel sounds return. Then begin clear liquids and advance diet as tolerated and as ordered. Expect sodium and cholesterol restrictions. Explain that this diet can help reduce the risk of recurrent arterial occlusion.

Transmyocardial revascularization

Transmyocardial revascularization (TMR) uses a high-energy laser to create channels from the epicardial surface into the left ventricular chamber. The purpose of the TMR is to increase perfusion directly to the heart muscle. This is performed on patients who are poor candidates for CABG and whose symptoms are not responding to other medical treatments.

Heart transplantation

Heart transplantation involves the replacement of a person's heart with a donor heart. It's the treatment of choice for patients with end-stage cardiac disease that have a poor prognosis, estimated survival of 6 to 12 months, and poor quality of life. A heart transplant candidate typically has uncontrolled symptoms and no other surgical options.

A heart transplant is the treatment of choice for those with end-stage cardiac disease, a poor prognosis, 6 to 12 months survival, and a poor quality of life.

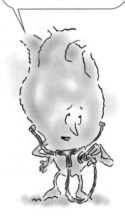

No guarantee

Transplantation doesn't guarantee a cure. Serious postoperative complications include infection and tissue rejection. Most patients experience one or both of these complications postoperatively.

Rejection and infection

Rejection typically occurs in the first 6 weeks after surgery. The patient is treated with monoclonal antibodies and potent immunosuppressants. The resulting immunosuppression places the patient at risk for life-threatening infection.

Nursing considerations

- Provide emotional support to the patient and his family. Begin to address their fears by discussing the procedure, possible complications, and the impact of transplantation and a prolonged recovery period on the patient's life.
- After surgery, maintain reverse isolation.
- Administer immunosuppressants and monitor the patient closely for signs of infection. Transplant recipients may exhibit subtle signs because immunosuppressants mask obvious signs.
- Monitor vital signs every 15 minutes until stabilized and assess the patient for signs of hemodynamic compromise, such as hypotension, decreased cardiac output, and shock.

Administer volume replacement to maintain CVP.

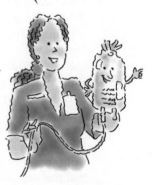

- If necessary, administer nitroprusside during the first 24 to 48 hours to control blood pressure. An infusion of dopamine can improve contractility and renal perfusion.
- Volume replacement with normal saline, plasma expanders, or blood products may be necessary to maintain CVP.
- A patient with elevated PAP may receive prostaglandin E to produce pulmonary vasodilation and reduce right ventricular afterload.
- Monitor ECG for rhythm disturbances.
- Maintain the chest tube drainage system at the prescribed negative pressure. Regularly assess for hemorrhage or sudden cessation of drainage.
- Continually assess the patient for signs of tissue rejection (decreased electrical activity on the ECG, right axis shift, atrial arrhythmias, conduction defects, weight gain, lethargy, ventricular failure, jugular vein distention, and increased T-cell count).
- Keep in mind that the effects of denervated heart muscle or denervation (in which the vagus nerve is cut during heart transplant surgery) makes such drugs as edrophonium (Tensilon) and anticholinergics (such as atropine) ineffective.

Valve surgery

To prevent heart failure, a patient with valvular stenosis or insufficiency accompanied by severe, unmanageable symptoms may require valve replacement (with a mechanical or prosthetic valve), valvular repair, or commissurotomy. (See *Types of valve surgery*, page 226.)

Why valve surgery?

Because of the high pressure generated by the left ventricle during contraction, stenosis and insufficiency most commonly affect the mitral and aortic valves. Other indications for valve surgery depend on the patient's symptoms and affected valve:

- In aortic insufficiency, the patient undergoes valve replacement after symptoms—palpitations, dizziness, dyspnea on exertion, angina, and murmurs—have developed or if the chest X-ray and ECG reveal left ventricular hypertrophy.
- In aortic stenosis, which may be asymptomatic, the practitioner may recommend valve replacement if cardiac catheterization reveals significant stenosis.
- In mitral stenosis, surgery is indicated if the patient develops fatigue, dyspnea, hemoptysis, arrhythmias, pulmonary hypertension, or right ventricular hypertrophy.
- In mitral insufficiency, surgery is usually done when the patient's symptoms—dyspnea, fatigue, and palpitations—interfere with ADLs or if insufficiency is acute, as in papillary muscle rupture.

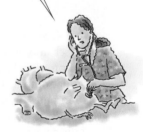

To prevent heart failure, a patient may need a valve replacement or other type of surgical repair.

Types of valve surgery

When a patient with valve disease develops severe symptoms, surgery may be necessary. Several surgical procedures are available.

Commissurotomy

During commissurotomy, the surgeon incises fused mitral valve leaflets and removes calcium deposits to improve valve mobility.

Valve repair

Valve repair includes resection or patching of valve leaflets, stretching or shortening of chordae tendineae, or placing a ring in a dilated annulus (annuloplasty). Valve repair is done to avoid the complications associated with the use of prosthetic valves.

Valve replacement

Valvular replacement involves replacement of the patient's diseased valve with a mechanical or biologic valve.

In the Ross procedure, the patient's own pulmonic valve is excised and used to replace the diseased aortic valve. An allograft from a human cadaver is then used to replace the pulmonic valve. Advantages of this procedure include the potential for the pulmonary autograft to grow when used in children, anticoagulation isn't necessary, and the increased durability of the replaced valves.

Minimally invasive valve surgery

Minimally invasive valve surgery can be performed without a large median sternotomy incision to repair or replace aortic and mitral valves. Port access techniques may also be used for mitral valve surgery using endovascular cardiopulmonary bypass. Advantages of these types of surgery include a less invasive procedure, shorter hospital stays, fewer postoperative complications, reduced costs, and smaller incisions.

Nursing considerations

Provide these care measures after valve surgery.

- Closely monitor the patient's hemodynamic status for signs of compromise. Watch especially for severe hypotension, decreased cardiac output, and shock. Check and record vital signs every 15 minutes until his condition stabilizes. Frequently assess heart sounds; report distant heart sounds or new murmurs, which may indicate prosthetic valve failure.
- Monitor the ECG continuously for disturbances in heart rate and rhythm, such as bradycardia, atrial fibrillation, ventricular tachycardia, and heart block. Such disturbances may signal injury of the conduction system, which may occur during valve surgery from proximity of the atrial and mitral valves to the AV node. Arrhythmias may also result from myocardial irritability or ischemia, fluid and electrolyte imbalance, hypoxemia, or hypothermia. If you detect serious abnormalities, notify the practitioner and be prepared to assist with temporary epicardial pacing.

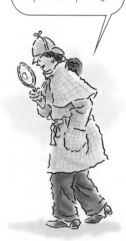

If you detect serious abnormalities in the patient's heart rate and rhythm, be ready to assist with temporary epicardial pacing.

- Take steps to maintain the patient's MAP between 70 and 100 mm Hg. Also, monitor PAP and left atrial pressure as ordered.
- Frequently assess the patient's peripheral pulses, capillary refill time, and skin temperature and color and auscultate for heart sounds. Evaluate tissue oxygenation by assessing breath sounds, chest excursion, and symmetry of chest expansion. Report any abnormalities.
- Check ABG values every 2 to 4 hours and adjust ventilator settings as needed.
- Maintain chest tube drainage at the prescribed negative pressure (usually −10 to −40 cm H_2O for adults). Assess chest tubes frequently for signs of hemorrhage, excessive drainage (greater than 200 ml/hour), and a sudden decrease or cessation of drainage.
- As ordered, administer analgesic, anticoagulant, antibiotic, antiarrhythmic, inotropic, and pressor medications as well as I.V. fluids and blood products. Monitor intake and output and assess for electrolyte imbalances, especially hypokalemia. When anticoagulant therapy begins, evaluate its effectiveness by monitoring prothrombin time and International Normalized Ratio daily.
- Throughout the patient's recovery period, observe carefully for complications.
- After weaning from the ventilator and removing the ET tube, promote chest physiotherapy. Start the patient on incentive spirometry and encourage him to cough, turn frequently, and deep breathe.

Vascular repair

Vascular repair may be needed to treat patients with:
- vessels damaged by arteriosclerotic or thromboembolic disorders trauma, infections, or congenital defects
- vascular obstructions that severely compromise circulation
- vascular disease that doesn't respond to drug therapy or nonsurgical treatments such as balloon catheterization
- life-threatening dissecting or ruptured aortic aneurysms
- limb-threatening acute arterial occlusion.

Repair review

Vascular repair methods include aneurysm resection, grafting, embolectomy, vena caval filtering, and endarterectomy. The surgery used depends on the type, location, and extent of vascular occlusion or damage. (See *Types of vascular repair*, page 228.)

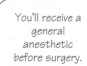

You'll receive a general anesthetic before surgery.

Nursing considerations
Provide care measures before and after vascular repair surgery.

Types of vascular repair

There are several surgical options to repair damaged or diseased vessels. Some of these options are aortic aneurysm repair, vena caval filter insertion, embolectomy, and bypass grafting.

Aortic aneurysm repair

Aortic aneurysm repair is done to remove an aneurysmal segment of the aorta. The surgeon first makes an incision to expose the aneurysm site. The patient is placed on a cardiopulmonary bypass machine, if necessary. The surgeon then clamps the aorta. The aneurysm is resected, and the damaged portion of the aorta is repaired.

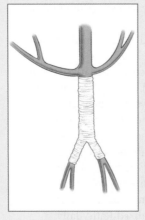

Embolectomy

An embolectomy is done to remove an embolism from an artery. During this procedure, the surgeon inserts a balloon-tipped indwelling catheter into the artery and passes it through the thrombus (top). He then inflates the balloon and withdraws the catheter to remove the thrombus (bottom).

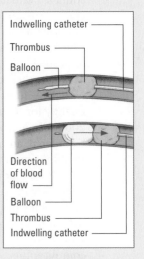

Indwelling catheter
Thrombus
Balloon
Direction of blood flow
Balloon
Thrombus
Indwelling catheter

Vena caval filter insertion

A vena caval filter is inserted to trap emboli in the vena cava, preventing them from reaching the pulmonary vessels. A vena caval filter or umbrella is inserted transvenously by catheter. After in place in the vena cava, the umbrella or filter traps emboli but allows venous blood flow.

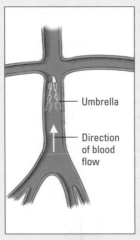

Umbrella
Direction of blood flow

Bypass grafting

Bypass grafting is used to bypass an arterial obstruction resulting from arteriosclerosis. After exposing the affected artery, the surgeon anastomoses a synthetic or autogenous graft to divert blood flow around the occluded arterial segment. The autogenous graft may be a vein or an artery harvested from elsewhere in the patient's body. A femoropopliteal bypass is depicted.

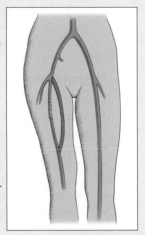

Before surgery
- Make sure the patient and his family understand the doctor's explanation of the surgery and possible complications.
- Tell the patient that he'll receive a general anesthetic and will awaken from the anesthetic in the CCU or PACU. Explain that he'll have an I.V. line in place, ECG electrodes for continuous cardiac monitoring,

and possibly an arterial line or a PA catheter to provide continuous pressure monitoring. He may also have a urinary catheter in place to allow accurate output measurement. If appropriate, explain that he'll be intubated and placed on mechanical ventilation.

Flow check

- Before surgery, perform a complete vascular assessment. Take vital signs to provide a baseline. Evaluate the strength and sound of the blood flow and the symmetry of the pulses and note bruits. Record the temperature of the extremities; their sensitivity to motor and sensory stimuli; and pallor, cyanosis, or redness. Rate peripheral pulse volume and strength on a scale of 0 (pulse absent) to 4 (bounding and strong pulse) and check capillary refill time by blanching the fingernail or toenail; normal refill time is less than 3 seconds.
- As ordered, instruct the patient to restrict food and fluids for at least 8 hours before surgery.

Be on guard!

- If the patient is awaiting surgery for aortic aneurysm repair, be on guard for signs and symptoms of acute dissection or rupture. Note especially sudden severe pain in the chest, abdomen, or lower back; severe weakness; diaphoresis; tachycardia; or a precipitous drop in blood pressure. If any of these occur, notify the practitioner immediately.

After surgery
- Check and record the patient's vital signs every 15 minutes until his condition stabilizes, then every 30 minutes for 1 hour, and hourly thereafter for 2 to 4 hours. Report hypotension and hypertension immediately.
- Auscultate heart, breath, and bowel sounds and report abnormal findings. Monitor the ECG for abnormalities in heart rate or rhythm. Also monitor other pressure readings and carefully record intake and output.
- Check the patient's dressing regularly for excessive bleeding.
- Assess the patient's neurologic and renal function and report abnormalities.
- Provide analgesics, as ordered, for incisional pain.
- Frequently assess peripheral pulses, using Doppler ultrasonography if palpation is difficult. Check all extremities bilaterally for muscle strength and movement, color, temperature, and capillary refill time.

Watch those wounds!

- Change dressings and provide incision care as ordered. Position the patient to avoid pressure on grafts and to reduce edema. Administer antithrombotics, as ordered, and monitor appropriate laboratory values to evaluate effectiveness.

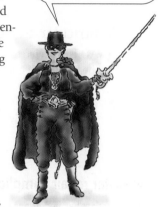

If your patient's awaiting surgery for aortic aneurysm repair, be on guard for signs and symptoms of acute dissection or rupture.

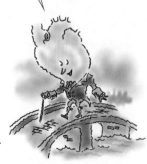

Remember, early ambulation can help prevent complications of immobility. I think I'll take the long way home!

- Assess for complications and immediately report relevant signs and symptoms. (See *Vascular repair complications*.)
- As the patient's condition improves, take steps to wean him from the ventilator if appropriate. To promote good pulmonary hygiene, encourage the patient to cough, turn, and breathe deep frequently.
- Assist the patient with ROM exercises, as ordered, to prevent thrombus formation. Assist with early ambulation to prevent complications of immobility.

VAD isn't so bad . . . it takes the pressure off me and keeps the blood flowing.

Ventricular assist device insertion

A VAD is a device that's implanted to provide support to a failing heart. A VAD consists of:
- a blood pump
- cannulas
- pneumatic or electrical drive console.

Vascular repair complications

After a patient has undergone vascular repair surgery, monitor for these potential complications.

Complication	Signs and symptoms
Pulmonary infection	• Fever • Cough • Congestion • Dyspnea
Infection	• Redness • Warmth • Drainage • Increased pain • Fever
Renal dysfunction	• Low urine output • Elevated BUN and serum creatinine levels
Occlusion	• Reduced or absent peripheral pulses • Paresthesia • Severe pain • Cyanosis
Hemorrhage	• Hypotension • Tachycardia • Restlessness and confusion • Shallow respirations • Abdominal pain • Increased abdominal girth

More output, less work

VADs are designed to decrease the heart's workload and increase cardiac output in patients with ventricular failure.

A temporary diversion

A VAD is commonly used while a patient waits for a heart transplant. In a surgical procedure, blood is diverted from a ventricle to an artificial pump. This pump, which is synchronized to the patient's ECG, then functions as the ventricle. (See *VAD: Help for a failing heart.*)

That's shocking!

VADs are also indicated for use in patients with cardiogenic shock that doesn't respond to maximal pharmacologic therapy or inability to be weaned from cardiopulmonary bypass.

VAD: Help for a failing heart

A VAD, which is commonly called a *bridge to transplant*, is a mechanical pump that relieves the workload of the ventricle as the heart heals or until a donor heart is located.

Implantable

The typical VAD is implanted in the upper abdominal wall. An inflow cannula drains blood from the left ventricle into a pump, which then pushes the blood into the aorta through the outflow cannula.

Pump options

VADs are available as continuous flow (axial flow) or pulsatile pumps. A continuous flow pump fills continuously and returns blood to the aorta at a constant rate. A pulsatile pump may work in one of two ways: It may fill during systole and pump blood into the aorta during diastole, or it may pump irrespective of the patient's cardiac cycle.

Many types of VAD systems are available. The illustrations below show a pulsatile pump and a continuous flow pump. Each has an external controller and a reserve power pack.

Potential complications

Despite the use of anticoagulants, the VAD may cause thrombi formation, leading to pulmonary embolism or stroke. Other complications may include heart failure, bleeding, cardiac tamponade, or infection.

Pulsatile pump

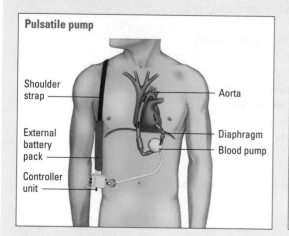

Shoulder strap — Aorta

External battery pack —

Controller unit —

— Diaphragm
Blood pump

Continous flow pump

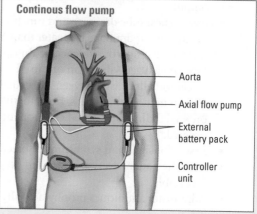

— Aorta

— Axial flow pump

— External battery pack

— Controller unit

Right or left?

A VAD is used to provide systemic or pulmonary support, or both:

- A right ventricular assist device (RVAD) provides pulmonary support by diverting blood from the failing right ventricle to the VAD, which then pumps the blood to the pulmonary circulation by way of the VAD connection to the pulmonary artery.
- With a left ventricular assist device (LVAD), blood flows from the left ventricle to the VAD, which then pumps blood back to the body by way of the VAD connection to the aorta.
- When RVAD and LVAD are used, biventricular support is provided.

Nursing considerations

Follow these care measures before and after insertion of a VAD.

Before insertion

- Prepare the patient and his family for insertion, reinforcing explanations about the device, its purpose, and what to expect after insertion.
- Make sure that informed consent is obtained.
- Continue close patient monitoring, including continuous ECG, pulmonary artery and hemodynamic status, and intake and output.

After insertion

- Assess the patient's cardiovascular status at least every 15 minutes until stable and then hourly. Monitor blood pressure and hemodynamic parameters, including cardiac output and cardiac index, ECG, and peripheral pulses.
- Inspect the incision and dressing at least every hour initially and then every 2 to 4 hours as indicated by the patient's condition.
- Monitor urine output hourly and maintain I.V. fluid therapy as ordered. Watch for signs of fluid overload or decreasing urine output.
- Assess chest tube drainage and function frequently. Notify the practitioner if drainage is greater than 150 ml over 2 hours. Auscultate lungs for evidence of abnormal breath sounds. Evaluate oxygen saturation or mixed venous oxygen saturation levels and administer oxygen as needed and ordered.
- Obtain hemoglobin levels, hematocrit, and coagulation studies as ordered. Administer blood component therapy as indicated and ordered.
- Assess for signs and symptoms of bleeding.
- Turn the patient every 2 hours and begin ROM exercises when he's stable.
- Administer antibiotics prophylactically if ordered.

> After VAD insertion, watch for signs of fluid overload or decreasing urine output. Your patient's fluid status can be most revealing after surgery.

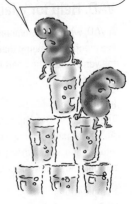

Balloon catheter treatments

Balloon catheter treatments of cardiovascular system disorders include IABP counterpulsation, balloon valvuloplasty, and percutaneous transluminal coronary angioplasty (PTCA).

IABP counterpulsation

IABP counterpulsation temporarily reduces left ventricular workload and improves coronary perfusion.

What for?

IABP counterpulsation may benefit patients with:
- cardiogenic shock
- septic shock
- intractable angina before surgery
- intractable ventricular arrhythmias
- ventricular septal or papillary muscle ruptures
- acute MI with left ventricular failure.

It's also used for patients who suffer pump failure before, during, or after cardiac surgery and serves as a bridge to other treatments, such as VAD, CABG, or heart transplant.

How so?

The doctor may perform balloon catheter insertion at the patient's bedside as an emergency procedure or in the operating room. (See *Understanding a balloon pump*, page 234.)

Nursing considerations
- Explain to the patient that the doctor is going to place a catheter in the aorta to help his heart pump more easily. Tell him that, while the catheter is in place, he can't sit up, bend his knee, or flex his hip more than 45 degrees.
- Attach the patient to a continuous ECG monitor and make sure he has an arterial line, a PA catheter, and a peripheral I.V. line in place.
- Gather a surgical tray for percutaneous catheter insertion, heparin, normal saline solution, the IABP catheter, and the pump console. Connect the ECG monitor to the pump console. Then prepare the femoral site.
- After the IABP catheter is inserted, select either the ECG or arterial waveform to regulate inflation and deflation of the balloon. With the ECG waveform, the pump inflates the balloon in the middle of the T wave (diastole) and deflates with the R wave (before systole). With the arterial waveform, the

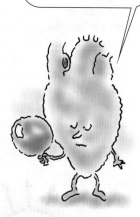

IABP counterpulsation temporarily reduces left ventricular workload and improves coronary perfusion.

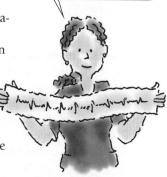

With IABP catheterization, balloon inflation and deflation is carefully timed to coincide with either the ECG or arterial waveform.

Understanding a balloon pump

An IABP consists of a polyurethane balloon attached to an external pump console by means of a large-lumen catheter. It's inserted percutaneously through the femoral artery and positioned in the descending aorta just distal to the left subclavian artery and above the renal arteries.

This external pump works in precise counterpoint to the left ventricle, inflating the balloon with helium early in diastole and deflating it just before systole. As the balloon inflates, it forces blood toward the aortic valve, thereby raising pressure in the aortic root and augmenting diastolic pressure to improve coronary perfusion. It also improves peripheral circulation by forcing blood through the brachiocephalic, common carotid, and subclavian arteries arising from the aortic trunk.

The balloon deflates rapidly at the end of diastole, creating a vacuum in the aorta. This reduces aortic volume and pressure, thereby decreasing the resistance to left ventricular ejection (afterload). This decreased workload, in turn, reduces the heart's oxygen requirements and, combined with the improved myocardial perfusion, helps prevent or diminish myocardial ischemia.

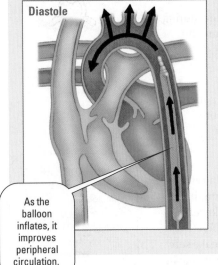

Diastole

As the balloon inflates, it improves peripheral circulation.

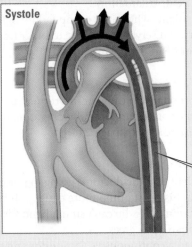

Systole

As the balloon deflates, afterload is decreased, which helps decrease myocardial ischemia.

upstroke of the arterial wave triggers balloon inflation. (See *Timing IABP counterpulsation*.)

- Frequently assess the insertion site. Don't elevate the head of the bed more than 45 degrees to prevent upward migration of the catheter and occlusion of the left subclavian artery. If the balloon occludes the artery, you may see a diminished left radial pulse, and the patient may report dizziness. Incorrect balloon placement may also cause flank pain or a sudden decrease in urine output.

Timing IABP counterpulsation

IABP counterpulsation is synchronized with either the ECG or arterial waveform. Ideally, balloon inflation should begin just after the aortic valve closes—at the dicrotic notch on the arterial waveform. Deflation should occur just before systole.

Proper timing is crucial

Early inflation can damage the aortic valve by forcing it closed, whereas late inflation permits most of the blood emerging from the ventricle to flow past the balloon, reducing pump effectiveness.

Late deflation increases the resistance against which the left ventricle must pump, possibly causing cardiac arrest.

Arterial waveforms

The illustration below depicts how IABP counterpulsation boosts peak diastolic pressure and lowers peak systolic and end-diastolic pressures.

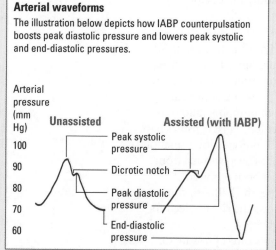

How timing affects waveforms

The arterial waveforms below show correctly and incorrectly timed balloon inflation and deflation.

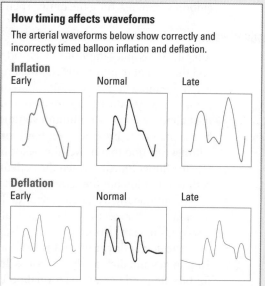

- Assess distal pulses, color, temperature, and capillary refill of the patient's extremities every 15 minutes for the first 4 hours after insertion. After 4 hours, assess hourly for the duration of IABP therapy.
- Watch for signs of thrombus formation, such as a sudden weakening of pedal pulses, pain, and motor or sensory loss.
- If indicated, apply antiembolism stockings.
- Encourage active ROM exercises every 2 hours for the arms, the unaffected leg, and the affected ankle.
- Maintain adequate hydration to help prevent thrombus formation.
- If bleeding occurs, apply direct pressure and notify the doctor.
- Assess the catheter insertion site every 2 hours.

- Assess the patient's cardiovascular and respiratory status at least every 4 hours. If possible, place the IABP on standby to eliminate any extraneous sounds.
- Administer anticoagulants as ordered to help prevent thrombus formation.

Warning!

- An alarm on the console may indicate a gas leak from a damaged catheter or ruptured balloon. If the alarm sounds or you see blood in the catheter, shut down the pump console and immediately place the patient in Trendelenburg's position to prevent an embolus from reaching the brain. Then notify the doctor.

Ready to wean

- After the signs and symptoms of left-sided heart failure diminish, and the patient requires only minimal drug support, the doctor begins weaning him from IABP counterpulsation. This may be accomplished by reducing the frequency of pumping or decreasing the balloon volume; a minimum volume or pumping ratio must be maintained to prevent thrombus formation. Most consoles have a flutter function that moves the balloon to prevent clot formation. Use the flutter function when the patient has been weaned from counterpulsation but the catheter hasn't yet been removed.
- To discontinue the IABP, the doctor deflates the balloon, clips the sutures, removes the catheter, and allows the site to bleed for 5 seconds to expel clots.
- After the doctor discontinues the IABP, apply direct pressure for 30 minutes and then apply a pressure dressing. Evaluate the site for bleeding and hematoma formation hourly for the next 4 hours.

Percutaneous balloon valvuloplasty

Performed in the cardiac catheterization lab, this procedure aims to improve valvular function by enlarging the orifice of a stenotic heart valve caused by a congenital defect, calcification, rheumatic fever, or aging. It involves introducing a small balloon valvuloplasty catheter through the skin at the femoral vein. (See *Percutaneous balloon valvuloplasty.*)

When surgery isn't the answer

While the treatment of choice for valvular heart disease remains surgery, percutaneous balloon valvuloplasty offers an alternative for individuals considered poor surgical candidates. Unfortunately, elderly patients with aortic disease commonly experience restenosis 1 to 2 years after undergoing valvuloplasty.

Percutaneous balloon valvuloplasty

During valvuloplasty, a surgeon inserts a small balloon catheter through the skin at the femoral vein and advances it until it reaches the affected valve. The balloon is then inflated, forcing the valve opening to widen.

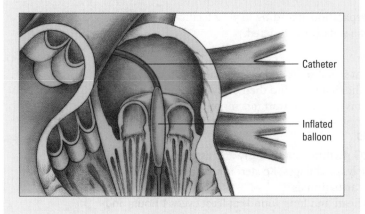

Catheter

Inflated balloon

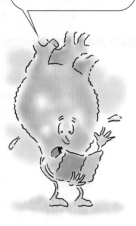

Woah! " . . . Misshapen valves, pieces of calcified valves breaking off, severe damage to valve leaflets . . . " And these are the decreased risks compared with more invasive procedures?

Those complicit complications

Despite the decreased risks as compared with some more invasive procedures, balloon valvuloplasty can lead to complications, including:

- worsening valvular insufficiency as a result of misshaping the valve so that it doesn't close completely
- pieces of the calcified valve breaking off, which may travel to the brain or lungs and cause an embolism
- severe damage to the delicate valve leaflets, requiring immediate surgery to replace the valve (rare)
- bleeding and hematoma formation at the arterial puncture site.

Nursing considerations

Provide these care measures before and after percutaneous balloon valvuloplasty.

Before the procedure

- Explain that a catheter will be inserted into an artery in the patient's groin.
- Reassure the patient that, even though he'll be awake during the procedure, he will receive sedation.

Check 'em all off

- Check the patient's history for allergies; if he has had allergic reactions to shellfish, iodine, or contrast media, notify the practitioner.

- Make sure that the results of coagulation studies, CBC, serum electrolyte studies, blood typing and crossmatching, BUN, and serum creatinine are available.
- Obtain baseline vital signs and assess peripheral pulses.
- Apply ECG electrodes and insert an I.V. line if one isn't already in place.
- Perform skin preparation according to your facility's policy.
- Give the patient a sedative as ordered.

After the procedure
- Assess the patient's vital signs and oxygen saturation every 15 minutes for the first hour and then every 30 minutes for 4 hours, unless his condition warrants more frequent checking.

Rhythms, sounds, and pulses

- Monitor his ECG rhythm continuously and assess hemodynamic parameters closely for changes. Be alert for the development of any new cardiac arrhythmias.
- Assess patient's heart and lung sounds at least every 4 hours and notify the practitioner for the development of any new murmurs or signs of valve failure.
- Assess peripheral pulses distal to the catheter insertion site as well as the color, sensation, temperature, and capillary refill time of the affected extremity.

Black and blue or bleeding

- Assess the catheter insertion site for hematoma, ecchymosis, and hemorrhage. If bleeding occurs, locate the artery and apply manual pressure; then notify the practitioner.
- Monitor the patient's neurologic status for any changes and report them to the practitioner immediately.

PTCA

A type of percutaneous coronary intervention, PTCA is a nonsurgical way to open coronary vessels narrowed by arteriosclerosis. It's usually used with cardiac catheterization to assess the stenosis and efficacy of angioplasty. It can also be used as a visual tool to direct the balloon-tipped catheter through a vessel's area of stenosis.

PTCA for pain

In PTCA, a balloon-tipped catheter is inserted into a narrowed coronary artery. This procedure, performed in the cardiac catheterization laboratory under local anesthesia, relieves pain due to angina and myocardial ischemia. (See *Understanding angioplasty.*)

Understanding angioplasty

PTCA is used to open an occluded coronary artery without opening the chest. This illustration shows what happens during the procedure.

First, the doctor threads the catheter. When angiography shows the guide catheter positioned at the occlusion site, the doctor carefully inserts a smaller double-lumen balloon catheter through the guide catheter and directs the balloon through the occlusion.

After the balloon is directed through the occlusion, the balloon is inflated, resulting in arterial stretching and plaque fracture. The balloon may need to be inflated and deflated several times until successful dilation occurs.

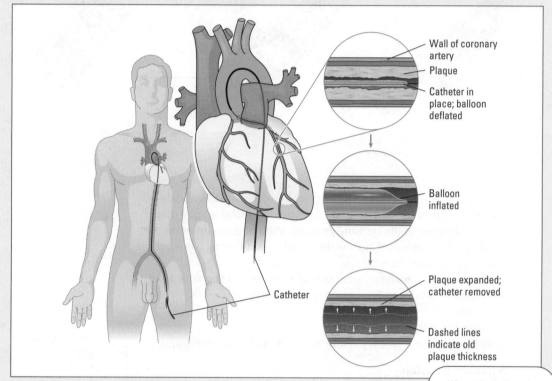

Wall of coronary artery

Plaque

Catheter in place; balloon deflated

Balloon inflated

Plaque expanded; catheter removed

Dashed lines indicate old plaque thickness

Catheter

Through one artery and into another

After coronary angiography confirms the presence and location of the occlusion, the doctor threads a guide catheter through the patient's femoral artery and into the coronary artery under fluoroscopic guidance.

Plaque, meet Balloon

When the guide catheter's position at the occlusion site is confirmed by angiography, the doctor carefully introduces a double-lumen balloon into the catheter and through the lesion, where a marked

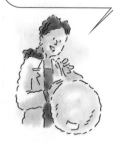

When the balloon is inflated, the plaque is compressed against the vessel wall, allowing coronary blood to flow more freely.

Coronary artery stents

An intravascular stent may be used to hold the walls of a vessel open. Some stents are coated with a drug that's slowly released to inhibit further aggregation of fibrin or clots.

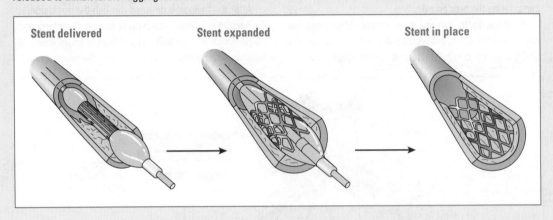

Stent delivered   Stent expanded   Stent in place

pressure gradient is obvious. The doctor alternately inflates and deflates the balloon until arteriography verifies successful arterial dilation and decrease in the pressure gradient. With balloon inflation, the plaque is compressed against the vessel wall, allowing coronary blood to flow more freely.

Placement of a coronary stent may also be done at the same time as an angioplasty. (See *Coronary artery stents*.)

Nursing considerations
Provide these care measures before and after cardiac catheterization.

Before the procedure
- Describe the procedure to the patient and his family and tell them it takes 1 to 4 hours to complete.
- Explain that a catheter will be inserted into an artery or a vein in the patient's groin and that he may feel pressure as the catheter moves along the vessel.
- Reassure the patient that although he'll be awake during the procedure, he'll be given a sedative. Instruct him to report any angina during the procedure.
- Explain that the doctor injects a contrast medium to outline the lesion's location. Warn the patient that he may feel a hot, flushing sensation or transient nausea during the injection.
- Check the patient's history for allergies; if he has had allergic reactions to shellfish, iodine, or contrast media, notify the doctor.

Instruct the patient to report any angina felt during cardiac catheterization.

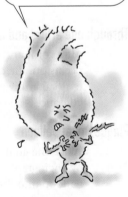

- Make sure the patient signs an informed consent form.
- Restrict food and fluids for at least 6 hours before the procedure.
- Make sure that the results of coagulation studies, CBC, serum electrolyte studies, blood typing and crossmatching, BUN, and serum creatinine are available.
- Obtain baseline vital signs and assess peripheral pulses.
- Apply ECG electrodes and insert an I.V. line if not already in place.
- Administer oxygen through a nasal cannula.
- Perform skin preparation according to your facility's policy.
- Give the patient a sedative as ordered.

After the procedure
- Assess the patient's vital signs and oxygen saturation every 15 minutes for the first hour and then every 30 minutes for 4 hours, unless his condition warrants more frequent checking. Monitor I.V. infusions, such as heparin or nitroglycerin, as indicated.
- Assess peripheral pulses distal to the catheter insertion site as well as the color, sensation, temperature, and capillary refill time of the affected extremity.
- Monitor ECG rhythm continuously and assess hemodynamic parameters closely for changes.
- Instruct the patient to remain in bed for 8 hours and to keep the affected extremity straight. Maintain sandbags in position if used to apply pressure to the catheter site. Elevate the head of the bed 15 to 30 degrees. If a hemostatic device was used to close the catheter insertion site, anticipate that the patient may be allowed out of bed in only a few hours.
- Assess the catheter site for hematoma, ecchymosis, and hemorrhage. If bleeding occurs, locate the artery and apply manual pressure; then notify the practitioner.
- Administer I.V. fluids as ordered (usually 100 ml/hour) to promote excretion of the contrast medium. Be sure to assess for signs of fluid overload.
- After the catheter is removed, apply direct pressure for at least 10 minutes and monitor the site often.
- Document the patient's tolerance of the procedure and status after it, including vital signs, hemodynamic parameters, appearance of catheter site, ECG findings, condition of the extremity distal to the insertion site, complications, and necessary interventions.

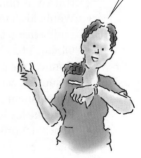

After the catheter is removed, apply direct pressure for at least 10 minutes.

Other therapy

Other treatments for cardiovascular disorders include synchronized cardioversion, defibrillation, and pacemaker insertion.

Synchronized cardioversion

Cardioversion (synchronized countershock) is an elective or emergency procedure used to correct tachyarrhythmias (such as atrial tachycardia, atrial flutter, atrial fibrillation, and symptomatic ventricular tachycardia). It's also the treatment of choice for patients with arrhythmias that don't respond to drug therapy.

Electrifying experience

In synchronized cardioversion, an electric current is delivered to the heart to correct an arrhythmia. Compared with defibrillation, it uses much lower energy levels and is synchronized to deliver an electric charge to the myocardium at the peak R wave. (See *Choosing the correct cardioversion energy level*.)

The procedure causes immediate depolarization, interrupting reentry circuits (abnormal impulse conduction that occurs when cardiac tissue is activated two or more times, causing reentry arrhythmias) and allowing the SA node to resume control.

Synchronizing the electrical charge with the R wave ensures that the current won't be delivered on the vulnerable T wave and disrupt repolarization. Thus, it reduces the risk that the current will strike during the relative refractory period of a cardiac cycle and induce ventricular fibrillation.

Nursing considerations
- Describe the procedure to the patient and make sure an informed consent is obtained.
- Withhold all food and fluids for 6 to 12 hours before the procedure. If cardioversion is urgent, withhold food beginning as soon as possible.
- Obtain a baseline 12-lead ECG.
- Connect the patient to a pulse oximeter and blood pressure cuff.
- Ensure I.V. access.
- If the patient is awake, administer a sedative as ordered.
- Place the leads on the patient's chest and assess his cardiac rhythm.
- Attach defibrillation pads to the chest wall; position the pads so that one pad is to the right of the sternum, just below the clavicle, and the other is at the fifth or sixth intercostal space in the left anterior axillary line.

Choosing the correct cardioversion energy level

When choosing an energy level for cardioversion, try the lowest energy level first. If the arrhythmia isn't corrected, repeat the procedure using the next energy level. Repeat this procedure until the arrhythmia is corrected or until the highest energy level is reached. The initial energy dose used for cardioversion is:
- 100 joules (biphasic and monophasic) for unstable regular ventricular tachycardia with a pulse
- 120 to 200 (biphasic) or 200 (monophasic) joules for atrial fibrillation
- 50 to 100 joules (biphasic and monophasic) for atrial flutter and other supraventricular tachycardia.

Ready to jolt

- Turn on the defibrillator and select the ordered energy level, usually between 50 and 100 joules.
- Activate the synchronized mode by depressing the synchronizer switch.
- Check that the machine is sensing the R wave correctly.
- Charge the machine.
- Instruct other personnel to stand clear of the patient and the bed to avoid the risk of an electric shock.

Letting the sparks fly

- Discharge the current by pushing the DISCHARGE or SHOCK button.
- If cardioversion is unsuccessful, repeat the procedure two or three times, as ordered, gradually increasing the energy with each additional countershock.
- If normal rhythm is restored, continue to monitor the patient and provide supplemental ventilation as long as needed.
- If the patient's cardiac rhythm changes to ventricular fibrillation, switch the mode from synchronized to defibrillate and defibrillate the patient immediately after charging the machine.
- Remember to reset the SYNC MODE on the defibrillator after each synchronized cardioversion. Resetting this switch is necessary because most defibrillators automatically reset to an unsynchronized mode.
- Document the use of synchronized cardioversion, the rhythm before and after cardioversion, medication given, amperage used, and how the patient tolerated the procedure.

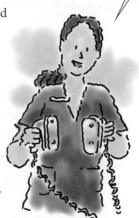

In defibrillation, an electric current is directed through the patient's heart.

Defibrillation

In defibrillation, an electric current is directed through the patient's heart. The current causes the myocardium to depolarize, which in turn encourages the SA node to resume control of the heart's electrical activity. (See *Biphasic defibrillators*, page 244.)

The electrodes delivering the current may be placed on the patient's chest or, during cardiac surgery, directly on the myocardium.

Biphasic defibrillators

Monophasic defibrillators deliver a single current of electricity that travels in one direction between the two pads on the patient's chest. A large amount of electrical current is required for effective monophasic defibrillation. Biphasic defibrillators are now more popular in hospitals. Pad placement is the same as with the monophasic defibrillator. The difference is that during biphasic defibrillation, the electrical current discharged from the pads travels in a positive direction for a specified duration and then reverses and flows in a negative direction for the remaining time of the electrical discharge.

Energy efficient
The biphasic defibrillator delivers two currents of electricity and lowers the defibrillation threshold of the heart muscle, making it possible to successfully defibrillate ventricular fibrillation with smaller amounts of energy.

Adjustable
The biphasic defibrillator is able to adjust for differences in impedance or the resistance of the current through the chest. This reduces the number of shocks needed to terminate ventricular fibrillation.

Less myocardial damage
Because the biphasic defibrillator requires lower energy levels and fewer shocks, damage to the myocardial muscle is reduced. Biphasic defibrillators used at the clinically appropriate energy level may be used for defibrillation and, in the synchronized mode, for synchronized cardioversion.

Act early and quickly

Because some arrhythmias, such as ventricular fibrillation, can cause death if not corrected, the success of defibrillation depends on early recognition and quick treatment.

In addition to treating ventricular fibrillation, defibrillation may also be used to treat ventricular tachycardia that doesn't produce a pulse or polymorphic ventricular tachycardia with a pulse.

Nursing considerations
- Assess the patient to determine if he lacks a pulse. Call for help and perform cardiopulmonary resuscitation (CPR) until the defibrillator and other emergency equipment arrive. (See *Automated external defibrillator.*)
- Connect the monitoring leads of the defibrillator to the patient and assess his cardiac rhythm in two leads.
- Expose the patient's chest and apply the self-adhesive, pre-gelled conductive pads at the proper positions. (See *Defibrillator pad placement*, page 246.)
- Turn on the defibrillator and, if performing external defibrillation, set the energy level at 200 joules (biphasic) or 360 joules (monophasic) for an adult patient.

Automated external defibrillator

An automated external defibrillator (AED) has a cardiac rhythm analysis system. The AED interprets the patient's cardiac rhythm and gives the operator step-by-step directions on how to proceed if defibrillation is indicated. Most AEDs have a "quick-look" feature that allows visualization of the rhythm with the paddles before electrodes are connected.

Computer-assisted system

The AED is equipped with a microcomputer that senses and analyzes a patient's heart rhythm at the push of a button. It then audibly or visually prompts you to deliver a shock.

All models have the same basic functions but offer different operating options. For example, all AEDs communicate directions by displaying messages on a screen, giving voice commands, or both. Some AEDs simultaneously display a patient's heart rhythm.

All devices record your interactions with the patient during defibrillation, either on a cassette tape or in a solid state memory module. Some AEDs have an integral printer for immediate event documentation.

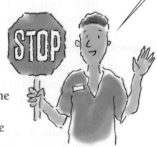

Before discharging the defibrillator, tell everyone to stand clear of the patient and the bed.

Charging and shocking once . . .

- Charge the unit by pressing the charge button located on the machine.
- Reassess the patient's cardiac rhythm in two leads.
- If the patient remains in a shockable rhythm, instruct all personnel to stand clear of the patient and the bed. Also make a visual check to make sure everyone is clear of the patient and the bed.
- Discharge the current by pressing the appropriate button on the defibrillator.
- Continue with 2 minutes of CPR. Reassess for a pulse and cardiac rhythm. Give supplemental oxygen and begin administering appropriate medications such as epinephrine.

. . . then again

- If necessary, after the initial shock and two rounds of CPR, prepare to defibrillate a second time at the same joules. Announce that you're preparing to defibrillate and follow the procedure described previously.
- Continue CPR.
- If the patient still has no pulse after the first two cycles of defibrillation and CPR, consider possible causes for failure of the patient's rhythm to convert, such as acidosis and hypoxia.
- If defibrillation restores a normal rhythm, assess the patient. Obtain baseline ABG levels and a 12-lead ECG. Provide

Defibrillator pad placement

Here's a guide to correct pad placement for defibrillation.

Anterolateral placement

For anterolateral placement, position one pad to the right of the upper sternum, just below the right clavicle, and the other over the fifth or sixth intercostal space at the left anterior axillary line.

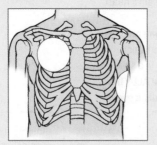

Anteroposterior placement

For anteroposterior placement, position the anterior pad directly over the heart at the precordium, to the left of the lower sternal border. Place the posterior pad under the patient's body beneath the heart and immediately below the scapula (but not on the vertebral column).

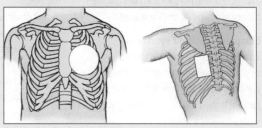

supplemental oxygen, ventilation, and medications as needed. Prepare the defibrillator for immediate reuse.

Document everything

- Document the procedure, including the patient's ECG rhythms before and after defibrillation; the number of times defibrillation was performed; the voltage used during each attempt; whether a pulse returned; the dosage, route, and time of any drugs administered; whether CPR was used; how the airway was maintained; and the patient's outcome.
- If the patient has recurrent episodes of ventricular tachycardia or ventricular fibrillation, the insertion of an implantable cardioverter-defibrillator (ICD) may be necessary. (See *Implantable cardioverter-defibrillator*.)

Permanent pacemaker insertion

A permanent pacemaker is a self-contained device surgically implanted in a pocket under the patient's skin. This is usually done in an operating room or cardiac catheterization laboratory.

Permanent pacemakers function in the demand mode, allowing the patient's heart to beat on its own but preventing it from falling below a preset rate.

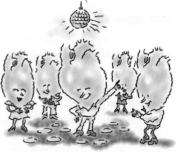

A permanent pacemaker prevents my rate from falling below a preset level so I can keep on dancing.

Implantable cardioverter-defibrillator

An ICD is implanted to continually monitor a patient's heart for bradycardia, ventricular tachycardia, and ventricular fibrillation. The device also administers either shocks or paced beats. Some ICDs can provide biventricular pacing or administer therapy for atrial fibrillation.

ICDs are generally indicated when drug therapy, surgery, or catheter ablation fails to prevent the patient's dangerous arrhythmia.

What it is

An ICD system consists of a programmable pulse generator and one or more lead wires. The pulse generator is a small battery-powered computer that monitors the heart's electrical signals and delivers electrical therapy when an abnormal rhythm is identified.

It also stores information on the heart's activity before, during, and after an arrhythmia, along with tracking which treatment was delivered and the outcome of that treatment. Many devices also store electrograms (electrical tracings similar to ECGs). With an interrogation device, a practitioner can retrieve this information to evaluate ICD function and battery status and to adjust ICD system settings.

How it's programmed

When caring for a patient with an ICD, it's important to know how the device is programmed. This information

is available through a status report that can be obtained and printed when the practitioner or specially trained technician interrogates the device. This involves placing a specialized piece of equipment over the implanted pulse generator to retrieve pacing function.

If the patient experiences an arrhythmia or if the device delivers a therapy, the program information is used to evaluate the functioning of the device. Program information includes:
* type and model of ICD
* status of the device (on or off)
* detection rates
* therapies that will be delivered (pacing, antitachycardia pacing, cardioversion, and defibrillation).

What you should know

* If the patient experiences cardiac arrest, initiate CPR and advanced cardiac life support.
* If the ICD delivers a shock while you're performing chest compressions, you may feel a slight shock. Wear gloves to eliminate this.
* It's safe to also externally defibrillate a patient with an ICD as long as the paddles aren't placed directly over the pulse generator. The anteroposterior paddle position is preferred.

And the nominees for insertion are . . .

Permanent pacemakers are indicated for patients with:
* persistent bradycardia
* complete heart block
* congenital or degenerative heart disease
* Stokes-Adams syndrome
* Wolff-Parkinson-White syndrome
* sick sinus syndrome.

Setting the pace

Pacing electrodes can be placed in the atria, ventricles, or both chambers (atrioventricular sequential or dual chamber). Biventricular pacemakers are also available for cardiac resynchronization therapy in some patients with heart failure. (See *Understanding pacemaker codes*, page 248.)

Understanding pacemaker codes

The capabilities of pacemakers are described by a five-letter coding system, although typically only the first three letters are used.

First letter	Second letter	Third letter	Fourth letter	Fifth letter
The first letter identifies which heart chambers are paced. Here are the letters used to signify these options: • V = ventricle • A = atrium • D = dual (ventricle and atrium) • O = none.	The second letter signifies the heart chamber where the pacemaker senses the intrinsic activity: • V = ventricle • A = atrium • D = dual • O = none.	The third letter shows the pacemaker's response to the intrinsic electrical activity it senses in the atrium or ventricle: • T = triggers pacing • I = inhibits pacing • D = dual; can be triggered or inhibited depending on the mode and where intrinsic activity occurs • O = none; the pacemaker doesn't change its mode in response to sensed activity.	The fourth letter describes rate modulation, also known as *rate responsiveness* or *rate-adaptive pacing*: • R = rate modulation (a sensor adjusts the programmed paced heart rate in response to patient activity) • O = none (rate modulation is unavailable or disabled).	The fifth letter is rarely used but specifies the location or absence of multisite pacing: • O = none (no multisite pacing is present) • A = atrium or atria (multisite pacing in the atrium or atria is present) • V = ventricle or ventricles (multisite pacing in the ventricle or ventricles is present) • D = dual site (dual site pacing in both the atria and ventricles is present).

The most common pacing codes are VVI for single-chamber pacing and DDD for dual-chamber pacing. To keep the patient healthy and active, some pacemakers are designed to increase the heart rate with exercise.

Nursing considerations

Provide care measures before and after pacemaker placement. Nursing responsibilities during surgical placement involve monitoring ECG and maintaining sterile technique.

Before surgery
• Explain the procedure to the patient.
• Before pacemaker insertion, clip the hair on the patient's chest from the axilla to the midline and from the clavicle to the nipple line on the side selected by the doctor.
• Establish an I.V. line.

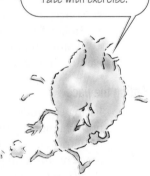

Good news for active patients! Some pacemakers are designed to increase the heart rate with exercise.

- Obtain baseline vital signs and a baseline ECG.
- Provide sedation as ordered.

After surgery
- Monitor the patient's ECG to check for arrhythmias and to ensure correct pacemaker functioning.
- Check the dressing for signs of bleeding and infection.
- Change the dressing according to facility policy.
- Check vital signs and LOC every 15 minutes for the first hour, every hour for the next 4 hours, then every 4 hours.
- Provide the patient with an identification card that lists the pacemaker type and manufacturer, serial number, pacemaker rate setting, date implanted, and the doctor's name.

Temporary pacemaker insertion

A temporary pacemaker is usually inserted in an emergency. The device consists of an external, battery-powered pulse generator and a lead or electrode system.

Temporary pacemakers typically come in three types, including:
1. transcutaneous
2. transvenous
3. epicardial.

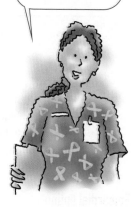

Transcutaneous pacing is used only until transvenous pacing is established.

Dire straits

In a life-threatening situation, a transcutaneous pacemaker is the best choice. This device works by sending an electrical impulse from the pulse generator to the patient's heart by way of two electrodes, which are placed on the front and back of the patient's chest.

Transcutaneous pacing is quick and effective, but it's used only until the doctor can institute transvenous pacing.

More comfortable and more reliable

Besides being more comfortable for the patient, a transvenous pacemaker is more reliable than a transcutaneous pacemaker.

Transvenous pacing involves threading an electrode catheter through a vein into the patient's right atrium or right ventricle. The electrode is attached to an external pulse generator that can provide an electrical stimulus directly to the endocardium. (See *Temporary transvenous pacemaker*, page 250.)

Transvenous pacemaker basics

Indications for a temporary transvenous pacemaker include:
- management of bradycardia
- presence of tachyarrhythmias
- other conduction system disturbances.

Temporary transvenous pacemaker

Transvenous pacing provides a more reliable pacing beat. This type of pacing is more comfortable for the patient because the pacing wire is inserted in the heart via a major vein.

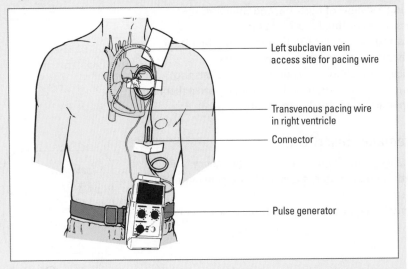

Left subclavian vein access site for pacing wire

Transvenous pacing wire in right ventricle

Connector

Pulse generator

The purpose of temporary transvenous pacemaker insertion is:
- to maintain circulatory integrity by providing for standby pacing in case of sudden complete heart block
- to increase heart rate during periods of symptomatic bradycardia
- occasionally, to control sustained supraventricular or ventricular tachycardia.

Epicardial option

During cardiac surgery, the surgeon may insert electrodes through the epicardium of the right ventricle and, if he wants to institute AV sequential pacing, the right atrium. From there, the electrodes pass through the chest wall, where they remain available if temporary pacing becomes necessary. This is called *epicardial pacing*. It uses the same equipment as temporary or transvenous pacers; it is done only after surgery.

Pacemaker no-no's

Among the contraindications to pacemaker therapy are electromechanical dissociation and ventricular fibrillation.

Nursing considerations

- Teach measures to prevent microshock; warn the patient not to use any electrical equipment that isn't grounded.
- Use other safety measures such as placing a plastic cover (supplied by the manufacturer) over the pacemaker controls to avoid an accidental setting change. If the patient needs emergency defibrillation, make sure the pacemaker can withstand the procedure. If you're unsure, disconnect the pulse generator to avoid damage.
- When using a transcutaneous pacemaker, don't place the electrodes over a bony area because bone conducts current poorly. With a female patient, place the anterior electrode under the patient's breast but not over her diaphragm.
- If the doctor inserts the transvenous pacer wire through the brachial or femoral vein, immobilize the patient's arm or leg to avoid putting stress on the pacing wires.
- After insertion of any temporary pacemaker, assess the patient's vital signs, skin color, LOC, and peripheral pulses to determine the effectiveness of the paced rhythm. Perform a 12-lead ECG to serve as a baseline and then perform additional ECGs daily or with clinical changes. Also, if possible, obtain a rhythm strip before, during, and after pacemaker placement; anytime the pacemaker settings are changed; and whenever the patient receives treatment because of a complication due to the pacemaker.
- Continuously monitor the ECG reading, noting capture, sensing, rate, intrinsic beats, and competition of paced and intrinsic rhythms. If the pacemaker is sensing correctly, the sense indicator on the pulse generator should flash with each beat.
- Record the date and time of pacemaker insertion, the type of pacemaker, the reason for insertion, and the patient's response. Note the pacemaker settings. Document any complications and the interventions taken.
- If the patient has epicardial pacing wires in place, clean the insertion site and change the dressing daily. At the same time, monitor the site for signs of infection. Always keep the pulse generator nearby in case pacing becomes necessary.

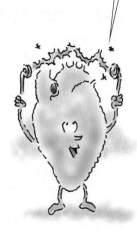

Teach measures to prevent microshock such as using only electrical equipment that's grounded.

Cardiovascular system disorders

Common cardiovascular disorders include acute coronary syndromes, aneurysms, cardiac arrhythmias, cardiac tamponade, cardiogenic shock, cardiomyopathy, heart failure, hypertensive crisis, pericarditis, and valvular heart disease.

Acute coronary syndromes

Patients with acute coronary syndromes have some degree of coronary artery occlusion. The degree of occlusion defines whether the acute coronary syndrome is:
- unstable angina
- non-ST-segment elevation myocardial infarction (NSTEMI)
- ST-segment elevation myocardial infarction (STEMI).

Plaque's place

The development of any acute coronary syndrome begins with a rupture or erosion of plaque—an unstable and lipid-rich substance. The rupture results in platelet adhesions, fibrin clot formation, and activation of thrombin.

What causes it

Patients with certain risk factors appear to face a greater likelihood of developing an acute coronary syndrome. These factors include:
- family history of heart disease
- obesity
- smoking
- high-fat, high-carbohydrate diet
- sedentary lifestyle
- menopause
- stress
- diabetes
- hypertension
- hyperlipoproteinemia.

How it happens

An acute coronary syndrome most commonly results when a thrombus progresses and occludes blood flow. (An early thrombus doesn't necessarily block blood flow.) The effect is an imbalance in myocardial oxygen supply and demand.

Degree and duration

The degree and duration of blockage dictate the type of infarct that occurs:

- If the patient has unstable angina, a thrombus partially occludes a coronary vessel. This thrombus is full of platelets. The partially occluded vessel may have distal microthrombi that cause necrosis in some myocytes.
- If smaller vessels infarct, the patient is at higher risk for MI, which may progress to NSTEMI. Usually, only the innermost layer of the heart is damaged.
- STEMI results when reduced blood flow through one of the coronary arteries causes myocardial ischemia, injury, and necrosis. The damage extends through all myocardial layers.

What to look for

A patient with angina typically experiences:

- burning
- squeezing
- crushing tightness in the substernal or precordial chest that may radiate to the left arm, neck, jaw, or shoulder blade.

A woman thing?

Any patient may experience atypical chest pain, but it's more common in women. (See *Atypical chest pain in women*.)

It hurts when I do this

Angina most frequently follows physical exertion but may also follow emotional excitement, exposure to cold, or a large meal. Angina is commonly relieved by nitroglycerin and rest. It's less severe and shorter lived than the pain of acute MI.

Four forms

Angina has four major forms:

1. stable—predictable pain, in frequency and duration, which can be relieved with nitrates and rest
2. unstable—increased pain, which is easily induced
3. Prinzmetal's or a variant—pain from unpredictable coronary artery spasm
4. microvascular—angina-like chest pain due to impairment of vasodilator reserve in a patient with normal coronary arteries.

Atypical chest pain in women

Women with CAD may experience typical chest pain but commonly experience atypical chest pain, vague chest pain, or a lack of chest pain. They're more likely than men to experience a toothache or pain in the arm, shoulder, jaw, neck, throat, back, breast, or stomach.

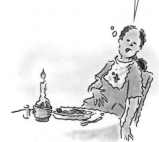

Angina can occur after exercise, excitement, exposure to cold, or a large meal.

My, my, MI pain

A patient with MI experiences severe, persistent chest pain that isn't relieved by rest or nitroglycerin. He may describe pain as crushing or squeezing. The pain is usually substernal but may radiate to the left arm, jaw, neck, or shoulder blades.

And many more

Other signs and symptoms of MI include:
- a feeling of impending doom
- fatigue
- nausea and vomiting
- shortness of breath
- cool extremities
- perspiration
- anxiety
- hypotension or hypertension
- palpable precordial pulse
- muffled heart sounds.

> Besides physical signs and symptoms, a patient with MI may report a feeling of impending doom or anxiety.

What tests tell you

These tests are used to diagnose CAD:
- ECG during an anginal episode shows ischemia. Serial 12-lead ECGs may be normal or inconclusive during the first few hours after an MI. Abnormalities include serial ST-segment depression in NSTEMI and ST-segment elevation and Q waves, representing scarring and necrosis, in STEMI. (See *Locating myocardial damage.*)
- Coronary angiography reveals coronary artery stenosis or obstruction and collateral circulation and shows the condition of the arteries beyond the narrowing.
- Myocardial perfusion imaging with thallium-201 during treadmill exercise discloses ischemic areas of the myocardium, visualized as "cold spots."
- With MI, serial serum cardiac marker measurements show elevated CK, especially the CK-MB isoenzyme (the cardiac muscle fraction of CK), troponin T and I, myoglobin, and IMA.
- C-reactive protein (CRP) levels help measure cardiac risk. Patients with chest pain and a higher CRP level have an increased risk of CAD. The PLAC test is a new test that also helps identify patients at a higher risk for CAD.
- With STEMI, echocardiography shows ventricular wall dyskinesia.

> For patients with angina, the goal is to reduce oxygen demand or increase oxygen supply.

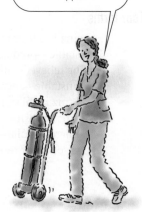

How it's treated

For patients with angina, the goal of treatment is to reduce myocardial oxygen demand or increase oxygen supply.

Locating myocardial damage

After you've noted characteristic lead changes of an acute MI, use this chart to identify the areas of damage. Match the lead changes in the second column with the affected wall in the first column and the artery involved in the third column. Column four shows reciprocal lead changes.

Wall affected	Leads	Artery involved	Reciprocal changes
Anterior	V_2 to V_4	Left coronary artery, left anterior descending (LAD) artery	II, III, aV_F
Anterolateral	I, aV_L, V_3 to V_6	LAD artery, circumflex artery	II, III, aV_F
Anteroseptal	V_1 to V_4	LAD artery	None
Inferior (diaphragmatic)	II, III, aV_F	Right coronary artery	I, aV_L
Lateral	I, aV_L, V_5, V_6	Circumflex artery, branch of left coronary artery	II, III, aV_F
Posterior	V_8, V_9	Right coronary artery, circumflex artery	V_1 to V_4
Right ventricular	V_{4R}, V_{5R}, V_{6R}	Right coronary artery	None

These treatments are used to manage angina:
- Nitrates reduce myocardial oxygen consumption.
- Beta-adrenergic blockers may be administered to reduce the workload and oxygen demands of the heart.
- If angina is caused by coronary artery spasm, calcium channel blockers may be given.
- Antiplatelet drugs minimize platelet aggregation and the danger of coronary occlusion.
- Antilipemic drugs can reduce elevated serum cholesterol or triglyceride levels.
- Obstructive lesions may necessitate CABG or PTCA. Other alternatives include laser angioplasty, minimally invasive surgery, atherectomy, or stent placement.

MI relief

The goals of treatment for MI are to relieve pain, stabilize heart rhythm, revascularize the coronary artery, preserve myocardial tissue, and reduce cardiac workload.

Here are some guidelines for treatment:
- Thrombolytic therapy should be started within 6 hours of the onset of symptoms (unless contraindications exist). Thrombolytic therapy involves administration of streptokinase (Streptase), alteplase (Activase), or reteplase (Retavase).

- PTCA or stent placements are options for opening blocked or narrowed arteries. Primary percutaneous coronary intervention is the preferred method in management of acute MI. In a patient presenting with STEMI, the patient's coronary artery should be opened with percutaneous coronary intervention within 90 minutes or with a target time of less than 60 minutes.
- Oxygen is administered to increase oxygenation of the blood.
- Nitroglycerin is administered sublingually to relieve chest pain, unless systolic blood pressure is less than 90 mm Hg or heart rate is less than 50 or greater than 100 beats/minute.

Heartache

- Morphine is administered as analgesia because pain stimulates the sympathetic nervous system, leading to an increase in heart rate and vasoconstriction.
- Aspirin and antiplatelet drugs are administered to inhibit platelet aggregation.
- I.V. heparin is given to patients who have received tissue plasminogen activator to increase the chances of patency in the affected coronary artery.
- Lidocaine, transcutaneous pacing patches (or a transvenous pacemaker), defibrillation, or epinephrine may be used if arrhythmias are present.
- Physical activity is limited for the first 12 hours to reduce cardiac workload, thereby limiting the area of necrosis.
- I.V. nitroglycerin is administered for 24 to 48 hours in patients without hypotension, bradycardia, or excessive tachycardia, to reduce afterload and preload and relieve chest pain.
- Glycoprotein IIb/IIIa inhibitors (such as abciximab [ReoPro]) are administered to patients with continued unstable angina or acute chest pain, or following invasive cardiac procedures, to reduce platelet aggregation.
- I.V. beta-adrenergic blocker is administered early to patients with evolving acute MI; it's followed by oral therapy to reduce heart rate and contractibility and reduce myocardial oxygen requirements.
- ACE inhibitors are administered to those with evolving MI with ST-segment elevation or left bundle-branch block to reduce afterload and preload and prevent remodeling.
- Laser angioplasty, atherectomy, or stent placement may be initiated.
- Lipid-lowering drugs are administered to patients with elevated LDL and cholesterol levels.

> Physical activity is limited for the first 12 hours after MI to reduce the cardiac workload and limit necrosis. Time to catch some Z's!

What to do

- During anginal episodes, monitor blood pressure and heart rate. Take an ECG before administering nitroglycerin or other nitrates. Record duration of pain, amount of medication required to relieve it, and accompanying symptoms.

CCU, ECG, and more!

- On admission to the coronary care unit, monitor and record the patient's ECG, blood pressure, temperature, and heart and breath sounds. Also, assess and record the severity, location, type, and duration of pain.
- Obtain a 12-lead ECG and assess heart rate and blood pressure when the patient experiences acute chest pain.
- Monitor the patient's hemodynamic status closely. Be alert for indicators suggesting decreased cardiac output, such as decreased blood pressure, increased heart rate, increased PAP, increased PAWP, decreased cardiac output measurements, and decreased right atrial pressure.
- Assess urine output hourly.
- Monitor the patient's oxygen saturation levels and notify the practitioner if oxygen saturation falls below 90%.
- Check the patient's blood pressure after giving nitroglycerin, especially the first dose.
- During episodes of chest pain, monitor ECG, blood pressure, and PA catheter readings (if applicable) to determine changes.
- Frequently monitor ECG rhythm strips to detect heart rate changes and arrhythmias.
- Obtain serial measurements of cardiac enzyme levels as ordered.
- Watch for crackles, cough, tachypnea, and edema, which may indicate impending left-sided heart failure. Carefully monitor daily weight, intake and output, respiratory rate, serum enzyme levels, ECG waveforms, and blood pressure. Auscultate for S_3 or S_4 gallops.
- Prepare the patient for reperfusion therapy as indicated.
- Administer and titrate medications as ordered. Avoid giving I.M. injections; I.V. administration provides more rapid symptom relief.

I need a break

- Organize patient care and activities to allow rest periods. If the patient is immobilized, turn him often and use intermittent compression devices. Gradually increase the patient's activity level as tolerated.
- Provide a clear liquid diet until nausea subsides. Anticipate a possible order for a low-cholesterol, low-sodium diet without caffeine.
- Provide a stool softener to prevent straining during defecation.

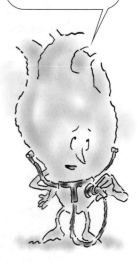

During episodes of chest pain, monitor ECG, blood pressure, and PA catheter readings for changes.

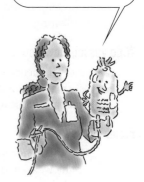

Remember, I.V. administration of medications provides more rapid relief of the patient's MI symptoms.

Aortic aneurysm

An aortic aneurysm is a localized outpouching or an abnormal dilation in a weakened arterial wall. Aortic aneurysm typically occurs in the aorta between the renal arteries and the iliac branches, but the abdominal, thoracic, or ascending arch of the aorta may be affected.

What causes it

The exact cause of an aortic aneurysm is unclear, but several factors place a person at risk, including:
- advanced age
- history of hypertension
- smoking
- atherosclerosis
- connective tissue disorders
- diabetes
- trauma.

How it happens

Aneurysms arise from a defect in the middle layer of the arterial wall (tunica media, or medial layer). Once the elastic fibers and collagen in the middle layer are damaged, stretching and segmental dilation occur. As a result, the medial layer loses some of its elasticity, and it fragments. Smooth muscle cells are lost, and the wall thins.

Thin and thinner

The thinned wall may contain calcium deposits and atherosclerotic plaque, making the wall brittle. As a person ages, the elastin in the wall decreases, further weakening the vessel. If hypertension is present, blood flow slows, resulting in ischemia and additional weakening.

Wide vessel, slow flow

After an aneurysm begins to develop, lateral pressure increases, causing the vessel lumen to widen and blood flow to slow. Over time, mechanical stressors contribute to elongation of the aneurysm.

Blood forces

Hemodynamic forces may also play a role, causing pulsatile stresses on the weakened wall and pressing on the small vessels that supply nutrients to the arterial wall. In aortic aneurysms, this causes the aorta to become bowed and tortuous.

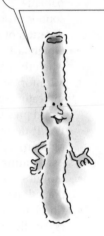

An aortic aneurysm arises from a defect in the middle layer of the arterial wall that causes stretching and segmental dilation, loss of elasticity, and arterial wall thinning.

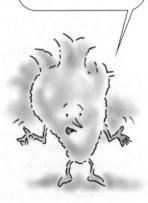

Most patients with aortic aneurysms are asymptomatic until an enlarging aneurysm compresses surrounding tissue.

What to look for

Most patients with aortic aneurysms are asymptomatic until the aneurysms enlarge and compress surrounding tissue.

A large aneurysm may produce signs and symptoms that mimic those of MI, renal calculi, lumbar disc disease, and duodenal compression.

When symptoms arise

Usually, if the patient exhibits symptoms, it's because of rupture, expansion, embolization, thrombosis, or pressure from the mass on surrounding structures. Rupture is more common if the patient also has hypertension or if the aneurysm is larger than 6 cm.

Thoracic aortic aneurysm

If the patient has a suspected thoracic aortic aneurysm, assess for:
- complaints of substernal pain possibly radiating to the neck, back, abdomen, or shoulders
- hoarseness or coughing
- difficulty swallowing
- difficulty breathing
- unequal blood pressure and pulse when measured in both arms
- aortic insufficiency murmur.

Acute expansion

When there's an acute expansion of a thoracic aortic aneurysm, assess for:
- severe hypertension
- neurologic changes
- a new murmur of aortic sufficiency
- right sternoclavicular lift
- jugular vein distention
- tracheal deviation.

Abdominal aortic aneurysm

The patient with an abdominal aortic aneurysm may experience:
- dull abdominal pain
- lower back pain that's unaffected by movement
- gastric or abdominal fullness
- pulsating mass in the periumbilical area (if the patient isn't obese)
- systolic bruit over the aorta on auscultation of the abdomen
- hypotension (with aneurysm rupture).

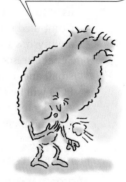

Some of the classic symptoms of a thoracic aortic aneurysm include substernal pain, hoarseness or coughing, difficulty swallowing, difficulty breathing, aortic murmur, and unequal blood pressure and pulses when measured in both arms.

What tests tell you

No specific laboratory test to diagnose an aortic aneurysm exists. However, these tests may be helpful:

- If blood is leaking from the aneurysm, leukocytosis and a decrease in hemoglobin and hematocrit may be noted.

Telltale TEE

- TEE allows visualization of the thoracic aorta. It's commonly combined with Doppler flow studies to provide information about blood flow.
- Abdominal ultrasonography or echocardiography can be used to determine the size, shape, and location of the aneurysm.
- Anteroposterior and lateral X-rays of the chest or abdomen can be used to detect aortic calcification and widened areas of the aorta.
- Computed tomography (CT) scan and MRI can disclose the aneurysm's size and effect on nearby organs.
- Serial ultrasonography at 6-month intervals reveals any growth of small aneurysms.
- ECG will be absent of any signs of MI.
- Aortography is used in determining the aneurysm's approximate size and patency of the visceral vessels.

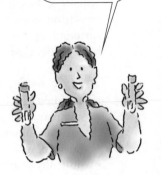

Unless blood is leaking from the aneurysm, there's no specific laboratory test to aid the diagnosis.

How it's treated

Aneurysm treatment usually involves surgery and appropriate drug therapy. Aortic aneurysms usually require resection and replacement of the aortic section using a vascular or Dacron graft. However, keep these points in mind:

- If the aneurysm is small and produces no symptoms, surgery may be delayed, with regular physical examination and ultrasonography performed to monitor its progression.
- Large or symptomatic aneurysms are at risk for rupture and need immediate repair.
- Endovascular grafting may be an option for a patient with an abdominal aortic aneurysm. This procedure, which can be done using local or regional anesthesia, is a minimally invasive procedure whereby the walls of the aorta are reinforced to prevent expansion and rupture of the aneurysm.
- Medications to control blood pressure, relieve anxiety, and control pain are also prescribed.

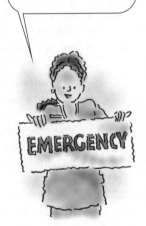

Rupture of an aortic aneurysm is a medical emergency requiring prompt treatment.

Rush to respond to rupture

Rupture of an aortic aneurysm is a medical emergency requiring prompt treatment, including:

- resuscitation with fluid and blood replacement
- I.V. propranolol to reduce myocardial contractility

- I.V. nitroprusside to reduce blood pressure and maintain it at 90 to 100 mm Hg systolic
- analgesics to relieve pain
- an arterial line and indwelling urinary catheter to monitor the patient's condition preoperatively.

What to do

- Assess the patient's vital signs, especially blood pressure, every 2 to 4 hours or more frequently, depending on the severity of his condition. Monitor blood pressure and pulse in extremities and compare findings bilaterally. If the difference in systolic blood pressure exceeds 10 mm Hg, notify the practitioner immediately.
- Assess cardiovascular status frequently, including heart rate, rhythm, ECG, and cardiac enzyme levels. MI can occur if an aneurysm ruptures along the coronary arteries.
- Obtain blood samples to evaluate kidney function by assessing BUN, creatinine, and electrolyte levels. Measure intake and output, hourly if necessary, depending on the patient's condition.
- Monitor CBC for evidence of blood loss, including decreased hemoglobin, hematocrit, and red blood cell (RBC) count.
- Send blood to the laboratory to be typed and crossmatched in case the patient needs a blood transfusion.
- If the patient's condition is acute, obtain an arterial sample for ABG analysis, as ordered, and monitor cardiac rhythm. Assist with arterial line insertion to allow for continuous blood pressure monitoring. Assist with insertion of a PA catheter to assess hemo-dynamic balance.
- Administer ordered medications to control aneurysm progression. Provide analgesics to relieve pain, if present.
- Observe the patient for signs of rupture, which may be imme-diately fatal. Watch closely for any signs of acute blood loss: decreasing blood pressure; increasing pulse and respiratory rates; cool, clammy skin; restlessness; and decreased LOC.

Rupture response

- If rupture occurs, insert a large-bore I.V. catheter, begin fluid resuscitation, and administer nitroprusside I.V. as ordered, usually to maintain a MAP of 70 to 80 mm Hg. Also administer propranolol I.V. (to reduce left ventricular ejection velocity) as ordered until the heart rate ranges from 60 to 80 beats per minute. Expect to administer additional doses every 4 to 6 hours until oral medications can be used.
- If the patient is experiencing acute pain, administer morphine I.V. as ordered.
- Prepare the patient for emergency surgery.

After surgery

- Administer nitroprusside or nitroglycerin and titrate to maintain a normotensive state.
- Provide analgesics to relieve pain.
- Administer anticoagulants, such as heparin, to help prevent formation of thrombi.
- Continue to monitor ECG for changes. Assess the patient's hemodynamic status at least every 4 hours; he may have a decreased CVP, PAP, and PAWP.
- Administer I.V. fluids as ordered.
- Monitor the patient for signs of bleeding, such as hypotension and decreased hemoglobin and hematocrit.
- Perform meticulous pulmonary hygiene measures, including suctioning, chest physiotherapy, and deep breathing.
- Assess urine output hourly.
- Maintain NG tube patency to ensure gastric decompression.
- Assist with serial Doppler examination of all extremities to evaluate the adequacy of vascular repair and presence of embolization.
- Assess for signs of poor arterial perfusion, such as pain, paresthesia, pallor, pulselessness, paralysis, and poikilothermy (coldness).

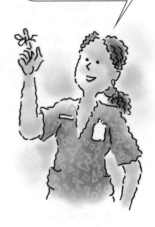

Remember the six signs of poor arterial perfusion: pain, paresthesia, pallor, pulselessness, paralysis, and poikilothermy.

Cardiac arrhythmias

In cardiac arrhythmia, abnormal electrical conduction or automaticity changes heart rate and rhythm.

Asymptomatic to catastrophic

Cardiac arrhythmias vary in severity, from those that are mild, asymptomatic, and require no treatment (such as sinus arrhythmia, in which heart rate increases and decreases with respiration) to catastrophic ventricular fibrillation, which requires immediate resuscitation.

Organized by origin and effects

Cardiac arrhythmias are generally classified according to their origin (ventricular or supraventricular). Their effect on cardiac output and blood pressure, partially influenced by the site of origin, determines their clinical significance. Lethal arrhythmias, such as ventricular tachycardia and ventricular fibrillation, are a major cause of sudden cardiac death.

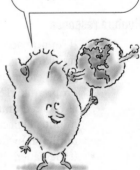

Arrhythmias are generally classified according to their point of origin—either ventricular or supraventricular.

What causes it

Common causes of cardiac arrhythmias include:
- congenital defects
- myocardial ischemia or infarction
- organic heart disease
- drug toxicity
- degeneration of the conductive tissue
- connective tissue disorders
- electrolyte imbalances
- cellular hypoxia
- hypertrophy of the heart muscle
- acid–base imbalances
- emotional stress.

How it happens

Cardiac arrhythmias may result from:
- enhanced or depressed automaticity
- altered conduction pathways
- abnormal electrical conduction.

What to look for

When a patient presents with a history of symptoms suggestive of cardiac arrhythmias, or has been treated for a cardiac arrhythmia, be alert for:
- reports of precipitating factors, such as exercise, smoking, sleep, emotional stress, exposure to heat or cold, caffeine intake, position changes, or recent illnesses
- attempts to alleviate the symptoms, such as coughing, rest, medications, or deep breathing
- reports of sensing the heart's rhythm, such as palpitations, irregular beating, skipped beats, or rapid or slow heart rate.

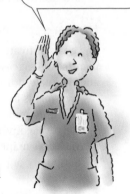

Listen to the patient's reports of precipitating factors, attempts to alleviate symptoms, and description of sensing the heart's rhythm.

A matter of degree

Physical examination findings vary depending on the arrhythmia and the degree of hemodynamic compromise.

Circulatory failure along with an absence of pulse and respirations is found with asystole, ventricular fibrillation, and sometimes with ventricular tachycardia.

That's not all

Additional findings may include:
- pallor
- cold and clammy extremities
- reduced urine output
- dyspnea

- hypotension
- weakness
- chest pains
- dizziness
- syncope
- anxiety
- fatigue
- auscultation of S_3.

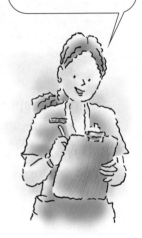

A patient may present with many of the telltale signs of arrhythmia, but a 12-lead ECG is the standard test for identifying the exact type of cardiac arrhythmia he has.

What tests tell you

- A 12-lead ECG is the standard test for identifying cardiac arrhythmias. A 15-lead ECG (in which additional leads are applied to the right side of the chest) or an 18-lead ECG (in which additional leads are also added to the posterior scapular area) may be done to provide more definitive information about the patient's right ventricle and posterior wall of the left ventricle. (See *Understanding cardiac arrhythmias*, pages 266 to 271.)
- Laboratory testing may reveal electrolyte abnormalities, hypoxemia or acid–base abnormalities (with ABG analysis), or drug toxicities as the cause of arrhythmias.
- Exercise testing may reveal exercise-induced arrhythmias.
- Electrophysiologic testing may be used to identify the mechanism of an arrhythmia and location of accessory pathways and to assess the effectiveness of antiarrhythmic drugs.

How it's treated

The goals of treatment are to return pacer function to the sinus node, increase or decrease ventricular rate to normal, regain AV synchrony, and maintain normal sinus rhythm.

Treatments to correct abnormal rhythms include therapy with:

- antiarrhythmic drugs
- electrical conversion with defibrillation and cardioversion
- Valsalva's maneuver
- temporary or permanent placement of a pacemaker to maintain heart rate
- ICD if indicated
- surgical removal or cryotherapy of an irritable ectopic focus to prevent recurring arrhythmias
- management of the underlying disorder such as correction of hypoxia.

What to do

Care for the patient experiencing a cardiac arrhythmia as follows:

- Evaluate the patient's ECG regularly for arrhythmia and assess hemodynamic parameters as indicated. Document arrhythmias and notify the practitioner immediately.

- When life-threatening arrhythmias develop, rapidly assess the patient's LOC, pulse and respiratory rates, and hemodynamic parameters. Monitor his ECG continuously. Be prepared to initiate CPR if indicated.
- Administer oxygen to help improve myocardial oxygen supply.
- Administer analgesics, as appropriate, and help the patient decrease anxiety.
- Assess the patient for predisposing factors, such as fluid and electrolyte imbalance, and signs of drug toxicity, especially with digoxin.
- Administer medications as ordered; monitor for adverse effects; and monitor vital signs, hemodynamic parameters (as appropriate), and appropriate laboratory studies. Prepare to assist with or perform cardioversion or defibrillation if indicated.
- If you suspect drug toxicity, report it to the practitioner immediately and withhold the next dose.
- If a temporary pacemaker needs to be inserted, make sure that a fresh battery is installed to avoid temporary pacemaker malfunction and carefully secure the external catheter wires and the pacemaker box.
- After pacemaker insertion, monitor the patient's pulse rate regularly and watch for signs of pacemaker failure and decreased cardiac output.

Cardiac tamponade

Cardiac tamponade is a rapid, unchecked increase in pressure in the pericardial sac. This compresses the heart, impairs diastolic filling, and reduces cardiac output.

Pericardial pressure

The increase in pressure usually results from blood or fluid accumulation in the pericardial sac. Even a small amount of fluid (50 to 100 ml) can cause a serious tamponade if it accumulates rapidly.

If fluid accumulates rapidly, cardiac tamponade requires emergency lifesaving measures to prevent death. A slow accumulation and increase in pressure may not produce immediate symptoms because the fibrous wall of the pericardial sac can gradually stretch to accommodate as much as 1 to 2 L of fluid.

What causes it

Cardiac tamponade may result from:
- idiopathic causes (such as Dressler's syndrome)
- effusion (from cancer, bacterial infections, tuberculosis, and, rarely, acute rheumatic fever)
- hemorrhage due to trauma (such as gunshot or stab wounds of the chest)

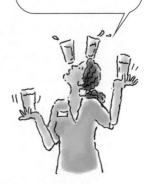

A patient with cardiac tamponade may not have immediate syptoms if fluid accumulates slowly. The fibrous wall of the pericardial sac can stretch gradually to accomodate as much as 1 to 2 L of fluid. That's a lot to handle!

(Text continues on page 272.)

Understanding cardiac arrhythmias

Here's an outline of many common cardiac arrhythmias and their features, causes, and treatments. Use a normal ECG strip, if available, to compare normal cardiac rhythm configurations with the rhythm strips shown here.

Characteristics of normal sinus rhythm include:
- ventricular and atrial rates of 60 to 100 beats per minute
- regular and uniform QRS complexes and P waves
- PR interval of 0.12 to 0.20 second
- QRS duration <0.12 second
- identical atrial and ventricular rates, with constant PR intervals.

Arrhythmia	Features
Sinus tachycardia 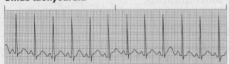	• Atrial and ventricular rhythms regular • Rate >100 beats/minute; rarely, >160 beats/minute • Normal P waves preceding each QRS complex
Sinus bradycardia 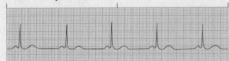	• Atrial and ventricular rhythms regular • Rate <60 beats/minute • Normal P waves preceding each QRS complex
Paroxysmal supraventricular tachycardia 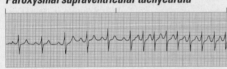	• Atrial and ventricular rhythms regular • Heart rate >160 beats/minute; rarely exceeds 250 beats/minute • P waves regular but aberrant; difficult to differentiate from preceding T waves • P waves preceding each QRS complex • Sudden onset and termination of arrhythmia
Atrial flutter 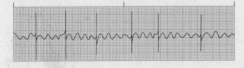	• Atrial rhythm regular; rate 250 to 400 beats per minute • Ventricular rate variable, depending on degree of AV block (usually 60 to 100 beats per minute) • No P waves; atrial activity appears as flutter waves (f waves); sawtooth configuration common in lead II • QRS complexes are uniform in shape but often irregular in rhythm.

Causes	Treatment
• Normal physiologic response to fever, exercise, anxiety, pain, dehydration; may also accompany shock, left-sided heart failure, hyperthyroidism, anemia, hypovolemia, pulmonary embolism, and anterior wall MI • May also occur with atropine, epinephrine, isoproterenol (Isuprel), aminophylline, caffeine, alcohol, cocaine, amphetamine, and nicotine use	• Correction of underlying cause • Beta-adrenergic blockers or calcium channel blocker
• Normal, in well-conditioned heart, as in an athlete, or during sleep • Increased intracranial pressure, vagal stimulation, vomiting, sick sinus syndrome, hypothyroidism, inferior wall MI, and hypothermia • May also occur with calcium channel blockers, beta-adrenergic blocker, digoxin (Lanoxin), and morphine use	• Correction of underlying cause • For low CO, dizziness, weakness, altered LOC, or low blood pressure; advanced cardiac life support (ACLS) protocol for administration of atropine • Temporary or permanent pacemaker • Dopamine (Intropin) or epinephrine infusion
• Stress, hypoxia, hypokalemia, cardiomyopathy, MI, valvular disease, Wolff-Parkinson-White syndrome, cor pulmonale, hyperthyroidism, anxiety, hypoxia, rheumatic heart disease • May also occur with digoxin toxicity; use of caffeine, marijuana, central nervous system stimulants, nicotine, or alcohol	• If patient is unstable, immediate cardioversion • If patient is stable, vagal stimulation, Valsalva's maneuver, and carotid sinus massage or adenosine • After rhythm converts, use calcium channel blockers or beta-adrenergic blockers.
• Heart failure, tricuspid or mitral valve disease, pulmonary embolism, cor pulmonale, pericarditis, and hyperthyroidism • May also occur with digoxin toxicity or alcohol use	• If patient is unstable with a ventricular rate >150 beats/minute, immediate cardioversion • If patient is stable, follow ACLS protocol for cardioversion and drug therapy, which may include calcium channel blockers, beta-adrenergic blockers, amiodarone, or digoxin. • Anticoagulation therapy may also be necessary. • Radio frequency ablation to control rhythm

(continued)

Understanding cardiac arrhythmias *(continued)*

Arrhythmia	Features
Atrial fibrillation 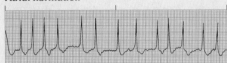	• Atrial rhythm grossly irregular; rate >400 beats/minute • Ventricular rhythm grossly irregular • QRS complexes of uniform configuration and duration • PR interval indiscernible • No P waves, atrial activity appears as erratic, irregular, baseline fibrillatory waves (f waves)
Junctional rhythm 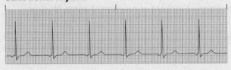	• Atrial and ventricular rhythms regular; atrial rate 40 to 60 beats per minute; ventricular rate usually 40 to 60 beats per minute (60 to 100 beats per minute is accelerated junctional rhythm) • P waves preceding, hidden within (absent), or after QRS complex; usually inverted if visible • PR interval (when present) <0.12 second • QRS complex configuration and duration normal, except in aberrant conduction
First-degree AV block 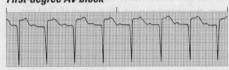	• Atrial and ventricular rhythms regular • PR interval >0.20 second • P wave precedes QRS complex. • QRS complex normal
Second-degree AV block *Mobitz I (Wenckebach)* 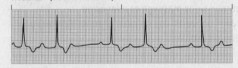	• Atrial rhythm regular • Ventricular rhythm irregular • Atrial rate exceeds ventricular rate. • PR interval progressively longer with each cycle until QRS complex disappears (dropped beat); PR interval shorter after dropped beat
Second-degree AV block *Mobitz II* 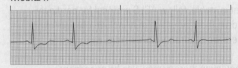	• Atrial rhythm regular • Ventricular rhythm regular or irregular, with varying degree of block • PR interval constant for conducted beats • P waves normal size and shape, but some aren't followed by a QRS complex

(continued)

Causes	Treatment
• Heart failure, chronic obstructive pulmonary disease, thyrotoxicosis, pericarditis, ischemic heart disease, pulmonary embolus, hypertension, mitral stenosis, atrial irritation, or complication of coronary bypass or valve replacement surgery • May also occur with nifedipine, digoxin, or alcohol use	• If patient is unstable with a ventricular rate >150 beats/minute, immediate cardioversion • If patient is stable, follow ACLS protocol and drug therapy, which may include calcium channel blockers, beta-adrenergic blockers, amiodarone, or digoxin. • Anticoagulation therapy may also be necessary. • In some patients with refractory atrial fibrillation uncontrolled by drugs, radio frequency catheter ablation
• MI or ischemia, hypoxia, vagal stimulation, and sick sinus syndrome • Valve surgery • May also occur with digoxin toxicity	• Correction of underlying cause • Atropine for symptomatic slow rate • Pacemaker insertion if patient doesn't respond to drugs • Discontinuation of digoxin if appropriate
• May be seen in healthy persons • MI or ischemia, hyperkalemia, complication of coronary bypass or valve surgery • May also occur with digoxin toxicity; use of beta-adrenergic blockers, calcium channel blockers, or amiodarone	• Correction of underlying cause • Possibly atropine if severe symptomatic bradycardia develops • Cautious use of digoxin, calcium channel blockers, and beta-adrenergic blockers
• Inferior wall MI, cardiac surgery, conduction system defects, and vagal stimulation • May also occur with digoxin toxicity; use of beta-adrenergic blockers or calcium channel blockers	• Treatment of underlying cause • Temporary pacemaker for symptomatic bradycardia (atropine usually not helpful) • Discontinuation of digoxin if appropriate
• Severe CAD, anterior wall MI, acute myocarditis, hypertension, conduction system defects, and complication of cardiac surgery	• Temporary or permanent pacemaker • Dopamine, or epinephrine for symptomatic bradycardia (atropine usually not helpful)

(continued)

Understanding cardiac arrhythmias *(continued)*

Arrhythmia	Features
Third-degree AV block *(complete heart block)* 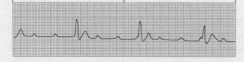	• Atrial rhythm regular • Ventricular rhythm regular and rate slower than atrial rate • No relation between P waves and QRS complexes • No constant PR interval • QRS duration normal (junctional pacemaker) or wide and bizarre (ventricular pacemaker)
Premature ventricular contraction (PVC) 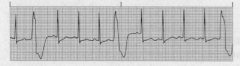	• Atrial rhythm regular • Ventricular rhythm may be regular except for aberrant beats. • QRS complex premature, usually followed by a complete compensatory pause • QRS complex wide and distorted, usually >0.12 second; conducted in opposite direction • Premature QRS complexes occurring alone, in pairs, or in threes, alternating with normal beats; focus from one or more sites • Ominous when clustered, multifocal, with R wave on T pattern
Ventricular tachycardia 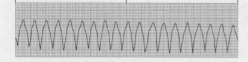	• Ventricular rate 100 to 250 beats per minute, rhythm usually regular • QRS complexes wide, bizarre, and independent of P waves • P waves not discernible • May start and stop suddenly
Ventricular fibrillation 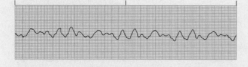	• Ventricular rhythm and rate chaotic and rapid • QRS complexes wide and irregular; no visible P waves
Asystole 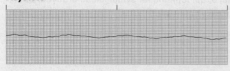	• No atrial or ventricular rate or rhythm • No discernible P waves, QRS complexes, or T waves

Causes	Treatment
• Inferior or anterior wall MI, hypoxia, postoperative complication of cardiac surgery, postprocedure complication of radiofrequency ablation in or near AV nodal tissue, and potassium imbalance • May also occur with digoxin toxicity	• Atropine, dopamine, or epinephrine for symptomatic bradycardia • Temporary or permanent pacemaker
• Heart failure; old or acute MI, ischemia, or contusion; myocardial irritation by ventricular catheter or a pacemaker; hypokalemia; hypocalcemia; hypomagnesemia; cardiomyopathy; hypoxia; and acidosis • May also occur with drug toxicity (digoxin, aminophylline, epinephrine, isoproterenol, or dopamine) • Caffeine, tobacco, or alcohol use • Psychological stress, anxiety, pain, or exercise	• If warranted, procainamide, amiodarone, or lidocaine I.V. • Treatment of underlying cause • Discontinuation of drug causing toxicity • Potassium chloride I.V. if PVC induced by hypokalemia • Magnesium sulfate I.V. if PVC induced by hypomagnesemia
• Myocardial ischemia, MI, or aneurysm; CAD; mitral valve prolapse; cardiomyopathy; ventricular catheters; hypokalemia; hypocalcemia; hypomagnesemia; myocardial reperfusion; acidosis; and hypoxia • May also occur with digoxin, procainamide, epinephrine, or quinidine toxicity • Anxiety	• If pulseless, initiate CPR; follow ACLS protocol for defibrillation, administration of epinephrine or vasopressin followed by amiodarone (lidocaine may be considered if amiodarone isn't available), and advanced airway placement; magnesium sulfate only for torsades de pointes • If regular wide-complex QRS rhythm (monomorphic) present, administer adenosine (follow ACLS protocol); if drug is unsuccessful, cardioversion • If polymorphic (irregular) ventricular tachycardia present, immediate defibrillation • ICD if recurrent ventricular tachycardia
• Myocardial ischemia, MI, untreated ventricular tachycardia, R-on-T phenomenon, hypokalemia, hypomagnesemia, hypoxemia, alkalosis, electric shock, and hypothermia • May also occur with digoxin, epinephrine, or tricyclic antidepressant toxicity	• CPR; follow ACLS protocol for defibrillation, ET intubation, and administration of epinephrine or vasopressin, and amiodarone • ICD if risk for recurrent ventricular fibrillation
• Myocardial ischemia, MI, heart failure, hypoxia, hypokalemia, severe acidosis, shock, ventricular arrhythmia, AV block, pulmonary embolism, heart rupture, hyperkalemia • May also occur with cocaine overdose	• Continue CPR and follow ACLS protocol for ET intubation and administration of epinephrine or vasopressin.

- hemorrhage due to nontraumatic causes (such as anticoagulant therapy in patients with pericarditis or rupture of the heart or great vessels)
- viral or postirradiation pericarditis
- chronic renal failure requiring dialysis
- drug reaction from procainamide, hydralazine, minoxidil, isoniazid (INH), penicillin, or daunorubicin (Cerubidine)
- connective tissue disorders (such as rheumatoid arthritis, systemic lupus erythematosus, rheumatic fever, vasculitis, and scleroderma)
- acute MI.

How it happens

In cardiac tamponade, accumulation of fluid in the pericardial sac causes compression of the heart chambers. This compression obstructs blood flow into the ventricles and reduces the amount of blood that can be pumped out of the heart with each contraction. (See *Understanding cardiac tamponade*.)

Understanding cardiac tamponade

The pericardial sac, which surrounds and protects the heart, is composed of several layers:
- The fibrous pericardium is the tough outermost membrane.
- The inner membrane, called the *serous membrane*, consists of the visceral and parietal layers.
- The visceral layer clings to the heart and is also known as the *epicardial layer* of the heart.
- The parietal layer lies between the visceral layer and the fibrous pericardium.

- The pericardial space—between the visceral and parietal layers—contains 10 to 30 ml of pericardial fluid. This fluid lubricates the layers and minimizes friction when the heart contracts.

In cardiac tamponade, shown below to the right, blood or fluid fills the pericardial space, compressing the heart chambers, increasing intracardiac pressure, and obstructing venous return. As blood flow into the ventricles decreases, so does CO. Without prompt treatment, low CO can be fatal.

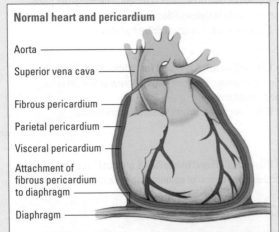

Normal heart and pericardium

- Aorta
- Superior vena cava
- Fibrous pericardium
- Parietal pericardium
- Visceral pericardium
- Attachment of fibrous pericardium to diaphragm
- Diaphragm

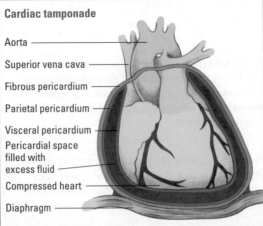

Cardiac tamponade

- Aorta
- Superior vena cava
- Fibrous pericardium
- Parietal pericardium
- Visceral pericardium
- Pericardial space filled with excess fluid
- Compressed heart
- Diaphragm

What to look for

Cardiac tamponade has three classic features known as *Beck's triad*:
1. elevated CVP with jugular vein distention
2. muffled heart sounds
3. drop in systolic blood pressure.

That's not all

Other signs include:
*   narrowed pulse pressure
*   orthopnea
*   anxiety
*   restlessness
*   jugular vein distention with inspiration
*   mottling
*   clear breath sounds (this helps distinguish cardiac tamponade from heart failure).

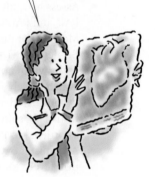

In cardiac tamponade, a chest X-ray reveals a widened mediastinum and enlarged cardiac silhouette.

What tests tell you

*   Chest X-ray shows a slightly widened mediastinum and an enlarged cardiac silhouette.
*   ECG may show low-amplitude QRS complex and electrical alternans, an alternating beat-to-beat change in amplitude of the P wave, QRS complex, and T wave. Generalized ST-segment elevation is noted in all leads. An ECG is used to rule out other cardiac disorders; it may reveal changes produced by acute pericarditis.
*   PA catheterization discloses increased CVP, right ventricular diastolic pressure, PAWP, and decreased cardiac output/cardiac index.
*   Echocardiography may reveal pericardial effusion with signs of right ventricular and atrial compression.
*   CT scan or MRI may be used to identify pericardial effusions or pericardial thickening caused by constrictive pericarditis.

How it's treated

The goal of treatment is to relieve intrapericardial pressure and cardiac compression by removing accumulated blood or fluid. This can be done three different ways:
1. pericardiocentesis (needle aspiration of the pericardial cavity)
2. surgical creation of an opening, called a *pericardial window*
3. insertion of a drain into the pericardial sac to drain the effusion.

When pressure's low

If the patient is hypotensive, trial volume loading with crystalloids such as I.V. normal saline solution may be used to maintain systolic blood pressure. An inotropic drug, such as dobutamine, may be necessary to improve myocardial contractility until fluid in the pericardial sac can be removed.

Additional treatments

Additional treatment may be necessary, depending on the cause. Examples of such causes and treatments are:

- traumatic injury—blood transfusion or a thoracotomy to drain reaccumulating fluid or to repair bleeding sites
- heparin-induced tamponade—administration of the heparin antagonist protamine sulfate
- warfarin-induced tamponade—vitamin K administration
- renal failure–induced tamponade—hemodialysis.

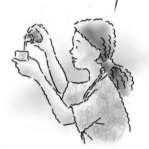

To correct heparin-induced tamponade, administer the heparin antagonist protamine sulfate.

What to do

- Monitor the patient's cardiovascular status frequently, at least every hour, noting extent of jugular vein distention, quality of heart sounds, and blood pressure.
- Assess hemodynamic status, including CVP, right atrial pressure, PAP, and PAWP and determine cardiac output.
- Monitor for pulsus paradoxus.
- Be alert for ST-segment and T-wave changes on ECG. Note rate and rhythm and report evidence of any arrhythmias.
- Watch closely for signs of increasing tamponade, increasing dyspnea, and arrhythmias and report immediately.
- Infuse I.V. solutions and inotropic drugs, such as dobutamine, as ordered to maintain the patient's blood pressure.
- Administer oxygen therapy as needed and assess oxygen saturation levels. Monitor the patient's respiratory status for signs of respiratory distress, such as severe tachypnea and changes in the patient's LOC. Anticipate the need for ET intubation and mechanical ventilation if the patient's respiratory status deteriorates.
- Prepare the patient for pericardiocentesis or thoracotomy.

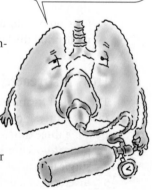

Administer oxygen and monitor for respiratory distress. And by all means, anticipate the need for ET and mechanical ventilation if the patient's respiratory status deteriorates.

Under pressure

- If the patient has trauma-induced tamponade, assess for other signs of trauma and institute appropriate care, including the use of colloids, crystalloids, and blood component therapy under pressure or by rapid volume infuser if massive fluid replacement is needed; administration of protamine sulfate for heparin-induced tamponade; and vitamin K administration for warfarin-induced tamponade.

- Assess renal function status closely, monitoring urine output every hour and notifying the practitioner if output is less than 0.5 mg/kg/hour.
- Monitor capillary refill time, LOC, peripheral pulses, and skin temperature for evidence of diminished tissue perfusion.

Cardiogenic shock

Cardiogenic shock is a condition of diminished cardiac output that severely impairs tissue perfusion. It's sometimes called *pump failure*.

Shocking stats

Cardiogenic shock is a serious complication in nearly 15% of all patients hospitalized with acute MI. It typically affects patients whose area of infarction involves 40% or more of left ventricular muscle mass; in such patients, mortality may exceed 85%.

What causes it

Cardiogenic shock can result from any condition that causes significant left ventricular dysfunction with reduced cardiac output, such as:
- MI (most common)
- myocardial ischemia
- papillary muscle dysfunction
- cardiomyopathy
- chronic or acute heart failure
- acidosis.

Other offenders

Other causes include myocarditis and depression of myocardial contractility after cardiac arrest and prolonged cardiac surgery.

Mechanical abnormalities of the ventricle, such as acute mitral or aortic insufficiency or an acutely acquired ventricular septal defect or ventricular aneurysm, may also result in cardiogenic shock.

How it happens

Regardless of the cause, here's what happens:
- Left ventricular dysfunction initiates a series of compensatory mechanisms that attempt to increase cardiac output and, in turn, maintain vital organ function.
- As cardiac output falls, baroreceptors in the aorta and carotid arteries initiate responses in the sympathetic nervous system. These

responses, in turn, increase heart rate, left ventricular filling pressure, and afterload to enhance venous return to the heart.

- These compensatory responses initially stabilize the patient but later cause the patient to deteriorate as the oxygen demands of the already compromised heart increase.

Lower and lower output

- The events involved in cardiogenic shock comprise a vicious cycle of low cardiac output, sympathetic compensation, myocardial ischemia, and even lower cardiac output.

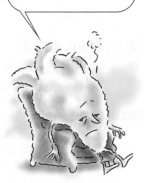

Compensatory mechanisms that increase cardiac output eventually cause the patient to deteriorate because of increased oxygen demands.

What to look for

Cardiogenic shock produces signs of poor tissue perfusion, such as:
- cold, pale, clammy skin
- drop in systolic blood pressure to 30 mm Hg below baseline or a sustained reading below 90 mm Hg that isn't attributable to medication
- tachycardia
- rapid respirations
- oliguria (urine output less than 20 ml/hour)
- anxiety
- confusion
- narrowing pulse pressure
- crackles heard in lungs
- neck vein distention
- S_3, faint heart sounds, and possibly a holosystolic murmur.

What tests tell you

- PAP monitoring reveals increased CVP, PAP, PAWP, and SVR, reflecting an increase in left ventricular end-diastolic pressure (preload) and heightened resistance to left ventricular emptying (afterload) caused by ineffective pumping and increased peripheral vascular resistance. Thermodilution catheterization reveals a reduced cardiac index.
- Invasive arterial pressure monitoring shows systolic arterial pressure less than 90 mm Hg caused by impaired ventricular ejection.
- ABG analysis may show metabolic and respiratory acidosis and hypoxia.
- ECG demonstrates possible evidence of acute MI, ischemia, or ventricular aneurysm and arrhythmias.

They tell me the signs of cardiogenic shock are as clear as the stars on a cloudless night, so I'm looking . . . looking . . . still looking . . .

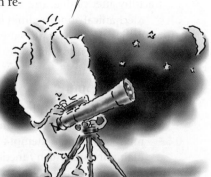

- Echocardiography is used to determine left ventricular function and reveals valvular abnormalities.
- Serum enzyme measurements display elevated levels of CK, aspartate aminotransferase, and alanine aminotransferase, which indicate MI or ischemia and suggest heart failure or shock. CK-MB (an isoenzyme of CK that occurs in cardiac tissue) and troponin isoenzyme levels may confirm acute MI.
- Brain natriuretic peptide (BNP) levels are elevated, indicating ventricular overload.
- Cardiac catheterization and echocardiography may reveal other conditions that can lead to pump dysfunction and failure, such as cardiac tamponade, papillary muscle infarct or rupture, ventricular septal rupture, pulmonary emboli, venous pooling (associated with venodilators and continuous or intermittent positive-pressure breathing), hypovolemia, and acute heart failure.

How it's treated

The goal of treatment is to enhance cardiovascular status by increasing cardiac output, improving myocardial perfusion, and decreasing cardiac workload. Treatment consists of administering a combination of cardiovascular drugs and mechanical-assist techniques.

Treatment ABCs

Treatment begins with these measures:
- maintaining a patent airway; preparing for intubation and mechanical ventilation if the patient develops respiratory distress
- supplemental oxygen to increase oxygenation
- continuous cardiac monitoring to detect changes in heart rate and rhythm; administration of antiarrhythmics, as necessary
- initiating and maintaining at least two I.V. lines with large-gauge needles for fluid and drug administration
- I.V. fluids, crystalloids, colloids, or blood products, as necessary, to maintain intravascular volume.

Cardiovascular drugs
Drug therapy may include I.V. dopamine, phenylephrine, or norepinephrine to increase blood pressure and blood flow to kidneys. Inamrinone or dobutamine—inotropic agents that increase myocardial contractility and cardiac output—are commonly used.

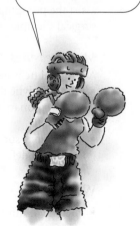

Initiate and maintain at least two I.V. lines with large-gauge needles to deliver the old one-two punch—I.V. fluids and cardiovascular drugs.

Decrease resistance and pressure

A vasodilator, nitroglycerin or nitroprusside, may be used with a vasopressor to further improve cardiac output by decreasing afterload (SVR) and reducing left ventricular end-diastolic pressure (preload). However, the patient's blood pressure must be adequate to support nitroprusside therapy and must be monitored closely.

Overloaded and out of control

Diuretics also may be used to reduce preload (PAWP) in patients with fluid volume overload. Antiarrhythmics may also be used to prevent or control arrhythmias that may reduce cardiac output.

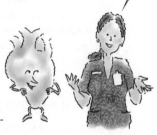

Improved ventricular ejection significantly improves cardiac output.

Mechanical assistance

Treatment may also include mechanical assistance by IABP to improve coronary artery perfusion and decrease cardiac workload. The IABP is inserted through the femoral artery into the descending thoracic aorta. The balloon inflates during diastole to increase coronary artery perfusion pressure and deflates before systole (before the aortic valve opens) to reduce resistance to ejection (afterload) and therefore reduce cardiac workload.

Improved ventricular ejection significantly improves cardiac output. Subsequent vasodilation in the peripheral vessels leads to lower preload volume and reduced workload of the left ventricle. This is because of decreasing SVR.

End-stage effort

When drug therapy and IABP insertion fail, a VAD may be inserted to assist the pumping action of the heart. When all other medical and surgical therapies fail, heart transplantation may be considered.

More measures

Additional treatment measures for cardiogenic shock may include:
- thrombolytic therapy or coronary artery revascularization to restore coronary artery blood flow, if cardiogenic shock is due to acute MI
- emergency surgery to repair papillary muscle rupture or ventricular septal defect, if either is the cause of cardiogenic shock.

What to do

- Begin I.V. infusions of normal saline solution using a large-bore (14G to 18G) catheter, which allows easier administration of later blood transfusions.

- Administer oxygen by facemask or artificial airway to ensure adequate oxygenation of tissues. Adjust the oxygen flow rate to a higher or lower level, as ABG measurements indicate. Many patients need 100% oxygen, and some require 5 to 15 cm H_2O of positive end-expiratory or continuous positive airway pressure ventilation.

Monitor, record, and then monitor more

- Monitor and record blood pressure, pulse, respiratory rate, and peripheral pulses every 1 to 5 minutes until the patient stabilizes. Monitor cardiac rhythm continuously. Systolic blood pressure less than 80 mm Hg usually results in inadequate coronary artery blood flow, cardiac ischemia, arrhythmias, and further complications of low cardiac output.
- Using a PA catheter, closely monitor CVP, PAP, PAWP, SVR, and cardiac output. High CVP and PAWP readings indicate heart failure, increased SVR, decreased cardiac output, and decreased cardiac index and should be reported immediately.

Watch all those fluids

- Determine how much fluid to give by checking blood pressure, urine output, CVP, or PAWP. Whenever the fluid infusion rate is increased, watch for signs of fluid overload, such as an increase in PAWP. If the patient is hypovolemic, preload may need to be increased, typically accomplished with I.V. fluids. However, I.V. fluids must be given cautiously, being increased gradually while hemodynamic parameters are closely monitored. In this situation, diuretics aren't given.
- Insert an indwelling urinary catheter to measure hourly urine output. If output is less than 30 ml/hour in adults, increase the fluid infusion rate but watch for signs of fluid overload such as an increase in PAWP. Notify the practitioner if urine output doesn't improve.
- Administer a diuretic, such as furosemide, as ordered, to decrease preload and improve stroke volume and cardiac output.
- Monitor ABG values, CBC, and electrolyte levels. Expect to administer sodium bicarbonate by I.V. push if the patient is acidotic. Administer electrolyte replacement therapy as ordered.
- During therapy, assess skin color and temperature and note any changes. Cold, clammy skin may be a sign of continuing peripheral vascular constriction, indicating progressive shock.

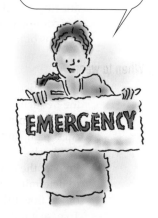

Report a high PAWP immediately. It indicates heart failure, increased systemic vascular resistance, decreased cardiac output, and decreased cardiac index.

Don't move!

- If your patient is on the IABP, move him as little as possible. Never flex the patient's "ballooned" leg at the hip because this may displace or fracture the catheter. Never place the patient in a sitting position for any reason (including chest X-rays) while the balloon is inflated; the balloon will tear through the aorta and result in immediate death.
- During use of the IABP, assess pedal pulses and skin temperature and color to ensure adequate peripheral circulation. Check the dressing over the insertion site frequently for bleeding and change it according to facility protocol. Also check the site for hematoma or signs of infection and culture any drainage.

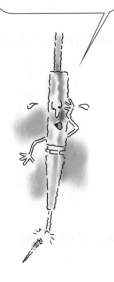

Never flex the patient's "ballooned" leg at the hip—I may become displaced or break.

When to wean

- If the patient becomes hemodynamically stable, gradually reduce the frequency of balloon inflation to wean him from the IABP.
- When weaning the patient from the IABP, watch for ECG changes, chest pain, and other signs of recurring cardiac ischemia as well as for shock.
- Prepare the patient for possible emergency cardiac catheterization to determine eligibility for PTCA or CABG to reperfuse (restore blood flow to) areas with reversible injury patterns.
- To ease emotional stress, plan care measures to allow frequent rest periods and provide as much privacy as possible. Allow family members to visit and comfort the patient as much as possible.

Cardiomyopathy

Cardiomyopathy generally refers to disease of the heart muscle fibers. It takes three main forms:
1. dilated
2. hypertrophic
3. restrictive (extremely rare).

Cardiomyopathy is the second most common direct cause of sudden death; CAD is first. Because dilated cardiomyopathy usually isn't diagnosed until its advanced stages, the prognosis is generally poor.

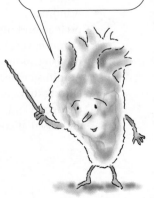

I'm sorry to report that dilated cardiomyopathy usually isn't diagnosed until it's advanced, so the prognosis is generally poor.

What causes it

Most patients with cardiomyopathy have idiopathic, or primary, disease, but some cases are secondary to identifiable causes. Hypertrophic cardiomyopathy is almost always inherited as a non-sex-linked autosomal dominant trait.

Males and blacks are at greatest risk for cardiomyopathy; other risk factors include hypertension, pregnancy, viral infections, and alcohol use.

How it happens

The disease course in cardiomyopathy depends on the special type, as outlined here.

Dilated cardiomyopathy

Dilated cardiomyopathy primarily affects systolic function. It results from extensively damaged myocardial muscle fibers. Consequently, contractility in the left ventricle decreases.

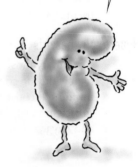

In dilated cardiomyopathy, I try to help maintain cardiac output by retaining water and sodium.

Poor compensation

As systolic function declines, stroke volume, ejection fraction, and cardiac output decrease. As end-diastolic volumes increase, pulmonary congestion may occur. The elevated end-diastolic volume is a compensatory response to preserve stroke volume despite a reduced ejection fraction.

The sympathetic nervous system is also stimulated to increase heart rate and contractility.

Kidneys kick in

The kidneys are stimulated to retain sodium and water to maintain cardiac output, and vasoconstriction occurs as the renin-angiotensin system is stimulated. When these compensatory mechanisms can no longer maintain cardiac output, the heart begins to fail.

Detrimental dilation

Left ventricular dilation occurs as venous return and SVR increase. The stretching of the left ventricle eventually leads to mitral insufficiency. Subsequently, the atria also dilate, as more work is required to pump blood into the full ventricles. Cardiomegaly is a consequence of dilation of the atria and ventricles. Blood pooling in the ventricles increases the risk of emboli.

Hypertrophic cardiomyopathy

Hypertrophic cardiomyopathy primarily affects diastolic function. The features of hypertrophic cardiomyopathy include:
- asymmetrical left ventricular hypertrophy
- hypertrophy of the intraventricular septum
- rapid, forceful contractions of the left ventricle
- impaired relaxation
- obstruction of left ventricular outflow.

Fouled-up filling

The hypertrophied ventricle becomes stiff, noncompliant, and unable to relax during ventricular filling. Consequently, ventricular filling is reduced and left ventricular filling pressure rises, causing increases in left atrial and pulmonary venous pressures and leading to venous congestion and dyspnea.

The increase in venous pressures and venous congestion leads to tachycardia, which causes a decrease in left ventricular filling time. Reduced ventricular filling during diastole and obstruction to ventricular outflow lead to low cardiac output.

Hypertrophy hazards

If papillary muscles become hypertrophied and don't close completely during contraction, mitral insufficiency occurs. Moreover, intramural coronary arteries are abnormally small and may not be sufficient to supply the hypertrophied muscle with enough blood and oxygen to meet the increased needs of the hyperdynamic muscle.

Restrictive cardiomyopathy

Restrictive cardiomyopathy is characterized by stiffness of the ventricle caused by left ventricular hypertrophy and endocardial fibrosis and thickening. The ability of the ventricle to relax and fill during diastole is reduced. Furthermore, the rigid myocardium fails to contract completely during systole. As a result, cardiac output decreases.

What to look for

Generally, for patients with dilated or restrictive cardiomyopathy, the onset is insidious. As the disease progresses, exacerbations and hospitalizations are frequent regardless of the type of cardiomyopathy.

Dilated cardiomyopathy

For a patient with dilated cardiomyopathy, signs and symptoms may be overlooked until left-sided heart failure occurs. Be sure to evaluate the patient's current condition and then compare it with that over the past 6 to 12 months. Signs and symptoms of dilated cardiomyopathy may include:
- shortness of breath, orthopnea, dyspnea on exertion, fatigue
- peripheral edema, hepatomegaly, jugular vein distention
- tachycardia, palpitations
- pansystolic murmur associated with mitral and tricuspid insufficiency

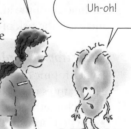

Unfortunately, signs and symptoms may be overlooked until left-sided heart failure occurs.

Uh-oh!

- S_3 and S_4 gallop rhythms
- irregular pulse if atrial fibrillation exists
- crackles in lungs.

Hypertrophic cardiomyopathy

Signs and symptoms vary widely among patients with hypertrophic cardiomyopathy. The presenting symptom is commonly syncope or sudden cardiac death. Other possible signs and symptoms include:
- angina
- dyspnea and orthopnea
- fatigue
- systolic ejection murmur along the left sternal border and apex
- ventricular arrhythmias
- irregular pulse with atrial fibrillation, palpitations
- S_4 and possible S_3 gallop rhythms, split S_2 heart sound.

Restrictive cardiomyopathy

A patient with restrictive cardiomyopathy presents with signs of heart failure and other signs and symptoms, including:
- fatigue and weakness
- dyspnea
- orthopnea
- chest pain
- hepatomegaly
- peripheral edema
- S_3 or S_4 gallop rhythms
- systolic murmurs
- heart blocks.

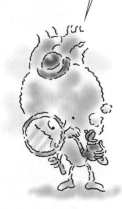

Oh, dear! The first clue to hypertrophic cardiomyopathy may be syncope or sudden cardiac death.

What tests tell you

These tests are used to diagnose cardiomyopathy:

Dilated cardiomyopathy
- Chest X-ray shows an enlarged heart and pulmonary edema.
- An ECG will show biventricular enlargement and, commonly, atrial fibrillation.
- Echocardiogram will show decreased ventricular movement and ejection fraction. It will also demonstrate an increase in atrial and ventricular chamber size and abdomen wall motion. It may also demonstrate mitral valve insufficiency.
- Hemodynamic monitoring will show an increased PAWP and PAP and a decreased cardiac output/cardiac index. In late stages, the CVP may also be elevated.

Hypertrophic cardiomyopathy

- Chest X-ray shows an enlarged heart with pronounced left atrial dilation. Pulmonary congestion may also be seen.
- An ECG will show left atrial enlargement and left ventricular hypertrophy. ST and T-wave changes may be seen. Atrial fibrillation and ventricular arrhythmias, such as ventricular tachycardia and ventricular fibrillation, are also common.
- An echocardiogram will show an enlarged left atrium and hypertrophy of the intraventricular septum. Left ventricular outflow narrowing, if present, can also be seen. Abnormal wall motion may also be present.
- Cardiac catheterization with heart biopsy can provide definitive diagnosis.

Restricted cardiomyopathy

- Chest X-ray shows an enlarged heart and pulmonary edema.
- An ECG will demonstrate low QRS complex voltage. AV heart blocks are commonly seen.
- Echocardiogram will show atrial enlargement. The walls of the ventricles will be thickened but the interior chamber size will be decreased.
- Hemodynamic monitoring will show increased PAP and PAWP. Left and right end-diastolic pressures will also be elevated.

How it's treated

There's no known cure for cardiomyopathy. Treatment is individualized based on the type of cardiomyopathy and the patient's condition.

Dilated cardiomyopathy

For a patient with dilated cardiomyopathy, treatment may involve:

- management of the underlying cause, if it's known
- ACE inhibitors and ARBs to reduce afterload through vasodilation and increase cardiac output
- diuretics, taken with ACE inhibitors, to reduce fluid retention
- digoxin, for patients not responding to ACE inhibitor and diuretic therapy, to improve myocardial contractility
- hydralazine and isosorbide dinitrate, in combination, to produce vasodilation
- beta-adrenergic blockers for patients with mild or moderate heart failure
- antiarrhythmics, such as amiodarone, used cautiously to control arrhythmias
- cardioversion to convert atrial fibrillation to sinus rhythm

- pacemaker insertion to correct arrhythmias
- anticoagulants to reduce the risk of emboli
- revascularization, such as CABG surgery, if dilated cardiomyopathy is due to ischemia
- valvular repair or replacement, if dilated cardiomyopathy is due to valve dysfunction
- lifestyle modifications such as smoking cessation; low-fat, low-sodium diet; physical activity; and abstinence from alcohol
- heart transplantation in patients resistant to medical therapy
- inotropes, such as dobutamine, to improve myocardial contractility and improve heart failure.

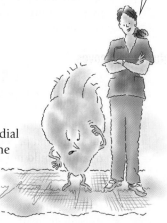

If the patient's condition doesn't improve with medical measures, a heart transplant may be needed.

Hypertrophic cardiomyopathy

For a patient with hypertrophic cardiomyopathy, treatment may involve:
- beta-adrenergic blockers to slow the heart rate, reduce myocardial oxygen demands, and increase ventricular filling by relaxing the obstructing muscle, thereby increasing cardiac output
- antiarrhythmic drugs, such as amiodarone, to reduce arrhythmias
- cardioversion to treat atrial fibrillation
- anticoagulation to reduce the risk for systemic embolism with atrial fibrillation
- verapamil and diltiazem to reduce ventricular stiffness and elevated diastolic pressures
- ablation of the AV node and implantation of a dual-chamber pacemaker (controversial), in patients with obstructive hypertrophic cardiomyopathy and ventricular tachycardias, to reduce the outflow gradient by altering the pattern of ventricular contraction
- ICD to correct ventricular arrhythmias
- ventricular myotomy or myectomy (resection of the hypertrophied septum) to ease outflow tract obstruction and relieve symptoms
- mitral valve replacement to correct mitral insufficiency
- heart transplantation for intractable symptoms.

Restrictive cardiomyopathy

For a patient with restrictive cardiomyopathy, treatment may involve:
- management of the underlying cause such as administering deferoxamine to bind iron in restrictive cardiomyopathy due to hemochromatosis
- digoxin, diuretics, and a restricted sodium diet to ease the symptoms of heart failure, although no therapy exists for patients with restricted ventricular filling
- oral vasodilators to control intractable heart failure.

What to do

- Administer drugs, as ordered, to promote adequate heart function.
- Assess hemodynamic status every 2 hours or more frequently, if necessary.
- Monitor intake and output closely and obtain daily weights; institute fluid restrictions as ordered.
- Institute continuous cardiac monitoring to evaluate for arrhythmias.

No sudden moves

- Assess the patient for possible adverse drug reactions, such as orthostatic hypotension associated with use of vasodilators, diuretics, or ACE inhibitors. Urge the patient to change positions slowly.
- Be aware that patients with hypertrophic cardiomyopathy should not receive medication that may decrease preload (diuretics, nitrates) or dopamine or digoxin because the increase in myocardial contractility may worsen the outflow obstruction.
- Auscultate heart and lung sounds, being alert for S_3 and S_4 heart sounds or murmurs, or crackles, rhonchi, and wheezes indicative of heart failure. Monitor vital signs for changes, especially a heart rate greater than 100 beats/minute, respiratory rate greater than 20 breaths per minute, and a systolic blood pressure less than 90 mm Hg, all of which suggest heart failure.
- Assist the patient with ADLs to decrease oxygen demand.

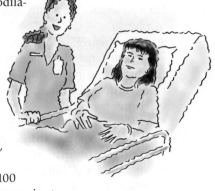

Assess for orthostatic hypotension, a possible adverse effect with some cardiac medications. Urge the patient to change positions slowly.

Oxygen orders

- Administer supplemental oxygen as ordered. Assess for changes in LOC, such as restlessness or decreased responsiveness, indicating diminished cerebral perfusion. If the patient has a PA catheter in place, evaluate mixed venous oxygen saturation levels; if not, monitor oxygen saturation levels using pulse oximetry.
- Organize care to promote periods of rest for the patient.
- Prepare the patient, as indicated, for insertion of pacemaker, ICD, IABP, or cardiac transplantation.

Heart failure

Heart failure occurs when the heart can't pump enough blood to meet the metabolic needs of the body. The American Heart

Association and American College of Cardiology developed a classification system for heart failure staging patients from stage A to D based on physical examination, diagnostic tests, and clinical symptoms.

Heart failure results in intravascular and interstitial volume overload and poor tissue perfusion. An individual with heart failure experiences reduced exercise tolerance, a reduced quality of life, and a shortened life span.

What causes it

The most common cause of heart failure is CAD, but it also occurs in infants, children, and adults with congenital and acquired heart defects.

How it happens

Heart failure may be classified into four general categories:
1. left-sided heart failure
2. right-sided heart failure
3. systolic dysfunction
4. diastolic dysfunction.

When the left loses its faculties

Left-sided heart failure is a result of ineffective left ventricular contractile function.

As the pumping ability of the left ventricle fails, cardiac output drops. Blood is no longer effectively pumped out into the body; it backs up into the left atrium and then into the lungs, causing pulmonary congestion, dyspnea, and activity intolerance.

If the condition persists, pulmonary edema and right-sided heart failure may result. Common causes include:
- left ventricular infarction
- hypertension
- aortic and mitral valve stenosis.

When right goes wrong

Right-sided heart failure results from ineffective right ventricular contractile function. The most common cause for right-sided heart failure is left-sided heart failure; however, it can result from a right ventricular MI.

When blood isn't pumped effectively through the right ventricle to the lungs, blood backs up into the right atrium and into the peripheral circulation. The patient gains weight and develops peripheral edema and engorgement of the kidney and other organs.

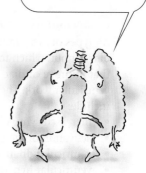

Uh-oh! Blood backs up into the left atrium and then into the lungs when the left ventricle can't pump well.

Blame it on the left

Right-sided heart failure may be due to an acute right ventricular infarction or a pulmonary embolus. However, the most common cause is profound backward flow due to left-sided heart failure.

Other causes of right-sided heart failure include:
- arrhythmias
- volume overload
- mitral and pulmonic valve stenosis
- cardiomyopathy.

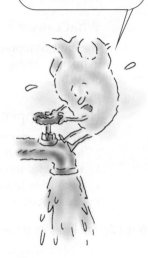

The most common cause of right-sided heart failure is profound backward flow due to left-sided heart failure. Does anybody know a good plumber?

Just can't pump enough

Systolic dysfunction occurs when the left ventricle can't pump enough blood out to the systemic circulation during systole and the ejection fraction falls. Consequently, blood backs up into the pulmonary circulation and pressure increases in the pulmonary venous system. Cardiac output decreases; weakness, fatigue, and shortness of breath may occur.

Causes of systolic dysfunction include:
- MI
- dilated cardiomyopathy
- arrhythmias
- aortic valve insufficiency
- acute rheumatic fever.

It all goes to swell from here.

Diastolic dysfunction occurs when the ability of the left ventricle to relax and fill during diastole is reduced and the stroke volume falls. Therefore, higher volumes are needed in the ventricles to maintain cardiac output. Consequently, pulmonary congestion and peripheral edema develop.

Diastolic dysfunction may occur as a result of left ventricular hypertrophy, hypertension, cardiomyopathy, MI, or cardiac tamponade.

This type of heart failure is less common than that due to systolic dysfunction, and treatment isn't as clear.

Compensatory mechanisms

All types of heart failure eventually lead to reduced cardiac output, which triggers compensatory mechanisms that improve cardiac output at the expense of increased ventricular work. The compensatory mechanisms include:
- increased sympathetic activity
- activation of the renin-angiotensin-aldosterone system
- ventricular dilation
- ventricular hypertrophy.

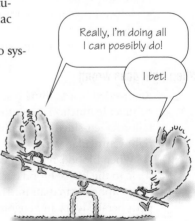

Really, I'm doing all I can possibly do!

I bet!

Increased sympathetic activity

Increased sympathetic activity—a response to decreased cardiac output and blood pressure—enhances peripheral vascular resistance, contractility, heart rate, and venous return. Signs of increased sympathetic activity, such as cool extremities and clamminess, may indicate impending heart failure.

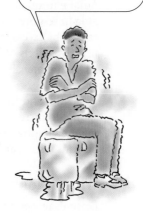

Such signs as cool extremities and clamminess may indicate impending heart failure.

Renin-angiotensin-aldosterone system

Increased sympathetic activity also restricts blood flow to the kidneys, causing them to secrete renin which, in turn, converts angiotensinogen to angiotensin I, which then becomes angiotensin II—a potent vasoconstrictor. Angiotensin causes the adrenal cortex to release aldosterone, leading to sodium and water retention and an increase in circulating blood volume.

This renal mechanism is helpful; however, if it persists unchecked, it can aggravate heart failure, as the heart struggles to pump against the increased volume.

Ventricular dilation

In ventricular dilation, an increase in end-diastolic ventricular volume (preload) causes increased stroke work and stroke volume during contraction. This stretches cardiac muscle fibers so that the ventricle can accept the increased volume. Eventually, the muscle becomes stretched beyond optimum limits and contractility declines.

Ventricular hypertrophy

In ventricular hypertrophy, an increase in ventricular muscle mass allows the heart to pump against increased resistance to the outflow of blood, improving cardiac output. However, this increased muscle mass also increases the myocardial oxygen requirements.

In heart failure, my job is to help the atria and ventricles control vasoconstriction and volume overload by releasing potent counterregulatory substances called prostaglandins. I guess you could call me a hero of sorts.

Compromising situation

An increase in the ventricular diastolic pressure necessary to fill the enlarged ventricle may compromise diastolic coronary blood flow, limiting the oxygen supply to the ventricle and causing ischemia and impaired muscle contractility.

Counterregulatory substances

In heart failure, counterregulatory substances—prostaglandins, atrial natriuretic factor, and BNP—are produced in an attempt to reduce the negative effects of volume overload and vasoconstriction caused by the compensatory mechanisms.

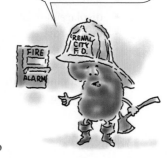

Kidneys' contributions

The kidneys release the prostaglandins prostacyclin and prostaglandin E2, which are potent vasodilators. These vasodilators also act to reduce volume overload produced by the renin-angiotensin-aldosterone system by inhibiting sodium and water reabsorption by the kidneys.

Counteracting hormones

Atrial natriuretic factor is a hormone that's secreted mainly by the atria in response to stimulation of the stretch receptors in the atria caused by excess fluid volume. This hormone works to counteract the negative effects of sympathetic nervous system stimulation and the renin-angiotensin-aldosterone system by producing vasodilation and diuresis.

BNP is another hormone that's secreted by the ventricle in response to increased ventricular pressures. BNP works in the same manner as atrial natriuretic factor to help counteract the sympathetic nervous system and the renin-angiotensin-aldosterone system.

What to look for

Learn to recognize the signs and symptoms of both right- and left-sided heart failure to ensure that your patient receives attention promptly.

Left-sided heart failure
Look for these early and later signs of disease.

Early bird specials

Early signs and symptoms of left-sided heart failure include:
- dyspnea
- orthopnea
- paroxysmal nocturnal dyspnea
- fatigue
- nonproductive cough.

Late night leftovers

Later clinical manifestations of left-sided heart failure may include:
- crackles on auscultation
- hemoptysis
- displacement of the PMI toward the left anterior axillary line
- tachycardia
- S_3 heart sound
- S_4 heart sound
- cool, cyanotic skin
- confusion.

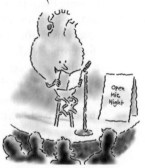

No need to tear up the floorboards to uncover the telltale signs of left- and right-sided heart failure. They're all written here for our edification.

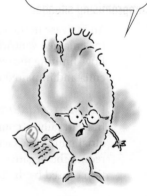

There's no doubt about it . . . I'm failing!

Right–sided heart failure

Look for these clinical manifestations of right-sided heart failure:
- neck vein distention
- hepatojugular reflux and hepatomegaly
- right upper quadrant pain
- anorexia and nausea
- nocturia
- weight gain
- pitting edema
- ascites or anasarca
- S_3 heart sound.

What tests tell you

These tests are used to diagnose heart failure:
- Chest X-ray shows increased pulmonary vascular markings, interstitial edema, or pleural effusion and cardiomegaly.
- ECG may indicate hypertrophy, ischemic changes, or infarction and may also reveal tachycardia.
- Laboratory testing may reveal abnormal liver function, elevated BUN and creatinine levels, and elevated BNP levels. (See *BNP: A potent predictor*.)
- ABG analysis may reveal hypoxemia from impaired gas exchange and respiratory alkalosis because the patient blows off more carbon dioxide as respiratory rate increases in compensation.
- Echocardiography may reveal left ventricular hypertrophy, dilation, and abnormal contractility.

Weighing the evidence

BNP: A potent predictor

It has been shown that elevated levels of B-type natriuretic peptide (BNP) can predict sudden death in patients with heart failure. In a follow-up study, researchers sought to determine the best predictors of mortality by comparing BNP levels with other established mortality predictors: peak oxygen consumption, BUN levels, systolic blood pressure, and pulmonary capillary wedge pressure. They analyzed data from 1,215 congestive heart failure patients and determined that BNP was the most robust predictor of mortality. They concluded that analyzing BNP levels could be useful in determining the urgency and timing of cardiac transplantation.

Source: Sachdeva, A., Horwich, T. B., & Fonarow, G. C. (2010). Comparison of usefulness of each of five predictors of mortality and urgent transplantation in patients with advanced heart failure. *American Journal of Cardiology, 106*(6), 830–835.

- Pulmonary artery monitoring typically demonstrates elevated PAP and PAWP, left ventricular end-diastolic pressure and decreased cardiac output/cardiac index in left-sided heart failure, and elevated right atrial pressure or CVP in right-sided heart failure.
- Radionuclide ventriculography may reveal an ejection fraction less than 40%; in diastolic dysfunction, the ejection fraction may be normal.

How it's treated

The goal of therapy is to improve pump function. Correction of heart failure may involve:

- treatment of the underlying cause, if it's known
- diuretics to reduce fluid volume overload, venous return, and preload
- ACE inhibitors for patients with left ventricle dysfunction to reduce production of angiotensin II, resulting in preload and afterload reduction
- beta-adrenergic blockers in patients with mild to moderate heart failure caused by left ventricular systolic dysfunction to prevent remodeling
- digoxin for patients with heart failure due to left ventricular systolic dysfunction to increase myocardial contractility, improve cardiac output, reduce the volume of the ventricle, and decrease ventricular stretch
- diuretics, nitrates, morphine, and oxygen to treat pulmonary edema
- administration of synthetic BNP medications, such as nesiritide (Natrecor), to help increase contractility
- lifestyle modifications to reduce symptoms of heart failure, such as weight loss, if obese; limited sodium (to 2 g/day) and alcohol intake; reduced fat intake; smoking cessation; stress reduction; and development of an exercise program
- CABG surgery or angioplasty for patients with heart failure due to CAD
- heart transplantation in patients receiving aggressive medical treatment but still experiencing limitations or repeated hospitalizations
- other surgery or invasive procedures, such as cardiomyoplasty, insertion of an IABP, partial left ventriculectomy, use of a mechanical VAD, and implantation of an ICD or a biventricular pacemaker.

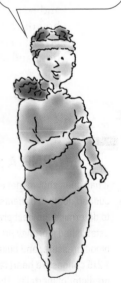

Teach your patient about lifestyle changes that can reduce symptoms of heart failure.

What to do

- Place the patient in Fowler's position to maximize chest expansion and give supplemental oxygen, as ordered, to ease his breathing. Monitor oxygen saturation levels and ABGs as indicated. If respiratory status deteriorates, anticipate the need for ET intubation and mechanical ventilation.

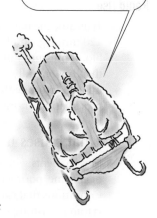

If the patient's respiratory status takes a downhill slide, be ready to institute intubation and mechanical ventilation.

Feel the rhythm

- Institute continuous cardiac monitoring and notify the practitioner of changes in rhythm and rate. If the patient develops tachycardia, administer beta-adrenergic blockers as ordered; if atrial fibrillation is present, administer anticoagulants or antiplatelet agents as ordered to prevent thrombus formation.
- If the patient develops a new arrhythmia, obtain a 12-lead ECG immediately.
- Monitor hemodynamic status, including cardiac output, cardiac index, and pulmonary and systemic vascular pressures closely, at least hourly, noting trends. If available, institute continuous cardiac output monitoring.
- Administer medications as ordered. Check apical heart rate before administering digoxin.
- Assess respiratory status frequently, at least every 1 to 2 hours. Auscultate lungs for abnormal breath sounds, such as crackles, wheezes, and rhonchi. Encourage coughing and deep breathing.
- Obtain daily weights and observe for peripheral edema.
- Assess hourly urine output. Also, monitor fluid intake, including I.V. fluids.
- Frequently monitor BUN and serum creatinine; liver function studies; and serum potassium, sodium, chloride, magnesium, and BNP levels daily.

Check the patient's apical heart rate before you administer digoxin.

Event planner

- Organize all activities to provide maximum rest periods. Assess for signs of activity intolerance, such as increased shortness of breath, chest pain, increased arrhythmias, heart rate greater than 120 beats/minute, and ST-segment changes, and have the patient stop activity.
- To prevent deep vein thrombosis caused by vascular congestion, assist the patient with ROM exercises. Enforce bed rest and apply antiembolism stockings or intermittent compression devices.
- Prepare the patient for surgical intervention or insertion of IABP or ICD if indicated.

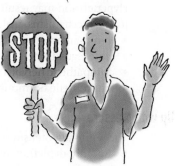

Hypertensive crisis

A hypertensive emergency, commonly called *hypertensive crisis*, refers to the abrupt, acute, and marked increase in blood pressure from the patient's baseline that ultimately leads to acute and rapidly progressing end-organ damage.

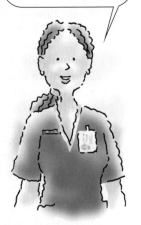

Hypertensive crisis typically strikes patients with long histories of chronic, poorly controlled, or untreated hypertension.

Rapid rise

Typically, the patient's diastolic blood pressure is greater than 120 mm Hg, and his MAP is greater than 150 mm Hg. The increased blood pressure value, although important, is probably less important than how rapidly the blood pressure increases. Arterial lines will be utilized to titrate therapy to the desired result of tissue perfusion and preservation of organ function.

What causes it

Most patients who develop hypertensive crisis have long histories of chronic, poorly controlled, or untreated primary hypertension. Conditions that cause secondary hypertension, such as pheochromocytoma, Cushing's syndrome, or autonomic dysreflexia, may also be responsible.

How it happens

Arterial blood pressure is a product of total peripheral resistance and cardiac output:
- Cardiac output is increased by conditions that increase heart rate, stroke volume, or both.
- Peripheral resistance is increased by factors that increase blood viscosity or reduce the lumen size of vessels, especially the arterioles.

Faulty mechanisms

Hypertension may result from a disturbance in one of the body's intrinsic mechanisms, including:
- renin-angiotensin system
- autoregulation
- sympathetic nervous system
- antidiuretic hormone.

Up with pressure

The renin-angiotensin system increases blood pressure in these ways:
- Sodium depletion, reduced blood pressure, and dehydration stimulate renin release.

- Renin reacts with angiotensinogen, a liver enzyme, and converts it to angiotensin I, which increases preload and afterload.
- Angiotensin I converts to angiotensin II in the lungs; angiotensin II is a potent vasoconstrictor that targets the arterioles.
- Circulating angiotensin II increases preload and afterload by stimulating the adrenal cortex to secrete aldosterone. This increases blood volume by conserving sodium and water.

Maintaining flow

In autoregulation, several intrinsic mechanisms together change an artery's diameter to maintain tissue and organ perfusion despite fluctuations in systemic blood pressure.

These mechanisms include stress relaxation and capillary fluid shifts:

- In stress relaxation, blood vessels gradually dilate when blood pressure increases, reducing peripheral resistance.
- In capillary fluid shift, plasma moves between vessels and extravascular spaces to maintain intravascular volume.

Taking control

Sympathetic nervous system mechanisms control blood pressure. When blood pressure decreases, baroreceptors in the aortic arch and carotid sinuses decrease their inhibition of the medulla's vasomotor center.

Consequent increases in sympathetic stimulation of the heart by norepinephrine increases cardiac output by:

- strengthening the contractile force
- raising the heart rate
- augmenting peripheral resistance by vasoconstriction.

Stress can also stimulate the sympathetic nervous system to increase cardiac output and peripheral vascular resistance. The release of antidiuretic hormone can regulate hypotension by increasing reabsorption of water by the kidney. In reabsorption, blood plasma volume increases, thus raising blood pressure. In hypertensive crisis, one or more of these regulating mechanisms is disrupted.

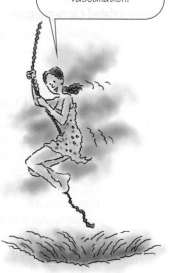

This is serious trouble! Hypertensive crisis can result in hypertensive encephalopathy because of cerebral vasodilation.

Strain for the brain

Hypertensive crisis can result in hypertensive encephalopathy because of cerebral vasodilation from an inability to maintain autoregulation. Blood flow increases, causing an increase in pressure and subsequent cerebral edema. This increase in pressure damages the intimal and medial lining of the arterioles.

What to look for

Your assessment of a patient in hypertensive crisis almost always reveals a history of hypertension that's poorly controlled or hasn't been treated. Signs and symptoms may include:
- severe, throbbing headache
- vomiting
- irritability
- confusion
- blurred vision or diplopia
- dyspnea on exertion, orthopnea, or paroxysmal nocturnal dyspnea
- angina
- possible left ventricular heave palpated at the mitral valve area
- S_4 heart sound
- acute retinopathy with retinal exudates.

Check the head

If the patient has hypertensive encephalopathy, you may note:
- decreased LOC
- disorientation
- seizures
- focal neurologic deficits, such as hemiparesis, and unilateral sensory deficits
- papilledema
- temporary vision loss.

Kidney-related consequences

If the hypertensive emergency has affected the kidneys, you may note reduced urine output as well as elevated BUN and creatinine levels.

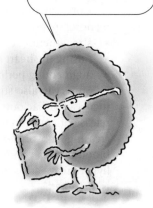

Hypertensive crisis may affect the kidneys, causing reduced urine output and elevated BUN and creatinine levels.

What tests tell you

- Blood pressure measurement confirms the diagnosis of hypertensive emergency. Blood pressure measurement, obtained several times at an interval of at least 2 minutes, reveals an elevated diastolic pressure greater than 120 mm Hg.
- If there's renal involvement, BUN may be greater than 20 mg/dl and serum creatinine level may be greater than 1.3 mg/dl.
- ECG may reveal ischemic changes or left ventricular hypertrophy.
- Echocardiography may reveal increased wall thickness with or without an increase in left ventricular size.
- Chest X-ray may reveal enlargement of the cardiac silhouette with left ventricular dilation or pulmonary congestion and pleural effusions with heart failure.

- Urinalysis results may be normal unless there's renal impairment; then specific gravity is low (less than 1.010); hematuria, casts, and proteinuria may also be found. If the patient's condition is due to a disease condition, such as pheochromocytoma, a 24-hour urine test reveals increases in vanillylmandelic acid and urinary catecholamines.
- Renal ultrasound may reveal renal artery stenosis.
- CT or MRI of the brain may show cerebral edema or hemorrhage.

How it's treated

Treatment is focused immediately on reducing the patient's blood pressure with I.V. antihypertensive therapy. However, care must be taken not to reduce the patient's blood pressure too rapidly because the patient's autoregulatory control is impaired.

Slow pressure cuts

The current recommendation is to reduce the blood pressure by no more than 25% of the MAP over the first 2 hours. Further reductions should occur over the next several days.

More measures

- Sodium nitroprusside given as an I.V. infusion and titrated according to the patient's response is the drug of choice. It has a rapid onset of action, and its effects cease within 1 to 5 minutes of stopping the drug. Thus, if the patient's blood pressure drops too low, stopping the drug almost immediately allows the blood pressure to increase.
- Other agents that may be used include labetalol, nitroglycerin (the drug of choice for treating hypertensive emergency when myocardial ischemia, acute MI, or pulmonary edema is present), and hydralazine (specifically indicated for treating hypertension in pregnant women with preeclampsia).
- Lifestyle changes may include weight reduction, smoking cessation, exercise, and dietary changes.
- After the acute episode is controlled, maintenance pharmacotherapy to control blood pressure plays a key role.

What to do

- Immediately obtain the patient's blood pressure.
- If not already in place, institute continuous cardiac and arterial pressure monitoring to assess blood pressure directly; determine the patient's MAP.
- Assess ABGs. Monitor the patient's oxygen saturation level using pulse oximetry; if you're monitoring the patient hemodynamically,

assess mixed venous oxygen saturation. Administer supplemental oxygen, as ordered, based on the findings.

- Administer I.V. antihypertensive therapy as ordered; if using nitroprusside, wrap the container in foil to protect it from the light and titrate the dose based on specified target ranges for systolic and diastolic pressures. Immediately stop the drug if the patient's blood pressure drops below the target range.
- Monitor blood pressure every 1 to 5 minutes while titrating drug therapy, then every 15 minutes to 1 hour as the patient's condition stabilizes.
- Continuously monitor ECGs and institute treatment as indicated if arrhythmias occur. Auscultate the patient's heart, noting signs of heart failure, such as S_3 or S_4 heart sounds.
- Assess the patient's neurologic status every hour initially and then every 4 hours as the patient's condition stabilizes.
- Monitor urine output every hour and notify the practitioner if output is less than 0.5 ml/kg/hour. Evaluate BUN and serum creatinine levels for changes and monitor daily weights.
- Obtain serum thiocyanate levels after 48 hours of therapy and then regularly thereafter while the patient is receiving nitroprusside.
- Administer other antihypertensives as ordered. As the patient's condition stabilizes, expect to begin oral antihypertensive therapy while gradually weaning I.V. drugs to prevent hypotension. If the patient is experiencing fluid overload, administer diuretics as ordered.
- Assess the patient's vision and report changes, such as increased blurred vision, diplopia, or loss of vision.
- Administer analgesics as ordered for headache; keep your patient's environment quiet, with low lighting.

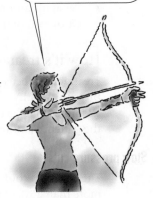

If the patient's blood pressure drops below the target range, stop I.V. hypertensive therapy.

Pericarditis

Pericarditis is an inflammation of the pericardium, the fibroserous sac that envelops, supports, and protects the heart. It occurs in acute and chronic forms. Acute pericarditis can be fibrinous or effusive, with purulent, serous, or hemorrhagic exudate. Chronic constrictive pericarditis is characterized by dense fibrous pericardial thickening.

What causes it

Pericarditis may result from:
- idiopathic factors (most common in acute pericarditis)
- bacterial, fungal, or viral infection (infectious pericarditis)

- neoplasms (primary disease or metastases from lungs, breasts, or other organs)
- high-dose radiation to the chest
- uremia
- hypersensitivity or autoimmune disease, such as acute rheumatic fever (the most common cause of pericarditis in children), systemic lupus erythematosus, and rheumatoid arthritis
- previous cardiac injury, such as MI (Dressler's syndrome), trauma, or surgery (postcardiotomy syndrome) that leaves the pericardium intact but causes blood to leak into the pericardial cavity
- drugs, such as hydralazine, procainamide, or daunorubicin.

How it happens

Here's what happens in pericarditis:
- Pericardial tissue damaged by bacteria or other substances results in the release of chemical mediators of inflammation (prostaglandins, histamines, bradykinins, and serotonin) into the surrounding tissue, thereby initiating the inflammatory process.
- Friction occurs as the inflamed pericardial layers rub against each other.
- Histamines and other chemical mediators dilate vessels and increase vessel permeability. Vessel walls then leak fluids and protein (including fibrinogen) into tissues, causing extracellular edema.
- Macrophages already present in the tissue begin to phagocytize the invading bacteria and are joined by neutrophils and monocytes.
- After several days, the area fills with an exudate composed of necrotic tissue and dead and dying bacteria, neutrophils, and macrophages.
- Eventually, the contents of the cavity autolyze and are gradually reabsorbed into healthy tissue.
- Pericardial effusion develops if fluid accumulates in the pericardial cavity.
- Cardiac tamponade results when there's a rapid accumulation of fluid in the pericardial space, compressing the heart and preventing it from filling during diastole, and resulting in a drop in cardiac output.
- Chronic constrictive pericarditis develops if the pericardium becomes thick and stiff from chronic or recurrent pericarditis, encasing the heart in a stiff shell and preventing the heart from properly filling during diastole. This causes an increase in both left- and right-sided filling pressures, leading to a drop in stroke volume and cardiac output.

Pericardial effusion develops if fluid accumulates in the pericardial cavity. Oh my!

What to look for

- The patient with acute pericarditis typically complains of sharp, sudden pain, usually starting over the sternum and radiating to the neck, shoulders, back, and arms. The pain is usually pleuritic, increasing with deep inspiration and decreasing when the patient sits up and leans forward. This decrease occurs because leaning forward pulls the heart away from the diaphragmatic pleurae of the lungs. A pericardial friction rub may be heard over the left lateral sternal border.

Cardiac complications

- Pericardial effusion, the major complication of acute pericarditis, may produce effects of heart failure, such as dyspnea, orthopnea, and tachycardia. It may also produce ill-defined substernal chest pain and a feeling of chest fullness.
- If fluid accumulates rapidly, cardiac tamponade may occur, causing pallor, clammy skin, hypotension, pulsus paradoxus, jugular vein distention, and, eventually, cardiovascular collapse and death.
- Chronic constrictive pericarditis causes a gradual increase in systemic venous pressure and produces symptoms similar to those of chronic right-sided heart failure, including fluid retention, ascites, and hepatomegaly.

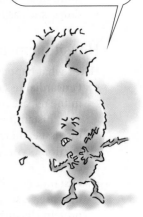

That hurts! A patient with acute pericarditis typically reports sharp, sudden pain, usually starting over the sternum and radiating to the neck, shoulders, back, and arms.

What tests tell you

These tests are used to diagnose pericarditis:
- ECG may reveal diffuse ST-segment elevation in the limb leads and most precordial leads that reflect the inflammatory process. Upright T waves are present in most leads. QRS segments may be diminished when pericardial effusion exists. Arrhythmias, such as atrial fibrillation and sinus arrhythmias, may occur. In chronic constrictive pericarditis, there may be low-voltage QRS complexes, T-wave inversion or flattening, and P mitral waves (wide P waves) in leads I, II, and V_6.
- Laboratory testing may reveal an elevated erythrocyte sedimentation rate as a result of the inflammatory process or a normal or elevated white blood cell (WBC) count, especially in infectious pericarditis; BUN may point to uremia as a cause of pericarditis. CRP levels may be elevated, indicating inflammation.
- Blood cultures may be used to identify an infectious cause.
- Antistreptolysin-O titers may be positive if pericarditis is due to rheumatic fever.
- Purified protein derivative skin test may be positive if pericarditis is due to tuberculosis.

- Echocardiography may show an echo-free space between the ventricular wall and the pericardium and reduced pumping action of the heart. It may also help identify if a pleural effusion is present. It may also help identify a pleural effusion.
- Chest X-rays may be normal with acute pericarditis. The cardiac silhouette may be enlarged, with a water bottle shape caused by fluid accumulation, if pleural effusion is present.

How it's treated

Treatment for a patient with pericarditis is done to:

- relieve symptoms
- prevent or correct pericardial effusion and cardiac tamponade
- manage the underlying disease.

> You should really be in an upright position to relieve dyspnea and chest pain.

Bed rest and drug therapy

In idiopathic pericarditis, post MI pericarditis, and postthoracotomy pericarditis, treatment is twofold, including:

- bed rest as long as fever and pain persist
- administration of NSAIDs to relieve pain and reduce inflammation.

If symptoms continue, the practitioner may prescribe corticosteroids to provide rapid and effective relief. Corticosteroids must be used cautiously because pericarditis may recur when drug therapy stops.

Further treatments

When infectious pericarditis results from disease of the left pleural space, mediastinal abscesses, or septicemia, the patient requires antibiotics, surgical drainage, or both.

If cardiac tamponade develops, the doctor may perform emergency pericardiocentesis and may inject antibiotics directly into the pericardial sac.

Heavy-duty treatments

Recurrent pericarditis may necessitate partial pericardiectomy, which creates a window that allows fluid to drain into the pleural space. In constrictive pericarditis, total pericardiectomy may be necessary to permit the heart to fill and contract adequately.

What to do

- Maintain the patient on bed rest until fever and pain diminish. Assist the patient with bathing if necessary. Provide a bedside commode to reduce myocardial oxygen demand.

- Place the patient in an upright position to relieve dyspnea and chest pain. Auscultate lung sounds at least every 2 hours. Administer supplemental oxygen as needed based on oxygen saturation or mixed venous oxygen saturation levels.
- Administer analgesics to relieve pain and NSAIDs, as ordered, to reduce inflammation. Administer steroids if the patient fails to respond to NSAIDs.
- If your patient has a PA catheter, monitor hemodynamic status. Assess the patient's cardiovascular status frequently, watching for signs of cardiac tamponade.
- Administer antibiotics on time to maintain consistent drug levels in the blood.
- Institute continuous cardiac monitoring to evaluate for changes in ECG. Look for the return of ST segments to baseline with T-wave flattening by the end of the first 7 days.
- Keep a pericardiocentesis set available if pericardial effusion is suspected and prepare the patient for pericardiocentesis as indicated.
- Provide appropriate postoperative care, similar to that given after cardiothoracic surgery.

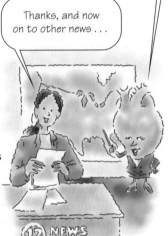

Look for a return of ST segments to baseline levels with T-waves flattening by the end of the week, Joy.

Thanks, and now on to other news . . .

Valvular heart disease

In valvular heart disease, three types of mechanical disruption can occur:
1. stenosis, or narrowing, of the valve opening
2. incomplete closure of the valve
3. prolapse of the valve.

What causes it

Valvular heart disease in children and adolescents most commonly results from congenital heart defects. In adults, rheumatic heart disease is a common cause.

Other causes are grouped according to the type of valvular heart disease and include the following:

Mitral insufficiency
- Hypertrophic cardiomyopathy
- Papillary muscle dysfunction
- Left ventricle dilation from left ventricle failure

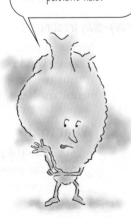

Valvular heart diseases are categorized according to the specific valves (mitral, aortic, or pulmonic) and type of disorder (stenosis or insufficiency) the patient has.

Mitral stenosis
- Endocarditis
- Left atrium tumors
- Mitral annulus calcification

Aortic insufficiency
- Calcification
- Endocarditis
- Hypertension
- Drugs, especially appetite suppressants

Aortic stenosis
- Calcification

Pulmonic stenosis
- Carcinoid syndrome

How it happens

Valvular heart disease may result from numerous conditions, which vary and are different for each type of valve disorder. Pathophysiology of valvular heart disease varies according to the valve and the disorder.

Mitral insufficiency

In mitral insufficiency, blood from the left ventricle flows back into the left atrium during systole, causing the atrium to enlarge to accommodate the backflow. As a result, the left ventricle also dilates to accommodate the increased volume of blood from the atrium and to compensate for diminishing cardiac output.

Ventricular hypertrophy and increased end-diastolic pressure result in increased PAP, eventually leading to left-sided and right-sided heart failure.

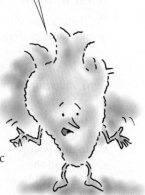

Although the pathophysiology varies with the type of valve and specific disorder, the end result seems to be the same—some form of heart failure and pulmonary involvement.

Mitral stenosis

In mitral stenosis, the valve narrows as a result of valvular abnormalities, fibrosis, or calcification. This obstructs blood flow from the left atrium to the left ventricle. Consequently, left atrial volume and pressure increase and the chamber dilates.

Greater resistance to blood flow causes pulmonary hypertension, right ventricular hypertrophy, and right-sided heart failure. Also, inadequate filling of the left ventricle produces low cardiac output.

Aortic insufficiency

In aortic insufficiency, blood flows back into the left ventricle during diastole, causing fluid overload in the ventricle which, in turn, dilates and hypertrophies. The excess volume causes fluid overload in the left atrium and, finally, the pulmonary system. Left-sided heart failure and pulmonary edema eventually result.

Aortic stenosis

In aortic stenosis, elevated left ventricular pressure tries to overcome the resistance of the narrowed valvular opening. The added workload increases the demand for oxygen, and diminished cardiac output causes poor coronary artery perfusion, ischemia of the left ventricle, and left-sided heart failure.

Pulmonic stenosis

In pulmonic stenosis, obstructed right ventricular outflow causes right ventricular hypertrophy in an attempt to overcome resistance to the narrow valvular opening. The ultimate result is right-sided heart failure.

What to look for

The history and physical examination findings vary according to the type of valvular defects.

Mitral insufficiency

Signs and symptoms of mitral insufficiency include:
- orthopnea
- dyspnea
- fatigue
- angina (rare)
- palpitations
- right-sided heart failure (jugular vein distention, peripheral edema, hepatomegaly)
- systolic murmur
- split S_2, S_3, and S_4 heart sounds.

Mitral stenosis

Signs and symptoms of mitral stenosis include:
- dyspnea on exertion, paroxysmal nocturnal dyspnea, orthopnea
- fatigue, weakness
- right-sided heart failure
- crackles on auscultation
- palpitations
- loud S_1 and S_2
- middiastolic murmur.

Aortic insufficiency

Signs and symptoms of aortic insufficiency include:
- dyspnea
- cough
- left-sided heart failure
- pulsus biferiens (rapidly rising and collapsing pulses)
- blowing diastolic murmur or S_3
- chest pain with exertion
- crackles on auscultation.

Aortic stenosis

Signs and symptoms of aortic stenosis include:
- dyspnea and paroxysmal nocturnal dyspnea
- fatigue
- syncope
- angina
- palpitations and cardiac arrhythmias
- left-sided heart failure
- systolic murmur at the base of the carotids
- chest pain with exertion
- split S_1 and S_2.

Pulmonic stenosis

Although a patient with pulmonic stenosis may be asymptomatic, possible signs and symptoms include:
- dyspnea on exertion
- right-sided heart failure
- systolic murmur.

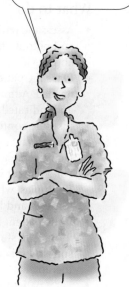

Be aware that a patient with pulmonic stenosis may have no symptoms at all.

What tests tell you

The diagnosis of valvular heart disease can be based on the results of:
- cardiac catheterization
- chest X-rays
- echocardiography
- ECG.

How it's treated

Treatments for patients with valvular heart disease commonly include:
- digoxin, a low-sodium diet, diuretics, vasodilators, and especially ACE inhibitors to correct left-sided heart failure
- oxygen administration in acute situations to increase oxygenation

- anticoagulants to prevent thrombus formation around diseased or replaced valves
- prophylactic antibiotics before and after surgery or dental care to prevent endocarditis
- nitroglycerin to relieve angina in conditions such as aortic stenosis
- beta-adrenergic blockers or digoxin to slow the ventricular rate in atrial fibrillation or atrial flutter
- cardioversion to convert atrial fibrillation to sinus rhythm
- open or closed commissurotomy to separate thick or adherent mitral valve leaflets
- balloon valvuloplasty to enlarge the orifice of a stenotic mitral, aortic, or pulmonic valve
- annuloplasty or valvuloplasty to reconstruct or repair the valve in mitral insufficiency
- valve replacement with a prosthetic valve for mitral and aortic valve disease.

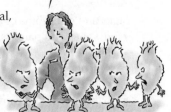

Treatment for valvular heart disease typically includes giving various combinations of medications and, in some cases, valve repair or replacement.

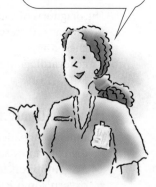

Watch those valves. If the patient has mitral stenosis, observe closely for signs and symptoms of pulmonary dysfunction, emboli, and adverse reactions to drug therapy.

What to do

- Assess the patient's vital signs, ABG values, pulse oximetry, intake and output, daily weights, blood chemistry studies, chest X-rays, and ECG.
- Place the patient in an upright position to relieve dyspnea if needed. Administer oxygen to prevent tissue hypoxia as needed and indicated by ABGs and pulse oximetry.
- Institute continuous cardiac monitoring to evaluate for arrhythmias; if any occur, administer appropriate therapy according to facility policy and the practitioner's order.
- For a patient with aortic insufficiency, observe the ECG for arrhythmias, which can increase the risk of pulmonary edema, and for fever and infection.
- If the patient has mitral stenosis, watch closely for signs of pulmonary dysfunction caused by pulmonary hypertension, tissue ischemia caused by emboli, and adverse reactions to drug therapy.
- For a patient with mitral insufficiency, observe for signs and symptoms of left-sided heart failure, pulmonary edema, and adverse reactions to drug therapy.

Quick quiz

1. The nurse obtains a rhythm strip on a patient who has had a myocardial infarction and makes the following analysis: P wave not apparent, ventricular rate 170, RR interval not measurable with a wide and distorted QRS complex. The nurse interprets this rhythm as:

    A. Sinus bradycardia
    B. Junctional escape rhythm
    C. Atrial fibrillation
    D. Ventricular tachycardia

Answer: D. The key variables when evaluating this rhythm is that there are no P waves present, and the QRS complex is wide and distorted.

2. A patient with dilated cardiomyopathy has developed atrial fibrillation that is unresponsive to drug therapy. The nurse anticipates the patient may need teaching about:

    A. Cardiac catheterization
    B. Insertion of an implantable cardioverter-defibrillator
    C. Electrical cardioversion
    D. Lifestyle modifications

Answer: C. After assessing for blood clots, there is a potential the patient could be a candidate for electrical cardioversion. The patient will also need to be anticoagulated with Coumadin to ensure no complications of emboli arise from the arterial fibrillation.

3. Which action should the nurse take first when preparing a patient for cardioversion with stable supraventricular tachycardia who is alert and oriented?

    A. Turn the synchronizer to the "off" position.
    B. Start a peripheral I.V. and ensure patency.
    C. Set the defibrillator to 300 joules.
    D. Place the patient on 100% nonrebreather.

Answer: B. A peripheral I.V. is needed in case the cardioversion puts the patient in a potential lethal dysrhythmia. It will also be needed to administer sedative medications.

4. Which parameter is often measured in right-sided heart failure to ensure appropriate fluid volume status within the patient?

    A. CVP
    B. Left-ventricular end-diastolic pressure
    C. PAWP
    D. Cardiac output

Answer: A. CVP is elevated in right-sided heart failure and is directly related to preload.

5. A patient whose cardiac monitor shows sinus bradycardia at the rate of 55 beats/minute; upon assessment, the nurse finds the patient is apneic with no palpable pulses. What should the nurse do first?
    A. Defibrillate.
    B. Give 100% oxygen per nonrebreather.
    C. Administer epinephrine.
    D. Start CPR and initiate a code blue.

Answer: D. The patient is in pulseless electrical activity and will need immediate lifesaving interventions. The nurse will need to start CPR and call a code blue.

Scoring

☆☆☆ If you answered all five questions correctly, you're all heart! (You'd have to be to make it through this cardiovascular workout!)

☆☆ If you answered four questions correctly, take heart. You have all the blood and gumption you need to succeed.

☆ If you answered fewer than four questions correctly, have yourself a heart-to-heart, then try again. You'll do better next time.

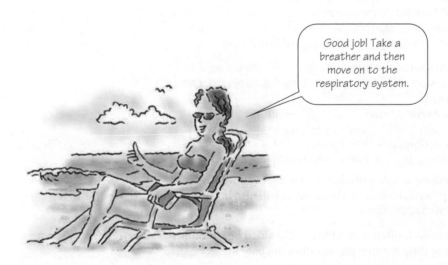

Good job! Take a breather and then move on to the respiratory system.

Suggested References

Jacobs, A. K., Antman, E. M., Faxon, D. P., Gregory, T., & Solis, P. (2007). Development of symptoms of care for ST-elevation myocardial infarction patients: Executive summary. *Circulation, 116*, 217–230.

Kushner, F. G., Hand, M., Smith, S. C., Jr., King, S. B., III, Anderson, J. L., Antman, E. M., . . . Williams, D. O. (2009). 2009 Focused updates: ACC/ACH guidelines for the management of patients with ST-elevation myocardial infarction and ACC/AHA/SCAI guidelines on percutaneous coronary intervention: A report of the American College of Cardiology Foundation/American Heart Association Task Force on Practice Guidelines. *Journal of the American College of Cardiology, 54*(23), 2205–2241.

Meaney, P. A., Bobrow, B. J., Mancini, M. E., Christenson, J., de Caen, A. R., Bhanji, F., . . . Leary, M. (2013). Cardiopulmonary resuscitation quality: Improving cardiac resuscitation outcomes both inside and outside the hospital— A concensus statement from the American Heart Association. *Circulation, 128*, 417–435.

Skillings, K., & Curtis, B. (2010). Tracheal tube cuff care. In D. J. Lynn-McHale Wiegand (Ed.), *AACN procedure manual for critical care* (6th ed., pp. 88–95). Philadelphia, PA: Saunders.

Sole, M. L., Klein, D. G., & Moseley, M. J. (Eds.). (2013). *Introduction to critical care nursing* (6th ed.). St. Louis, MO: Elsevier.

Storm, J. B., & Libby, P. (2011). Atherosclerosis. In L. S. Lilly (Ed.), *Pathophysiology of heart disease: A collaborative project of medical students and faculty* (5th ed., pp. 113–134). Philadelphia, PA: Lippincott Williams & Wilkins.

Wright, R. S., Anderson, J. L., Adams, C. D., Bridges, C. R., Casey, D. E., Jr., Ettinger, S. M., . . . Zidar, J. P. (2011). 2011 ACCF/AHA focused update of the guidelines for the management of patients with unstable angina/non–ST-elevation myocardial infarction: A report of the American College of Cardiology Foundation/American Heart Association Task Force on Practice Guidelines. *Journal of American College of Cardiology, 57*(19), 215–367.

Chapter 5

Respiratory system

Just the facts

In this chapter, you'll learn:

◆ structure and function of the respiratory system

◆ assessment of the respiratory system

◆ diagnostic tests and procedures for the respiratory system

◆ respiratory disorders and treatments.

Understanding the respiratory system

The respiratory system delivers oxygen to the bloodstream and removes excess carbon dioxide from the body.

Respiratory system structures

The structures of the respiratory system include the airways and lungs, bony thorax, and respiratory muscles. (See *A close look at the respiratory system*.)

Airways and lungs

The airways of the respiratory system consist of two parts: the upper and lower airways. The two lungs are parts of the lower airway and share space in the thoracic cavity with the heart and great vessels, trachea, esophagus, and bronchi.

Upper airway

The upper airway warms, filters, and humidifies inhaled air and then sends it to the lower airway. It also contains the structures that enable a person to make sounds. Upper airway structures include the nasopharynx (nose), oropharynx (mouth), laryngopharynx, and larynx.

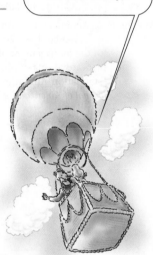

What a system the body has going! The upper airways warm, filter, and humidify air before sending it to the lower airways.

A close look at the respiratory system

Get to know the basic structures and functions of the respiratory system so you can perform a comprehensive respiratory assessment and identify abnormalities. The major structures of the upper and lower airways are illustrated below. An alveolus, or acinus, is shown in the inset.

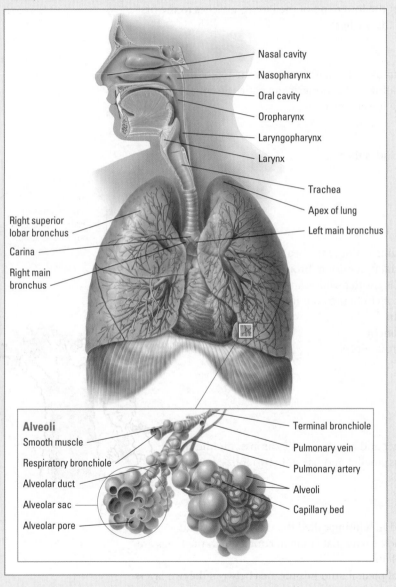

Nasal cavity

Nasopharynx

Oral cavity

Oropharynx

Laryngopharynx

Larynx

Trachea

Apex of lung

Left main bronchus

Right superior lobar bronchus

Carina

Right main bronchus

Alveoli

Smooth muscle

Respiratory bronchiole

Alveolar duct

Alveolar sac

Alveolar pore

Terminal bronchiole

Pulmonary vein

Pulmonary artery

Alveoli

Capillary bed

In the zone

The larynx, which is located at the top of the trachea, houses the vocal cords. It's the transition point between the upper and lower airways.

The larynx is composed of nine cartilage segments. The largest is the shield-shaped thyroid cartilage. The cricoid cartilage, which is the only complete ring at the lower end of the larynx, attaches to the first cartilaginous ring of the trachea.

To flap and protect

The epiglottis is a flap of tissue that closes over the top of the larynx when the patient swallows. This protects the patient from aspirating food or fluid into the lower airways.

Lower airway

The lower airway includes the:
- trachea
- bronchi
- lungs.

Lowdown on lower airway

The lower airway begins with the trachea, which divides at the carina to form the right and left mainstem bronchi of the lungs. The right mainstem bronchus is shorter, wider, and more vertical than the left.

The mainstem bronchi branch out in the lungs, forming the:
- segmental bronchi
- subsegmental bronchi
- nonrespiratory bronchioles
- respiratory bronchioles
- alveolar ducts
- alveoli.

Lungs and lobes

The right lung is larger and has three lobes: upper, middle, and lower. The left lung is smaller and has only two lobes: upper and lower.

Plenty of pleura

Each lung is wrapped in a lining called the *visceral pleura*, and all areas of the thoracic cavity that come in contact with the lungs are lined with parietal pleura.

A small amount of pleural fluid fills the area between the two layers of the pleura. This allows the layers to slide smoothly over each other as the chest expands and contracts. The parietal pleura also contain nerve endings that transmit pain signals when inflammation occurs.

> The mainstem bronchi branch out in the lungs to form smaller airways.

All about alveoli

The alveoli are the gas exchange units of the lungs. The lungs in a typical adult contain about 300 million alveoli.

Alveoli consist of type I and type II epithelial cells:

- Type I cells form the alveolar walls, through which gas exchange occurs.
- Type II cells produce surfactant, a lipoprotein that coats the alveoli. During inspiration, the alveolar surfactant allows the alveoli to expand uniformly. During expiration, the surfactant prevents alveolar collapse.

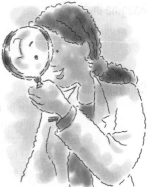

Hundreds of millions of tiny alveoli conduct gas exchange in the lungs.

In circulation

Oxygen-depleted blood enters the lungs from the pulmonary artery of the right ventricle, then flows through the main pulmonary arteries into the smaller vessels of the pleural cavities and the main bronchi, through the arterioles, and eventually, to the capillary networks in the alveoli.

Trading gases

Gas exchange (oxygen and carbon dioxide diffusion) takes place in the alveoli. After passing through the pulmonary capillaries, oxygenated blood flows through progressively larger vessels, enters the main pulmonary veins, and finally, flows into the left atrium. (See *Tracking pulmonary circulation*.)

Tracking pulmonary circulation

The right and left pulmonary arteries carry deoxygenated blood from the right side of the heart to the lungs. These arteries divide to form distal branches called *arterioles*, which terminate as a concentrated capillary network in the alveoli and alveolar sac, where gas exchange occurs.

Venules—the end branches of the pulmonary veins—collect oxygenated blood from the capillaries and transport it to larger vessels, which carry it to the pulmonary veins. The pulmonary veins enter the left side of the heart, where oxygenated blood is distributed throughout the body.

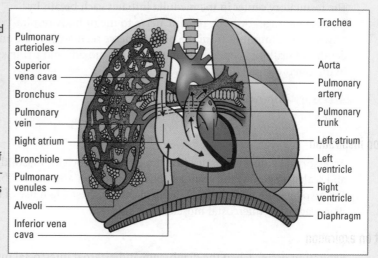

Bony thorax

The bony thorax is composed of:
- clavicles
- sternum
- scapula
- 12 sets of ribs
- 12 thoracic vertebrae.

Imagine that!

Parts of the thorax and some imaginary vertical lines on the chest are used to describe the locations of pulmonary assessment findings. (See *Respiratory assessment landmarks.*)

Can you take a ribbing?

Ribs are made of bone and cartilage and allow the chest to expand and contract during each breath. All ribs are attached to vertebrae. The first seven ribs also are attached directly to the sternum. The 8th, 9th, and 10th ribs are attached to the ribs above them. The 11th and 12th ribs are called *floating ribs* because they aren't attached to any other bones in the front.

Respiratory muscles

The primary muscles used in breathing are the diaphragm and the external intercostal muscles. These muscles contract when the patient inhales and relax when the patient exhales.

Brain–breath connection

The respiratory center in the medulla initiates each breath by sending messages over the phrenic nerve to the primary respiratory muscles. Impulses from the phrenic nerve regulate the rate and depth of breathing, depending on the carbon dioxide and pH levels in the cerebrospinal fluid.

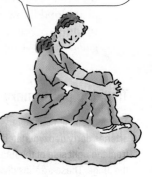

Ho-hum. The diaphragm and the external intercostal muscles contract on inhalation and relax on exhalation.

Accessory inspiratory muscles
Here's how other muscles assist in breathing:

In on inspiration

Accessory inspiratory muscles (the trapezius, sternocleidomastoid, and scalenes) elevate the scapula, clavicle, sternum, and upper ribs. This expands the front-to-back diameter of the chest when use of the diaphragm and intercostal muscles isn't effective.

Out on expiration

Expiration occurs when the diaphragm and external intercostal muscles relax. If the patient has an airway obstruction, he may also use the abdominal muscles and internal intercostal muscles to exhale. (See *Understanding the mechanics of breathing*, page 316.)

Respiratory assessment landmarks

Use these figures to find the common landmarks used in respiratory assessment.

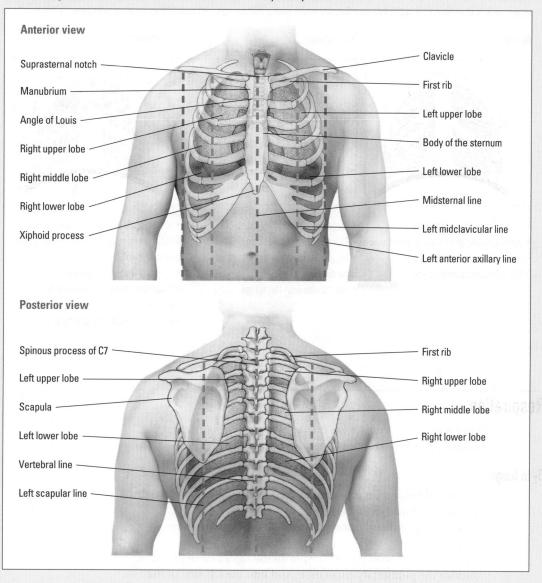

Anterior view

Suprasternal notch

Manubrium

Angle of Louis

Right upper lobe

Right middle lobe

Right lower lobe

Xiphoid process

Clavicle

First rib

Left upper lobe

Body of the sternum

Left lower lobe

Midsternal line

Left midclavicular line

Left anterior axillary line

Posterior view

Spinous process of C7

Left upper lobe

Scapula

Left lower lobe

Vertebral line

Left scapular line

First rib

Right upper lobe

Right middle lobe

Right lower lobe

Understanding the mechanics of breathing

Mechanical forces, such as movement of the diaphragm and intercostal muscles, drive the breathing process. In these depictions, a plus sign ($+$) indicates positive pressure and a minus sign ($-$) indicates negative pressure.

At rest	Inhalation	Exhalation
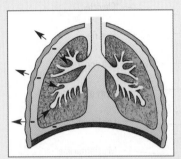	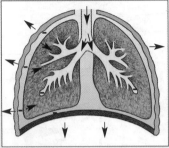	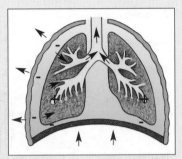

- Inspiratory muscles relax.
- Atmospheric pressure is maintained in the tracheobronchial tree.
- No air movement occurs.

- Inspiratory muscles contract.
- The diaphragm descends.
- Negative alveolar pressure is maintained.
- Air moves into the lungs.

- Inspiratory muscles relax, causing the lungs to recoil to their resting size and position.
- The diaphragm ascends.
- Positive alveolar pressure is maintained.
- Air moves out of the lungs.

Respiration

Effective respiration requires gas exchange in the lungs (external respiration) and in the tissues (internal respiration).

O₂ to lungs

Three external respiration processes are needed to maintain adequate oxygenation and acid–base balance:
1. Ventilation (gas distribution into and out of the pulmonary airways)
2. Pulmonary perfusion (blood flow from the right side of the heart, through the pulmonary circulation, and into the left side of the heart)
3. Diffusion (gas movement from an area of greater to lesser concentration through a semipermeable membrane).

O_2 to tissues

Internal respiration occurs only through diffusion, when the red blood cells (RBCs) release oxygen and absorb carbon dioxide.

Ventilation and perfusion

Gravity affects oxygen and carbon dioxide transport in a positive way by causing more unoxygenated blood to travel to the lower and middle lung lobes than to the upper lobes. That's why ventilation and perfusion differ in various parts of the lungs.

> Gas exchange is most efficient where perfusion and ventilation match.

Match game

Areas where perfusion and ventilation are similar have a ventilation-perfusion ($\dot{V}/\dot{Q}$) match; gas exchange is most efficient in such areas.

For example, in normal lung function, the alveoli receive air at a rate of about 4,000 cc/minute, while the capillaries supply blood to the alveoli at a rate of about 5 L/minute, creating a $\dot{V}/\dot{Q}$ ratio of 4:5 or 0.8. (See *Understanding ventilation and perfusion*, page 318.)

Mismatch mayhem

A $\dot{V}/\dot{Q}$ mismatch, resulting from $\dot{V}/\dot{Q}$ dysfunction or altered lung mechanics, causes most of the impaired gas exchange in respiratory disorders.

Ineffective gas exchange between the alveoli and pulmonary capillaries can affect all body systems by changing the amount of oxygen delivered to living cells. Ineffective gas exchange causes three outcomes:

- *Shunting* (reduced ventilation to a lung unit) causes unoxygenated blood to move from the right side of the heart to the left side of the heart and into systemic circulation. Shunting may result from a physical defect that allows unoxygenated blood to bypass fully functioning alveoli. It may also result when airway obstruction prevents oxygen from reaching an adequately perfused area of the lung. Common causes of shunting include acute respiratory distress syndrome (ARDS), atelectasis, pneumonia, and pulmonary edema.
- *Dead-space ventilation* (reduced perfusion to a lung unit) occurs when alveoli don't have adequate blood supply for gas exchange

Understanding ventilation and perfusion

Effective gas exchange depends on the relationship between ventilation and perfusion, or the ($\dot{V}/\dot{Q}$) ratio. The diagrams below show what happens when the ($\dot{V}/\dot{Q}$) ratio is normal and abnormal.

Normal ventilation and perfusion

When ventilation and perfusion are matched, unoxygenated blood from the venous system returns to the right side of the heart and through the pulmonary artery to the lungs, carrying carbon dioxide (CO_2). The arteries branch into the alveolar capillaries. Gas exchange takes place in the alveolar capillaries.

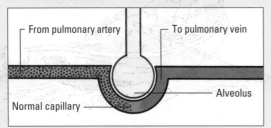

Inadequate perfusion (dead-space ventilation)

When the ($\dot{V}/\dot{Q}$) ratio is high, as shown here, ventilation is normal but alveolar perfusion is reduced or absent. Note the narrowed capillary, indicating poor perfusion. This commonly results from a perfusion defect, such as pulmonary embolism or a disorder that decreases cardiac output.

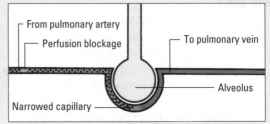

Inadequate ventilation (shunt)

When the ($\dot{V}/\dot{Q}$) ratio is low, pulmonary circulation is adequate but not enough oxygen is available to the alveoli for normal diffusion. A portion of the blood flowing through the pulmonary vessels doesn't become oxygenated.

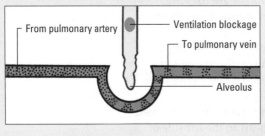

Inadequate ventilation and perfusion (silent unit)

A silent unit indicates an absence of ventilation and perfusion to the lung area. A silent unit may help compensate for a ($\dot{V}/\dot{Q}$) balance by delivering blood flow to better ventilated lung areas.

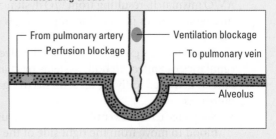

KEY ▨ Blood with CO_2 ▨ Blood with O_2 ▨ Blood with CO_2 and O_2

to occur, such as with pulmonary emboli and pulmonary infarction.
- A *silent unit* (a combination of shunting and dead-space ventilation) occurs when little or no ventilation and perfusion are present, such as in cases of pneumothorax and severe ARDS.

Oxygen transport

Most oxygen collected in the lungs binds with hemoglobin to form oxyhemoglobin; however, a small portion of it dissolves in the plasma. The portion of oxygen that dissolves in the plasma can be measured as the partial pressure of arterial oxygen (PaO_2) in blood.

Riding the RBC express

After oxygen binds to hemoglobin, RBCs carry it by way of the circulatory system to tissues throughout the body. Internal respiration occurs by cellular diffusion when RBCs release oxygen and absorb the carbon dioxide produced by cellular metabolism. The RBCs then transport the carbon dioxide back to the lungs for removal during expiration.

Acid–base balance

Because carbon dioxide is 20 times more soluble than oxygen, it dissolves in the blood, where most of it forms bicarbonate (a base) and smaller amounts form carbonic acid.

Acid–base controller

The lungs control bicarbonate levels by converting bicarbonate to carbon dioxide and water for excretion. In response to signals from the medulla, the lungs can change the rate and depth of ventilation. This controls acid–base balance by adjusting the amount of carbon dioxide that's lost.

In metabolic alkalosis, which results from excess bicarbonate retention, the rate and depth of ventilation decrease so that carbon dioxide is retained. This increases carbonic acid levels.

In metabolic acidosis (resulting from excess acid retention or excess bicarbonate loss), the lungs increase the rate and depth of ventilation to exhale excess carbon dioxide, thereby reducing carbonic acid levels.

> Poorly functioning lungs can produce acid–base imbalances.

Off balance

Inadequately functioning lungs can produce acid–base imbalances. For example, *hypoventilation* (reduced rate and depth of ventilation) results in carbon dioxide retention, causing respiratory acidosis. Conversely, *hyperventilation* (increased rate and depth of ventilation) leads to increased exhalation of carbon dioxide and causes respiratory alkalosis.

Respiratory assessment

Respiratory assessment is a critical nursing responsibility. Conduct a thorough assessment to detect both obvious and subtle respiratory changes.

History

Build your patient's health history by asking short, open-ended questions. Conduct the interview in several short sessions if you have to, depending on the severity of your patient's condition. Ask his family to provide information if your patient can't.

Respiratory disorders may be caused or exacerbated by obesity, smoking, environmental, and workplace conditions so be sure to ask about these conditions.

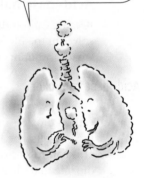

Respiratory disorders may be caused or worsened by obesity, smoking, environmental and workplace conditions.

Current health status

Begin by asking why your patient is seeking care. Because many respiratory disorders are chronic, ask how the patient's latest acute episode compares with previous episodes and what relief measures are helpful and unhelpful.

Chronic complaint department

Patients with respiratory disorders commonly report such complaints as:
- shortness of breath
- cough
- sputum production
- wheezing
- chest pain
- sleep disturbance.

Shortness of breath

Assess your patient's shortness of breath by asking him to rate his usual level of dyspnea on a scale of 0 to 10, in which 0 means no dyspnea and 10 means the worst he has experienced. Then ask him to rate his current level of dyspnea. Other scales grade dyspnea as it relates to activity, such as climbing a set of stairs or walking a city block. (See *Grading dyspnea.*)

In addition to using a severity scale, ask these questions: What do you do to relieve the shortness of breath? How well does it usually work?

Grading dyspnea

To assess dyspnea as objectively as possible, ask your patient to briefly describe how various activities affect his breathing. Then, document his response using this grading system:

- *Grade 0*: not troubled by breathlessness except with strenuous exercise
- *Grade 1*: troubled by shortness of breath when hurrying on a level path or walking up a slight hill
- *Grade 2*: walks more slowly on a level path (because of breathlessness) than people of the same age or has to stop to breathe when walking on a level path at his own pace
- *Grade 3*: stops to breathe after walking about 100 yards (91 m) on a level path
- *Grade 4*: too breathless to leave the house or breathless when dressing or undressing.

Pillow talk

A patient with *orthopnea* (shortness of breath when lying down) tends to sleep with his upper body elevated. Ask this patient how many pillows he uses. The answer reflects the severity of the orthopnea. For instance, a patient who uses three pillows can be said to have "three-pillow orthopnea."

> The number of pillows you need to sleep indicates the severity of your orthopnea.

Cough

Ask the patient with a cough these questions: At what time of day do you cough most often? Is the cough productive? Has it changed recently (if chronic)? If so, how? What makes the cough better? What makes it worse?

Sputum

If a patient produces sputum, ask him to estimate the amount produced in teaspoons or some other common measurement. Also ask these questions: What's the color and consistency of the sputum? Has it changed recently (if chronic)? If so, how? Do you cough up blood? If so, how much and how often?

Wheezing

If a patient wheezes, ask these questions: When does wheezing occur? What makes you wheeze? Do you wheeze loudly enough for others to hear it? What helps stop your wheezing?

Chest pain

If the patient has chest pain, ask these questions: Where is the pain? What does it feel like? Is it sharp, stabbing, burning, or aching? Does it move to another area? How long does it last? What causes it? What makes it better?

Pain provocations

Chest pain due to a respiratory problem is usually the result of pleural inflammation, inflammation of the costochondral junctions, or soreness of chest muscles because of coughing. It may also be the result of indigestion. Less common causes of pain include rib or vertebral fractures caused by coughing or osteoporosis.

Sleep disturbance

Sleep disturbances may be related to obstructive sleep apnea (OSA) or another sleep disorder requiring additional evaluation. Some important questions are "do you feel rested in the morning" and "do breathing problems cause you to awaken at night."

Daytime drowsiness

If the patient complains of being drowsy or irritable in the daytime, ask these questions: How many hours of continuous sleep do you get at night? Do you wake up often during the night? Does your family complain about your snoring or restlessness? Do you fall asleep easily during the day?

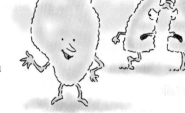

Previous health status

Look at the patient's health history, being especially watchful for:
- a smoking habit
- exposure to secondhand smoke
- allergies
- previous surgeries
- respiratory diseases, such as pneumonia, asthma, and tuberculosis (TB).

Ask about current immunizations, such as a flu shot or pneumococcal vaccine. Also determine if the patient uses any respiratory equipment, such as oxygen or nebulizers, at home.

Family history

Ask the patient if he has a family history of cancer, sickle cell anemia, heart disease, or chronic illness, such as asthma or emphysema. Determine whether the patient lives with anyone who has an infectious disease, such as TB or influenza.

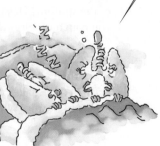

Lifestyle patterns

Ask about the patient's workplace because some jobs, such as coal mining and construction work, expose workers to substances that can cause lung disease.

Also ask about the patient's home, community, and other environmental factors that may influence how he deals with his respiratory problems. For example, you may ask questions about interpersonal relationships, stress management, and coping methods. Ask about the patient's sex habits and drug use, which may be connected with acquired immunodeficiency syndrome–related pulmonary disorders.

Physical examination

In most cases, you should begin the physical examination after you take the patient's history. However, you may not be able to take a complete history if the patient develops an ominous sign such as acute respiratory distress. If your patient is in respiratory distress, establish the priorities of your nursing assessment, progressing from the most critical factors (airway, breathing, and circulation [the ABCs]) to less critical factors. (See *Emergency respiratory assessment*, page 324.)

Four steps

Use a systematic approach to detect subtle and obvious respiratory changes. The four steps for conducting a physical examination of the respiratory system are:
- inspection
- palpation
- percussion
- auscultation.

Back, then front

Examine the back first, using inspection, palpation, percussion, and auscultation. Always compare one side with the other. Then examine the front of the chest using the same sequence. The patient can lie back when you examine the front of the chest if that's more comfortable for him.

Making introductions

Before you begin the physical examination, make sure the room is well lit and warm. Introduce yourself to the patient and explain why you're there.

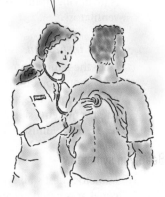

Examine the back first and always compare one side with the other, following a systematic sequence of inspection, palpation, percussion, and auscultation.

Emergency respiratory assessment

If your patient is in acute respiratory distress, immediately assess the ABCs—airway, breathing, and circulation. If these are absent, call for help and start cardiopulmonary resuscitation.

Next, quickly check for signs of impending crisis by asking yourself these questions:

• Is the patient having trouble breathing?
• Is the patient using accessory muscles to breathe? If chest excursion is less than the normal 1⅛" to 2⅜" (3 to 6 cm), look for evidence that the patient is using accessory muscles when he breathes, including shoulder elevation, intercostal muscle retraction, and use of scalene and sternocleidomastoid muscles.
• Has the patient's level of consciousness (LOC) diminished?

• Is he confused, anxious, or agitated?
• Does he change his body position to ease breathing?
• Does his skin look pale, diaphoretic, or cyanotic?

Setting priorities
If your patient is in respiratory distress, establish priorities for your nursing assessment. Don't assume the obvious. Note positive and negative factors, starting with the most critical factors (the ABCs) and progressing to less critical factors.

If you don't have time to go through each step of the nursing process, make sure you gather enough data to answer vital questions. A single sign or symptom has many possible meanings, so gather a group of findings to assess the patient and develop interventions.

Inspection

Make a few observations about the patient as soon as you enter the room and include these observations in your assessment. Note the patient's position in the bed. Does he appear comfortable? Is he sitting up or lying quietly or shifting about? Does he appear anxious? Is he having trouble breathing? Does he require oxygen? Is he on a ventilator?

Chest inspection

Help the patient into an upright position, if possible. Ideally, the patient should be undressed from the waist up or clothed in a hospital gown. Inspect the patient's chest configuration, tracheal position, chest symmetry, skin condition, and nostrils (for flaring) and look for accessory muscle use.

Beauty in symmetry

Look for chest wall symmetry. Both sides of the chest should appear equal at rest and expand equally as the patient inhales. The diameter

> Your first observations of the patient are important parts of the assessment.

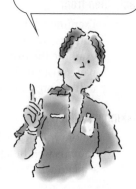

of the chest, from front to back, should be about one-half of the width of the chest.

A new angle

Also, look at the angle between the ribs and the sternum at the point immediately above the xiphoid process. This angle, the costal angle, should be less than 90 degrees in an adult. The angle is larger if the chest wall is chronically expanded because of an enlargement of the intercostal muscles, as can happen with chronic obstructive pulmonary disease (COPD).

Muscles in motion

When the patient inhales, his diaphragm should descend and the intercostal muscles should contract. This dual motion causes the abdomen to push out and the lower ribs to expand laterally. (See *Types of breathing*.)

When the patient exhales, his abdomen and ribs return to their resting positions. The upper chest shouldn't move much. Accessory muscles may hypertrophy, indicating frequent use. This may be normal in some athletes, but for most patients, it indicates a respiratory problem, especially when the patient purses his lips and flares his nostrils when breathing.

Chest wall abnormalities

Inspect for chest wall abnormalities, keeping in mind that a patient with a deformity of the chest wall might have completely normal lungs that are cramped in the chest. The patient might have a smaller-than-normal lung capacity and limited exercise tolerance.

Barrels, pigeons, and curves

Common abnormalities include:

* *Barrel chest*—A barrel chest looks like the name implies; it's abnormally round and bulging. Barrel chest may be normal in infants and elderly patients. In other patients, barrel chest occurs as a result of COPD due to lungs that have lost their elasticity. The patient typically uses accessory muscles to breathe and easily becomes breathless. Also note kyphosis of the thoracic spine.
* *Pigeon chest*—A patient with pigeon chest, or pectus carinatum, has a chest with a sternum that protrudes beyond the front of the abdomen. The displaced sternum increases the front-to-back diameter of the chest but is a minor deformity that doesn't require treatment.
* *Funnel chest*—A patient with funnel chest, or pectus excavatum, has a funnel-shaped depression on all of or part of the sternum.

Types of breathing

Men, children, and infants usually use abdominal, or diaphragmatic, breathing. Athletes and singers do as well. Most women, however, usually use chest, or intercostal, breathing.

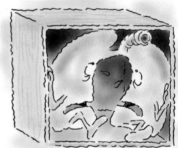

Hey, I'm pretty cramped in here!

This may cause disruptions in respiratory or cardiac function. Compression of the heart and great vessels may cause murmurs.

- *Thoracic kyphoscoliosis*—The patient's spine curves to one side and the vertebrae are rotated. Because the rotation distorts lung tissues, it may be more difficult to assess respiratory status.

> The rate, rhythm, and quality of respirations are key indicators of respiratory function.

Raising a red flag

Watch for paradoxical, or uneven, movement of the patient's chest wall. Paradoxical movement may appear as an abnormal collapse of part of the chest wall when the patient inhales or an abnormal expansion when the patient exhales. In either case, such uneven movement indicates a loss of normal chest wall function.

Breathing rate and pattern

Assess your patient's respiratory function by determining the rate, rhythm, and quality of respirations.

Count on it

Adults normally breathe at a rate of 12 to 20 breaths per minute. To determine the patient's respiratory rate, count for a full minute, or longer if you note abnormalities. Don't tell the patient what you're doing or he might alter his natural breathing pattern.

The respiratory pattern should be even, coordinated, and regular, with occasional sighs. The normal ratio of inspiration to expiration (I:E ratio) is about 1:2.

> As your patient's body temperature increases with fever, respiratory rate also increases.

Abnormal respiratory patterns

Identifying abnormal respiratory patterns can be a great help in understanding the patient's respiratory status and overall condition.

Tachypnea

Tachypnea is a respiratory rate greater than 20 breaths per minute; the depth may be normal or shallow. It's commonly seen in patients with restrictive lung disease, pain, sepsis, obesity, anxiety, and respiratory distress. Fever is another possible cause. The respiratory rate may increase by 4 breaths per minute for every 1°F (0.6°C) increase in body temperature.

Bradypnea

Bradypnea is a respiratory rate below 10 breaths per minute. It's commonly noted just before a period of apnea or full respiratory arrest.

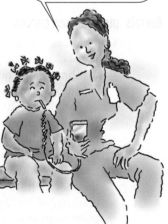

Depressed CNS

Patients with bradypnea might have central nervous system (CNS) depression as a result of excessive sedation, tissue damage, diabetic coma, or any situation in which the brain's respiratory center is depressed. Increased intracranial pressure and metabolic alkalosis may also cause bradypnea. Note that the respiratory rate is usually slower during sleep.

Apnea

Apnea is the absence of breathing. Periods of apnea may be short and occur sporadically, such as in Cheyne-Stokes respirations or other abnormal respiratory patterns. This condition may be life-threatening if periods of apnea last long enough and should be addressed immediately.

Hyperpnea

Hyperpnea is characterized by deep breathing with either a normal or increased rate. It occurs during exercise or due to fever, hypoxia, or acid–base imbalances.

Kussmaul's respirations

Kussmaul's respirations are rapid and deep, with sighing breaths. This type of breathing occurs in patients with metabolic acidosis, especially when associated with diabetic ketoacidosis, as the respiratory system tries to lower the carbon dioxide level in the blood and restore it to normal pH.

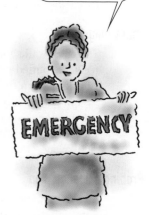

Address long periods of apnea immediately! They may be life-threatening.

Cheyne-Stokes respirations

Cheyne-Stokes respirations have a regular cycle of change in the rate and depth of breathing. Respirations are initially shallow but gradually become deeper and deeper before becoming shallow again followed by a period of apnea, lasting 20 to 60 seconds, and the cycle starts again. This respiratory pattern is seen in patients with heart failure, kidney failure, or CNS damage. Cheyne-Stokes respirations can be a normal breathing pattern during sleep in elderly patients.

Biot's respirations

Biot's respirations involve rapid deep breaths that alternate with abrupt periods of apnea. They're an ominous sign of severe CNS damage.

Inspecting related structures

Inspect the patient's skin for pallor, cyanosis, and diaphoresis.

Don't be blue

Skin color varies considerably among patients, but a patient with a bluish tint to his skin, nail beds, and mucous membranes is considered cyanotic. Cyanosis, which occurs when oxygenation to the tissues is poor, is a late sign of hypoxemia.

Finger findings

When you inspect the fingers, assess for clubbing, a sign of long-standing respiratory or cardiac disease. The fingernail normally enters the skin at an angle of less than 180 degrees. When clubbing occurs, the angle is greater than or equal to 180 degrees.

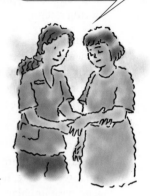

Inspect the fingers for clubbing—a sign of long-standing respiratory or cardiac disease.

Palpation

Palpation of the chest provides some important information about the respiratory system and the processes involved in breathing. (See *Palpating the chest.*)

Leaky lungs

The chest wall should feel smooth, warm, and dry. Crepitus, which feels like puffed-rice cereal crackling under the skin, indicates that air is leaking from the airways or lungs.

If a patient has a chest tube, you may find a small amount of subcutaneous air around the insertion site. If the patient has no chest tube, or the area of crepitus is getting larger, alert the practitioner right away.

Probing palpation pain

Gentle palpation shouldn't cause the patient pain. If the patient complains of chest pain, try to find a painful area on the chest wall. Here's a guide to assessing some types of chest pain:
- Painful costochondral joints are typically located at the midclavicular line or next to the sternum.
- A rib or vertebral fracture is quite painful over the fracture.
- Sore muscles may result from protracted coughing.
- A collapsed lung can cause pain in addition to dyspnea.

Feeling for fremitus

Palpate for tactile fremitus (palpable vibrations caused by the transmission of air through the bronchopulmonary system). Fremitus is decreased over areas where pleural fluid collects, when the patient speaks softly, and with pneumothorax, atelectasis, and emphysema.

Fremitus is increased normally over the large bronchial tubes and abnormally over areas in which alveoli are filled with fluid or exudates, as happens in pneumonia. (See *Checking for tactile fremitus*, page 330.)

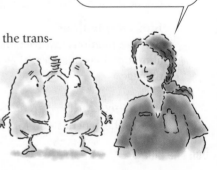

You're positive you haven't been sneaking anymore late-night crispy rice cereal snacks? You're starting to feel more crackly to me.

Palpating the chest

To palpate the chest, place the palm of your hand (or hands) lightly over the thorax, as shown below left. Palpate for tenderness, alignment, bulging, and retractions of the chest and intercostal spaces. Assess the patient for crepitus, especially around drainage sites. Repeat this procedure on the patient's back.

Next, use the pads of your fingers, as shown below right, to palpate the front and back of the thorax. Pass your fingers over the ribs and any scars, lumps, lesions, or ulcerations. Note the skin temperature, turgor, and moisture. Also note tenderness and bony or subcutaneous crepitus. The muscles should feel firm and smooth.

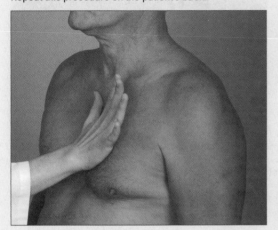

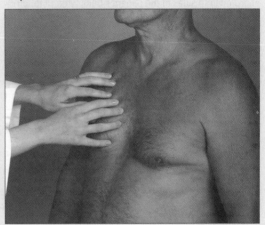

Evaluating symmetry

To evaluate your patient's chest wall symmetry and expansion, place your hands on the front of the chest wall with your thumbs touching each other at the second intercostal space. As the patient inhales deeply, watch your thumbs. They should separate simultaneously and equally to a distance several centimeters away from the sternum.

Repeat the measurement at the fifth intercostal space. You may take the same measurement on the back of the chest near the 10th rib.

Warning signs

The patient's chest may expand asymmetrically if he has:
- pleural effusion
- atelectasis
- pneumonia
- pneumothorax.

> Asymmetry or abnormal chest expansion may be warning signs of diseases and disorders.

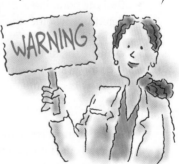

Checking for tactile fremitus

When you check the back of the thorax for tactile fremitus, ask the patient to fold his arms across his chest, as shown here. This movement shifts the scapulae out of the way.

What to do

Check for tactile fremitus by lightly placing your open palms on both sides of the patient's back without touching his back with your fingers, as shown. Ask the patient to repeat "ninety-nine" loud enough to produce palpable vibrations. Then palpate the front of the chest using the same hand positions.

What the results mean

Vibrations that feel more intense on one side than the other indicate tissue consolidation on that side. Less intense vibrations may indicate emphysema, pneumothorax, or pleural effusion. Faint or no vibrations in the upper posterior thorax may indicate bronchial obstruction or a fluid-filled pleural space.

Chest expansion may be decreased at the level of the diaphragm if the patient has:
- emphysema
- respiratory depression
- diaphragm paralysis
- atelectasis
- obesity
- ascites.

Percussion

Percuss the chest to:
- find the boundaries of the lungs
- determine whether the lungs are filled with air, fluid, or solid material
- evaluate the distance the diaphragm travels between the patient's inhalation and exhalation. (See *Percussing the chest.*)

Sites and sounds

Listen for normal, resonant sounds over most of the chest. In the left front chest wall from the third or fourth intercostal space at the sternum to the third or fourth intercostal space at the midclavicular line, listen for a dull sound; that's the space

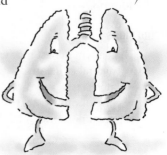

And you thought I was just filled with hot air!

Percussing the chest

To percuss the chest, hyperextend the middle finger of your left hand if you're right-handed or the middle finger of your right hand if you're left-handed.

Place your hand firmly on the patient's chest. Use the tip of the middle finger of your dominant hand—your right hand if you're right-handed, left hand if you're left-handed—to tap on the middle finger of your other hand just below the distal joint (as shown here).

The movement should come from the wrist of your dominant hand, not your elbow or upper arm. Keep the fingernail you use for tapping short so you don't hurt yourself. Follow the standard percussion sequence over the front and back chest walls.

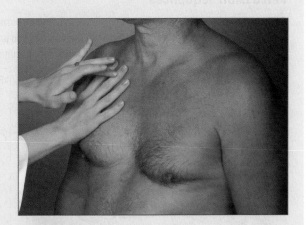

occupied by the heart. With careful percussion, you can identify the borders of the heart when lung tissue is normal. Resonance resumes at the sixth intercostal space. The sequence of sounds in the back is slightly different. (See *Percussion sequences*, page 332.)

Warning sounds

When you hear hyperresonance during percussion, it means you've found an area of increased air in the lung or pleural space. Expect to hear hyperresonance in your patients with:

- pneumothorax
- acute asthma
- *bullous emphysema* (large holes in the lungs from alveolar destruction).

When you hear abnormal dullness, it means you've found areas of decreased air in the lungs. Expect abnormal dullness in the presence of:

- pleural fluid
- consolidation atelectasis
- tumor.

Detecting diaphragm movement

Percussion also allows you to assess how much the diaphragm moves during inspiration and expiration. The normal diaphragm descends 1⅛″ to 1⅞″ (3 to 5 cm) when the patient inhales. The diaphragm doesn't move as far in patients with emphysema, respiratory depression, diaphragm paralysis, atelectasis, obesity, or ascites.

Hyperresonance indicates increased air in the lung or pleural space; dullness is a sign of decreased air in the lungs. I hear that!

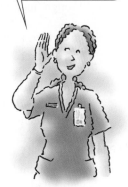

Percussion sequences

Follow these percussion sequences to distinguish between normal and abnormal sounds in the patient's lungs. Compare sound variations from one side with the other as you proceed. Carefully describe abnormal sounds you hear and note their locations. (Follow the same sequence for auscultation.)

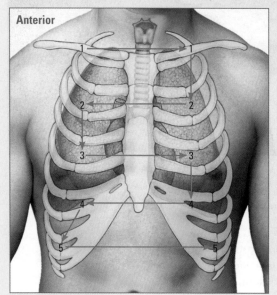

Anterior

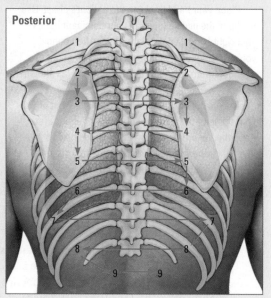

Posterior

Auscultation

As air moves through the bronchi, it creates sound waves that travel to the chest wall. The sound produced by breathing changes as air moves from larger to smaller airways. Sounds also change if they pass through fluid, mucus, or narrowed airways.

Auscultation preparation

Auscultation sites are the same as percussion sites. Listen to a full cycle of inspiration and expiration at each site, using the diaphragm of the stethoscope. Ask the patient to breathe through his mouth if it doesn't cause discomfort; nose breathing alters the pitch of breath sounds.

When things get hairy

If the patient has abundant chest hair, mat it down with a damp washcloth so the hair doesn't make sounds that could be mistaken for crackles.

> Can't decide between the mouth and the nose? When auscultating, have the patient breathe through his mouth, if possible. Nose-breathing can change the pitch of breath sounds.

Be firm

To auscultate for breath sounds, press the diaphragm side of the stethoscope firmly against the skin. Remember that if you listen through clothing or chest hair, breath sounds won't be heard clearly, and you may hear unusual and deceptive sounds.

Normal breath sounds

During auscultation, listen for four types of breath sounds over normal lungs. (See *Locations of normal breath sounds*.)

Here's a rundown of the normal breath sounds and their characteristics:

- Tracheal breath sounds, heard over the trachea, are harsh and discontinuous. They occur when the patient inhales or exhales.
- Bronchial breath sounds, usually heard next to the trachea just above or below the clavicle, are loud, high-pitched, and discontinuous. They're loudest when the patient exhales.
- Bronchovesicular sounds are medium-pitched and continuous. They're best heard over the upper third of the sternum and between the scapulae when the patient inhales or exhales.
- Vesicular sounds, heard over the rest of the lungs, are soft and low-pitched. They're prolonged during inhalation and shortened during exhalation. (See *Qualities of normal breath sounds*.)

Interpreting breath sounds

Classify each breath sound you auscultate by its intensity, pitch, duration, characteristic, and location. Note whether it occurs during inspiration, expiration, or both.

Locations of normal breath sounds

These photographs show the locations of different types of normal breath sounds.

Anterior thorax

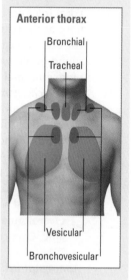

Posterior thorax

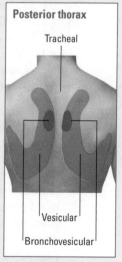

Qualities of normal breath sounds

Use this chart as a quick reference for the qualities of normal breath sounds.

Breath sound	Quality	Inspiration–expiration ratio	Location
Tracheal	Harsh, high-pitched	I < E	Over trachea
Bronchial	Loud, high-pitched	I > E	Next to trachea
Bronchovesicular	Medium in loudness and pitch	I = E	Next to sternum, between scapula
Vesicular	Soft, low-pitched	I > E	Remainder of lungs

Inspect the unexpected

Breath sounds heard in an unexpected area are abnormal. For instance, if you hear bronchial sounds where you expect to hear vesicular sounds, the area you're auscultating might be filled with fluid or exudates, as in pneumonia. The vesicular sounds you expect to hear in those areas are absent because no air is moving through the small airways.

> Breath sounds heard in an unexpected area are abnormal. Pardon me, but did you just say something?

Vocal fremitus

Vocal fremitus is the sound produced by chest vibrations as the patient speaks. Abnormal transmission of voice sounds can occur over consolidated areas because sound travels well through fluid. There are three common abnormal voice sounds:

- *Bronchophony*—Ask the patient to say "ninety-nine" or "blue moon." Over normal tissue, the words sound muffled, but over consolidated areas, the words sound unusually loud.
- *Egophony*—Ask the patient to say "E." Over normal lung tissue, the sound is muffled, but over consolidated areas, it sounds like the letter A.
- *Whispered pectoriloquy*—Ask the patient to whisper "1, 2, 3." Over normal lung tissue, the numbers are almost indistinguishable. Over consolidated tissue, the numbers sound loud and clear.

Abnormal breath sounds

Because solid tissue transmits sound better than air or fluid, breath sounds (as well as spoken or whispered words) are louder than normal over areas of consolidation. If pus, fluid, or air fills the pleural space, breath sounds are quieter than normal. If a foreign body or secretions obstruct a bronchus, breath sounds are diminished or absent over lung tissue distal to the obstruction.

Adventitious sounds

Adventitious sounds are abnormal no matter where you hear them in the lungs. (See *Abnormal breath sounds*.)

There are five types of adventitious breath sounds:

1. *Crackles* are intermittent, nonmusical, and brief crackling sounds caused by collapsed or fluid-filled alveoli popping open that are heard primarily when the patient inhales. They're classified as either fine or coarse and usually don't clear with coughing. If they do, they're most likely caused by secretions. (See *Types of crackles*, page 336.)
2. *Wheezes* are high-pitched sounds heard first when a patient exhales. They're caused by narrowed airways. As the severity of the

block increases, they may also be heard on inspiration. Patients may wheeze as a result of asthma, infection, or airway obstruction from a tumor or foreign body. (See *When wheezing stops*, page 336.)

3. *Rhonchi* are low-pitched, snoring, rattling sounds that occur primarily when a patient exhales, although they may also be heard when the patient inhales. Rhonchi usually change or disappear with coughing. The sounds occur when fluid partially blocks the large airways. Rhonchi can be heard with conditions such as COPD and pneumonia.

4. *Stridor* is a loud, high-pitched crowing sound that's heard, usually without a stethoscope, during inspiration. It's caused by an obstruction in the upper airway and requires immediate attention. Stridor can be heard in conditions such as croup, foreign body, or vocal cord edema after extubation.

5. *Pleural friction rub* is a low-pitched, grating, rubbing sound heard when the patient inhales and exhales. Pleural inflammation causes the two layers of pleura to rub together. The patient may complain of pain in areas where the rub is heard.

Diagnostic tests

If your patient's history and the physical examination findings reveal evidence of pulmonary dysfunction, diagnostic testing is done to identify and evaluate the dysfunction. These tests include:
- blood and sputum studies
- endoscopy and imaging
- pulmonary angiography
- bedside testing procedures.

Prepping the patient

Diagnostic testing may be routine for you, but it can be frightening to the patient. Take steps to prepare the patient and his family for each procedure and monitor the patient during and after the procedure.

Some tests can be performed at the bedside in the critical care unit. Many others, however, must be performed in the imaging department; in these cases, you may need to accompany unstable patients who require monitoring.

Blood and sputum studies

Blood and sputum studies include arterial blood gas (ABG) analysis and sputum analysis.

Abnormal breath sounds

Here's a quick guide to assessing abnormal breath sounds:

• *Crackles*— intermittent, nonmusical, crackling sounds heard during inspiration; classified as fine or coarse; common in elderly people when small sections of the alveoli don't fully aerate and secretions accumulate during sleep; alveoli reexpand or pop open when the patient takes deep breaths upon awakening

• *Wheezes*— high-pitched sounds caused by blocked airflow; heard on exhalation

• *Rhonchi*— low-pitched snoring or rattling sounds; heard primarily on exhalation

• *Stridor*—loud, high-pitched sound heard during inspiration

• *Pleural friction rub*—low-pitched, grating sound heard during inspiration and expiration; accompanied by pain.

Types of crackles

Here's how to differentiate fine crackles from coarse crackles, a critical distinction when assessing the lungs.

Fine crackles

These characteristics distinguish fine crackles:
• They occur when the patient stops inhaling.
• They're usually heard in lung bases.
• They sound like a piece of hair being rubbed between the fingers or like Velcro being pulled apart.
• They occur in restrictive diseases, such as pulmonary fibrosis, asbestosis, silicosis, atelectasis, heart failure, and pneumonia.

Coarse crackles

These characteristics distinguish coarse crackles:
• They occur when the patient starts to inhale and may be present when the patient exhales.
• They may be heard through the lungs and even at the mouth.
• They sound more like bubbling or gurgling as air moves through secretions in the larger airways.
• They occur in COPD, pneumonia with severe congestion, pulmonary edema, and in severely ill patients who can't cough.

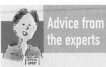

Advice from the experts

When wheezing stops

If you no longer hear wheezing in a patient having an acute asthma attack, the attack may be far from over. When bronchospasm and mucosal swelling become severe, little air can move through the airways. As a result, wheezing stops.

If all other assessment criteria—labored breathing, prolonged expiratory time, and accessory muscle use—point to acute bronchial obstruction (a medical emergency), maintain the patient's airway and give oxygen and medications as ordered to relieve the obstruction. The patient may begin to wheeze again when the airways open more.

ABG analysis

ABG analysis enables evaluation of gas exchange in the lungs by measuring the partial pressures of gases dissolved in arterial blood.

The ABCs of ABGs

Arterial blood is used because it reflects how much oxygen is available to peripheral tissues. Together, ABG values tell the story of how well a patient is ventilating and whether he's developing acidosis or alkalosis.

Here's a summary of commonly assessed ABG values and what the findings indicate:
- pH measurement of the hydrogen ion (H^+) concentration is an indication of the blood's acidity or alkalinity.
- Partial pressure of arterial carbon dioxide ($PaCO_2$) reflects the adequacy of ventilation of the lungs.
- PaO_2 reflects the body's ability to pick up oxygen from the lungs.
- Bicarbonate (HCO_3^-) level reflects the activity of the kidneys in retaining or excreting bicarbonate.
- Oxygen saturation (SaO_2) is the percentage of hemoglobin saturated with oxygen at the time of measurement. (See *Normal ABG values*.)

Interpreting ABG values

Here's an interpretation of possible ABG values:

- A Pao_2 value greater than 100 mm Hg reflects more than adequate supplemental oxygen administration. A value less than 80 mm Hg indicates hypoxemia.
- An Sao_2 value less than 95% represents decreased saturation and may contribute to a low Pao_2 value.
- A pH value above 7.45 (alkalosis) reflects an H^+ deficit; a value below 7.35 (acidosis) reflects an H^+ excess.

A sample scenario

Suppose you find a pH value greater than 7.45, indicating alkalosis. Investigate further by checking the $Paco_2$ value, which is known as the *respiratory parameter*. This value reflects how efficiently the lungs eliminate carbon dioxide. A $Paco_2$ value below 35 mm Hg indicates respiratory alkalosis and hyperventilation.

Next, check the HCO_3^- value, called the *metabolic parameter*. An HCO_3^- value greater than 26 mEq/L indicates metabolic alkalosis.

Likewise, a pH value below 7.35 indicates acidosis. A $Paco_2$ value above 45 mm Hg indicates respiratory acidosis; an HCO_3^- value below 22 mEq/L indicates metabolic acidosis.

See-saw systems

The respiratory and metabolic systems work together to keep the body's acid–base balance within normal limits. If respiratory acidosis develops, for example, the kidneys compensate by conserving bicarbonate. That's why you expect to see an above normal HCO_3^- value.

Similarly, if metabolic acidosis develops, the lungs compensate by increasing the respiratory rate and depth to eliminate carbon dioxide. (See *Understanding acid–base disorders*, page 338.)

Nursing considerations

- In most critical care units, a doctor, respiratory therapist, or specially trained critical care nurse draws ABG samples, usually from an arterial line if the patient has one. If a percutaneous puncture must be done, the site must be chosen carefully. The most common site is the radial artery, but the brachial or femoral arteries can be used. When a radial artery is used, an Allen's test is done before drawing the sample to determine whether the ulnar artery can provide adequate circulation to the hand, in case the radial artery is damaged. (See *Performing Allen's test*, page 339.)

Normal ABG values

ABG values provide information about the blood's acid–base balance and oxygenation.

Normal values are:
- pH—7.35 to 7.45
- $Paco_2$—35 to 45 mm Hg
- Pao_2—80 to 100 mm Hg
- HCO_3^-—22 to 26 mEq per L
- Sao_2—95% to 100%.

The respiratory and metabolic systems work together to maintain acid–base balance.

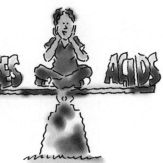

Understanding acid–base disorders

This chart provides an overview of selected acid–base disorders.

Disorder and ABG findings	Possible causes	Signs and symptoms
Respiratory acidosis (excess CO_2 retention) pH <7.35 HCO_3^- >26 mEq/L (if compensating) Partial pressure of arterial CO_2 ($Paco_2$) >45 mm Hg	• CNS depression from drugs, injury, or disease • Respiratory arrest • Hypoventilation from pulmonary, cardiac, or neuromuscular disease	*Early*: tachycardia, tachypnea *Late*: bradypnea, confusion, hypotension, lethargy, coma (very late sign)
Respiratory alkalosis (excess CO_2 excretion) pH >7.45 HCO_3^- <22 mEq/L (if compensating) $Paco_2$ <35 mm Hg	• Hyperventilation from anxiety, pain, or improper ventilator settings • Respiratory stimulation by drugs, disease, or fever • Gram-negative bacteremia • Pulmonary embolism	Paresthesias, confusion, light-headedness, anxiety, palpitations
Metabolic acidosis (bicarbonate loss, acid retention) pH <7.35, HCO_3^- <22 mEq/L, $Paco_2$ <35 mm Hg (if compensating)	• HCO_3^- depletion from severe diarrhea • Excessive production of organic acids from endocrine disorders, shock, or drug intoxication • Inadequate excretion of acids from renal disease • Diabetic ketoacidosis	Fruity breath, headache, lethargy, nausea, vomiting, abdominal pain, tremors, confusion, coma (if severe)
Metabolic alkalosis (bicarbonate retention, acid loss) pH >7.45, HCO_3^- >26 mEq/L, $Paco_2$ >45 mm Hg (if compensating)	• Loss of hydrochloric acid from prolonged vomiting or gastric suctioning • Loss of potassium from increased renal excretion (as in diuretic therapy) or steroids • Excessive alkali ingestion • Hepatic disease	Slow breathing, hypertonic muscles, twitching, confusion, tetany, seizures, dizziness, coma (if severe)

- After obtaining the sample, apply pressure to the puncture site for 5 minutes and tape a gauze pad firmly in place. Regularly monitor the site for bleeding and check the arm for signs of complications, such as swelling, discoloration, pain, numbness, and tingling. (See *Obtaining an ABG sample*, page 340.)
- Note whether the patient is breathing room air or oxygen. If the patient is on oxygen via nasal cannula, document the number of liters. If the patient is receiving oxygen by mask or mechanical ventilation, document the fraction of inspired oxygen (Fio_2).
- Examples of conditions that can interfere with test results are failure to properly heparinize the syringe before drawing a blood sample or exposing the sample to air. Venous blood in the sample may lower

Performing Allen's test

Before obtaining an ABG sample from the radial artery, make sure you perform Allen's test to assess the patient's collateral arterial blood supply:
• Rest the patient's arm on the mattress or bedside stand and support his wrist with a rolled towel. Have him clench his fist. Then, using your index and middle fingers, press on the radial and ulnar arteries. Hold this position for a few seconds.
• Without removing your fingers from the patient's arteries, ask him to unclench his first and hold his hand in a relaxed position. His palm will be blanched because pressure from your fingers has impaired normal blood flow.
• Release pressure on the patient's ulnar artery. If his hand becomes flushed, which indicates blood filling the vessels, you can safely proceed with the radial artery puncture. If his hand doesn't become flushed, perform the test on the other arm.

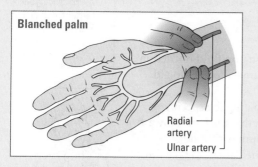

Blanched palm

Radial artery
Ulnar artery

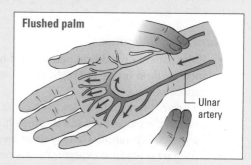

Flushed palm

Ulnar artery

PaO_2 levels and elevate $PaCO_2$ levels. Make sure you remove all air bubbles in the sample syringe because air bubbles also alter results.
• Make sure the sample of arterial blood is kept cold, preferably on ice, and delivered as soon as possible to the laboratory for analysis. Some chemical reactions that alter findings continue to take place after the blood is drawn; rapid cooling and analysis of the sample minimizes this.

Sputum analysis

Sputum analysis assesses sputum specimens (the material expectorated from a patient's lungs and bronchi during deep coughing) to diagnose respiratory disease, identify the cause of pulmonary infection (including viral and bacterial causes), identify abnormal lung cells, identify malignancies, and manage lung disease.

Under the microscope

Sputum specimens are stained and examined under a microscope and, depending on the patient's condition, sometimes cultured. Culture and sensitivity testing is used to identify a specific microorganism and its antibiotic sensitivities. A negative culture may suggest a viral infection.

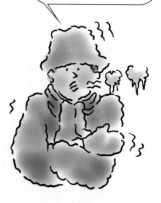

Keep it cold and be quick! Deliver the chilled arterial blood sample ASAP for analysis!

Obtaining an ABG sample

Follow the steps below to obtain a sample for ABG analysis:
• After performing Allen's test, perform a cutaneous arterial puncture (or, if an arterial line is in place, draw blood from the arterial line).
• Use a heparinized blood gas syringe to draw the sample.
• Eliminate all air from the sample, place it on ice immediately, and transport it for analysis.

• Apply pressure to the puncture site for 3 to 5 minutes. If the patient is receiving anticoagulants or has a coagulopathy, hold the puncture site for 10 to 15 minutes or until the bleeding has stopped.
• Tape a gauze pad firmly over the puncture site. If the puncture site is on the arm, don't tape the entire circumference because this may restrict circulation.

Nursing considerations
• If the patient's condition permits and he isn't on fluid restriction, increase fluid intake the night before sputum collection to aid expectoration.
• To prevent foreign particles from contaminating the specimen, instruct the patient not to eat, brush his teeth, or use mouthwash before expectorating. He may rinse his mouth with water.
• When he is ready to expectorate, instruct the patient to take three deep breaths and force a deep cough.
• Before sending the specimen to the laboratory, make sure it's sputum, not saliva. Saliva has a thinner consistency and more bubbles (froth) than sputum.

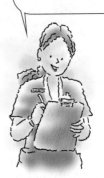

Instruct your patient not to eat, brush his teeth, or use mouthwash before sputum collection.

Endoscopy and imaging

Endoscopy and imaging tests include bronchoscopy, chest X-ray, magnetic resonance imaging (MRI), thoracic computed tomography (CT) scan, and $\dot{V}/\dot{Q}$ scan.

Bronchoscopy

Bronchoscopy allows direct visualization of the larynx, trachea, and bronchi through a fiberoptic bronchoscope, a slender flexible tube with mirrors and a light at its distal end. The flexible fiberoptic bronchoscope is preferred to metal because it's smaller, allows a better view for the bronchi, and carries less risk for trauma.

To remove and evaluate

The purpose of a bronchoscopy is to:
• remove foreign bodies, malignant or benign tumors, mucus plugs, or excessive secretions from the tracheobronchial tree and control massive hemoptysis

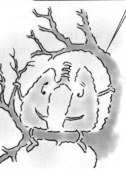

Bronchoscopy allows removal of tissue or foreign bodies from the tracheobronchial tree.

- pass brush biopsy forceps or a catheter through the bronchoscope to obtain specimens for cytologic evaluation.

Nursing considerations
- Before bronchoscopy, collect the patient's history. A physical examination is performed; preprocedure studies may include a chest X-ray, ABG analysis, and clotting studies.

Head to the suite

- The patient usually goes to a procedure suite for the bronchoscopy. In some cases—such as when the patient is on a ventilator—it may be performed at the bedside. Explain the procedure to the patient and his family and answer their questions.
- The patient may be premedicated with atropine to dry secretions and a mild sedative or antianxiety agent such as midazolam (Versed) to help him relax. Before insertion of the bronchoscope, a topical anesthetic is applied to the oropharynx, nasopharynx, larynx, vocal cords, and trachea to suppress the cough reflex and prevent gagging.
- The practitioner introduces the bronchoscope tube through the patient's nose or mouth into the airway. Various ports on the bronchoscope allow for suctioning, oxygen administration, and biopsies during the procedure. Monitor vital signs, oxygen saturation levels with pulse oximetry, and heart rhythm throughout the procedure.
- After the procedure, the patient is positioned on his side or may have the head of the bed elevated 30 degrees until the gag reflex returns. Assess respiratory status and monitor vital signs, oxygen saturation levels, and heart rhythm. Report signs and symptoms of respiratory distress, such as dyspnea, laryngospasm, or hypoxemia.
- Monitor cardiac status frequently for changes in heart rate or rhythm. Report any tachycardia or evidence of arrhythmia.

Hold the fries

- If the patient isn't intubated, assess for return of the gag, cough, and swallow reflexes. Maintain nothing-by-mouth status until these reflexes return. Explain to the patient that temporary hoarseness or sore throat may occur after the procedure and that gargle or lozenges may be ordered to ease discomfort.
- Obtain a chest X-ray as ordered to detect pneumothorax and evaluate lung status.
- Keep resuscitative equipment available during the procedure and for 24 hours afterward.

Chest X-ray

During chest radiography (commonly known as *chest X-ray*), X-ray beams penetrate the chest and react on specially sensitized film. Because normal pulmonary tissue is radiolucent, such abnormalities as infiltrates, foreign bodies, fluid, and tumors appear dense on the film.

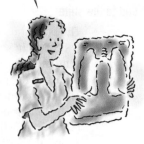

A chest X-ray is most useful when it's compared with previous films, allowing changes to be detected.

More is better

A chest X-ray is most useful when compared with the patient's previous films, allowing the practitioner to detect changes.

By themselves, chest X-rays may not provide definitive diagnostic information. For example, they may not reveal mild to moderate obstructive pulmonary disease. However, they can show the location and size of lesions and can also be used to identify structural abnormalities that influence ventilation and diffusion.

X-ray vision

Examples of abnormalities visible on X-ray include:
- pneumothorax
- fibrosis
- atelectasis
- infiltrates
- tumors.

Nursing considerations
- When a patient in the critical care unit can't be moved, chest X-ray is commonly performed at the bedside. Explain to the patient that someone will help him to a sitting position while a cold, hard film plate is placed behind his back. If testing is done in the radiology department, you may need to accompany the patient. The patient usually lies on a stretcher or X-ray table and is asked to take a deep breath and to hold it for a few seconds while the X-ray is taken. Instruct the patient to remain still for those few seconds.

Advise the patient that each required X-ray will take only a few seconds but that he must remain still and hold his breath during that time.

Minimal exposure

- Provide reassurance that the amount of radiation exposure is minimal. Facility personnel leave the area when the technician takes the X-ray because they're potentially exposed to radiation many times per day.
- Make sure that female patients of childbearing age wear a lead apron. Males should have protection for the testes.

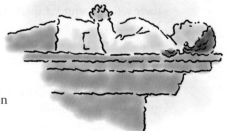

Magnetic resonance imaging

MRI is a noninvasive test that employs a powerful magnet, radio waves, and a computer. It's used to diagnose respiratory disorders by providing high-resolution, cross-sectional images of lung structures and by tracing blood flow.

A view that's see-through

The greatest advantage of MRI is that it enables one to "see through" bone and delineate fluid-filled soft tissue in great detail, without using ionizing radiation or contrast media. It's used to distinguish tumors from other structures such as blood vessels.

Nursing considerations
- All metal objects must be removed from the patient before entering the scanning room. (See *MRI and metals don't mix.*)
- If the patient is claustrophobic, sedation may be ordered before the test. You or another nurse generally accompanies the patient to the MRI suite.
- Tell the patient that he'll be asked to lie on a table that slides into an 8' (2.4 m) tunnel inside the magnet. Some facilities can perform open MRIs, which are more tolerable for patients who are claustrophobic. The test usually takes 15 to 30 minutes.
- Instruct the patient to breathe normally but not to talk or move during the test, to avoid distorting the results.
- Explain that the machinery is noisy, with sounds ranging from an incessant ping to a loud bang. The patient may feel claustrophobic or bored. Encourage him to relax and to concentrate on breathing or a favorite subject or image.

Thoracic computed tomography scans

Thoracic CT scan provides cross-sectional views of the chest by passing an X-ray beam from a computerized scanner through the body at different angles and depths. A contrast agent is sometimes used to highlight blood vessels and allow greater visual discrimination.

The two major types of thoracic CT are helical CT and axial CT. In a helical CT (the most commonly used type), the X-ray tube rotates in a spiral fashion around the patient and generates an X-ray beam, which is picked up by detectors. In an axial CT (used for high-resolution CT scanning of the lungs), rotation is circular.

CT in 3-D

Thoracic CT scan provides a three-dimensional image of the lung, allowing the doctor to assess abnormalities in the configuration of the trachea or major bronchi and evaluate masses or lesions, such as tumors and abscesses, and abnormal lung shadows.

MRI and metals don't mix

Before your patient undergoes MRI, make sure he doesn't have a pacemaker or surgically implanted joint, pin, clip, valve, or pump containing metal. Such objects could be attracted to the strong MRI magnet.

Ask your patient whether he has ever worked with metals or has ever had metal in his eyes. Some facilities have a checklist that covers all pertinent questions regarding metals, clips, pins, pacemakers, and other devices. If he has such an object or device, the test can't be done.

Nursing considerations

- Confirm that the patient isn't allergic to iodine or shellfish. A patient with these allergies may have an adverse reaction to the contrast medium.
- If a contrast medium is used, explain that it's injected into the existing I.V. line or that a new line may be inserted.
- Explain to the patient that he may feel flushed or notice a metallic or salty taste in his mouth when the contrast medium is injected.
- Explain that the CT scanner circles around the patient for 10 to 30 minutes, depending on the procedure, and that the equipment may make him feel claustrophobic.
- Instruct the patient to lie still during the test.
- Inform the patient that the contrast medium may discolor his urine for 24 hours.
- Encourage oral fluid intake to flush the contrast medium out of the patient's system, unless it's contraindicated or the patient is on nothing-by-mouth status. The practitioner may write an order to increase the rate of I.V. fluid infusion.

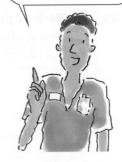

Remember to get plenty of fluid into your patient's system to flush the contrast medium.

Ventilation-perfusion scan

A $\dot{V}/\dot{Q}$ scan is used to:
- evaluate $\dot{V}/\dot{Q}$ mismatch
- detect pulmonary emboli
- evaluate pulmonary function, especially in patients with marginal lung reserves.
    Although it's less reliable than pulmonary angiography, $\dot{V}/\dot{Q}$ scanning carries fewer risks.

Two-tined test

A $\dot{V}/\dot{Q}$ scan has two parts:
1. During the ventilation portion of the test, the patient inhales the contrast medium gas; ventilation patterns and adequacy of ventilation are noted on the scan.
2. During the perfusion scan, the contrast medium is injected I.V. and the pulmonary blood flow to the lungs is visualized.

A caveat

$\dot{V}/\dot{Q}$ scans aren't commonly used for patients on mechanical ventilators because the ventilation portion of the test is difficult to perform. (Pulmonary angiography is the preferred test for a critically ill patient with a suspected pulmonary embolus.)

Nursing considerations

- Explain the test to the patient and his family, telling them who performs the test and where it's done.

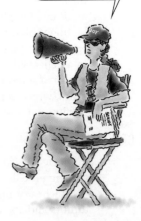

Take two! A $\dot{V}/\dot{Q}$ scan is a two-part test.

- Like pulmonary angiography, a V̇/Q̇ scan requires the injection of a contrast medium. Confirm that the patient doesn't have an allergy to the contrast material.
- Explain to the patient that the test has two parts. During the ventilation portion, a mask is placed over his mouth and nose and the patient breathes in the contrast medium gas mixed with air while the scanner takes pictures of his lungs. For the perfusion portion, the patient is placed in a supine position on a movable table as the contrast medium is injected into the I.V. line while the scanner again takes pictures of the lungs.
- After the procedure, maintain bed rest as ordered and monitor the patient's vital signs, oxygen saturation levels, and heart rhythm.
- Monitor for adverse reactions to the contrast medium, which may include restlessness, tachypnea and respiratory distress, tachycardia, urticaria, and nausea and vomiting. Keep emergency equipment nearby in case of a reaction.

Pulmonary angiography

Pulmonary angiography, also called *pulmonary arteriography*, allows radiographic examination of the pulmonary circulation.

After injecting a radioactive contrast dye through a catheter inserted into the pulmonary artery or one of its branches, a series of X-rays is taken to detect blood flow abnormalities, possibly caused by emboli or pulmonary infarction.

More reliable, more risks

Pulmonary angiography yields more reliable results than a V̇/Q̇ scan but carries higher risks for certain conditions, such as cardiac arrhythmias (especially ventricular arrhythmias due to myocardial irritation from passage of the catheter through the heart chambers). It may be the preferred test, especially if the patient is on a ventilator.

Nursing considerations
- Explain the procedure to the patient and his family and answer their questions. Tell him who performs the test, where it's done, and how long it takes.

Preprocedure patient preparation
- Confirm that the patient isn't allergic to shellfish or iodine. Notify the practitioner if the patient has such an allergy because the patient may have an adverse reaction to the contrast medium. Diphenhydramine (Benadryl) and prednisone (Deltasone) may be administered, as ordered, before the test to reduce the risk for a reaction to the dye.
- Preprocedure testing should include evaluation of renal function (by serum creatinine levels and blood urea nitrogen [BUN] levels)

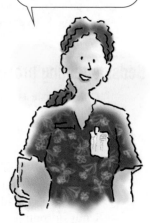

Pulmonary angiography may be preferred over V̇/Q̇ scanning, especially if your patient is on a ventilator.

and potential risk of bleeding (by prothrombin time, partial thromboplastin time [PTT], and platelet count). Notify the practitioner of abnormal results.

- Instruct the patient to lie still for the procedure.
- Explain that he'll probably feel a flushed sensation in his face as the dye is injected.

Postprocedure procedures

- Maintain bed rest, as ordered, and monitor the patient's vital signs, oxygen saturation levels, and heart rhythm.
- Keep a femoral compression device over the injection site as ordered.
- After the procedure, check the pressure dressing for signs of bleeding. Monitor the patient's peripheral pulse in the arm or leg used for catheter insertion (mark the site); check the temperature, color, and sensation of the extremity; and compare with the opposite side.
- Unless contraindicated, encourage the patient to drink more fluids to flush the dye or contrast medium from his system or increase the I.V. flow rate as ordered.
- Check serum creatinine and BUN levels after the procedure because the contrast medium can cause acute renal failure.
- Monitor for adverse reactions to the contrast medium, which may include restlessness, tachypnea and respiratory distress, tachycardia, facial flushing, urticaria, and nausea and vomiting. Keep emergency equipment nearby in case of a reaction.

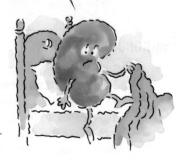

Maintain the patient on bed rest and be sure to check serum creatinine and BUN levels because the contrast medium can cause acute renal failure.

Bedside testing procedures

Diagnostic tests used at the bedside to evaluate respiratory function include pulse oximetry, mixed venous oxygen saturation (SvO_2), and end-tidal carbon dioxide ($ETCO_2$) monitoring.

Pulse oximetry

Pulse oximetry is a relatively simple procedure used to monitor arterial oxygen saturation noninvasively. It's performed either intermittently or continuously.

Shedding light on the subject

In this procedure, two diodes send red and infrared light through a pulsating arterial vascular bed such as the one in the fingertip.

A photodetector (also called a *sensor* or *transducer*) slipped over the finger measures the transmitted light as it passes through the vascular bed, detects the relative amount of color absorbed by arterial blood, and calculates the saturation without interference from the venous blood, skin, or connective tissue. The percentage expressed is the ratio of oxygen to hemoglobin. (See *A closer look at pulse oximetry*.)

Note denotation

In pulse oximetry, arterial oxygen saturation values are usually denoted with the symbol SpO_2. Arterial oxygen saturation values, which are measured invasively via ABG analysis, are denoted by the symbol SaO_2.

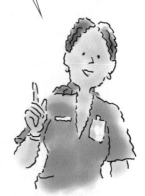

Place the sensor over a finger or other site so that the light beams and sensors are opposite each other.

Nursing considerations

- Place the sensor over the finger or other site, such as the toe, bridge of the nose, or earlobe, so that the light beams and sensors are opposite each other.
- Protect the sensor from exposure to strong light, such as fluorescent lighting, because it interferes with results. Check the sensor site frequently to make sure the device is in place and to examine the skin for abrasion and circulatory impairment.
- The pulse oximeter displays the patient's pulse rate and oxygen saturation reading. The pulse rate on the oximeter must correspond to the patient's actual pulse. If the rates don't correspond, the saturation reading can't be considered accurate. You may need to reposition the sensor to obtain an accurate reading.
- Rotate the sensor site at least every 4 hours, or according to the manufacturer's instructions and your facility's policy for site rotation, to avoid skin irritation and circulatory impairment.
- If oximetry is done properly, the oxygen saturation readings are usually within 2% of ABG values. A normal reading is 95% to 100%.

Poisoning precludes pulse oximetry

- Pulse oximetry isn't used when carbon monoxide (CO) poisoning is suspected because the oximeter doesn't differentiate between oxygen and CO bound to hemoglobin. An ABG analysis should be performed in such cases.

A closer look at pulse oximetry

Oximetry may be intermittent or continuous and is used to monitor arterial oxyhemoglobin saturation. Normal oxyhemoglobin saturation levels are 95% to 100% for adults. Lower levels may indicate hypoxemia and warrant intervention.

Interfering factors

Certain factors can interfere with the accuracy of oximetry readings. For example, an elevated bilirubin level may falsely lower oxyhemoglobin saturation readings, whereas elevated carboxyhemoglobin or methemoglobin levels can falsely elevate oxyhemoglobin saturation readings.

Certain intravascular substances, such as lipid emulsions and dyes, can also prevent accurate readings. Other interfering factors include excessive light (such as from phototherapy or direct sunlight), excessive patient movement, excessive ear pigment, dark skin color, hypothermia, hypotension, and vasoconstriction.

Some acrylic nails and certain colors of nail polish (blue, green, black, and brown-red) may also interfere with readings.

Mixed venous oxygen saturation monitoring

SvO_2 reflects the oxygen saturation level of venous blood. It's determined by measuring the amount of oxygen extracted and used or consumed by the body's tissues.

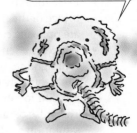

The patient's SvO_2 level reflects the amount of oxygen extracted by the body's tissues. Hey, we all have needs!

SvO_2 indications

In a healthy adult, an SvO_2 level between 60% and 80% indicates adequate tissue perfusion.

Decreased values less than 60% indicate increased oxygen extraction by the tissues. A decrease in oxygen delivery or an increase in tissue demands can cause this.

Increased values greater than 80% may occur in states of increased oxygen delivery or may indicate decreased oxygen extraction by the tissues (when tissue hypoxia exists despite the availability of oxygen).

Drawing from the right location

Ideally, the SvO_2 sample is obtained from the most distal port of the pulmonary artery (PA) catheter, which contains the ideal mix of all venous blood in the heart. Samples may be drawn from a central catheter if a PA catheter isn't available.

A calculating catheter

Continuous SvO_2 monitoring is done using the SvO_2 or oximetric PA catheter. This specialized PA catheter calculates oxygen saturation of hemoglobin by measuring the wavelengths of reflected light through fiberoptic bundles.

The information is exhibited on a bedside computer and may be displayed numerically and graphically. The manufacturer's instructions for catheter calibration must be followed to ensure accurate readings.

Follow the manufacturer's instructions for catheter calibration to ensure accurate readings.

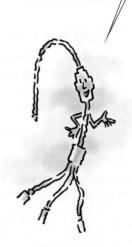

Nursing considerations

- Explain the procedure to the patient and his family. Make sure they understand the expected outcomes and risks of the procedure related to catheter placement, pneumothorax, cardiac arrhythmias, and infection.
- If you assist with catheter insertion, monitor the patient's vital signs and heart rhythm as you assess for changes in ventilatory function.
- Apply a sterile dressing or sterile transparent dressing over the catheter insertion site. Follow your facility's policy for changing the dressing and pulmonary artery monitoring system (tubing and solution).
- Document the date and time of catheter insertion, initial SvO_2 readings, and any changes in the patient's condition. Monitor the pulmonary artery pressure (PAP) and SvO_2 readings and document hourly or according to your facility's policy. (See *Normal and abnormal SvO_2 waveforms*, page 350.)

- Closely monitor the patient's hemodynamic status. Troubleshoot the catheter for problems that can interfere with accurate testing, such as loose connections, balloon rupture, or clot formation on the tip of the catheter.

End-tidal carbon dioxide monitoring

$ETCO_2$ is used to measure the carbon dioxide concentration at end expiration. An $ETCO_2$ monitor may be a separate monitor or part of the patient's bedside hemodynamic monitoring system.

Indications for $ETCO_2$ monitoring include:
- monitoring patency of the airway in acute airway obstruction and apnea and respiratory function
- early detection of changes in carbon dioxide production and elimination with hyperventilation therapy, or hypercapnia or hyperthermia states
- assessing effectiveness of interventions such as mechanical ventilation or neuromuscular blockade used with mechanical ventilation and prone positioning
- effectiveness of cardiopulmonary resuscitation (CPR) in emergency situations.

In–lightened

In $ETCO_2$ monitoring, a photodetector measures the amount of infrared light absorbed by the airway during inspiration and expiration. (Light absorption increases along with the carbon dioxide concentration.) The monitor converts these data to a carbon dioxide value and a corresponding waveform, or capnogram if capnography is used. (See *Understanding $ETCO_2$ monitoring*, page 351.)

Crunching the numbers

Values are obtained by monitoring samples of expired gas from an endotracheal (ET) tube or an oral or nasopharyngeal airway. Although the values are similar, the $ETCO_2$ values are usually 2 to 5 mm Hg lower than the $PaCO_2$ value.

Capnograms and $ETCO_2$ monitoring reduce the need for frequent ABG sampling.

Nursing considerations
- Explain the procedure to the patient and his family.
- Assess the patient's respiratory status, vital signs, oxygen saturation, and $ETCO_2$ readings. Observe waveform quality and trends of $ETCO_2$ readings and observe for suddenly increased readings (which may indicate hypoventilation, partial airway obstruction, or respiratory depressant effects from drugs) or decreased readings (due to complete airway obstruction, dislodged ET tube, or ventilator malfunction). Notify the practitioner of a 10% increase or decrease in readings.

Normal and abnormal SvO$_2$ waveforms

This tracing represents a stable, normal SvO$_2$ level: higher than 60% and lower than 80%. Note the relatively constant line.

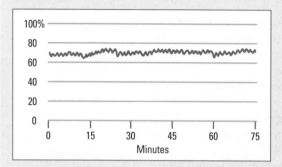

This waveform shows typical changes in the SvO$_2$ level as a result of various activities.

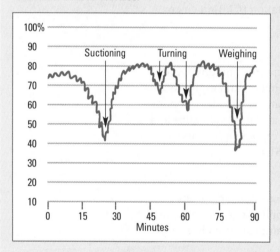

This tracing represents the patient's response to a muscle relaxant.

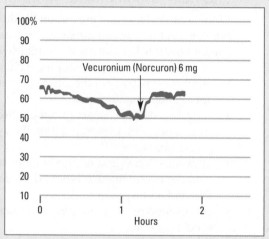

This waveform shows the patient's response to changes in ventilator settings. Note that increasing the positive end-expiratory pressure (PEEP) causes an increase in SvO$_2$; therefore, the FIO$_2$ can be decreased.

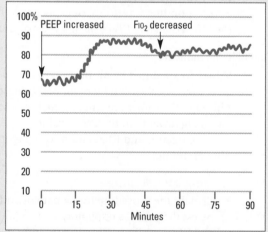

Understanding ETco₂ monitoring

The optical portion of an ETco₂ monitor contains an infrared light source, a sample chamber, a special CO_2 filter, and a photodetector.

In ETco₂ monitoring, the infrared light passes through the sample chamber and is absorbed in varying amounts, depending on the amount of CO_2 the patient just exhaled. The photodetector measures CO_2 content and relays this information to the microprocessor in the monitor, which displays the CO_2 value and waveform.

Capnogram reading

The CO_2 waveform, or capnogram, produced in ETco₂ monitoring reflects the course of CO_2 elimination during exhalation. A normal capnogram (shown below) consists of several segments, which reflect the various stages of exhalation and inhalation.

Normally, any gas eliminated from the airway during early exhalation is dead-space gas that hasn't undergone exchange at the alveolocapillary membrane. Measurements taken during this period contain no CO_2. As exhalation continues, CO_2 concentration increases sharply and rapidly. The sensor now detects gas that has undergone exchange, producing measurable quantities of CO_2.

The final stages of alveolar emptying occur during late exhalation. During the alveolar plateau phase, CO_2 concentration increases gradually because alveolar emptying is relatively constant.

The point at which the ETco₂ value is derived is the end of exhalation, when CO_2 concentration peaks. However, this value doesn't accurately reflect alveolar CO_2 if no alveolar plateau is present. During inhalation, the CO_2 concentration declines sharply to zero.

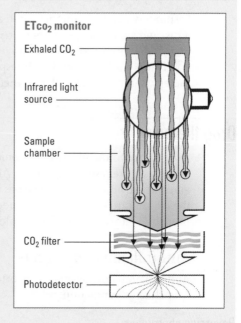

ETco₂ monitor

Exhaled CO_2

Infrared light source

Sample chamber

CO_2 filter

Photodetector

This peak that occurs during the end of exhalation indicates the point at which the ETco₂ value is derived.

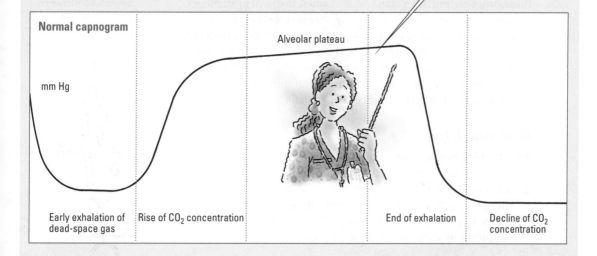

Normal capnogram

mm Hg

Alveolar plateau

Early exhalation of dead-space gas

Rise of CO_2 concentration

End of exhalation

Decline of CO_2 concentration

Treatments

Respiratory disorders interfere with airway clearance, breathing patterns, and gas exchange. If not corrected, they can adversely affect many other body systems and can be life-threatening.

Treatments for patients with respiratory disorders include drug therapy, surgery, and inhalation therapy.

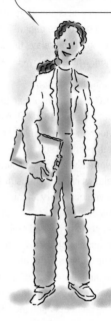

Notify the practitioner if there's a 10% increase or decrease in $ETco_2$ readings.

Drug therapy

Drugs are used for airway management in patients with such disorders as acute respiratory failure, ARDS, asthma, emphysema, and chronic bronchitis. Some types of drugs commonly seen in the critical care environment include anti-inflammatory agents, bronchodilators, neuromuscular blocking agents, and sedatives.

Anti-inflammatory agents

Anti-inflammatory agents (corticosteroids) are used to reduce bronchial inflammation.

Reversing obstruction

Corticosteroids are the most effective anti-inflammatory agents used to treat patients with reversible airflow obstruction. They work by suppressing immune responses and reducing inflammation.

Systemic drugs, such as dexamethasone, methylprednisolone (Medrol), and prednisone, are given to manage an acute respiratory event such as acute respiratory failure or exacerbation of COPD. These drugs are initially given I.V., and when the patient stabilizes, the dosage is tapered, and oral dosing may be substituted.

Patients with asthma commonly use inhaled steroids, such as beclomethasone (QVAR), budesonide (Pulmicort Flexhaler), flunisolide (AeroBid), fluticasone (Flovent), and triamcinolone (Azmacort). These agents also work by suppressing the immune response and reducing airway inflammation. (See *Understanding corticosteroids.*)

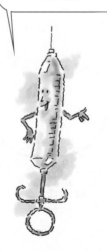

Systemic drugs are given I.V. at first, then tapered and delivered orally when the patient stabilizes.

Bronchodilators

Bronchodilators relax bronchial smooth muscles and are used to treat patients with bronchospasms. Here's how some types of bronchodilators are used:

- Short-acting inhaled beta$_2$-adrenergic agonists, such as albuterol (Proventil) and pirbuterol (Maxair), are used to relieve acute symptoms in asthma and bronchospasm.

Understanding corticosteroids

Use this table to learn about the indications, adverse reactions, and practice pointers associated with corticosteroids.

Drugs	Indications	Adverse reactions	Practice pointers
Systemic steroids • Dexamethasone • Methylprednisolone (Medrol) • Prednisone	• Anti-inflammatory for acute respiratory failure, ARDS, and COPD • Anti-inflammatory and immunosuppressor for asthma	• Heart failure • Arrhythmias • Edema • Circulatory collapse • Thromboembolism • Pancreatitis • Peptic ulcer • Insomnia • Hyperglycemia • Hypokalemia • Acute adrenal insufficiency	• Use cautiously in patients with recent myocardial infarction (MI), hypertension, renal disease, and GI ulcer. • Monitor blood pressure and blood glucose levels.
Inhaled steroids • Beclomethasone (QVAR) • Budesonide (Pulmicort) • Flunisolide (AeroBid) • Fluticasone (Flonase) • Triamcinolone (Azmacort)	• Long-term asthma control	• Hoarseness • Dry mouth • Wheezing • Bronchospasm • Oral candidiasis • Headache	• Don't use for treatment of acute asthma attack. • Use a spacer to improve the efficiency of drug delivery. • Rinse the patient's mouth after use to prevent oral fungal infection.

- Epinephrine acts on both alpha- and beta-adrenergic receptors. It's used to relieve anaphylactic, allergic, and other hypersensitivity reactions. Its beta-adrenergic effects relax bronchial smooth muscle and relieve bronchospasm.
- Anticholinergic agents, such as ipratropium (Atrovent) and tiotropium (Spiriva), act by inhibiting the action of acetylcholine at bronchial smooth muscle receptor sites and thus produce bronchodilation. (See *Understanding bronchodilators*, page 354.)

Neuromuscular blocking agents

Patients on mechanical ventilation may require neuromuscular blocking agents to eliminate spontaneous breathing efforts that can interfere with the ventilator's function. Neuromuscular blocking agents cause paralysis without altering the patient's LOC. (See *Understanding neuromuscular blocking agents*, pages 355 and 356.)

(Text continues on page 357.)

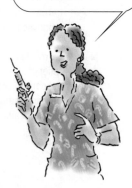

Epinephrine is used to relieve anaphylactic, allergic, and other hypersensitivity reactions.

Understanding bronchodilators

Use this table to learn about the indications, adverse reactions, and practice pointers associated with bronchodilators.

Drugs	Indications	Adverse reactions	Practice pointers
Beta₂-adrenergic agonists			
Albuterol	• Provide short-acting relief of acute symptoms with asthma and bronchospasm. • Prevent exercise-induced bronchospasm.	• Paradoxical bronchospasm • Tachycardia • Palpitations • Tremor • Hyperactivity	• Warn patient about possibility of paradoxical bronchospasm. If it occurs, stop drug and seek medical treatment. • Be aware that elderly patient may require a lower dose. • Monitor respiratory status, vital signs, and heart rhythm.
Epinephrine	• Relax bronchial smooth muscle by stimulating beta₂-adrenergic receptors; used for bronchospasm, hypersensitivity reaction, anaphylaxis, acute asthma	• Ventricular fibrillation • Palpitations • Tachycardia • Cerebral hemorrhage • Hypertension	• Use cautiously in elderly patients and those with long-standing asthma and emphysema with degenerative heart disease. • Monitor respiratory status, vital signs, and heart rhythm. • Be aware of contraindication in patients with angle-closure glaucoma, coronary insufficiency, and cerebral arteriosclerosis.
Pirbuterol	• Relieve acute symptoms with asthma and bronchospasm.	• Palpitations • Tachycardia • Tremor • Paradoxical bronchospasm • Restlessness • Irritability	• Warn patient about possibility of paradoxical bronchospasm. If it occurs, stop drug and seek medical treatment. • Be aware that elderly patient may require a lower dose. • Monitor respiratory status, vital signs, and heart rhythm.
Anticholinergic agents			
Ipratropium	• Provide short-acting relief of bronchospasm associated with chronic bronchitis and emphysema.	• Bronchospasm • Palpitations • Nervousness	• Because of delayed onset of bronchodilation, the drug isn't recommended for acute respiratory distress. • Use cautiously in patients with angle-closure glaucoma, bladder neck obstruction, and prostatic hypertrophy. • Monitor respiratory status, vital signs, and heart rhythm.
Tiotropium	• Provide long-acting relief of bronchospasm associated with COPD, chronic bronchitis, and emphysema.	• Cough • Upper respiratory tract infection • Pharyngitis	• Inform patient that drug is for maintenance treatment of COPD and not for immediate relief of breathing problems. • Watch for evidence of hypersensitivity (especially angioedema) and paradoxical bronchospasm. • Use cautiously in women who are pregnant or breastfeeding; patients with creatinine clearance of 50 ml/minute or less; or patients with angle-closure glaucoma, prostatic hyperplasia, or bladder neck obstruction.

Understanding neuromuscular blocking agents

Use this table to learn about the indications, adverse reactions, and practice pointers associated with neuromuscular blocking agents.

Drugs	Indications	Adverse reactions	Practice pointers
Succinylcholine	• Used as adjunct to anesthesia to induce skeletal muscle relaxation • Facilitate ET intubation and mechanical ventilation.	• Bradycardia, arrhythmias, cardiac arrest • Postoperative muscle pain • Respiratory depression, apnea, bronchoconstriction • Malignant hyperthermia, increased intraocular pressure, flushing • Anaphylaxis	• Be aware that the drug is contraindicated in patients with a history of malignant hyperthermia, acute angle-closure glaucoma, and penetrating eye injuries. • Monitor the patient for histamine release and resulting hypotension and flushing. • Be sure to have emergency resuscitation and ventilation equipment available.
Nondepolarizing			
Atracurium	• Used as adjunct to general anesthesia, to facilitate ET intubation, and to provide skeletal muscle relaxation during surgery or mechanical ventilation	• Flushing, bradycardia • Prolonged dose-related apnea • Anaphylaxis	• Keep in mind that the drug doesn't affect consciousness or relieve pain. Be sure to keep the patient sedated and administer analgesics, if appropriate. • Be aware that the drug has little or no effect on heart rate and doesn't counteract or reverse the bradycardia caused by anesthetics or vagal stimulation. Thus, bradycardia is seen more frequently with atracurium than with other neuromuscular blocking agents. Pretreatment with anticholinergics (atropine or glycopyrrolate) is advised. • Use this drug only if ET intubation, administration of oxygen under positive pressure, artificial respiration, and assisted or controlled ventilation are immediately available. • Use a peripheral nerve stimulator to monitor responses during critical care unit administration; it may be used to detect residual paralysis during recovery and to avoid atracurium overdose.

(continued)

Understanding neuromuscular blocking agents *(continued)*

Drugs	Indications	Adverse reactions	Practice pointers
Nondepolarizing *(continued)*			
Cisatracurium	• Used as adjunct to general anesthesia, to facilitate ET intubation, and to provide skeletal muscle relaxation during surgery or mechanical ventilation • Maintain neuromuscular blockade.	• Hypotension • Flushing	• Be aware that the drug isn't compatible with propofol injection or ketorolac injection for Y-site administration. It's acidic and may not be compatible with an alkaline solution having a pH greater than 8.5, such as barbiturate solutions for Y-site administration. Don't dilute in lactated Ringer's injection because of chemical instability. • Keep in mind that the drug isn't recommended for rapid sequence ET intubation because of its intermediate onset of action. • In patients with neuromuscular disease (myasthenia gravis and myasthenic syndrome), watch for possible prolonged neuromuscular block. • Monitor the patient's acid–base balance and electrolyte levels.
Pancuronium	• Used as adjunct to anesthesia to induce skeletal muscle relaxation and facilitate intubation and ventilation; weakens muscle contractions in induced seizures	• Residual muscle weakness • Prolonged, dose-related respiratory insufficiency or apnea • Allergic or idiosyncratic hypersensitivity reactions • Tachycardia	• If using succinylcholine, allow its effects to subside before giving pancuronium. • Don't mix this drug in the same syringe or give through same needle with barbiturates or other alkaline solutions. • Be aware that large doses may increase frequency and severity of tachycardia.
Vecuronium	• Used as adjunct to anesthesia, to facilitate intubation, and to provide skeletal muscle relaxation during surgery or mechanical ventilation	• Respiratory insufficiency or apnea • Skeletal muscle weakness	• Administer by rapid I.V. injection or I.V. infusion; don't give I.M. • Prepare for a recovery time that may double in patients with cirrhosis or cholestasis. • Assess baseline serum electrolyte levels, acid–base balance, and renal and hepatic function before administration.

Sedatives

Benzodiazepines, such as midazolam, lorazepam (Ativan), and propofol (Diprivan), are used for conscious sedation and preoperative sedation to reduce anxiety and awareness in patients undergoing diagnostic or surgical procedures.

These drugs are also used to relieve anxiety and promote sedation in patients on mechanical ventilators, especially those receiving neuromuscular blocking agents. Such agents cause paralysis without altering the patient's LOC, which—without sedation—is frightening for the patient. (See *Understanding sedatives*.)

Understanding sedatives

Use this table to learn about the indications, adverse reactions, and practice pointers associated with sedatives.

Drugs	Indications	Adverse reactions	Practice pointers
Lorazepam	• Anxiety • Status epilepticus • Insomnia • Premedication before operative procedures	• Drowsiness • Acute withdrawal syndrome (after sudden discontinuation in physically dependent patients) • Urine retention	• Be aware that the drug is contraindicated in patients with acute angle-closure glaucoma. • Use cautiously in patients with pulmonary, renal, or hepatic impairment and in elderly, acutely ill, or debilitated patients. • For I.V. administration, dilute lorazepam with an equal volume of a compatible diluent, such as dextrose 5% in water (D_5W), sterile water for injection, or normal saline solution. • Inject the drug directly into a vein or into the tubing of a compatible I.V. infusion, such as normal saline solution or D_5W solution. The rate of lorazepam I.V. injection shouldn't exceed 2 mg/minute. Have emergency resuscitative equipment and oxygen available when administering I.V. • Monitor liver function studies to prevent cumulative effects and to ensure adequate drug metabolism. • Keep in mind that parenteral administration of drug is more likely to cause apnea, hypotension, bradycardia, and cardiac arrest in elderly patients.
Midazolam	• Preoperative sedation (to induce sleepiness or drowsiness and relieve apprehension)	• Pain at injection site	• Be aware that the drug is contraindicated in patients with acute angle-closure glaucoma and in those experiencing shock, coma, or acute alcohol intoxication.

(continued)

Understanding sedatives *(continued)*

Drugs	Indications	Adverse reactions	Practice pointers
	• Conscious sedation before short diagnostic or endoscopic procedures	• Cardiac arrest • Nausea • Hiccups • Decreased respiratory rate • Apnea • Hypotension • Amnesia	• Use cautiously in patients with uncompensated acute illnesses, in elderly, or debilitated patients. • Closely monitor cardiopulmonary function; continuously monitor patients who have received midazolam to detect potentially life-threatening respiratory depression.
Midazolam	• Continuous infusion for sedation of intubated and mechanically ventilated patients as a component of anesthesia or during treatment in a critical care setting		• Have emergency respiratory equipment readily available. Laryngospasm and bronchospasm, although rare, may occur. • Be aware that solutions compatible with midazolam include D$_5$W, normal saline solution, and lactated Ringer's solution.
Propofol	• Induce and maintain anesthesia • Sedate mechanically ventilated patients	• Hypotension • Bradycardia • Hyperlipidemia • Apnea	• Keep in mind that the drug is contraindicated in patients hypersensitive to propofol or components of the emulsion, including soybean oil, egg lecithin, and glycerol. Because drug is administered as an emulsion, administer cautiously to patients with a disorder of lipid metabolism (such as pancreatitis, primary hyperlipoproteinemia, and diabetic hyperlipidemia). Use cautiously if the patient is receiving lipids as part of a total parenteral nutrition infusion; I.V. lipid dose may need to be reduced. Use cautiously in elderly or debilitated patients and in those with circulatory or seizure disorders. • Keep in mind that although the hemodynamic effects of drug can vary, its major effect in patients maintaining spontaneous ventilation is arterial hypotension (arterial pressure can decrease as much as 30%) with little or no change in heart rate and cardiac output. However, significant depression of cardiac output may occur in patients undergoing assisted or controlled positive pressure ventilation. • Don't mix propofol with other drugs or blood products. If it's to be diluted before infusion, use only D$_5$W and don't dilute to a concentration of less than 2 mg/ml. After dilution, drug appears to be more stable in glass containers than in plastic. • Change the infusion bottle and tubing every 12 hours.

Surgery

If drugs or other therapeutic modes fail to maintain the patient's airway patency and protect healthy tissues from disease, surgery may be necessary. Some types of respiratory surgeries are tracheotomy, chest tube insertion, thoracotomy, and lung transplant.

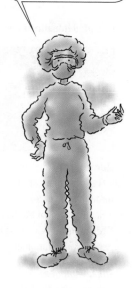

Surgery may be necessary if drugs or other treatment measures fail.

Tracheotomy

A tracheotomy is a surgical procedure to create an opening into the trachea, called a *tracheostomy*, which allows insertion of an indwelling tube to keep the patient's airway open. A tracheotomy is used to bypass an upper airway obstruction, facilitate removal of secretions, or permit long-term mechanical ventilation.

The tracheostomy tube may be made of plastic, polyvinyl chloride, or metal and comes in various sizes, lengths, and styles depending on the patient's needs. A patient receiving mechanical ventilation needs a cuffed tube to prevent backflow of air around the tube. A cuffed tracheostomy tube also prevents an unconscious or a paralyzed patient from aspirating food or secretions. (See *Comparing tracheostomy tubes*, page 360.)

Emergency or planned procedure

In emergency situations, such as laryngeal edema with anaphylactic shock or foreign body obstruction, tracheotomy may be done at the bedside. More commonly, it's a planned procedure that's done in an operating room when a patient is likely to need prolonged mechanical ventilation.

Nursing considerations

- Before an emergency tracheotomy, briefly explain the procedure to the patient as time permits and quickly obtain supplies or a tracheotomy tray.
- Before a scheduled tracheotomy, explain the procedure and the need for anesthesia to the patient and his family. If possible, mention whether the tracheostomy is permanent or temporary. Tell them the patient is monitored in the critical care unit before and after the procedure.
- Ensure that samples for ABG analysis and other diagnostic tests have been collected and that the patient or a responsible family member has signed a consent form.

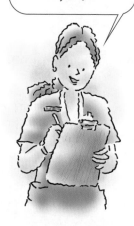

If your patient requires an emergency bedside tracheotomy, gather the necessary supplies or a tracheotomy tray quickly.

Afterward ward

- After the procedure, assess the patient's respiratory status, breath sounds, oxygen saturation level, vital signs, and heart rhythm. Note any crackles, rhonchi, wheezes, or diminished breath sounds.

Comparing tracheostomy tubes

Tracheostomy tubes are made of plastic or metal and come in uncuffed, cuffed, and fenestrated varieties. Tube selection depends on the patient's condition and the practitioner's preference. Make sure you're familiar with the advantages and disadvantages of these commonly used tracheostomy tubes.

Uncuffed (plastic or metal)

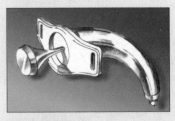

Advantages
* Free flow of air around tube and through larynx
* Reduced risk of tracheal damage
* Mechanical ventilation possible in patient with neuromuscular disease

Disadvantages
* Increased risk of aspiration in adults due to lack of cuff
* Adapter possibly needed for ventilation

Plastic cuffed (low pressure and high volume)

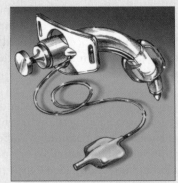

Advantages
* Disposable
* Cuff bonded to tube (won't detach accidentally inside trachea)
* Low cuff pressure that's evenly distributed against tracheal wall (no need to deflate periodically to lower pressure)
* Reduced risk of tracheal damage

Disadvantages
* Possibly more expensive than other tubes

Fenestrated

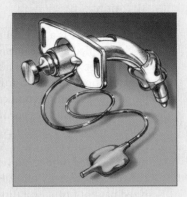

Advantages
* Speech possible through upper airway when external opening is capped and cuff is deflated
* Breathing by mechanical ventilation possible with inner cannula in place and cuff inflated
* Easy removal of inner cannula for cleaning

Disadvantages
* Possible occlusion of fenestration
* Possible dislodgment of inner cannula
* Cap removal necessary before inflating cuff

* Assess the patient for complications that can occur within the first 48 hours after tracheostomy tube insertion, including hemorrhage, edema into tracheal tissue causing airway obstruction, aspiration of secretions, hypoxemia, and introduction of air into surrounding tissue causing subcutaneous emphysema.
* Keep appropriate equipment at the bedside for immediate use in an emergency. (See *Emergency tracheostomy equipment.*)

Emergency tracheostomy equipment

Make sure you keep emergency tracheostomy equipment at the patient's bedside, including:
- sterile tracheal dilator or sterile hemostat
- sterile obturator that fits the tracheostomy tube
- extra sterile tracheostomy tube and obturator in the appropriate size
- suction equipment and supplies.

Keep the emergency equipment in full view in the patient's room at all times for easy access in case of emergency. Consider taping a wrapped, sterile tracheostomy tube to the head of the bed for easy access. If your patient coughs or pulls the tracheostomy tube out, you may use a sterile tracheal dilator to keep the stoma open and the airway patent until a new tube can be inserted.

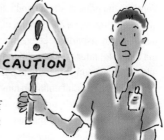

To avoid dislodging the tube, don't change your patient's tracheostomy ties unnecessarily.

- Perform tracheostomy care at least every 8 hours or as needed. Change the dressing as often as needed because a wet dressing with exudate or secretions predisposes the patient to skin excoriation, breakdown, and infection.
- Don't change the tracheostomy ties unnecessarily during the immediate postoperative period (usually 4 days) to avoid accidentally dislodging the tube.
- Document the procedure; the amount, color, and consistency of secretions; stoma and skin conditions; the patient's respiratory status; the duration of any cuff deflation, and cuff pressure readings with inflation. (See *Deflating and inflating a tracheostomy cuff*, page 362.)

Chest tube insertion

Chest tube insertion may be needed when treating patients with pneumothorax, hemothorax, empyema, pleural effusion, or chylothorax. The tube, which is inserted into the pleural space, allows blood, fluid, pus, or air to drain and allows the lung to reinflate.

Gotta have some negative pressure

After insertion, the chest tube is connected to a disposable chest tube drainage system. The system uses gravity and, possibly, suction to restore negative pressure and remove material that collected in the pleural cavity. Depending on the type of system, the wet or dry seal in the drainage system allows air and fluid to escape from the pleural cavity but doesn't allow air to reenter. The addition of suction

Deflating and inflating a tracheostomy cuff

During tracheostomy care, you may need to deflate and inflate a tracheostomy cuff. If so, gather a 10-ml syringe, stethoscope, and handheld resuscitation bag and follow these steps:

• Read the cuff manufacturer's instructions because cuff types and procedures vary widely.

• Confirm the patient's identity using two patient identifiers according to your facility's policy.

• Explain the procedure to him, provide privacy, and reassure him.

• Perform hand hygiene.

• Assess the patient's condition.

• Help the patient into semi-Fowler's position, if possible, or place him in a supine position with the head of the bed elevated as tolerated to prevent aspiration of secretions.

• Hyperoxygenate the patient and then suction the oropharyngeal cavity to prevent pooled secretions from descending into the trachea after cuff deflation.

• Remove the ventilation device or humidified oxygen.

• Insert a 10-ml syringe into the cuff pilot balloon. Ventilate the patient with a handheld resuscitation bag and slowly withdraw air from the cuff until a small leak is heard during inspiration. Leave the syringe attached to the tubing for later reinflation of the cuff. Slow deflation allows positive lung pressure to push secretions upward from the bronchi. Cuff deflation may also stimulate the patient's cough reflex, producing additional secretions.

• Reinflate the cuff using the minimal-leak technique or the minimal occlusive volume technique to help gauge the proper inflation point.

• If you're inflating the cuff using cuff pressure measurement, be careful not to exceed 25 mm Hg. If pressure exceeds 25 mm Hg, notify the doctor because you may need to change to a larger size tube, use higher inflation pressures, or permit a larger air leak.

• After you've inflated the cuff, remove the syringe.

• Reattach the ventilation device or humidified oxygen.

• Check for minimal leaks at the cuff seal. You shouldn't feel air coming from the patient's mouth, nose, or tracheostomy site, and a conscious patient shouldn't be able to speak.

• Observe the patient for adequate ventilation.

• Be alert for air leaks from the cuff itself. Suspect a leak if injection of air fails to inflate the cuff or increase cuff pressure, if you can't inject the amount of air you withdrew, if the patient can speak, if ventilation fails to maintain adequate respiratory movement with pressures or volumes previously considered adequate, or if air escapes during the ventilator's inspiratory cycle.

• Note the exact amount of air used to inflate the cuff to detect tracheomalacia if more air is consistently needed.

• Make sure that the patient is comfortable and can easily reach the call button and communication aids.

• Properly clean or dispose of all equipment, supplies, and trash according to your facility's policy.

• Remove your gloves and perform hand hygiene.

• Replenish any used supplies and make sure all necessary emergency supplies are at the bedside.

• Document the procedure.

increases the negative intrapleural pressure and helps overcome air leakage by improving the rate of airflow out of the patient and improving fluid removal.

Put a valve on it

A one-way flutter valve, such as the Heimlich valve, is sometimes used instead of a drainage system. The one-way valve is connected to the end of the chest tube and allows accumulated air to escape but not enter. This type of valve allows portability for patients who need long-term chest tube placement.

Nursing considerations

- Explain the procedure to the patient and his family. Make sure that an appropriate consent form is signed.
- Obtain baseline vital signs.
- Collect necessary equipment, including a thoracotomy tray and a drainage system. Prepare lidocaine (Xylocaine) for local anesthesia as directed. The practitioner will clean the insertion site with antiseptic solution. Set up the drainage system according to the manufacturer's instructions and place it at the bedside. (See *Closed chest drainage systems*.)
- Assess respiratory function and obtain vital signs and oxygen saturation levels immediately after insertion. Routinely assess chest tube function. Describe and record the amount of drainage at least every 8 hours. Notify the practitioner immediately if the amount of drainage is greater than 200 ml in 1 hour (indicates bleeding).

Closed chest drainage systems

There are three types of chest tube drainage systems: a water seal wet suction system, a water seal dry suction system, and a dry seal dry suction system.

Water seal wet suction system
A water seal wet suction system is a disposable plastic drainage system that contains three chambers. The drainage chamber is on the right and has three calibrated columns that display the amount of drainage collected. When the first column fills, drainage carries over into the second and, when that fills, into the third.

The water seal chamber is located in the center. The suction control chamber on the left is filled with water to achieve various suction levels. Rubber diaphragms are provided at the rear of the device to change the water level or remove samples of drainage. A positive pressure relief valve at the top of the water seal chamber vents excess pressure into the atmosphere, preventing pressure buildup.

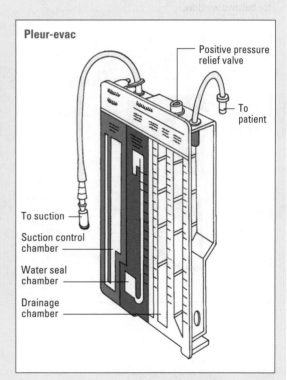

Pleur-evac

Positive pressure relief valve

To patient

To suction

Suction control chamber

Water seal chamber

Drainage chamber

(continued)

Closed chest drainage systems *(continued)*

Water seal dry suction system

A water seal dry suction system has two chambers and doesn't use water to control the amount of suction. A dry suction control regulator balances the suction force and the atmosphere. The drainage chamber is on the right and has three calibrated columns that display the amount of drainage collected. When the first column fills, drainage carries over into the second and, when that fills, into the third.

The water seal chamber is located on the bottom left. The rotary dry suction control regulator is located on the top left and is turned to the ordered suction mark. An indicator appears when the desired negative pressure is achieved. In some models, an orange float appears in an indicator window. Other models indicate that the correct amount of suction is being delivered when the bellows reach the calibrated triangular mark in the suction monitor bellows window.

Dry seal dry suction system

A dry seal dry suction system has two chambers: a drainage collection chamber and an air leak monitor. It doesn't use water to control the amount of suction or to provide a seal. It has a dry one-way valve for seal protection. A dry suction control regulator balances the suction force and the atmosphere. The drainage chamber is on the right and has three calibrated columns that display the amount of drainage collected. When the first column fills, drainage carries over into the second and, when that fills, into the third.

The air leak monitor is located on the bottom left. The rotary dry suction control regulator is located on the top left and is turned to the ordered suction mark. An indicator appears when the desired negative pressure is achieved. In some models, an orange float appears in an indicator window. Other models indicate that the correct amount of suction is being delivered when the bellows reach the calibrated triangular mark in the suction monitor bellows window.

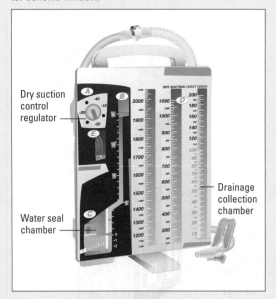

Dry suction control regulator

Water seal chamber

Drainage collection chamber

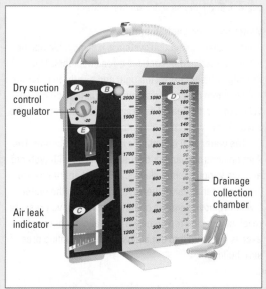

Dry suction control regulator

Air leak indicator

Drainage collection chamber

- Avoid creating dependent loops, kinks, or pressure in the tubing. Don't lift the drainage system above the patient's chest because fluid may flow back into the pleural space. (See *Checking for chest tube leaks*.) Clamping of chest tubes is no longer the recommended practice. If the chest tube becomes disconnected, it should be immediately attached to a new drainage system. If a drainage system is not readily available, the end of the tube (about 2 cm) should be inserted into sterile water. Sterile water should be kept at the bedside for emergencies.
- If the drainage collection chamber fills, replace it according to your facility's policy. To do so, double clamp the chest tube close to the insertion site (using two clamps facing in opposite directions), exchange the system, remove the clamps, and retape the connection.
- To prevent a tension pneumothorax (which can occur when clamping stops air and fluid from escaping), never leave the chest tube clamped for more than 1 minute.
- Notify the practitioner immediately if the patient develops cyanosis, rapid or shallow breathing, subcutaneous emphysema, chest pain, or excessive bleeding.

Thoracotomy

Thoracotomy, a surgical incision into the thoracic cavity, is done to locate and examine abnormalities, such as tumors, bleeding sites, or thoracic injuries; to perform a biopsy; or to remove diseased lung tissue. It's most commonly done to remove part or all of a lung to spare healthy lung tissue from disease.

Lung excisions

Types of lung excisions include pneumonectomy, lobectomy, segmental resection, and wedge resection:

Bye-bye lung

A *pneumonectomy* is the excision of an entire lung. It's usually performed to treat patients with bronchogenic cancer but may be used to treat those with TB, bronchiectasis, or lung abscess. Pneumonectomy is used only when a less radical approach would fail to remove all diseased tissue. After a pneumonectomy, chest cavity pressures stabilize, and over time, fluid fills the cavity where lung tissue was removed, preventing significant mediastinal shift.

One out of five lobes

A *lobectomy* is the removal of one of the five lung lobes. It's used to treat patients with bronchogenic cancer, TB, lung abscess,

> Thoracotomy is usually done to remove part or all of a lung.

Checking for chest tube leaks

When trying to locate a leak in your patient's chest tube system, try:
- briefly cross-clamping the tube at various points along its length, beginning at the tube's proximal end and working down toward the drainage system
- paying special attention to the seal around the connections
- pushing any loose connections back together and taping them securely.

Bubble may mean trouble

The bubbling of the system stops when a clamp is placed between an air leak and the water seal. If you clamp along the tube's entire length and the bubbling doesn't stop, you probably need to replace the drainage unit because it may be cracked.

emphysematous blebs, benign tumors, or localized fungal infections. After this surgery, the remaining lobes expand to fill the entire pleural cavity.

How do you like your resection?

A *segmental resection* is the removal of one or more lung segments. This procedure preserves more functional tissue than lobectomy; it's commonly used to treat patients with bronchiectasis.

A *wedge resection* is removal of a small portion of the lung without regard to segments. It preserves the most functional tissue of all the surgeries but is used only when the patient has a small, well-circumscribed lesion. Remaining lung tissue should be reexpanded.

Other thoracic surgeries

Here are some other types of thoracic surgeries:

- Exploratory thoracotomy is used to examine the chest and pleural space in evaluating chest trauma and tumors.
- Decortication is used to help reexpand the lung in a patient with empyema. It involves removing or stripping the thick, fibrous membrane covering the visceral pleura.
- Thoracoplasty is performed to remove part or all of one rib and to reduce the size of the chest cavity. It decreases the risk for mediastinal shift when TB has reduced lung volume.
- Bronchoplastic (sleeve) reduction involves the excision of one lobar bronchus along with part of the right or left bronchus. The distal bronchus is then reanastomosed to the proximal bronchus or trachea.
- Lung reduction surgery is used to treat patients with emphysema. Giant bullae are excised, thereby reducing lung volume and allowing compressed alveoli to reexpand.
- Video-assisted thoracic surgery is a minimally invasive technique used to treat patients with some pulmonary conditions, perform open lung biopsies, and to stage and diagnose some lung cancers.

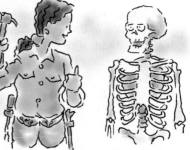

With thoracoplasty, part or all of a rib is removed to reduce the size of the chest cavity.

Nursing considerations

- Explain the procedure to the patient and his family. Tell them that after surgery, the patient may have a chest tube and oxygen delivery system in place.
- After thoracic surgery, assess vital signs, oxygen saturation levels, breath sounds, and cardiopulmonary and hemodynamic status. Monitor for cardiac arrhythmias. Atrial arrhythmias, especially atrial fibrillation, commonly occur after pneumonectomy due to pulmonary vasculature blood flow changes and atrial enlargement; patients may be treated prophylactically with cardiac glycosides.

- Monitor the chest tube insertion site and assess and record the amount and characteristics of drainage. Suction isn't used after a pneumonectomy, and the chest tube is attached to gravity drainage only.
- If the patient underwent a pneumonectomy, position him only on his operative side or his back until stabilized. This prevents fluid from draining into the unaffected lung if the sutured bronchus opens.
- Monitor for complications of thoracotomy, including hemorrhage, infection, tension pneumothorax, bronchopleural fistula, and empyema.

Lung transplantation

Lung transplantation involves the replacement of one or both lungs with that from a donor. COPD is the most common underlying disease that necessitates lung transplantation; others include cystic fibrosis, sarcoidosis, pulmonary hypertension, and pulmonary fibrosis.

So, who qualifies?

The qualifications for lung transplantation vary based on the underlying disease process. The patient must have significant pulmonary complications as well as other specific criteria.

Not gonna happen

Contraindications to lung transplantation have traditionally included the following:
- uncontrolled or untreatable pulmonary or extrapulmonary infection
- malignancy in the last 2 years
- significant dysfunction of other vital organs
- significant chest wall or spinal deformity
- active tobacco smoking
- drug or alcohol dependency
- unresolved psychosocial problems or noncompliance with medical therapy
- human immunodeficiency virus infection
- ongoing hepatitis B or C viral infection
- absence of a consistent or reliable social support system.

Other factors must be taken into account on an individual basis. These include ventilator dependence; nutritional status; previous cardiothoracic surgery; and such preexisting medical conditions as coronary artery disease, hypertension, diabetes mellitus, and osteoporosis, which would be aggravated by the medical regimen after transplantation.

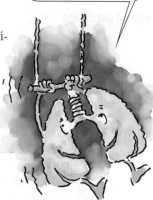

To qualify for lung transplantation, I thought I would have to jump through hoops, not swing from a trapeze. What gives?

TKO for transplant

Lung transplantation is performed under general anesthesia. Bilateral anterior thoracotomy incisions and a transverse sternotomy provide access to the thoracic cavity. After removal of the patient's lungs, the donor lungs are implanted with anastomoses to the patient's bronchus.

Cardiopulmonary bypass is commonly used during the transplantation procedure.

Complications

The major complication after lung transplantation is organ rejection, which occurs because the recipient's body responds to the implanted tissue as a foreign body and triggers an immune response. This leads to fibrosis and scar formation.

Secondary snags

Another major complication after lung transplantation is infection due to immunosuppressive therapy.

Other possible complications include hemorrhage and reperfusion edema. Long-term complications (typically occurring after 3 years) include obliterative bronchiolitis and posttransplant lymphoproliferative disorder. Either may be fatal.

Nursing considerations

Provide care before and after transplantation.

Educate and administer

- Answer all questions about the transplantation and what the patient can expect. Explain postoperative care (e.g., intubation), equipment used in the acute postoperative phase, and availability of analgesics for pain.
- Administer medications and obtain laboratory testing as ordered.

Keep on assessing

- Assess cardiopulmonary status frequently (every 5 to 15 minutes in the immediate postoperative period) until the patient is stabilized. Be alert for cardiac index less than 2.2, hypotension, fever higher than 99.5°F (37.5°C), crackles or rhonchi, and decreased oxygen saturation.
- Assess respiratory status and ventilatory equipment frequently and suction secretions as necessary. Expect frequent ABG analyses and daily chest X-rays to evaluate the patient's readiness to wean from the ventilator.
- Assess chest tube drainage for amount, color, and characteristics. Assess for bleeding. Notify the doctor according to the hospital's and surgeon's parameters for normal drainage.

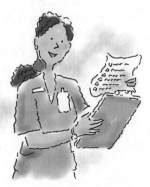

Check the patient's ABG levels and chest X-rays daily to determine if he can be weaned from the ventilator.

- Closely monitor fluid intake and output. If the patient becomes hemodynamically unstable, administer vasoactive and inotropic agents as ordered and titrate the dose to achieve the desired response.
- After extubation, assess the patient often for shortness of breath, tachypnea, dyspnea, malaise, and increased sputum production; these suggest acute rejection.
- After a single-lung transplantation, the newly implanted lung is denervated, but the patient's remaining lung continues to send messages to the brain indicating poor oxygenation. The patient may complain of shortness of breath and dyspnea even with oxygen saturation levels greater than 90%.
- Maintain strict infection control precautions such as meticulous hand washing.
- Inspect surgical dressings for bleeding in the early post-operative phase. Inspect the surgical incisions later for redness, swelling, and other signs of infection.

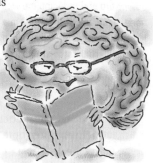

After a single-lung transplantation, the remaining lung continues to send messages to the brain that it's oxygen-starved, even though oxygen saturation is over 90%. I am feeling a bit Snack-ish!

Inhalation therapy

Inhalation therapy involves carefully controlled ventilation techniques to help the patient maintain optimal ventilation in case of respiratory failure. Techniques include ET intubation, mechanical ventilation and oxygen administration, and noninvasive positive pressure ventilation (NPPV). Proper weaning from ventilation techniques is also a part of inhalation therapy.

ET intubation

ET intubation involves insertion of a tube into the trachea through the mouth or nose to establish a patent airway. It protects patients from aspiration by sealing off the trachea from the digestive tract and permits removal of tracheobronchial secretions in patients who can't cough effectively. ET intubation also provides a route for mechanical ventilation and oxygen administration. ET intubation may be more difficult to accomplish in an obese patient. (See *Intubating an obese patient*, page 370.)

Too good to be true?

Drawbacks of ET intubation are that it bypasses normal respiratory defenses against infection, reduces cough effectiveness, may be uncomfortable, and prevents verbal communication.

Potential complications of ET intubation include:
- bronchospasm or laryngospasm
- aspiration of blood, secretions, or gastric contents
- tooth damage or loss
- injury to the lips, mouth, pharynx, or vocal cords

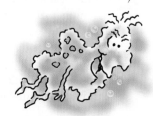

ET intubation bypasses normal respiratory defenses against infection. That's good news for me but bad news for the patient!

Intubating an obese patient

Laryngoscopy and ET tube placement can be difficult in obese patients. These patients may have altered upper airway anatomy resulting in a poor view of the glottis despite optimal laryngoscopic technique. In addition, short, thick necks may limit mobility and make it difficult to place the patient in the optimal sniffing position, which has traditionally been recommended to optimize glottic visualization during direct laryngoscopy. The ramped position may be more effective for an obese patient.

In preparation for intubation, place an obese patient in an upright or semi-upright position, depending on the degree of respiratory distress. An upright position improves respiratory function by allowing the diaphragm to fall downward and reducing the weight on the chest wall. If there's no contraindication, such as cervical spine precautions, place an obese patient in a ramped, or head-elevated, position for direct laryngoscopy. In the ramped position, blankets or commercially available beds are used to elevate the head and torso so that the external auditory meatus and the sternal notch are aligned horizontally.

- hypoxemia (if attempts at intubation are prolonged or oxygen delivery interrupted)
- tracheal stenosis, erosion, and necrosis
- cardiac arrhythmias.

Orotracheal intubation
With orotracheal intubation, the oral cavity is used as the route of insertion. It's preferred in emergency situations because it's easier and faster. However, maintaining exact tube placement is more difficult because the tube must be well secured to avoid kinking and prevent bronchial obstruction or accidental extubation. It's also uncomfortable for conscious patients because it stimulates salivation, coughing, and retching.

The right size

The typical size for an oral ET tube is 7.5 mm (indicates the size of the lumen) for women and 8 mm for men.

Not for everyone

Orotracheal intubation is contraindicated in patients with orofacial injuries, acute cervical spinal injury, and degenerative spinal disorders.

Nasal intubation
With nasal intubation, a nasal passage is used as the route of insertion. Nasal intubation is much less common than orotracheal intubation.

A conscious choice

Nasal intubation is usually more comfortable than oral intubation and is typically used for conscious patients who are at risk for imminent respiratory arrest or who have cervical spinal injuries. It's contraindicated for patients with facial or basilar skull fractures.

Difficult and damaging

Although it's more comfortable than oral intubation, nasal intubation is more difficult to perform. Because the tube passes blindly through the nasal cavity, it causes more tissue damage, increases the risk for infection by nasal bacteria introduced into the trachea, and increases the risk for pressure necrosis of the nasal mucosa.

Nursing considerations
- After securing the ET tube, reconfirm tube placement by noting bilateral breath sounds and $ETco_2$ readings. (See *Securing an ET tube.*)

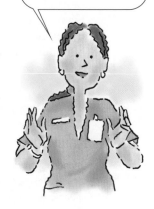

On the downside, nasal intubation is more difficult to do than oral intubation and causes more tissue damage.

Securing an ET tube

Secure an ET tube with an ET tube holder, as recommended by the American Heart Association and American Pediatric Association. Alternatively, tape the tube in place to prevent dislodgment.

Before securing an ET tube, make sure that the patient's face is clean, dry, and free from beard stubble. If possible, suction his mouth and dry the tube just before taping. Check the reference mark on the tube to ensure correct placement. After securing the ET tube, always check for bilateral breath sounds to ensure that it hasn't been displaced by manipulation.

When you're using an ET tube holder
- Made of hard plastic or of softer materials, an ET tube holder is a convenient way to secure an ET tube in place. The tube holder is available in adult and pediatric sizes, and some models may come with bite blocks attached. Place the strap around the patient's neck and secure around the tube with Velcro fasteners. Because each model is different, check with the manufacturers guidelines for correct placement and care.

When you're using tape
- Tear about 2' (60 cm) of tape, split both ends in half about 4" (10 cm), and place the tape adhesive side up on a flat surface.
- Tear another piece of tape about 10" (25 cm) long and place it adhesive side down in the center of the 2' piece.
- Slide the tape under the patient's neck and center it.
- Bring the right side of the tape up and wrap the top split end counterclockwise around the tube; secure the bottom split end beneath the patient's lower lip.
- Bring the left side of the tape up and wrap the bottom split piece clockwise around the tube; secure the top split above the patient's upper lip.

- Auscultate breath sounds and watch for bilateral chest movement to ensure correct tube placement and full lung ventilation.
- A chest X-ray will be ordered to confirm tube placement.
- Disposable $ETco_2$ detectors are used to confirm tube placement in emergency departments, postanesthesia care units, and critical care units that don't use continual $ETco_2$ monitoring. Follow the manufacturer's instructions for proper use of the device. Don't use the detector with a heated humidifier or nebulizer because humidity, heat, and moisture can interfere with the device. (See *Analyzing carbon dioxide levels.*)

Analyzing carbon dioxide levels

Depending on which $ETco_2$ detector you use, the meaning of color changes within the detector dome may differ. Here's a description of one type of detector, the Easy Cap detector, and what color changes mean:

- The rim of the Easy Cap is divided into four segments (clockwise from the top): CHECK, A, B, and C. The CHECK segment is solid-purple, signifying the absence of CO_2.
- The numbers in the other sections range from 0.03 to 5, indicating the percentage of exhaled CO_2. The color should fluctuate from purple during ventilation (section A) to yellow during inspiration (section C) at the end of expiration. This indicates that the $ETco_2$ levels are adequate (above 2%).
- An end-expiratory color change from C to the B range may be the first sign of hemodynamic instability.

- During CPR, an end-expiratory color change from the A or B range to the C range may mean the return of spontaneous ventilation.
- During prolonged cardiac arrest, inadequate pulmonary perfusion leads to inadequate gas exchange. The patient exhales little or no CO_2, so the color stays in the purple range even with proper intubation. Ineffective CPR also leads to inadequate pulmonary perfusion.

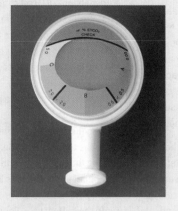

- Measure the distance from the edge of the lip to the end of the tube and document the distance on the flow sheet. If the tube has measurement markings on it, record the measurement where the tube exits at the lips. By periodically monitoring this mark, you can detect tube displacement.
- Follow standard precautions and suction through the ET tube as the patient's condition indicates to clear secretions and prevent mucus plugs from obstructing the tube. Hyperoxygenate the patient before and after suctioning to reduce suction-induced hypoxia. If available, use a closed tracheal suctioning system, which permits the ventilated patient to remain on the ventilator during suctioning. (See *Closed tracheal suctioning,* page 374.)

Mechanical ventilation

Mechanical ventilation involves the use of a machine to move air into a patient's lungs. Mechanical ventilators use either positive or negative pressure to ventilate patients.

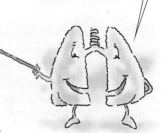

Mechanical ventilation uses a machine to move air into the patient's lungs.

When to ventilate

Indications for mechanical ventilation include:
- acute respiratory failure due to ARDS, pneumonia, acute exacerbations of COPD, pulmonary embolism, heart failure, trauma, tumors, or drug overdose
- respiratory center depression due to stroke, brain injury, or trauma
- neuromuscular disturbances caused by neuromuscular diseases, such as Guillain-Barré syndrome, multiple sclerosis, and myasthenia gravis; trauma, including spinal cord injury; or CNS depression.

Accentuate the positive

Positive pressure ventilators exert a positive pressure on the airway, which causes inspiration while increasing tidal volume (V_T). A high-frequency ventilator uses high respiratory rates and low V_T to maintain alveolar ventilation.

The inspiratory cycles of these ventilators may be adjusted for volume, pressure, or time:
- A volume-cycled ventilator, the type used most commonly, delivers a preset volume of air each time, regardless of the amount of lung resistance.

Closed tracheal suctioning

The closed tracheal suctioning system can ease removal of secretions and reduce patient complications. The system consists of a sterile suction catheter in a clear plastic sleeve. It permits the patient to remain connected to the ventilator during suctioning.

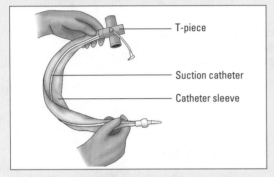

- T-piece
- Suction catheter
- Catheter sleeve

As a result, the patient can maintain the V_T, oxygen concentration, and PEEP delivered by the ventilator while being suctioned. In turn, this reduces the occurrence of suction-induced hypoxemia.

Another advantage of this system is a reduced risk of infection, even when the same catheter is used many times. The caregiver doesn't need to touch the catheter, and the ventilator circuit remains closed.

Performing the procedure

To perform the procedure, gather a closed suction control valve, a T-piece to connect the artificial airway to the ventilator breathing circuit, and a catheter sleeve that encloses the catheter and has connections at each end for the control valve and the T-piece. Then, follow these steps:
- Perform hand hygiene and put on gloves.
- Remove the closed suctioning system from its wrapping. Attach the control valve to the connecting tubing.
- Depress the thumb suction control valve and keep it depressed while setting the suction pressure to the desired level.
- Connect the T-piece to the ventilator breathing circuit, making sure that the irrigation port is closed, then connect the T-piece to the patient's ET or tracheostomy tube (as shown above right).

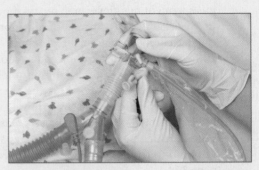

- Hyperoxygenate and hyperinflate the patient's lungs using the ventilator.
- With one hand keeping the T-piece parallel to the patient's chin, use the thumb and index finger of the other hand to advance the catheter through the tube and into the patient's tracheobronchial tree (as shown below).

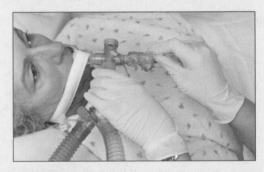

- If necessary, gently retract the catheter sleeve as you advance the catheter.
- While continuing to hold the T-piece and control valve, apply intermittent suction and withdraw the catheter until it reaches its fully extended length in the sleeve. Repeat the procedure as necessary.
- After you finish suctioning, flush the catheter by maintaining suction while slowly introducing normal saline solution or sterile water into the irrigation port.
- Place the thumb control valve in the off position.
- Dispose of and replace the suction equipment and supplies according to your facility's policy.
- Remove your gloves and perform hand hygiene.
- Change the closed suction system according to your facility's policy.

- A pressure-cycled ventilator generates flow until the machine reaches a preset pressure, regardless of the volume delivered or the time required to achieve the pressure.
- A time-cycled ventilator generates flow for a preset amount of time.

Several different modes of ventilatory control are found on the ventilator. The choice of mode depends on the patient's respiratory condition. (See *Ventilator modes*, page 376.)

Out goes the thorax, in flows the air

Negative pressure ventilators work by creating negative pressure, which pulls the thorax outward and allows air to flow into the lungs. They're used primarily to treat patients with slowly progressing neuromuscular disorders. Examples of such ventilators include the iron lung, the cuirass (chest shell), and the body wrap.

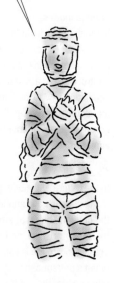

Negative pressure ventilators include the iron lung, the cuirass, and the body wrap.

Nursing considerations
- Provide emotional support to the patient during all phases of mechanical ventilation to reduce anxiety and promote successful treatment.
- Even if the patient is unresponsive, continue to explain all procedures and treatments.

Be alarmed

- Make sure the ventilator alarms are on at all times to alert you to potentially hazardous conditions and changes in the patient's status. If an alarm sounds and the problem can't be easily identified, disconnect the patient from the ventilator and use a handheld resuscitation bag to ventilate him. (See *Responding to ventilator alarms*, page 377.)
- Assess cardiopulmonary status frequently, at least every 2 to 4 hours or more often, if indicated. Assess vital signs and auscultate breath sounds. Monitor pulse oximetry or $ETco_2$ levels and hemodynamic parameters as ordered. Monitor intake and output and assess for fluid volume excess or dehydration.
- Be alert for the development of complications associated with mechanical ventilation. These complications include decreased cardiac output (especially with the use of PEEP), barotrauma, pneumothorax, atelectasis, oxygen toxicity, stress ulcers, and ventilator-associated pneumonia (VAP). (See *Preventing VAP*, page 378.)

Ventilator modes

Positive pressure ventilators are categorized as volume or pressure ventilators and have various modes and options.

Volume modes

Volume modes include controlled ventilation (CV) or controlled mandatory ventilation (CMV), assist-control (A/C) or assisted mandatory ventilation (AMV), and intermittent mandatory ventilation (IMV) or synchronized intermittent mandatory ventilation (SIMV).

CV or CMV

In the CV or CMV mode, the ventilator supplies all ventilation for the patient. The respiratory rate, V_T, inspiratory time, and PEEP are preset. This mode is usually used when a patient can't initiate spontaneous breaths, such as when he's paralyzed from a spinal cord injury or neuromuscular disease, or chemically paralyzed with neuromuscular blocking agents.

A/C or AMV

In the A/C or AMV mode, the basic respiratory rate is set along with the V_T, inspiratory time, and PEEP, but the patient is able to breathe faster than the preset rate. The sensitivity is set so that when the patient initiates a spontaneous breath, a full V_T is delivered, so that all breaths are the same V_T, whether triggered by the patient or delivered at the set rate. If the patient tires and his drive to breathe is

negated, the ventilator continues to deliver breaths at the preset rate.

IMV or SIMV

IMV and SIMV modes require preset respiratory rate, V_T, inspiratory time, sensitivity, and PEEP. Mandatory breaths are delivered at a set rate and V_T. In between the mandatory breaths, the patient can breathe spontaneously at his own rate and V_T. The V_T of these spontaneous breaths can vary because the breaths are determined by the patient's ability to generate negative pressure in his chest. With SIMV, the ventilator synchronizes the mandatory breaths with the patient's own inspirations.

Pressure modes

Pressure modes include pressure-support ventilation (PSV), pressure-controlled ventilation (PCV), pressure-controlled/inverse ratio ventilation (PC/IRV), and airway pressure release ventilation (APRV).

PSV

The PSV mode augments inspiration for a spontaneously breathing patient. The inspiratory pressure level, PEEP, and sensitivity are preset. When the patient initiates a breath, the breath is delivered at the preset pressure level and is maintained throughout inspiration. The patient determines the V_T, respiratory rate, and inspiratory time.

PCV

In PCV mode, inspiratory pressure, inspiratory time, respiratory rate, and PEEP are preset. V_T varies with the patient's airway pressure and compliance.

PC/IVR

PC/IVR combines pressure-limited ventilation with an inverse ratio of inspiration to expiration. In this mode, the inspiratory pressure, respiratory rate, inspiratory time (1:1, 2:1, 3:1, or 4:1), and PEEP are preset. PCV and PC/IRV modes may be used in patients with ARDS.

APRV

During APRV, a high continuous positive airway pressure (P high) is delivered for a long duration (T high) and then falls to a lower pressure (P low) for a shorter duration (T low). The transition from P high to P low deflates the lungs and eliminates CO_2. Conversely, the transition from P low to P high inflates the lungs. Alveolar recruitment is maximized by the high continuous positive airway pressure. Spontaneous breathing is allowed throughout the ventilation cycle, which results in a decreased requirement for sedation and neuromuscular blockade use. APRV mode may be used in patients with acute lung injury or ARDS.

Responding to ventilator alarms

This chart outlines the possible causes and the nursing interventions needed if a ventilator alarm sounds.

Signal	Possible cause	Interventions
Low-pressure alarm	ET tube disconnected from ventilator	Reconnect the tube to the ventilator.
	Tube displaced above vocal cords or tracheostomy tube extubated	Check the tube placement; reposition if needed. If extubation or displacement has occurred, ventilate the patient manually and call the practitioner immediately.
	Leaking V_T from low cuff pressure (from an underinflated or ruptured cuff or a leak in the cuff or one-way valve)	Listen for a whooshing sound around the tube, indicating an air leak. If you hear one, check the cuff pressure. If you can't maintain pressure, call the practitioner; he may need to insert a new tube.
	Ventilator malfunction	Disconnect the patient from the ventilator and ventilate him manually, if necessary. Obtain another ventilator.
	Leak in ventilator circuitry (from loose connection or hole in tubing, loss of temperature-sensitive device, or cracked humidification jar)	Make sure all connections are intact. Check for holes or leaks in the tubing and replace, if necessary. Check the humidification jar and replace, if cracked.
High-pressure alarm	Increased airway pressure or decreased lung compliance caused by worsening disease	Auscultate the lungs for evidence of increasing lung consolidation, barotrauma, or wheezing. Call the practitioner if indicated.
	Patient biting on oral ET tube	Insert a bite block if needed.
	Secretions in airway	Look for secretions in the airway. To remove them, suction the patient or have him cough.
	Condensate in large-bore tubing	Check tubing for condensate and remove any fluid.
	Intubation of right mainstem bronchus	Check tube position. If it has slipped, call the practitioner, who may need to reposition it.
	Patient coughing, gagging, or attempting to talk	If the patient fights the ventilator, the practitioner may order a sedative or neuromuscular blocking agent.
	Chest wall resistance	Reposition the patient to see if doing so improves chest expansion. If repositioning doesn't help, administer the prescribed analgesic.
	Failure of high-pressure relief valve	Have the faulty equipment replaced.
	Bronchospasm	Assess the patient for the cause. Report to the practitioner and treat the patient, as ordered.

Preventing VAP

VAP is a type of hospital-acquired pneumonia that develops more than 48 to 72 hours after ET intubation. In 2008, the Society of Healthcare Epidemiology of America and the Infectious Diseases Society of America issued practice recommendations to reduce the risk for VAP. In addition to minimizing mechanical ventilation, the recommendations included reducing colonization of the aerodigestive tract and preventing aspiration.

Key prevention strategies
• Perform hand hygiene before and after contact with patients.
• Perform hand hygiene before and after contact with the patient's respiratory equipment and items in the patient's room and after contact with respiratory secretions.
• Wear gloves whenever contact with respiratory secretions or contaminated objects is anticipated and perform hand hygiene before and after glove use.
• Avoid unnecessary antibiotics.
• Perform routine antiseptic mouth care.
• Prevent aspiration of contaminated secretions
• Elevate the head of the bed 30 to 45 degrees.
• Assess the patient's readiness for weaning and the appropriateness of spontaneous breathing trials daily.

• Extubate patients as soon as possible. Apply weaning protocols and optimal use of sedation.
• Remove condensate from ventilatory circuits before repositioning the patient. Keep the ventilatory circuit closed during condensate removal.
• Change the ventilatory circuit only when visibly soiled or malfunctioning.
• Use sterile water to rinse reusable respiratory equipment.
• Store and disinfect respiratory therapy equipment properly.
• Minimize gastric distension. Monitor the patient's tolerance of gastric feedings, auscultate for bowel sounds, and measure abdominal girth frequently. Measure residual gastric volume during continuous feedings and before each intermittent feeding to decrease the likelihood of gastric distension and aspiration.
• Limit the use of opioid and anticholinergic drugs.
• Decrease gastric acidity using stress ulcer prophylaxis.
• Institute a mobility protocol to decrease the amount of time spent on bed rest.
• Educate health care personnel who care for patients undergoing ventilation about VAP.

• Unless contraindicated, keep the head of the bed elevated and turn the patient from side to side every 1 to 2 hours to aid lung expansion and removal of secretions. Perform active or passive range-of-motion (ROM) exercises for all extremities to reduce the hazards of immobility.
• Place the call bell within the patient's reach and establish a method of communication (such as a communication board) because intubation and mechanical ventilation impair the patient's ability to speak.

- Administer a sedative or neuromuscular blocking agent, as ordered, to relax the patient or eliminate spontaneous breathing efforts that can interfere with the ventilator's action.

Be extra vigilant

- Remember that the patient receiving a neuromuscular blocking agent requires close observation because he can't breathe or communicate. In addition, if the patient is receiving a neuromuscular blocking agent, make sure he also receives a sedative and analgesia. Neuromuscular blocking agents cause paralysis without altering the patient's LOC. Reassure the patient and his family that the paralysis is temporary. Provide routine eye care and instill artificial tears because the patient can't blink.
- Make sure emergency equipment is readily available in case the ventilator malfunctions or the patient is extubated accidentally. If there's a problem with the ventilator, disconnect the patient from the ventilator and manually ventilate with 100% oxygen; use a handheld resuscitation bag connected to the ET or tracheostomy tube, troubleshoot the ventilator, and correct the problem. If you can't determine the cause, call for help and have the respiratory therapist evaluate the problem. (See *Understanding manual ventilation*, page 380.)

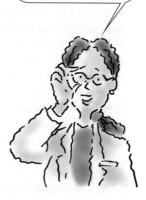

Stay alert! A patient receiving a neuromuscular blocking agent requires close observation because of his inability to breathe or communicate.

Weaning

The patient's body quickly comes to depend on artificial ventilation and must gradually be reintroduced to normal breathing.

Spontaneous strength

Successful weaning depends on a strong spontaneous respiratory effort, ABG levels within normal limits, a stable cardiovascular system, and sufficient respiratory muscle strength and LOC to sustain spontaneous breathing. Criteria must be individualized. Some patients may not meet all the weaning parameters, such as patients with chronic hypoxemia values, but may be ready for attempts at the discontinuation of mechanical ventilation.

Pressure-support ventilation may be used to help the patient build respiratory muscle strength before complete weaning from mechanical ventilation occurs.

Weaning methods

Several weaning methods are used:

- In *intermittent mandatory ventilation* (IMV), the number of breaths produced by the ventilator is gradually reduced, allowing the patient to breathe independently. Decreasing the number of breaths allows the patient to gradually increase his respiratory muscle strength and endurance.
- *Pressure-support ventilation* (PSV) may be used alone or as an adjunct to IMV in the weaning process. In this procedure, a set burst of pressure is applied during inspiration with the

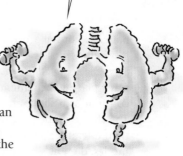

Understanding manual ventilation

A handheld resuscitation bag is an inflatable device that can be attached to a face mask or directly to a tracheostomy or an ET tube to allow manual delivery of oxygen or room air to the lungs of a patient who can't breathe by himself.

Although usually used in an emergency, manual ventilation can also be performed while the patient is disconnected temporarily from a mechanical ventilator, such as during a tubing change, during transport, or before suctioning. In such instances, the use of the handheld resuscitation bag maintains ventilation. Oxygen administration with a resuscitation bag can help improve a compromised cardiorespiratory system.

Ventilation guidelines
To manually ventilate a patient with an ET or tracheostomy tube, follow these guidelines:
• If oxygen is readily available, connect the handheld resuscitation bag to the oxygen. Attach one end of the tubing to the bottom of the bag and the other end to the nipple adapter on the flow meter of the oxygen source.

• Turn on the oxygen and adjust the flow rate according to the patient's condition.
• Before attaching the handheld resuscitation bag, suction the ET or tracheostomy tube to remove any secretions that may obstruct the airway.
• Remove the mask from the ventilation bag and attach the handheld resuscitation bag directly to the tube.
• Keeping your nondominant hand on the connection of the bag to the tube, use your dominant hand to compress the bag every 5 seconds to deliver approximately 1,000 cc of air.

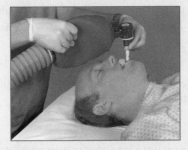

• Deliver breaths with the patient's own inspiratory effort (if any is present). Don't attempt to deliver a breath as the patient exhales.
• Observe the patient's chest to ensure that it rises and falls with each

compression. If ventilation fails to occur, check the connection and the patency of the patient's airway; if necessary, reposition his head and suction.
• Be alert for possible underventilation, which commonly occurs because the handheld resuscitation bag is difficult to keep positioned while ensuring an open airway. In addition, the volume of air delivered to the patient varies with the type of bag used and the hand size of the person compressing the bag. An adult with a small- or medium-sized hand may not consistently deliver 1,000 cc of air. For these reasons, have someone assist with the procedure if possible.
• Keep in mind that air is forced into the patient's stomach with manual ventilation, placing the patient at risk for aspiration of vomitus (possibly resulting in pneumonia) and gastric distention.
• Record the date and time of the procedure, reason and length of time the patient was disconnected from mechanical ventilation and received manual ventilation, any complications and the nursing action taken, and the patient's tolerance of the procedure.

patient's normal breathing pattern, allowing the patient to build respiratory muscle strength.
• *Spontaneous breathing trials* can be accomplished in one of three ways: placing the patient on minimum pressure support, using continuous positive airway pressure (CPAP), or using a T piece. The choice of the method is determined individually. If the patient tolerates a spontaneous breathing trial with any of these modes, then he's usually extubated.

Nursing considerations

- When weaning the patient, continue to observe for respiratory distress, fatigue, hypoxemia, or cardiac arrhythmias.
- Schedule weaning to comfortably and realistically fit into the patient's daily regimen, avoiding weaning during such times as meals, baths, or lengthy therapeutic procedures.
- Document the length of the weaning trial and the patient's toleration of the procedure.
- After the patient is successfully weaned and extubated, place him on the appropriate oxygen therapy. (See *Types of oxygen therapy*.)

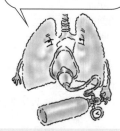

I'm fully weaned from the ventilation machine, but still dependent on oxygen. Not very stylish, but I'm not complaining.

Types of oxygen therapy

Various types of devices are used to deliver oxygen therapy. Regardless of the type, always assess the patient closely and check the results of pulse oximetry or ABG analysis 20 to 30 minutes after adjusting the flow rate.

Delivery device	Oxygen concentration administered	Administration guidelines
Nasal cannula	Low flow, 1 to 6 L per minute (24% to 44% Fio_2)	• Ensure patency of nostrils with flashlight; position prongs in nostrils. • Hook the cannula tubing behind the patient's ears and under his chin, sliding the adjuster upward under the chin to secure. • Alternatively position elastic strap over the patient's ears and around the back of his head; avoid applying too tightly, which can cause pressure on the facial structures and occlude the cannula. • Note that, with this device, oral breathers achieve the same oxygen delivery as nasal breathers. • Be aware that headache may occur if flow rate is greater than 6 L/minute. • If administering 4 L/minute or greater, add humidification to avoid over-drying of nasal mucous membranes.
Simple mask	6 to 12 L per minute (35% to 50% Fio_2)	• Ensure proper-fitting mask for the patient. • Place mask over the patient's nose, mouth, and chin, molding the flexible metal edge to the bridge of his nose. • Adjust elastic band around the patient's head to hold the mask firmly but comfortably in place. • If necessary, tape gauze pads to the mask over the patient's cheek area to make an airtight seal. • If the mask doesn't fit snugly, room air will dilute the oxygen, interfering with the delivery of the prescribed concentration. • Be aware that a minimum of 6 L/minute is required in all masks to flush CO_2 from it so that the patient doesn't rebreathe it.
Partial rebreather mask	6 to 10 L per minute (35% to 60% Fio_2)	• Follow the measures as for a simple mask with these additions: – Monitor the reservoir bag collapse; if it collapses more than slightly during inspiration, raise the flow rate until only a slight deflation is seen.

(continued)

Types of oxygen therapy *(continued)*

Delivery device	Oxygen concentration administered	Administration guidelines
Partial rebreather mask *(continued)*		– Keep in mind that marked or complete deflation indicates insufficient oxygen flow, which could lead to CO_2 accumulation in the mask. – Keep the reservoir bag from twisting or kinking. – Ensure free expansion of the bag by keeping it outside of the patient's gown and bedcovers.
Nonrebreather mask	6 to 10 L per minute (60% to 100% FIO_2)	• Be aware that this type of mask delivers the highest percentage of oxygen without intubation and mechanical ventilation. • Follow the measures as for a simple mask with these additions: – Make sure the mask fits snugly and the one-way valves are secure and functioning. – Watch for possible signs of CO_2 buildup due to a malfunctioning valve. – Monitor the deflation of the reservoir bag; if it collapses more than slightly during inspiration, raise the flow rate until only a slight deflation is seen. – Be aware that marked or complete deflation indicates insufficient oxygen flow, which could lead to CO_2 accumulation in the mask. – Keep the reservoir bag from twisting or kinking. – Ensure free expansion of the bag by keeping it outside of the patient's gown and bedcovers.
Venturi mask	4 to 10 L per minute (24% to 55% FIO_2); allows for precise concentration administration	• Follow the measures as for a simple mask with these additions: – Ensure that the proper device is used and that the oxygen flow rate is set at the amount specified on each mask. – Make sure that the Venturi valve is set for the desired FIO_2. – Ensure a snug but comfortably fitting mask; a loose fit or twisting, kinking, or blocked oxygen ports may alter the oxygen concentration being given.
Transtracheal oxygen	Variable	• Keep in mind that this catheter device supplies oxygen throughout the respiratory cycle. • After insertion, obtain a chest X-ray as ordered to confirm placement of the catheter. • Assess the patient for bleeding, respiratory distress, pneumothorax, pain, coughing, or hoarseness. • Don't use the catheter for approximately 1 week after insertion to reduce the risk of subcutaneous emphysema.
Aerosols	Variable; high-humidity oxygen that can be heated or cooled delivered by a jet nebulizer	• Be alert for condensation buildup in the tubing; empty the tubing at frequent intervals. • Ensure that condensate doesn't enter the trachea. • Monitor the tracheostomy tube's site (if the patient has one) for signs of irritation and pressure. • When using a high-output nebulizer, watch for signs of overhydration, pulmonary edema, crackles, and electrolyte imbalances.

Noninvasive positive pressure ventilation

NPPV refers to the administration of ventilatory support without the use of an invasive artificial airway such as an ET or tracheostomy tube. Instead, a noninvasive interface (nasal mask, face mask, or nasal pillow) is used along with a ventilator dedicated to noninvasive ventilation. (See *Types of noninvasive interfaces for NPPV.*) The modes of ventilation most commonly used are CPAP and bilevel positive airway pressure (BiPAP).

CPAP provides constant low-flow pressure into the airways to help hold the airway open, mobilize secretions, treat atelectasis, and, generally, ease the work of breathing. BiPAP delivers a preset inspiratory positive airway pressure (IPAP) and expiratory positive airway pressure (EPAP). The V_T correlates with the difference between the IPAP and the EPAP. Most BiPAP devices also permit a backup respiratory rate to be set.

Conditions that usually respond to NPPV include exacerbations of COPD that are complicated by hypercapnic acidosis, cardiogenic pulmonary edema, and hypoxemic respiratory failure. NPPV may also be helpful for preventing postextubation respiratory failure. The need for emergent intubation, coma, cardiac arrest, and respiratory arrest are absolute contraindications to NPPV use.

Relative contraindications include:
- inability to cooperate, protect the airway, or clear secretions
- nonrespiratory organ failure
- facial surgery, trauma, or deformity

Types of noninvasive interfaces for NPPV

Noninvasive interfaces used in NPPV are pictured below.

Nasal mask **Face mask** **Nasal pillow**

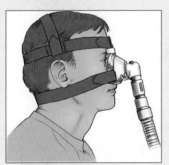 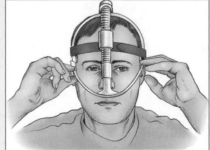 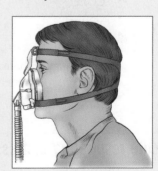

- high aspiration risk
- prolonged duration of mechanical ventilation anticipated
- recent esophageal anastomosis.
  Most complications due to NPPV are local and related to the tightly fitting mask. They include:
- local skin damage
- eye irritation, sinus pain, or sinus congestion
- mild gastric distention.
  Complications related to positive pressure ventilation, such as barotrauma and hemodynamic instability, are less common with NPPV than with invasive positive pressure ventilation.

Nursing considerations
- Closely monitor the patient's respiratory and hemodynamic status. Observe for signs and symptoms of respiratory distress and be prepared for intubation.
- Evaluate the patient's ability to tolerate the interface and troubleshoot equipment problems.
- If you're using a mask, cushion the forehead and the bridge of the nose before attaching the mask to decrease the risk for skin damage.
- Provide reassurance to the patient and his family to decrease their anxiety.

Respiratory system disorders

Common respiratory disorders you encounter in the critical care unit include:
- ARDS
- acute respiratory failure
- CO poisoning
- COPD
- OSA
- pneumonia
- pneumothorax
- pulmonary embolism
- pulmonary hypertension
- status asthmaticus.

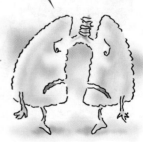

ARDS can quickly lead to acute respiratory failure, so know the clinical signs.

Acute respiratory distress syndrome

ARDS is a type of pulmonary edema not related to heart failure. ARDS may follow direct or indirect lung injury and can quickly lead to acute respiratory failure.

The three hallmark features of ARDS are:
1. bilateral patchy infiltrates on chest X-ray
2. no signs or symptoms of heart failure
3. no improvement in PaO_2 despite increasing oxygen delivery.

The prognosis for patients with ARDS varies depending on the cause and the patient's age and health status before developing ARDS.

What causes it

Some of the most common predisposing factors for ARDS are:
- sepsis
- lung injury from trauma such as chest contusion
- pulmonary embolism (air, fat, amniotic fluid, or thrombus)
- shock (any type)
- disseminated intravascular coagulation
- pancreatitis
- massive blood transfusions
- burns
- cardiopulmonary bypass
- drug overdose
- aspiration of stomach contents
- pneumonitis
- near drowning
- pneumonia
- inhalation of noxious gases (such as ammonia or chlorine).

How it happens

In ARDS, the tissues lining the alveoli and the pulmonary capillaries are injured either directly, by aspiration of gastric contents or inhalation of noxious gases, or indirectly, by chemical mediators released into the bloodstream in response to systemic disease.

Inflammation follows injury

The injured tissues release cytokines and other molecules that cause inflammation as white blood cells (WBCs) collect at the site and swelling occurs. The tissues become more permeable to fluid and proteins, and the hydrostatic pressure gradient between the alveoli and the capillaries is reversed.

Impaired exchange

Proteins and fluid begin to move from the capillaries into the alveoli. When this happens, gas exchange is impaired in the affected alveoli. As the process continues, the alveoli collapse (atelectasis), and gas exchange becomes impossible.

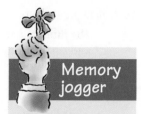

Memory jogger

To remember the progression of **ARDS**, use this mnemonic.

- **A**ssault to the pulmonary system
- **R**espiratory distress
- **D**ecreased lung compliance
- **S**evere respiratory failure

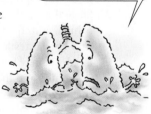

Fluid in the interstitial spaces, alveolar spaces, and small airways prevents air from moving into the lungs.

Ventilation prevention

The fluid that accumulates in the interstitial spaces, alveolar spaces, and small airways causes the lungs to stiffen, preventing air from moving into the lungs (ventilation).

Shunt stunts

As alveoli fill with fluid or collapse, the capillaries surrounding the alveoli fail to absorb oxygen. The body responds by shunting blood away from these alveoli, a process called *right-to-left shunting*.

Responses to the big buildup

As fluid builds up in the alveoli, the patient develops thick, frothy sputum and marked hypoxemia with increasing respiratory distress. As pulmonary edema worsens, inflammation leads to fibrosis, further impeding gas exchange.

Offline alkaline

Tachypnea due to respiratory distress causes alkalosis as carbon dioxide levels decrease. The body tries to compensate and to bring the blood pH back into the normal range through metabolic acidosis. The lack of oxygen also forces the body into anaerobic metabolism, which adds to the acidosis.

Unless gas exchange is restored and this process is reversed, acidosis worsens until all organ systems are affected and fail.

What to look for

ARDS occurs in four stages, each with these typical signs and symptoms:

1. Stage I involves dyspnea, especially on exertion. Respiratory and heart rates are normal to high. Auscultation may reveal diminished breath sounds, particularly when the patient is tachypneic. Stage I develops usually within the first 12 hours after the initial injury in response to decreasing oxygen levels in the blood.

2. Stage II is marked by greater respiratory distress. Respiratory rate is high, and the patient may use accessory muscles to breathe. He may appear restless, apprehensive, and mentally sluggish, or agitated. He may have a dry cough or frothy sputum. The heart rate is elevated and the skin is cool and clammy. Lung auscultation may reveal basilar crackles. Respiratory alkalosis is present on the ABG. The symptoms at this stage are sometimes incorrectly attributed to trauma.

3. Stage III involves obvious respiratory distress, with tachypnea, use of accessory breathing muscles, and decreased mental acuity. The patient exhibits tachycardia with arrhythmias (usually premature

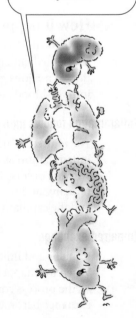

Uh-oh! Unless gas exchange is restored, increasing acidosis could be the downfall of all the organ systems.

Understanding ARDS

Here's how ARDS progresses:

1. Injury reduces normal blood flow to the lungs. Platelets aggregate and release histamine (H), serotonin (S), and bradykinin (B).

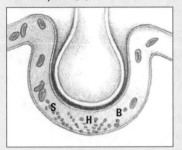

2. The released substances inflame and damage the alveolar capillary membrane, increasing capillary permeability. Fluids then shift into the interstitial space.

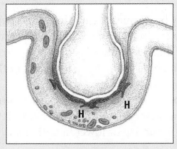

3. Capillary permeability increases, and proteins and fluids leak out, increasing interstitial osmotic pressure and causing pulmonary edema.

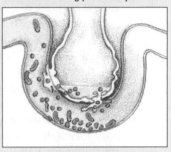

4. Decreased blood flow and fluids in the alveoli damage surfactant and impair the cell's ability to produce more. The alveoli then collapse, thus impairing gas exchange.

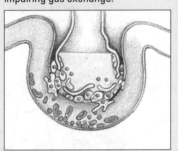

5. Oxygenation is impaired, but CO_2 easily crosses the alveolar capillary membrane and is expired. Blood oxygen and CO_2 levels are low.

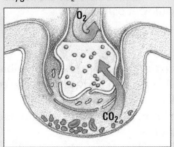

6. Pulmonary edema worsens and inflammation leads to fibrosis. Gas exchange is further impeded, resulting in an increase in CO_2 levels.

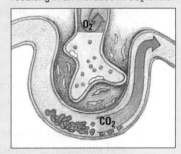

ventricular contractions) and labile blood pressure. The skin is pale and cyanotic. Auscultation may disclose diminished breath sounds, basilar crackles, and rhonchi. Respiratory acidosis is present on the ABG. This stage generally requires ET intubation and mechanical ventilation.

4. Stage IV is characterized by decreasing respiratory and heart rates. The patient's mental status nears loss of consciousness. The skin is cool and cyanotic. Breath sounds are severely diminished to absent. (See *Understanding ARDS*.)

What tests tell you

These test results are used to diagnose ARDS:

- ABG analysis initially shows decreased PaO_2 despite oxygen supplementation. Because of tachypnea, $PaCO_2$ is also decreased, causing an increase in blood pH (respiratory alkalosis).
- As ARDS worsens, $PaCO_2$ increases and pH decreases as the patient becomes acidotic. This is worsened by metabolic acidosis caused by a lack of oxygen that forces the body to switch to anaerobic metabolism.
- Initially, chest X-rays may be normal. Basilar infiltrates begin to appear in about 24 hours. In later stages, lung fields have a ground glass appearance and, eventually, as fluid fills the alveoli, white patches appear. These may eventually cover both lung fields entirely in later stages of ARDS.
- PA catheterization may be used to identify the cause of pulmonary edema through pulmonary artery wedge pressure (PAWP) measurement. PAWP is 19 mm Hg or lower in patients with ARDS.
- A differential diagnosis must be done to rule out cardiogenic pulmonary edema, pulmonary vasculitis, and diffuse pulmonary hemorrhage. Tests used to determine the causative agent may include sputum analysis, blood cultures, toxicology tests, and serum amylase levels (to rule out pancreatitis).

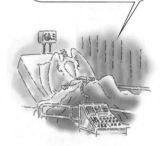

Patients with stage III ARDS generally require ET intubation and mechanical ventilation.

How it's treated

The goal of therapy is to correct the original cause, if possible, and provide enough oxygen to allow normal body processes to continue until the lungs begin to heal.

- Antibiotics and steroids may be administered to fight infection and minimize inflammation.
- Diuretics may be needed to reduce interstitial and pulmonary edema. In later stages of ARDS, however, vasopressors are usually prescribed to maintain blood pressure and blood supply to critical tissues.
- Respiratory support is most important. Humidified oxygen delivery through a tight-fitting mask and using CPAP may be adequate. ET intubation and mechanical ventilation are commonly required. PEEP may prevent alveolar collapse. High-frequency jet ventilation is sometimes used. Suctioning as necessary removes accumulated secretions from the tracheobronchial tree.
- Prone positioning may improve the patient's oxygenation. (See *Prone positioning.*)

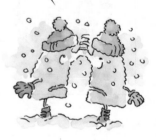

Either I'm entering the later stages of ARDS or we're in for one heck of a blizzard!

Prone positioning

Prone positioning (also known as *proning*) is a therapeutic maneuver to improve oxygenation and pulmonary function in patients with acute lung injury or ARDS. It involves physically turning a patient facedown, which shifts blood flow to regions of the lung that are better ventilated.

The criteria for prone positioning commonly include:
- acute onset of acute respiratory failure
- hypoxemia, specifically a partial pressure of arterial oxygen/fraction of inspired oxygen (PaO_2/FIO_2)
- ratio of 300 or less for acute lung injury or a PaO_2/FIO_2 ratio of 200 or less for ARDS
- radiologic evidence of diffuse bilateral pulmonary infiltrates.

Equipment innovations

Innovative equipment, such as a lightweight, cushioned frame that straps to the front of the patient before turning, minimizes the risks associated with moving patients and keeping them prone for several hours at a time.

With the right equipment, prone positioning may aid movement of the diaphragm by allowing the abdomen to expand more fully. It's usually used for 6 or more hours per day, for up to 10 days, until the patient's need for a high concentration of inspired oxygen resolves.

Patients with extrapulmonary ARDS (such as ARDS due to multiple traumas) respond well to prone positioning.

Pro-prone positioning

Prone positioning is indicated to support mechanically ventilated patients with ARDS, who require high concentrations of inspired oxygen. In patients who respond, prone positioning may correct severe hypoxemia and aid maintenance of adequate oxygenation (PaO_2 greater than 60%) in patients with acute lung injury, while avoiding ventilator-induced lung injury. It isn't clear whether patient's survival rates are increased.

No prone positioning

Prone positioning is contraindicated for patients whose heads can't be supported in a facedown position or who can't tolerate a head-down position. Relative contraindications include increased intracranial pressure, spinal instability, unstable bone fractures, multiple trauma, left-sided heart failure (nonpulmonary respiratory failure), shock, abdominal compartment syndrome, abdominal surgery, extreme obesity (weight greater than 300 lb [136.1 kg]), and pregnancy. Hemodynamically unstable patients (systolic blood pressure less than 90 mm Hg), despite aggressive fluid resuscitation and vasopressors, should be thoroughly evaluated before being placed in the prone position.

More meds

Additional medications are generally required when intubation and mechanical ventilation are instituted. Sedatives, including opioids and, sometimes, neuromuscular blocking agents, minimize restlessness and allow ventilation.

What to do

ARDS requires careful monitoring and supportive care. When your patient isn't intubated, watch carefully for signs of respiratory failure, which can happen quickly and necessitate intubation and mechanical ventilation.

- Assess the patient's respiratory status at least every 2 hours or more often, if indicated. Note respiratory rate, rhythm, and depth. Report the presence of dyspnea and accessory muscle use. Be alert for inspiratory retractions.

- Administer oxygen as ordered. Monitor FIO_2 levels.
- Auscultate lungs bilaterally for adventitious or diminished breath sounds. Inspect the color and character of sputum; clear, frothy sputum indicates pulmonary edema. To maintain PEEP, suction only as needed.
- Check ventilator settings often. Assess oxygen saturation continuously by pulse oximetry or SvO_2 by PA catheter. Monitor serial ABG levels; document and report changes in oxygen saturation as well as metabolic and respiratory acidosis and PaO_2 changes.

It's vital

- Monitor vital signs. Institute cardiac monitoring and observe for arrhythmias that may result from hypoxemia, acid–base disturbances, or electrolyte imbalance.
- Monitor the patient's LOC, noting confusion or mental sluggishness.
- Be alert for signs of treatment-induced complications, including arrhythmias, disseminated intravascular coagulation, GI bleeding, infection, malnutrition, paralytic ileus, pneumothorax, pulmonary fibrosis, renal failure, thrombocytopenia, and tracheal stenosis.
- Be alert for the development of multiple organ dysfunction syndrome. Monitor renal, GI, and neurologic system function.
- Give sedatives as ordered to reduce restlessness. Administer sedatives and analgesics at regular intervals if the patient on mechanical ventilation is receiving neuromuscular blocking agents.
- Provide routine eye care and instill artificial tears to prevent corneal drying and abrasion from the loss of the blink reflex in mechanically ventilated patients receiving neuromuscular blocking agents.
- Administer anti-infective agents as ordered if the underlying cause is sepsis or an infection.
- Place the patient in a comfortable position that maximizes air exchange, such as semi-Fowler's or high Fowler's position. A continuous rotation bed or prone positioning may be needed.

Take a break!

- Allow for periods of rest to prevent fatigue and reduce oxygen demand.
- If your patient has a PA catheter in place, know the desired PAWP level and check readings as indicated. Watch for decreasing SvO_2. Because PEEP may reduce cardiac output, check for hypotension, tachycardia, and decreased urine output.

- Evaluate the patient's serum electrolyte levels frequently as ordered. Measure urine output hourly to ensure adequate renal function. Monitor intake and output. Weigh the patient daily.
- Record caloric intake. Administer tube feedings and parenteral nutrition as ordered.
- Perform passive ROM exercises to maintain joint mobility. Provide meticulous skin care to prevent breakdown.

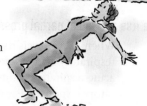

Place the patient in a comfortable position that maximizes air exchange, such as semi-Fowler's or high Fowler's position. This would not be comfortable!

Acute respiratory failure

Acute respiratory failure results when the lungs can't adequately oxygenate blood or eliminate carbon dioxide.

In patients with normal lung tissue, respiratory failure is indicated by a $PaCO_2$ above 50 mm Hg and a PaO_2 below 55 mm Hg. These limits don't apply to patients with chronic lung disease, such as COPD, who typically have consistently high carbon dioxide levels and low PaO_2.

What causes it

Conditions that cause alveolar hypoventilation, $\dot{V}/\dot{Q}$ mismatch, or right-to-left shunting can lead to respiratory failure. These include:
- acute COPD exacerbation
- aspiration pneumonia
- pneumonia
- obesity
- anesthesia
- pneumothorax
- atelectasis
- sleep apnea
- pulmonary edema
- pulmonary emboli
- CNS disease (such as myasthenia gravis, Guillain-Barré syndrome, and amyotrophic lateral sclerosis)
- head trauma
- CNS depressants.

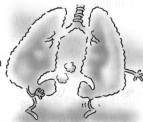

Uh-oh! When I can't oxygenate blood or remove carbon dioxide, acute respiratory failure results.

How it happens

Respiratory failure results from impaired gas exchange. Any condition associated with $\dot{V}/\dot{Q}$ mismatch caused by alveolar hypoventilation or intrapulmonary shunting can lead to acute respiratory failure if left untreated.

Poor ventilation

Alveolar hypoventilation occurs when respiratory effort is diminished or when airway obstruction leads to decreased airflow in the alveoli. This can occur with neuromuscular diseases or conditions that interfere with respiration.

Poor oxygenation

Blood that passes through the lungs but isn't oxygenated due to alveolar hypoventilation is known as *shunted blood*. Blood flow in the lung can be impaired by obstruction or hypovolemia. Obstruction is the most acute form and is most commonly caused by pulmonary emboli.

The rise and fall of partial pressures

When $PaCO_2$ levels rise above normal and pH drops below normal, respiratory acidosis develops. (PaO_2 levels also drop below normal in acute respiratory failure.) Other organ systems respond with compensatory responses. For example, the sympathetic nervous system triggers vasoconstriction, increases peripheral resistance, and increases the heart rate.

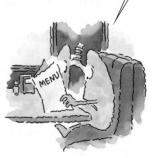

Let's see . . . nothing too acidic today. I'm lactic acid–intolerant, you know.

Lots of lactic acid

As tissue hypoxemia develops, tissues resort to anaerobic metabolism, which results in a buildup of lactic acid (a by-product of anaerobic metabolism) and thus metabolic acidosis. This takes longer to develop than respiratory acidosis, but the result is increasing acidity of the blood, which interferes with normal metabolism of all body systems.

What to look for

Your patient's history may reveal an underlying respiratory condition or an acute process leading to respiratory failure (such as asphyxia, drug overdose, or trauma).

Got no time

There's usually little time to collect a thorough history, and the patient typically can't give the history himself. His family members or medical records may be the main sources of such information.

Time is of the essence

Physical assessment findings vary, depending on the duration of the condition. Initially, the body responds with secretion of epinephrine.

Eventually, as the patient's condition worsens, epinephrine secretion has less effect.

On inspection, note ashen skin and cyanosis of the oral mucosa, lips, and nail beds. The patient may use accessory muscles of respiration to breathe and sit bolt upright or slightly hunched over. He may be agitated or highly anxious. In later stages, as the patient's level of mentation decreases due to hypoxemia, he may lie down and appear confused and disoriented.

If pneumothorax is present, you may observe asymmetrical chest movement. Tactile fremitus may be present as well.

Finding failure

Look for these physical signs of respiratory failure:
- Tachypnea increases the patient's respiratory rate so it's greater than the normal range of 16 to 20 breaths per minute.
- Tachycardia is a heart rate greater than 100 beats/minute. You may not see this in patients with heart disease who are taking medications that prevent tachycardia. The pulse may be strong and rapid initially but thready and irregular in later stages.
- Cold, clammy skin and frank diaphoresis are apparent, especially around the forehead and face.
- Percussion reveals hyperresonance in patients with COPD. In patients with atelectasis or pneumonia, percussion sounds are dull or flat.
- Lung auscultation usually reveals diminished breath sounds. In patients with pneumothorax, breath sounds are absent over the affected lung tissue. In other cases of respiratory failure, adventitious breath sounds, such as wheezes (in asthma) and rhonchi (in bronchitis), may be heard. If you auscultate crackles, suspect pulmonary edema as the cause of respiratory failure.

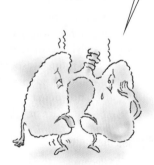

Tachypnea . . . tachycardia . . . cold, clammy skin, frank diaphoresis . . . I have all the classic signs of respiratory failure—or I'm just overreacting to news that I'm being audited by the IRS.

What tests tell you

- ABG analysis indicates early respiratory failure when Pao_2 is low (usually less than 60 mm Hg) and $Paco_2$ is high (greater than 45 mm Hg) and the HCO_3^- level is normal. The pH is also low. ABG levels in patients with COPD may be difficult to interpret, so compare them with earlier ABG values.
- Chest X-ray is used to identify pulmonary diseases, such as emphysema, atelectasis, pneumothorax, infiltrates, and effusions.
- Electrocardiogram (ECG) can demonstrate arrhythmias, commonly found with cor pulmonale and myocardial hypoxia.
- Pulse oximetry reveals a decreasing Spo_2 level.

- WBC count aids detection of an underlying infection. Blood cultures, sputum cultures, and Gram stain may also be used to identify pathogens.
- Abnormally low hemoglobin and hematocrit levels signal blood loss, indicating decreased oxygen carrying capacity.
- PA catheterization is used to distinguish pulmonary causes from cardiovascular causes of acute respiratory failure and to monitor the effects of treatment. Svo_2 levels less than 50% indicate impaired tissue oxygenation.

How it's treated

The primary goal of treatment is to restore adequate gas exchange. The secondary goal is to correct the underlying cause and development of respiratory failure.

Go to the O_2

Oxygen therapy is initiated immediately to optimize oxygenation of pulmonary blood. You may instruct the patient to try pursed-lip breathing to prevent alveolar collapse. If the patient can't breathe adequately on his own, ET intubation and mechanical ventilation are instituted. High-frequency or pressure ventilation is sometimes used to force airways open.

Oh, and drug therapy, too

Various drug therapies may be ordered:
- Reversal agents, such as naloxone (Narcan), are given if drug overdose is suspected.
- Bronchodilators are given to open airways.
- Antibiotics are given to combat infection.
- Corticosteroids may be given to reduce inflammation.
- Continuous I.V. solutions of positive inotropic agents may be given to increase cardiac output, and vasopressors may be given to induce vasoconstriction to improve or maintain blood pressure. Fluids are generally restricted to reduce cardiac workload and edema.
- Diuretics may be given to reduce fluid overload and edema.

Bypass the lungs

Recent studies indicate that extracorporeal membrane oxygenation (ECMO) may improve survival in patients with severe acute respiratory failure. (See *Understanding ECMO.*)

To prevent alveolar collapse, instruct the patient to try pursed-lip breathing. There will be no time for lipstick though.

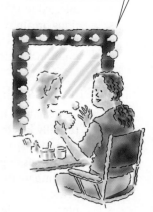

Understanding ECMO

ECMO is a type of prolonged mechanical cardiopulmonary support. During ECMO, blood is extracted from the vascular system and circulated outside the body by a mechanical pump. While outside the body, the blood passes through an oxygenator and heat exchanger. In the oxygenator, hemoglobin becomes fully saturated with oxygen while CO_2 is removed. The blood is then reinfused into the vascular system. Before initiating ECMO, the patient is anticoagulated with I.V. heparin.

Venovenous ECMO

There are two types of ECMO: venovenous (VV) and venoarterial (VA). During VV ECMO, blood is extracted from a large central vein and returned to the venous circulation. Venous cannulae are usually placed in the right common femoral vein (for drainage) and right internal jugular vein (for infusion). VV ECMO provides respiratory support without hemodynamic support and is generally used in acute respiratory failure.

Venoarterial ECMO

During VA ECMO, blood is extracted from a large central vein and returned to the arterial system, bypassing the heart and lungs. A venous cannula is usually placed in the right common femoral vein (for extraction), and an arterial cannula is usually placed into the right femoral artery (for infusion). VA ECMO can be used for respiratory or cardiac failure because it provides both respiratory and hemodynamic support.

Blood flow

Following cannulation, the patient is connected to the ECMO circuit and the blood flow is increased until appropriate respiratory and hemodynamic parameters are reached. After achieving the initial goals, maintain the blood flow at that rate. Continuous venous oximetry, which directly measures the oxyhemoglobin saturation of the blood in the venous limb of the ECMO circuit, facilitates frequent assessment and adjustments.

Because platelets are continuously consumed due to the sheer forces of extracorporeal flow and exposure to the foreign surface area, closely monitor the platelet count. Platelet transfusions may be required daily.

Readiness for discontinuation

Frequently evaluate a patient's readiness for discontinuation of ECMO. For patients with respiratory failure, improvements in radiographic appearance, pulmonary compliance, and arterial oxyhemoglobin saturation indicate that the patient may be ready to have ECMO discontinued. Before discontinuing ECMO permanently, perform one or more trials of taking the patient off ECMO.

ECMO complications

Complications associated with ECMO include:
- bleeding
- thromboembolism
- cannulation-related complications, including vessel perforation with hemorrhage, arterial dissection, distal ischemia, and incorrect location
- heparin-induced thrombocytopenia.

VA ECMO–specific complications include:
- pulmonary hemorrhage
- pulmonary infarction
- aortic thrombosis
- coronary or cerebral hypoxia.

What to do

- Assess the patient's respiratory status at least every 2 hours or more often, as indicated. Observe for a positive response to oxygen therapy, such as improved breathing, color, and oximetry and ABG values.
- Position the patient for optimal breathing effort when he isn't intubated. Put the call bell within easy reach to reassure the

patient and prevent unnecessary exertion when he needs to call the nurse.
- Maintain a normothermic environment to reduce the patient's oxygen demand.
- Monitor vital signs, heart rhythm, and fluid intake and output, including daily weights, to identify fluid overload (from I.V. fluids and medications) or impending dehydration (from aggressive diuretic therapy).
- After intubation, auscultate the lungs to check for accidental intubation of the esophagus or the mainstem bronchus. Be alert for aspiration, broken teeth, nosebleeds, and vagal reflexes causing bradycardia, arrhythmias, and hypotension.
- Don't suction too often without identifying the underlying cause of an equipment alarm. Use strict sterile technique during suctioning. ET intubation bypasses many of the body's normal barriers to infection, so the patient is at high risk during this procedure.
- Watch oximetry and capnography values because these are important indicators of changes in the patient's condition.
- Note the amount and quality of lung secretions and look for changes in the patient's status.
- Check cuff pressure on the ET tube to prevent erosion from an overinflated cuff. Normal cuff pressure is about 20 mm Hg.
- Provide a means of communication for patients who are intubated and alert. Institutions use different approaches based on signs and signals or communication boards. Explain all procedures to the patient and his family.

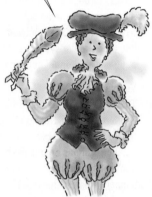

Be sure to provide a means of communication for patients who are intubated and alert.

Carbon monoxide poisoning

CO is an odorless, colorless, tasteless, nonirritating gas that can cause sudden illness and death. CO poisoning is responsible for up to 40,000 emergency department visits and 5,000 to 6,000 deaths per year, making it one of the leading causes of poisoning death in the United States.

What causes it

Common causes of CO poisoning include:
- smoke inhalation
- inhaling fumes from poorly functioning heating systems and improperly vented fuel-burning devices (such as kerosene heaters, charcoal grills, camping stoves, or gasoline-powered electrical generators)

- inhaling fumes from motor vehicles operating in such poorly ventilated areas as ice rinks, warehouses, and parking garages
- inhaling fumes from underground electrical cable fires, which can seep into adjacent buildings and homes
- inhaling or ingesting methylene chloride, an industrial solvent and a component of paint remover, which is metabolized to CO by the liver.

How it happens

CO diffuses rapidly across the pulmonary capillary membrane. RBCs pick up CO quicker than they pick up oxygen. If the air is filled with CO, the body may replace oxygen in blood with CO. This blocks oxygen from getting into the body.

What to look for

The most common symptoms of CO poisoning are headache, dizziness, weakness, nausea, vomiting, chest pain, and confusion. Unless suspected, CO poisoning can be difficult to diagnose because the symptoms mimic other illnesses. People who are sleeping or intoxicated can die from CO poisoning before ever experiencing symptoms. (See *Symptoms in children.*)

Severe CO toxicity can produce neurologic symptoms such as seizures, syncope, or coma and such cardiovascular and metabolic manifestations as myocardial ischemia, ventricular arrhythmias, pulmonary edema, and profound lactic acidosis.

What tests tell you

- Co-oximetry of an ABG sample or bedside pulse CO-oximetry reveals an elevated carboxyhemoglobin level.
- ABG analysis reveals normal Pao_2 levels.
- Complete blood count may reveal mild leukocytosis.
- Chest X-ray findings are usually normal.
- CT scan may reveal evidence of cerebral edema and focal lesions.
- MRI may reveal focal lesions and white matter demyelination.
- ECG may reveal sinus tachycardia.

How it's treated

Treatment is aimed at replacing the CO in the blood with oxygen as quickly as possible. The patient may receive 100% oxygen therapy until he's asymptomatic and carboxyhemoglobin levels are below 10%. Comatose patients, or those with severely impaired mental status, should be intubated and mechanically ventilated using 100% oxygen. For patients suffering from CO poisoning after smoke inhalation, it's important to consider concomitant cyanide toxicity,

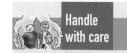

Handle with care

Symptoms in children

In young children, signs of CO poisoning may be more subtle and nonspecific than those in adults. Infants and toddlers may present with such complaints as fussiness or feeding difficulty as the sole manifestation of CO poisoning. Because of their higher oxygen use and higher minute ventilation, young children may develop signs and symptoms of CO poisoning before older children and adults who experience the same exposure.

which can further impair tissue oxygen use and worsen the degree of cellular hypoxia.

In some cases, hyperbaric oxygen therapy is recommended. With this therapy, the patient is placed in a full-body pressurized chamber. Inside the chamber, air pressure is more than twice as high as normal atmospheric pressure. This speeds the replacement of CO with oxygen in the blood.

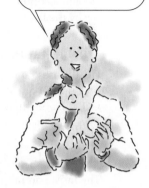

Comatose patients should be intubated and mechanically ventilated using 100% oxygen.

What to do

- Monitor carboxyhemoglobin levels as ordered.
- Assess respiratory, cardiovascular, and neurologic status often, as indicated by the patient's condition.
- Administer oxygen as ordered. Encourage coughing and deep breathing.
- Position the patient for optimal breathing effort.
- Institute cardiac monitoring to detect the development of arrhythmias secondary to hypoxemia.
- Maintain the patient on bed rest to decrease tissue oxygen demand.

Chronic obstructive pulmonary disease

COPD results from emphysema, chronic bronchitis, asthma, or a combination of these disorders. It's the most common chronic lung disease in the United States.

Out...

COPD is a chronic condition that can usually be managed on an outpatient basis even in advanced disease, when a patient may require continuous oxygen therapy.

...or in

Exacerbations of COPD that necessitate hospitalization are caused by various factors that place additional demand on the respiratory system, such as infection, heart failure, and exposure to allergens.

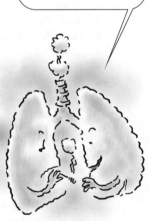

There's no getting around the fact that cigarette smoking or exposure to cigarette smoke is a leading cause of COPD—the most common chronic lung disease in the United States.

What causes it

Common causes of COPD include:
- cigarette smoking or exposure to cigarette smoke
- recurrent or chronic respiratory tract infections
- air pollution
- allergies.

Familial and hereditary factors, such as alpha$_1$-antitrypsin deficiency paired with cigarette smoking, are also responsible for emphysema.

How it happens

Patients with COPD have decreased gas exchange ability due to alveolar damage caused by exposure to smoke or chemical irritants over a long period.

Quit it!

Smoke inhalation impairs ciliary action and macrophage function and causes inflammation in the airways and increased mucus production. Early inflammatory changes may be reversed if the patient stops smoking before lung disease becomes extensive.

Air trap

In chronic bronchitis, mucus plugs and narrowed airways cause air trapping. Air trapping also occurs with asthma and emphysema. In emphysema, permanent enlargement of the acini is accompanied by destruction of the alveolar walls. Obstruction and air trapping result from tissue changes rather than mucus production.

Here's what happens in air trapping: Hyperinflation of the alveoli occurs on expiration. On inspiration, airways enlarge, allowing air to pass beyond the obstruction; on expiration, airways narrow and prevent gas flow.

Pressure pockets

As the alveolar walls are destroyed, they're no longer separate but coalesce into large air pockets that put additional pressure on surrounding tissues. This affects the lung's blood supply as well because it increases the pressure needed to push blood through the lungs. This form of high blood pressure is known as *pulmonary hypertension*.

Overwhelming work

Eventually, the high workload overwhelms the right side of the heart, and hypertrophy and right-sided failure (cor pulmonale) result. Patients commonly have supraventricular arrhythmias such as atrial fibrillation, which increase the danger of thrombus formation.

Because gas exchange is impaired, hypercapnia (Paco$_2$ above 40 mm Hg) becomes the norm for these patients. The respiratory center of the brain, which stimulates breathing when $Paco_2$ rises, becomes dependent instead on low Pao_2. This is an important consideration when oxygen is given for hypoxemia.

What to look for

Your patient most likely has a history of COPD and may be able to identify the precipitating cause (e.g., exposure to an allergen).

Tachy and not-so-tachy finds

Your patient is also likely to have tachycardia and an irregular heart rhythm as well as tachypnea and dyspnea on exertion. Fever may be present in the case of infection.

When you inspect the chest, you may notice that the anterolateral diameter is increased (barrel chest), and the patient may appear generally cachectic. He may be coughing, with copious sputum production, if he has chronic bronchitis, or he may be wheezing.

When you listen to breath sounds, listen for a prolonged expiratory phase, perhaps crackles or rhonchi, and generally some decreased air movement.

Time will tell

Patients with COPD have abnormal breath sounds to begin with, and it may be hard to tell at first what's baseline and what's newly abnormal. As you listen over several hours or days, abnormal breath sounds eventually become apparent.

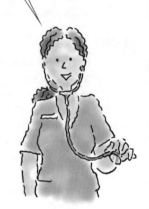

Your patient with COPD may have abnormal baseline breath sounds.

What tests tell you

Stable COPD patients exhibit these abnormal diagnostic test results, which may be considered their baseline values:
- Pulmonary function tests show increased residual volume, with decreased vital capacity and amount of air exhaled in the first second of expiration.
- Chest X-ray shows increased bronchovascular markings and over-aeration of the lungs. In advanced disease, the diaphragm is flattened and bronchovascular markings may be reduced.
- ABG analysis may show reduced Pao_2 and normal or increased $Paco_2$. In advanced COPD, it isn't uncommon for baseline $Paco_2$ levels to be 50 mm Hg or higher.
- ECG may show atrial arrhythmias and, in advanced disease, right ventricular hypertrophy.
- Blood count reveals elevated hemoglobin levels.

When it worsens

During an exacerbation, diagnostic tests may yield these additional results:
- ABG analysis shows PaO_2 below the patient's baseline. $PaCO_2$ may be low, normal, or high, depending on the patient's baseline.
- Chest X-ray may show infiltrates if pneumonia is present.
- ECG may show sinus tachycardia with supraventricular and, sometimes, ventricular arrhythmias.

How it's treated

Provide supportive treatments for your patients with COPD. Bronchodilators and membrane stabilizing aerosols are useful in maintaining open airways. Steroids may be given to reduce inflammation if necessary. In some cases, continuous oxygen supplementation is needed.

Address the effects, then treat the cause

During exacerbations, management is twofold. First, respiratory support is given to avoid respiratory failure and cardiac arrest. Equally important is treatment addressing the underlying cause of the exacerbation.
- Your patient may receive oxygen supplementation. Care must be taken when the baseline $PaCO_2$ level is high. The patient's respiratory center relies on low oxygen levels to stimulate breathing. Administer controlled oxygen therapy by monitoring ABG levels and patient assessments.
- If respiratory failure is imminent, ET intubation and mechanical ventilation are needed.
- Aerosolized bronchodilators, such as albuterol, are given to open airways.
- Epinephrine, a potent bronchodilator, may be given.
- Corticosteroids are given (usually by I.V.) to reduce inflammation.
- Diuretic agents may be given to reduce edema and cardiac workload.
- Antiarrhythmic medications may be given to control arrhythmias. The patient is usually put on continuous ECG monitoring for observation of the heart rate and rhythm.
- Antibiotics are given to treat or prevent infection.
- If pneumothorax is present, a chest tube may be inserted.

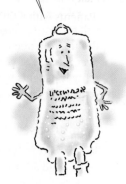

I.V. corticosteroids are given to reduce inflammation when COPD is exacerbated.

What to do

- Assess respiratory status; auscultate breath sounds; monitor oxygen saturation and ABG values; and observe for a positive response to oxygen therapy, such as improved breathing, color, or oximetry and ABG values. Anticipate the need for intubation and mechanical ventilation.

- Assess frequently and carefully. Changes can be subtle and rapid. Be sure to assess mental status because it's an early and sensitive indicator of respiratory status. New onset of confusion and agitation are red flags, as is lethargy.
- Monitor vital signs and heart rhythm and observe for arrhythmias, which may indicate hypoxemia, right-sided heart failure, or an adverse effect of bronchodilator use.
- Obtain laboratory tests as ordered and report results promptly.
- Offer emotional support. Keep the environment as calm as possible and the air temperature warm. The patient may not be able to speak easily because of shortness of breath, so explain what's happening and try to anticipate his needs.

Obstructive sleep apnea

OSA is a disorder characterized by recurrent episodes of upper airway obstruction and a reduction in ventilation. It's defined as cessation of breathing (apnea) during sleep usually caused by repetitive upper airway obstruction. OSA interferes with people's ability to obtain adequate rest, thus affecting memory, learning, and decision making.

OSA is an important disorder because patients are at increased risk for poor neurologic and cognitive performance and organ system dysfunction due to repeated arousals and hypoxemia during sleep over months to years. In addition, there's an increased risk for mortality if patients with cardiovascular risks aren't treated. (See *OSA and coronary artery disease.*)

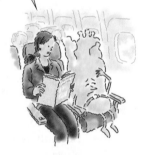

I'm just so tired all the time. I'm afraid I'm in trouble with this OSA!

What causes it

Risk factors for OSA include obesity, male gender, postmenopausal status, and advanced age. The major risk factor is obesity; a larger neck circumference and increased amounts of peripharyngeal fat narrow and compress the upper airway.

OSA affects approximately 9% of males and 4% of females and is more prevalent in blacks who are younger than age 35, compared to whites of the same age group.

Other associated factors include alterations in the upper airway, such as structural changes that contribute to the collapsibility of the upper airway. Current smokers (but not past smokers) are nearly three times more likely to have OSA than never smokers.

Weighing the evidence

OSA and coronary artery disease

There's increasing evidence that severe (but probably not mild) OSA is associated with cardiovascular morbidity related to coronary artery disease. In this prospective longitudinal epidemiologic study, 1,927 men and 2,495 women age 40 or older and free from coronary heart disease and heart failure at the time of baseline polysomnography were studied for a median of 8.7 years.

After adjusting for multiple risk factors, the researchers found that OSA was associated with an increased risk for heart failure in middle-aged and older men. They didn't find the same association in women of any age.

Source: Gottlieb, D. J., Yenokyan, G., Newman, A. B., O'Connor, G. T., Punjabi, N. M., Quan, S. F., . . . Shahar, E. (2010). Prospective study of obstructive sleep apnea and incident coronary heart disease and heart failure: The Sleep Heart Health Study. *Circulation, 122*(4), 352–360.

How it happens

The pharynx is a collapsible tube that can be compressed by the soft tissues and structures surrounding it. Upper airway patency is maintained by the bony and cartilaginous structures surrounding the naso- and oropharynx, plus 12 pairs of skeletal muscles. A patient with OSA has a reduced upper airway size due to excess surrounding soft tissue or a highly compliant airway. A reduced airway size, combined with diminished neural output to the upper airway muscles during sleep and at apnea onset, results in partial or complete upper airway collapse.

What to look for

Snoring and daytime sleepiness are the most common presenting complaints of OSA. Additional signs and symptoms include restless sleep, periods of silence terminated by loud snoring, poor concentration, nocturnal angina, and awakening with a sensation of choking, gasping, or smothering.

What tests tell you

Full-night, attended, in-laboratory polysomnography is considered the gold standard diagnostic test for OSA. Patterns of abnormalities in the following areas are identified:
- total sleep time
- sleep efficiency

- sleep stage percentage
- sleep stage latency
- arousals
- apneas
- hypopneas
- respiratory effort-related arousals
- indices that describe the frequency of abnormal respiratory events during sleep, including the apnea index, apnea hypopnea index, and respiratory disturbance index
- snoring
- body position
- oxyhemoglobin saturation
- limb movements.

How it's treated

Various treatments are used. Weight loss, sleep position, and avoidance of alcohol and medications that inhibit the CNS are the first steps. In more severe cases involving hypoxemia and severe hypercapnia, the treatment includes CPAP or BiPAP therapy with supplemental oxygen. CPAP is used to prevent airway collapse, whereas BiPAP makes breathing easier and results in a lower average airway pressure. Although these treatments are effective in management of OSA, compliance with treatment is a major concern.

Taking a bite out of OSA

There is an increasing number of oral appliances designed to protrude the mandible forward, such as mandibular advancement splints, or hold the tongue in a more anterior position, such as tongue-retaining devices. Either design holds the soft tissues of the oropharynx away from the posterior pharyngeal wall, thereby maintaining upper airway patency.

Surgical treatment appears to be most effective in patients who have mild OSA due to a severe, surgically correctable obstructing lesion. Simple tonsillectomy may be effective for patients with larger tonsils and low body mass index. Uvulopalatopharyngoplasty (UPPP) is one of the most common surgical procedures performed. It involves resection of the uvula, redundant retrolingual soft tissue, and palatine tonsillar tissue.

Laser-assisted and radiofrequency ablation are less invasive variants of UPPP. Other common surgical procedures for OSA include septoplasty, rhinoplasty, nasal turbinate reduction, nasal polypectomy, palatal advancement pharyngoplasty, tonsillectomy, adenoidectomy, palatal implants, tongue reduction (partial glossectomy, lingual tonsillectomy), and maxillomandibular advancement.

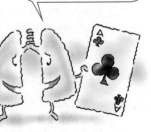

Surgery may be in the cards to correct OSA and improve breathing.

What to do

- Keep the patient's head of the bed elevated 30 to 45 degrees, avoid a supine position, and maintain a neutral head position and neck alignment to maintain a patent airway and improve oxygenation.
- Administer CPAP or BiPAP as ordered to reduce incidence of sleep apnea. Assess for any intolerance related to the procedure.
- Obtain a dietary consult to initiate weight loss program.
- Closely monitor respiratory and cardiovascular status closely after surgical treatment or correction for OSA.

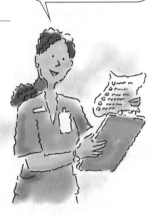

Frequent and careful assessment is the key to care because changes can be subtle and develop rapidly.

Pneumonia

Pneumonia is an acute infection of the lung parenchyma that commonly impairs gas exchange. More than 3 million cases of pneumonia are diagnosed yearly in the United States.

Those at risk

The prognosis is good for patients with pneumonia who are otherwise healthy. Debilitated patients are at much greater risk; bacterial pneumonia is a leading cause of death among such individuals. Pneumonia occurs in both sexes and in all ages, but older adults are at greater risk for developing it. (See *Pneumonia in older adults.*)

Handle with care

Pneumonia in older adults

Older adults are at greater risk for developing pneumonia because their weakened chest musculature reduces their ability to clear secretions. Those in long-term care facilities are especially susceptible.

Bacterial pneumonia is the most common type found in older adults; viral pneumonia is the second most common type. Aspiration pneumonia results from impaired swallowing ability and a diminished gag reflex due to stroke or prolonged illness.

And presenting . . .
An older adult with pneumonia may present with fatigue, slight cough, and a rapid respiratory rate. Pleuritic pain and fever may be present. An absence of fever doesn't mean absence of infection in an older adult; many older adults develop a subnormal body temperature in response to infection.

What starts it

Infectious agents may be bacterial, viral, mycoplasmal, rickettsial, fungal, protozoal, or mycobacterial.

Where it infects

Types of pneumonia based on location of the infection include:
- bronchopneumonia, involving distal airways and alveoli
- lobular pneumonia, involving part of a lobe
- lobar pneumonia, involving an entire lobe.

Get it here, there, or anywhere

Pneumonia may be classified as community-acquired, hospital-acquired (nosocomial), or aspiration pneumonia. (See *Types of pneumonia*, pages 407 and 408.)

Shared with the community

As the name implies, community-acquired pneumonia occurs in the community setting or within the first 48 hours of admission to a health care facility because of community exposure.

Not-so-comical pneumonia

Hospital-acquired pneumonia refers to the development of pneumonia 48 hours after admission to a health care facility. For example, development of pneumonia after ET intubation and placement on a ventilator can be a type of nosocomial pneumonia.

When location doesn't matter

Aspiration pneumonia can occur in the community or health care facility setting.

What causes it

Primary pneumonia results from inhalation of a pathogen, such as bacteria or virus. Examples are pneumococcal and viral pneumonia.

Secondary pneumonia may follow initial lung damage from a noxious chemical or other insult (superinfection) or may result from hematogenous spread of bacteria from a distant area.

Aspiration pneumonia results from inhalation of foreign matter, such as vomitus or food particles, into the bronchi. It's more common in elderly or debilitated patients; those receiving NG tube feedings; and those with an impaired gag reflex, poor oral hygiene, or a decreased LOC.

Yes, it's true. It's possible to develop pneumonia by acquiring an infection after being admitted to the hospital or any health care facility.

Yikes!

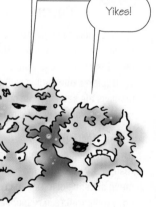

Types of pneumonia

Here's an overview of the various types of pneumonia, including their causative agents and common assessment findings.

Type	Causative agent	Assessment findings
Aspiration pneumonia	Chronic aspiration of gastric or oropharyngeal contents into trachea or lungs	• Fever • Crackles • Dyspnea • Hypotension • Tachycardia • Cyanosis • Chest X-ray with infiltrates
Community-acquired pneumonias		
Streptococcal pneumonia (pneumococcal pneumonia)	*Streptococcus pneumoniae*	• Sudden onset of single shaking chill • Fever 102° to 104°F (38.9° to 40°C) • History of previous upper respiratory infection • Pleuritic chest pain • Severe cough • Rust-colored sputum • Areas of consolidation on chest X-ray (usually lobar) • Elevated WBC count • Sputum culture possibly positive for gram-positive *S. pneumoniae*
Haemophilus influenzae pneumonia	*H. influenzae*	• Insidious onset • History of upper respiratory tract infection 2 to 6 weeks earlier • Fever • Chills • Dyspnea • Productive cough • Chest X-ray with infiltrates in one or more lobes

Type	Causative agent	Assessment findings
Community-acquired pneumonias (continued)		
Mycoplasma pneumonia	*Mycoplasma pneumoniae*	• Insidious onset • Sore throat • Ear pain • Headache • Low-grade fever • Pleuritic pain • Erythema rash • Dry cough • Myalgia
Viral pneumonia	Influenza virus, type A	• Initially beginning as upper respiratory infection • Cough (initially non-productive; later purulent sputum) • Low-grade fever • Chills • Malaise • Dyspnea • Frontal headache • Chest X-ray with diffuse bilateral bronchopneumonia radiating from hilus • Normal to slightly elevated WBC count • Fatigue
Legionnaires' disease	*Legionella pneumophila*	• Flulike symptoms • Malaise • Headache within 24 hours • Fever • Shaking chills • Fatigue • Mental confusion • Anorexia

(continued)

Types of pneumonia *(continued)*

Type	Causative agent	Assessment findings
Community-acquired pneumonias *(continued)*		
Legionnaires' disease *(continued)*		• Nausea, vomiting • Myalgia • Chest X-ray with patchy infiltrates, consolidation, and possible effusion
Hospital-acquired pneumonias		
Klebsiella pneumonia	*Klebsiella pneumoniae*	• Fever • Recurrent chills • Rusty, bloody viscous sputum • Cyanosis of lips and nail beds • Shallow grunting respirations • Severe pleuritic chest pain • Chest X-ray typically with consolidation in upper lobe • Elevated WBC count • Sputum culture and Gram stain possibly positive for gram-negative cocci *Klebsiella*

Type	Causative agent	Assessment findings
Hospital-acquired pneumonias *(continued)*		
Pseudomonas pneumonia	*Pseudomonas aeruginosa*	• Fever • Chills • Dyspnea • Cyanosis • Green foul-smelling sputum • Chest X-ray with diffuse consolidation
Staphylococcal pneumonia (may also be community-acquired)	*Staphylococcus aureus*	• Cough • Chills • High fever 102° to 104°F (38.9° to 40°C) • Pleuritic pain • Progressive dyspnea • Bloody sputum • Tachypnea • Hypoxemia • Chest X-ray with multiple abscesses and infiltrate; empyema • Elevated WBC count • Sputum culture and Gram stain possibly positive for gram-positive staphylococci

How it happens

The disease process varies among bacterial, viral, and aspiration pneumonia.

- In bacterial pneumonia, which can affect any part of the lungs, an infection initially triggers alveolar inflammation and edema. Capillaries become engorged with blood, causing stasis. As the alveolocapillary membrane breaks down, the alveoli fill with blood and inflammatory exudates, resulting in atelectasis.

- Viral pneumonia more commonly attacks bronchiolar epithelial cells, causing interstitial inflammation and desquamation. It then spreads to the alveoli. In advanced infection, a hyaline membrane may form, further compromising gas exchange.
- Aspiration pneumonia triggers similar inflammatory changes in the affected area and also inactivates surfactant over a large area, leading to alveolar collapse. Acidic gastric contents may directly damage the airways and alveoli, and small particles may cause obstruction. The resulting inflammation makes the lungs susceptible to secondary bacterial pneumonia.

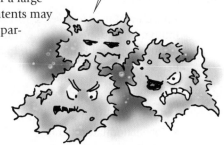

We get around! Bacterial pneumonia can move through the bloodstream to the lungs.

What to look for

Signs and symptoms of pneumonia include pleuritic chest pain, cough, shortness of breath, and fever.

Sounds, sights, and sensations

Your patient's cough may be dry, as in mycoplasma pneumonia, or very productive. The sputum may be creamy yellow, green, or rust-colored.

In advanced cases of all types of pneumonia, percussion reveals dullness over the affected area of the lung. Auscultation may disclose crackles, wheezes, or rhonchi over the affected areas as well as decreased breath sounds and decreased tactile fremitus.

What tests tell you

- Chest X-rays disclose infiltrates, confirming the diagnosis.
- Sputum specimen for Gram stain and culture and sensitivity testing may reveal inflammatory cells as well as bacterial cells.
- WBC count and differential may indicate the presence and type of infection. Elevated polymorphonucleocytes may indicate bacterial infection; in viral or mycoplasmal pneumonia, though, WBC count may not be elevated at all.
- ABG analysis may be done to determine the extent of respiratory compromise due to alveolar inflammation.
- Bronchoscopy or transtracheal aspiration allows the collection of material for cultures to identify the specific infectious organism. Pleural fluid may also be sampled for culture and Gram stain.
- Pulse oximetry may show a reduced oxygen saturation level and indicate the need for oxygen supplementation.

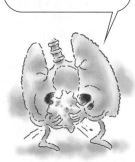

Oh, the pain of it all! The classic signs and symptoms of pneumonia are pleuritic chest pain, cough, shortness of breath, and fever. I've got them all!

How it's treated

Because the cause is commonly infectious and, in cases of secondary and aspiration pneumonia, bacterial secondary infections are a risk, antimicrobial therapy is started immediately. The type of antibiotic used depends on the infectious agent.

More oxygen, please

Your patient may receive oxygen supplementation, including ET intubation and mechanical ventilation in severe cases when respiratory arrest is imminent. In severe cases, PEEP may be needed to prevent alveolar collapse.

Add-ons

Other treatment measures include:
- bronchodilator therapy
- antitussives for cough
- high-calorie diet and adequate fluid intake
- bed rest
- analgesics to relieve pleuritic chest pain.

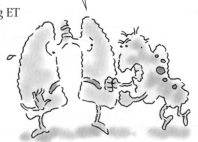

I hope they gave me the right antibiotic to fight off this microbe. He means business!

What to do

- Maintain a patent airway and oxygenation. Place the patient in Fowler's position to maximize chest expansion and give supplemental oxygen as ordered. Monitor oxygen saturation and ABG levels as ordered.
- Assess respiratory status often, at least every 2 hours. Auscultate the lungs for abnormal breath sounds, such as crackles, wheezes, or rhonchi. Encourage coughing and deep breathing.
- If your patient's respiratory status deteriorates, anticipate the need for ET intubation and mechanical ventilation.
- Adhere to standard precautions and institute appropriate transmission-based precautions, depending on the causative organism.
- Institute cardiac monitoring to detect the development of arrhythmias secondary to hypoxemia.
- Reposition your patient to maximize chest expansion, allow rest, and reduce discomfort and anxiety.
- Obtain ordered diagnostic tests and report results promptly.
- Administer drug therapy as ordered.
- Carefully monitor your patient's intake and output to allow early identification of dehydration, fluid overload, and accurate tracking of nutritional status.
- Determine if the patient is a candidate for the pneumococcal and influenza vaccines.

Pneumothorax

Pneumothorax is an accumulation of air in the pleural cavity that leads to partial or complete lung collapse. The amount of air trapped in the intrapleural space determines the degree of lung collapse. In some cases, venous return to the heart is impeded, causing a life-threatening condition called *tension pneumothorax*.

Pneumothorax can be classified as either traumatic or spontaneous. *Traumatic pneumothorax* may be further classified as open or closed. (Note that an open [penetrating] wound may cause closed pneumothorax.) *Spontaneous pneumothorax*, which is also considered closed, is most common in older patients with COPD but can occur in young, healthy patients as well.

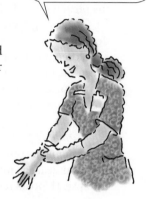

Adhere to standard precautions and other appropriate safety measures, depending on the causative organism.

What causes it

The causes of pneumothorax vary according to classification.

Traumatic pneumothorax

Causes of open pneumothorax include:
- penetrating chest injury (stab or gunshot wound)
- insertion of a central venous catheter
- chest surgery
- transbronchial biopsy
- thoracentesis or closed pleural biopsy.
Causes of closed pneumothorax include:
- blunt chest trauma
- air leakage from ruptured blebs
- rupture resulting from barotrauma caused by high intrathoracic pressures during mechanical ventilation
- tubercular or cancerous lesions that erode into the pleural space
- interstitial lung disease such as eosinophilic granuloma.

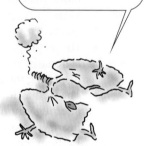

Accumulation of air in the pleural cavity can cause partial or complete lung collapse.

Spontaneous pneumothorax

Spontaneous pneumothorax is usually caused by the rupture of a subpleural bleb (a small cystic space) at the surface of a lung.

Tension pneumothorax

Causes of pneumothorax include:
- penetrating chest wound treated with an airtight dressing
- fractured ribs
- mechanical ventilation
- high-level PEEP that causes alveolar blebs to rupture
- chest tube occlusion or malfunction.

How it happens

The pathophysiology of pneumothorax also varies according to classification.

Traumatic pneumothorax

Open pneumothorax occurs when atmospheric air flows directly into the pleural cavity (under negative pressure). As the air pressure in the pleural cavity becomes positive, the lung on the affected side collapses, causing decreased total lung capacity. As a result, the patient develops a $\dot{V}/\dot{Q}$ imbalance that leads to hypoxia.

Closed pneumothorax occurs when an opening is created between the intrapleural space and the parenchyma of the lung. Air enters the pleural space from within the lung, causing increased pleural pressure and preventing lung expansion during inspiration.

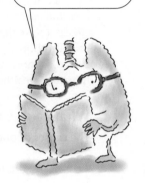

In my book, pneumothorax spells trouble for me.

Spontaneous pneumothorax

In spontaneous pneumothorax, the rupture of a subpleural bleb causes air leakage into the pleural spaces, which causes the lung to collapse. Hypoxia results from decreased total lung capacity, vital capacity, and lung compliance.

Tension pneumothorax

Tension pneumothorax results when air in the pleural space is under higher pressure than air in the adjacent lung. Here's what happens:
- Air enters the pleural space from the site of pleural rupture, which acts as a one-way valve. Thus, air enters the pleural space on inspiration but can't escape as the rupture site closes on expiration.
- More air enters with each inspiration, and air pressure begins to exceed barometric pressure.
- The air pushes against the recoiled lung, causing compression atelectasis, and pushes against the mediastinum, compressing and displacing the heart and great vessels.
- The mediastinum eventually shifts away from the affected side, affecting venous return and putting ever greater pressure on the heart, great vessels, trachea, and contralateral lung.

Without immediate treatment, this emergency can rapidly become fatal. (See *Understanding tension pneumothorax*.)

What to look for

Assessment findings depend on the severity of the pneumothorax. Spontaneous pneumothorax that releases a small amount of air into the pleural space may cause no signs and symptoms. Generally, tension pneumothorax causes the most severe respiratory signs and symptoms.

Understanding tension pneumothorax

In tension pneumothorax, air accumulates intrapleurally and can't escape. As intrapleural pressure increases, the lung on the affected side collapses.

On inspiration, the mediastinum shifts toward the unaffected lung, impairing ventilation.

On expiration, the mediastinal shift distorts the vena cava and reduces venous return.

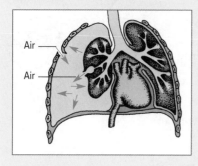

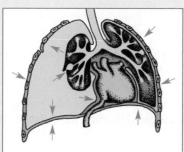

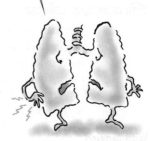

Depending on the severity of pneumothorax, your patient may have sudden, sharp pleuritic pain that exacerbates with movement, breathing, or coughing. Oh, that one hurt!

Every breath hurts

Your patient's history reveals sudden, sharp, pleuritic chest pain. The patient may report that chest movement, breathing, and coughing exacerbate the pain. He may also report shortness of breath.

Further findings

Inspection reveals asymmetric chest wall movement with overexpansion and rigidity on the affected side. The skin may be cool, clammy, and cyanotic. Palpation of the chest wall may reveal crackling beneath the skin (subcutaneous emphysema) and decreased vocal fremitus.

In addition, percussion may reveal hyperresonance on the affected side, auscultation may disclose decreased or absent breath sounds on the affected side, and vital signs may follow the pattern of respiratory distress seen with respiratory failure.

Did we mention the tension?

Tension pneumothorax also causes:
- hypotension and tachycardia due to decreased cardiac output
- tracheal deviation to the opposite side (a late sign)
- distended jugular veins due to high intrapleural pressure, mediastinal shift, and increased cardiovascular pressure.

What tests tell you

- Chest X-rays reveal air in the pleural space and a mediastinal shift that confirm pneumothorax.
- ABG analysis reveals hypoxemia, usually with elevated $Paco_2$ and normal bicarbonate ion levels in the early stages.
- ECG may reveal decreased QRS amplitude, precordial T-wave inversion, rightward shift of frontal QRS axis, and small precordial R voltage.

How it's treated

Treatment of pneumothorax depends on the cause and severity.

With trauma

Open or traumatic pneumothorax may necessitate surgical repair of affected tissues, followed by chest tube placement with an underwater seal.

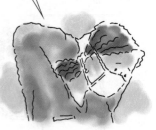

Open or traumatic pneumothorax may require surgical repair of affected tissues and chest tube placement. See you in the OR.

With less lung collapse

Spontaneous pneumothorax with less than 30% lung collapse, no signs of increased pleural pressure, and no dyspnea or indications of physiologic compromise may be corrected with:
- bed rest to preserve energy
- monitoring of vital signs to detect physiologic compromise
- oxygen administration to improve hypoxia
- aspiration of air from the intrapleural space with a large-bore needle attached to a syringe to restore negative pressure within the pleural space.

With more lung collapse

Greater than 30% lung collapse may necessitate other measures, such as:
- placing a chest tube in the second or third intercostal space in the midclavicular line to reexpand the lung by restoring negative intrapleural pressure
- connecting the chest tube to an underwater seal or low-pressure suction to reexpand the lung.

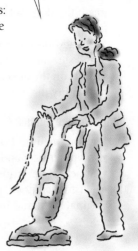

I don't think this is the kind of low-level suctioning they had in mind . . . Gotcha, dust bunnies!

With tension

Treatment for your patient with tension pneumothorax typically involves:
- immediate large-bore needle insertion into the pleural space through the second intercostal space to reexpand the lung, followed by insertion of a chest tube if large amounts of air escape through the needle after insertion
- analgesics to promote comfort and encourage deep breathing and coughing. (See *Combating tension pneumothorax.*)

Take charge!

Combating tension pneumothorax

Tension pneumothorax, the entrapment of air within the pleural space, can be fatal without prompt treatment.

What causes it?

An obstructed or dislodged chest tube is a common cause of tension pneumothorax. Other causes include blunt chest trauma or high-pressure mechanical ventilation. In such cases, increased positive pressure within the patient's chest cavity compresses the affected lung and the mediastinum, shifting them toward the opposite lung. This impairs venous return and cardiac output and may cause the lung to collapse.

Telltale signs

Suspect tension pneumothorax if the patient develops dyspnea, chest pain, an irritating cough, vertigo, syncope, or anxiety after a blunt chest trauma or if the patient has a chest tube in place. Is his skin cold, pale, and clammy? Are his respiratory and pulse rates unusually rapid? Does the patient have equal bilateral chest expansion?

If you note these signs and symptoms, palpate the patient's neck, face, and chest wall for subcutaneous emphysema and palpate his trachea for deviation from midline. Auscultate the lungs for decreased or absent breath sounds on one side. Then percuss them for hyperresonance. If you suspect tension pneumothorax, notify the practitioner immediately and help identify the cause.

What to do

- Assess the patient's respiratory status, including auscultation of bilateral breath sounds, at least every 1 to 2 hours. Monitor oxygen saturation levels closely for changes; obtain ABG analysis as ordered.
- Monitor hemodynamic parameters frequently as appropriate and indicated; anticipate the need for cardiac monitoring because hypoxemia can predispose the patient to arrhythmias.
- Watch for complications, signaled by pallor, gasping respirations, and sudden chest pain. Carefully monitor vital signs at least every hour for indications of shock, increasing respiratory distress, or mediastinal shift. If your patient's respiratory status deteriorates, anticipate the need for ET intubation and mechanical ventilation and assist as necessary.
- Assist with the chest tube insertion and connect to suction, as ordered. Monitor your patient for possible complications associated with chest tube insertion.
- Check chest tube devices frequently for drainage and proper functioning.
- Reposition your patient to promote comfort and drainage.

Pulmonary embolism

Pulmonary embolism is an obstruction of the pulmonary arterial bed. It occurs when a mass lodges in a pulmonary artery branch, partially or completely obstructing blood flow distal to it. This causes a ($\dot{V}/\dot{Q}$) mismatch, resulting in hypoxemia and intrapulmonary shunting.

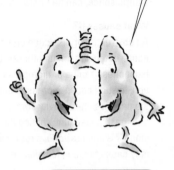

Pulmonary embolism causes a $\dot{V}/\dot{Q}$ mismatch that results in hypoxemia and intrapulmonary shunting.

What causes it

The most common source of pulmonary embolism is a dislodged thrombus that originated in the deep veins of the leg or, less commonly, in the pelvic, renal, or hepatic veins, or right side of the heart. Other emboli arise from fat, air, amniotic fluid, tumor cells, or a foreign object, such as a needle, catheter part, or talc (from drugs intended for oral administration that are injected I.V. by addicts).

Risky red flags

Risk factors for developing pulmonary embolism include:

- predisposing disorders, including lung disorders, cardiac disorders (valvular disease and arrhythmias, such as atrial fibrillation), infection, diabetes, history of thromboembolism, sickle cell disease, and polycythemia
- venous stasis in those who are on prolonged bed rest, immobile, obese, burn victims, older than age 40, or in orthopedic casts
- venous injury caused by surgery (especially of the legs, pelvis, abdomen, and thorax), long-bone or pelvic fractures, I.V. drug abuse, I.V. therapy, or manipulation or disconnection of central lines
- increased blood coagulability resulting from cancer, high-estrogen hormonal contraceptive use (particularly in women older than age 40 who smoke cigarettes), or pregnancy (which involves hypercoagulability, decreased mobility, edema, and decreased venous return).

A dislodged thrombus originating in the deep veins of the leg is the most common cause of a pulmonary embolism.

The skinny on fat and air

Fat embolism risk factors include osteomyelitis, long-bone fractures, burns, and adipose tissue or liver trauma. Risk factors for air embolism include cardiopulmonary bypass, hemodialysis, deep vein catheter insertion, and endoscopy.

How it happens

Here's what happens when pulmonary embolism develops:

- A thrombus forms as a result of trauma to the vascular wall, venous stasis, or hypercoagulability of the blood.
- Further trauma, clot dissolution, sudden muscle spasm, pressure changes, or a change in peripheral blood flow can cause the thrombus to loosen or fragment.
- After it's dislodged, the thrombus becomes an embolus and floats through the venous system to the right side of the heart and on to the pulmonary vasculature, where it lodges in a small vessel and occludes blood flow beyond the occlusion.
- A $\dot{V}/\dot{Q}$ mismatch results in hypoxemia that's commonly irreversible.

What to look for

Your patient's history may reveal a predisposing condition or another risk factor for pulmonary embolism.

The large and small of it

Other symptoms depend on the size of the embolus and if it's a fat or air embolism.

- A small embolism may not cause any signs or symptoms.
- An embolism that occludes less than 50% of the pulmonary artery bed may cause shortness of breath, anxiety, chest pain, S_3 or S_4 heart sound, and crackles on auscultation.
- An embolism that occludes more than 50% of the artery bed may cause a sense of impending doom, dyspnea, tachycardia, confusion, right-sided heart failure, hypotension, and pulseless electrical activity.
- A fat embolism may produce no symptoms for up to 24 hours. Symptoms may include restlessness, confusion, shortness of breath, petechiae on the chest, wheezing, and hypoxemia.
- An air embolism may cause palpitations, weakness, tachycardia, and hypoxia.

What tests tell you

$\dot{V}/\dot{Q}$ scan demonstrates a mismatch, indicating abnormal perfusion.

- Pulmonary angiography may reveal a pulmonary vessel filling defect or an abrupt vessel ending, indicating pulmonary embolism. Angiography is the definitive test for pulmonary embolus, even though the risk of test-related complications, such as cardiac arrhythmias, is high.

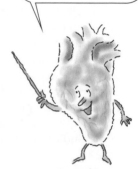

A dislodged thrombus, or an embolus, can float through the venous system to the heart and lungs and become stuck in a small vessel, occluding blood flow beyond that point.

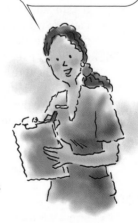

The signs and symptoms of pulmonary embolism vary with the size of the embolus and with other factors such as whether it's caused by a thrombus, fat, or air.

- A spiral CT is frequently used to diagnose a PE. The scanner rotates while it continuously takes pictures in slices. This develops into a three-dimensional picture that can visualize an emboli.
- ECG results distinguish pulmonary embolism from MI and show right axis deviation; right bundle branch block; tall, peaked P waves; depressed ST segments; T-wave inversions; and supraventricular arrhythmias.
- Chest X-ray is used to rule out other pulmonary diseases, but it's inconclusive within 1 to 2 hours of the embolic event. It may also indicate areas of atelectasis, an elevated diaphragm, pleural effusion, a prominent pulmonary artery, and, occasionally, the characteristic wedge-shaped infiltrate that suggests pulmonary infarction.
- ABG analysis reveals hypoxemia and possibly hypocapnia due to tachypnea.
- PA catheterization may reveal an elevated central venous pressure and PAP and a normal PAWP.
- MRI is used to identify the embolus or blood flow changes indicating an embolus.

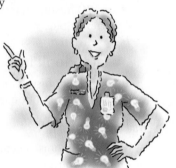

Pulmonary angiography is still the gold standard for diagnosing a pulmonary embolism, even though the risk of complications is high.

How it's treated

The goal of treatment is to allow adequate gas exchange until the obstruction can be removed or resolves on its own. Oxygen therapy is the primary treatment.

In addition to oxygen therapy, these treatment measures may be indicated:

- For patients with blood clots, anticoagulation with low-molecular-weight heparin, I.V. unfractionated heparin, subcutaneous unfractionated heparin, or subcutaneous fondaparinux (Arixtra) inhibits the formation of more thrombi. It's followed by warfarin (Coumadin) for 3 to 6 months, depending on risk factors.
- Patients with massive pulmonary embolism and shock may need fibrinolytic therapy with streptokinase (Streptase) or alteplase (Activase) to enhance fibrinolysis of the pulmonary emboli and remaining thrombi.
- Embolism from other sources may necessitate other therapy to dissolve the embolus, depending on its nature. Septic embolism, for example, calls for antibiotic therapy rather than anticoagulation.
- If hypotension occurs, vasopressors may be required to maintain blood pressure.

Surgical salvation

- Surgery is indicated for patients who can't take anticoagulants because of recent surgery or blood dyscrasia or who have recurrent emboli during anticoagulant therapy. Surgery, which shouldn't be performed without angiographic evidence of pulmonary embolism, consists of pulmonary embolectomy, pulmonary endarterectomy, or insertion of an inferior vena cava filter to filter blood returning to the heart and lungs.

What to do

- Monitor your patient's respiratory status, oxygen saturation, and breath sounds and administer oxygen therapy as ordered. If breathing is severely compromised, anticipate the need for ET intubation and mechanical ventilation.
- Monitor vital signs and heart rhythm to detect arrhythmias secondary to hypoxemia. Because many signs and symptoms of pulmonary embolism mimic those of MI, obtain a 12-lead ECG to rule out MI.
- Obtain laboratory tests as ordered and report results promptly.
- Monitor PTT regularly for patients on anticoagulation therapy. Effective heparin therapy increases PTT to about 2 to 2½ times normal.
- Keep antidotes for anticoagulants readily available. These include protamine sulfate for heparin and vitamin K for warfarin. Blood products may be needed in case of life-threatening bleeding.
- During anticoagulant therapy, assess your patient for epistaxis, petechiae, and other signs of abnormal bleeding. Apply pressure over venous puncture sites for 5 to 10 minutes and 15 to 20 minutes for arterial sites until bleeding stops. Avoid giving I.M. injections.
- Avoid giving aspirin and other nonsteroidal anti-inflammatory drugs (NSAIDs) if the patient is taking anticoagulants.
- Promote your patient's comfort by repositioning him often and administering analgesics for pain. Encourage leg movement if the patient is alert. Never massage the lower extremities.
- Monitor nutritional intake to ensure adequate calorie and fluid intake.
- Explain all procedures to the patient, even if his mentation is altered, and to the patient's family when present.

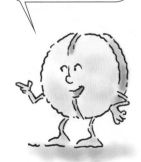

If your patient can't take anticoagulants or has recurrent emboli while on anticoagulant therapy, he may need an umbrella filter to prevent clots from traveling to the heart and lungs.

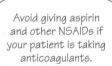

Avoid giving aspirin and other NSAIDs if your patient is taking anticoagulants.

Pulmonary hypertension

Pulmonary hypertension refers to chronically elevated mean PAP, over 25 mm Hg, at rest.

What causes it

Primary, or idiopathic, pulmonary hypertension has no known cause. It's most common in women between ages 20 and 40 and is usually fatal within 3 to 4 years. Mortality is highest in pregnant women.

Prefaced with heart or lung disease

Secondary pulmonary hypertension results from existing cardiac or pulmonary disease, or both. Cardiac causes include:
- left-sided heart failure
- ventricular septal defect
- patent ductus arteriosus.

    Pulmonary causes include COPD and vasoconstriction of the arterial bed due to hypoxemia and acidosis.

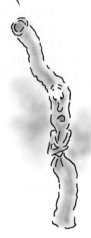

This vasoconstriction is for the birds. However, you'll find I can be most resistant when I want to be.

How it happens

In primary pulmonary hypertension, the intimal lining of the pulmonary arteries thickens, narrowing the lumen of the artery, impairing distensibility, and increasing vascular resistance.

    Alveolar hypoventilation can result from diseases causing alveolar destruction or diseases that prevent the chest wall from expanding sufficiently to allow air into the alveoli. The resulting decreased ventilation increases pulmonary vascular resistance.

    Hypoxemia resulting from the $\dot{V}/\dot{Q}$ mismatch causes vasoconstriction, further increasing vascular resistance and resulting in pulmonary hypertension.

Sans treatment

If a patient with pulmonary hypertension doesn't receive treatment, here's what happens:
- Hypertrophy occurs in the medial smooth muscle layer of the arterioles, worsening nondistensibility.
- Increased pressure in the lungs is transmitted to the right ventricle (which supplies the pulmonary artery).
- The ventricle becomes hypertrophic and eventually fails (cor pulmonale).
- Impaired distensibility due to hypertrophy can cause arrhythmias.

What to look for

Patients with pulmonary hypertension typically report increasing dyspnea on exertion, weakness, syncope, and fatigue.

Look, touch, and listen

Look for the signs of pulmonary hypertension, including:

- tachycardia
- tachypnea with mild exertion
- decreased blood pressure
- changes in mental status, from restlessness to agitation or confusion
- signs of right-sided heart failure, such as ascites and jugular vein distention
- an easily palpable right ventricular lift and a reduced carotid pulse
- possible peripheral edema
- decreased diaphragmatic excursion and respiration
- point of maximal impulse displaced beyond the midclavicular line
- systolic ejection murmur; a widely split S_2, and an S_3 or S_4 sound; or decreased breath sounds and loud, turbulent sounds heard on auscultation.

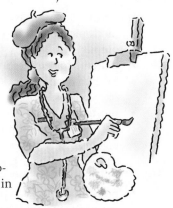

Let me paint a picture of a patient with pulmonary hypertension . . . someone who reports increasing dyspnea on exertion, weakness, syncope, and fatigue.

What tests tell you

- ABG analysis reveals hypoxemia.
- ECG changes commensurate with right ventricular hypertrophy include right axis deviation and tall or peaked P waves in inferior leads.
- PA catheterization reveals increased mean PAP above 25 mm Hg. It may also show an increased PAWP if the underlying cause is left atrial myxoma, mitral stenosis, or left-sided heart failure; otherwise, PAWP is normal.
- Pulmonary angiography is used to detect filling defects in pulmonary vasculature.
- Pulmonary function studies may show decreased flow rates and increased residual volume in underlying obstructive disease. In underlying restrictive disease, they may show reduced total lung capacity.
- Radionuclide imaging reveals abnormal right and left ventricular function.
- Echocardiography allows assessment of ventricular wall motion and possible valvular dysfunction. It's also used to identify right ventricular enlargement, abnormal septal configuration, and reduced left ventricular cavity size.
- Perfusion lung scanning may yield normal results or multiple patchy and diffuse filling defects not consistent with pulmonary embolism.

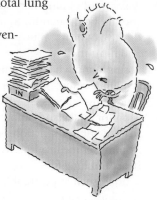

Don't forget me! Read up on how ECG changes indicate right ventricular hypertrophy.

How it's treated

Treatment measures include:

- oxygen therapy to correct hypoxemia
- fluid restriction to decrease preload and minimize workload of the right ventricle.
- Exercise training to improve peak oxygen consumption.
  In severe cases with irreversible changes, heart–lung transplantation may be necessary.

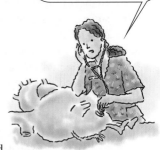

In severe cases with irreversible changes, heart–lung transplantation may be necessary.

Diverse drugs

Your patient may receive:

- inotropic medications such as digoxin to increase cardiac output
- diuretics to decrease intravascular volume and venous return
- calcium channel blockers to reduce myocardial workload and oxygen consumption
- prostanoids, such as epoprostenol (Flolan), treprostinil (Remodulin), or iloprost (Ventavis), and endothelin receptor antagonists, such as bosentan (Tracleer), ambrisentan (Letairis), or sitaxsentan (Thelin), to improve hemodynamic parameters and functional capacity
- phosphodiesterase type 5 inhibitors, such as sildenafil (Viagra, Revatio), tadalafil (Cialis, Adcirca), or vardenafil (Levitra), to improve pulmonary hemodynamics and exercise capacity
- bronchodilators to relax smooth muscles and increase airway patency
- anticoagulant therapy to reduce the risk for intrapulmonary thrombosis and thromboembolism.

What to do

- Assess cardiopulmonary status. Auscultate heart and breath sounds, being alert for S_3 heart sounds, murmurs, or crackles indicative of heart failure. Monitor vital signs, oxygen saturation, and heart rhythm.
- Assess hemodynamic status, including PAP and PAWP every 2 hours or more often, depending on the patient's condition, and report any changes.
- Monitor intake and output closely and obtain daily weights. Institute fluid restriction as ordered.
- Administer medications as ordered to promote adequate heart and lung function. Assess for potential adverse reactions, such as postural hypotension with diuretics.
- Administer supplemental oxygen as ordered and organize care to allow rest periods.

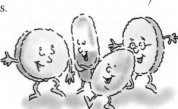

Administer drugs as ordered to promote adequate heart and lung function.

Status asthmaticus

Status asthmaticus is a life-threatening situation resulting from an acute asthma attack. It begins with impaired gas exchange and—without rapid intervention—may lead to respiratory failure and, eventually, death.

Asthma overview

Asthma is a chronic inflammatory airway disorder that causes episodic airway obstruction and hyperresponsiveness of the airway to multiple stimuli. It results from bronchospasms, increased mucus secretion, and mucosal edema. If left untreated or if the patient doesn't respond to drug therapy after 24 hours, status asthmaticus is diagnosed.

Making things worse

Asthma exacerbations are acute or subacute episodes of worsening shortness of breath, coughing, and wheezing, with measurable decreases in expiratory airflow.

What causes it

Many asthmatics, especially children, have intrinsic and extrinsic asthma.

Outside factors

Extrinsic, or *atopic*, asthma begins in childhood. Patients are typically sensitive to specific external allergens. Extrinsic allergens that can trigger an asthma attack include such elements as pollen, animal dander, house dust or mold, kapok or feather pillows, food additives containing sulfites, and other sensitizing substances.

Extrinsic asthma in childhood is commonly accompanied by other hereditary allergies, such as eczema and allergic rhinitis.

Factors within

Patients with *intrinsic*, or *nonatopic*, asthma react to internal, nonallergenic factors. Intrinsic factors that can trigger an asthma attack include emotional stress, fatigue, endocrine changes, temperature variations, humidity variations, exposure to noxious fumes, anxiety, coughing or laughing, and genetic factors.

Most episodes occur after a severe respiratory tract infection, especially in adults.

Irritants in the workplace

Many adults acquire an allergic form of asthma or exacerbation of existing asthma from exposure to agents in the workplace.

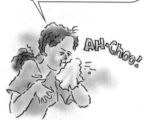

Extrinsic allergens, such as pollen and pet dander, can trigger an asthma attack.

AH-choo!

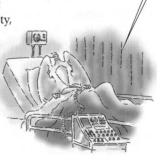

Most intrinsic asthma attacks in adults follow severe respiratory tract infection.

Such irritants as chemicals in flour, acid anhydrides, and excreta of dust mites in carpet are a few such agents that trigger asthma.

Genetic messes

Asthma is associated with two genetic influences, including:
- the ability to develop asthma because of an abnormal gene (atopy)
- the tendency to develop hyperresponsive airways (without atopy).

A potent mix

Environmental factors interact with inherited factors to cause asthmatic reactions with associated bronchospasms.

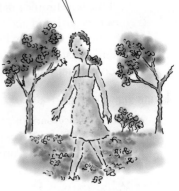

When exposed to antigens such as pollen, mast cells in the lung release histamine, which causes swelling in smooth muscles.

How it happens

Status asthmaticus begins with an asthma attack. In asthma, bronchial linings overreact to various stimuli, causing episodic smooth muscle spasms that severely constrict the airways. (See *Understanding asthma.*)

Here's how asthma develops into status asthmaticus:
- Immunoglobulin (Ig) E antibodies attached to histamine-containing mast cells and receptors on cell membranes initiate intrinsic asthma attacks.
- When exposed to an antigen, such as pollen, the IgE antibody combines with the antigen.
- On subsequent exposure to the antigen, mast cells degranulate and release mediators.
- Mast cells in the lung are stimulated to release histamine and the slow-reacting substance of anaphylaxis.
- Histamine attaches to receptor sites in the larger bronchi, where it causes swelling in smooth muscles.
- Mucous membranes become inflamed, irritated, and swollen. The patient may experience dyspnea, prolonged expiration, and an increased respiratory rate.
- Leukotrienes attach to receptor sites in the smaller bronchi and cause local swelling of the smooth muscle.
- Leukotrienes also cause prostaglandins to travel by way of the bloodstream to the lungs, where they enhance the effect of histamine. A wheeze may be audible during coughing; the higher the pitch, the narrower is the bronchial lumen.
- Histamine stimulates the mucous membranes to secrete excessive mucus, further narrowing the bronchial lumen.

As mucous membranes become inflamed, irritated, and swollen, the patient may experience dyspnea, prolonged expiration, and increased respiratory rate.

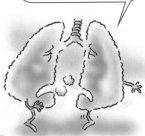

Understanding asthma

Asthma is an inflammatory disease of the airways. The inflammation causes hyper-responsiveness (to various stimuli) and bronchospasms. Here's how an asthma attack progresses:

1. Histamine attaches to receptor sites in larger bronchi, causing swelling of the smooth muscles.

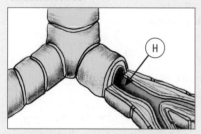

2. Leukotrienes attach to receptor sites in the smaller bronchi and cause swelling of smooth muscle there. Leukotrienes also cause prostaglandins to travel via the bloodstream to the lungs, where they enhance histamine's effects.

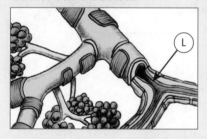

3. Histamine stimulates the mucous membranes to secrete excessive mucus, further narrowing the bronchial lumen. On inhalation, the narrowed bronchial lumen can still expand slightly; however, on exhalation, the increased intrathoracic pressure closes the bronchial lumen completely.

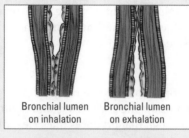

Bronchial lumen on inhalation   Bronchial lumen on exhalation

4. Mucus fills lung bases, inhibiting alveolar ventilation. Blood is shunted to alveoli in other parts of the lungs, but it still can't compensate for diminished ventilation.

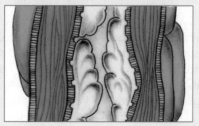

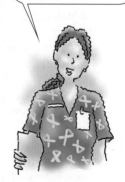

Histamine stimulates the secretion of excessive mucus, narrowing the bronchial lumen.

Got goblet?

- Goblet cells secrete viscous mucus that's difficult to cough up, resulting in coughing, rhonchi, increased-pitch wheezing, and increased respiratory distress. Mucosal edema and thickened secretions further block the airways.
- On inhalation, the narrowed bronchial lumen can still expand slightly, allowing air to reach the alveoli. On exhalation, increased intrathoracic pressure closes the bronchial lumen completely. Air enters but can't escape.

- When status asthmaticus occurs, hypoxemia worsens and expiratory rate and volume decrease even further.
- Obstructed airways impede gas exchange and increase airway resistance. The patient labors to breathe.
- As breathing and hypoxemia tire the patient, respiratory rate drops to normal, $Paco_2$ levels rise, and the patient hypoventilates from exhaustion.
- Respiratory acidosis develops as $Paco_2$ increases.
- The situation becomes life-threatening when no air is audible on auscultation (a silent chest) and $Paco_2$ rises to over 70 mm Hg.
- Without treatment, the patient experiences acute respiratory failure.

What to look for

An asthma attack may begin slowly or dramatically. Progressive cyanosis, confusion, and lethargy may indicate that the acute asthma attack has progressed to status asthmaticus.

What the patient reports

Typically, the patient reports exposure to a particular allergen followed by a sudden onset of dyspnea, wheezing, and tightness in the chest accompanied by a cough that produces thick clear or yellow sputum.

The patient may complain of feeling suffocated, appear visibly dyspneic, and be able to speak only a few words before pausing to catch his breath.

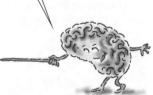

Your patient's mental status is a sensitive indicator of oxygen deprivation that may signal impending respiratory failure.

What you may find

Mental status is a sensitive indicator of oxygen deprivation, and the patient may initially be irritable or anxious. As hypoxemia progresses, the patient becomes confused and increasingly lethargic, a sign of impending respiratory failure.

The patient's heart rate is elevated and commonly irregular. Respiratory rate is also well above normal. When the patient begins to tire, his respiratory rate begins to slow, which may be another sign of impending respiratory failure if the patient is also confused and lethargic.

On inspection, you may see intercostal retractions. During an attack, the patient's face may appear pale and diaphoretic. The patient generally sits bolt upright or leans forward slightly.

On percussing the chest wall, you may find hyperresonance; palpation may reveal vocal fremitus.

Listen to the lungs

When you listen to the lungs, you may hear harsh respirations with inspiratory and expiratory wheezes and, possibly, reduced breath sounds over some areas of the lung. The expiratory phase of respiration is prolonged. Marked wheezing may develop due to increased edema and mucus in the lower airways.

Breath sounds and wheezing may suddenly stop (status) because of severe bronchoconstriction and edema.

What tests tell you

These tests are used to establish the diagnosis:
- Pulmonary function tests reveal decreased vital capacity and increased total lung and residual capacities during an acute attack. Peak and expiratory flow rate measurements are less than 60% of baseline.
- Pulse oximetry commonly shows that oxygen saturation is less than 90%.
- Chest X-ray may show hyperinflation with areas of atelectasis and flat diaphragm due to increased intrathoracic volume.
- ABG analysis reveals decreasing PaO_2 and increasing $PaCO_2$.
- ECG shows sinus tachycardia during an attack.
- Sputum analysis may indicate increased viscosity, mucus plugs, presence of Curschmann's spirals (casts of airways), Charcot-Leyden crystals, and eosinophils; culture may disclose causative organisms if infection is the trigger.
- A complete blood count with differential shows an increased eosinophil count secondary to inflammation and an elevated WBC count and granulocyte count if an acute infection is present.

How it's treated

In acute status asthmaticus, the patient is monitored closely for respiratory failure. Oxygen, bronchodilators, epinephrine, corticosteroids, and nebulizer therapies may be ordered. The patient may be intubated and placed on mechanical ventilation if $PaCO_2$ increases or if respiratory arrest occurs.

Addressing asthma

Correcting asthma typically involves:
- prevention by identifying and avoiding precipitating factors, such as environmental allergens or irritants
- desensitization to specific antigens if the stimuli can't be removed entirely, which decreases the severity of asthma attacks with future exposure
- bronchodilators (such as epinephrine, albuterol) to decrease bronchoconstriction, reduce bronchial airway edema, and increase pulmonary ventilation

- corticosteroids (such as methylprednisolone) to decrease bronchoconstriction, reduce bronchial airway edema, and increase pulmonary ventilation
- subcutaneous epinephrine to counteract the effects of mediators of an asthma attack
- mast cell stabilizers (cromolyn [Intal] and nedocromil [Tilade]) in patients with atopic asthma who have seasonal disease; when given prophylactically, they block the acute obstructive effects of antigen exposure by inhibiting the degranulation of mast cells, thereby preventing the release of chemical mediators responsible for anaphylaxis
- leukotriene-receptor modifiers (montelukast [Singulair] and zafirlukast [Accolate]) given prophylactically to help block the inflammatory actions in asthma.

Calling for high humidity

- humidified oxygen to correct dyspnea, cyanosis, and hypoxemia and to maintain an oxygen saturation greater than 90%
- mechanical ventilation, which is necessary if the patient doesn't respond to initial ventilatory support and drugs or develops respiratory failure
- relaxation exercises to increase circulation and aid recovery from an asthma attack.

What to do

- Conduct careful and frequent assessment of the patient's respiratory status, especially if the patient isn't intubated. Check the respiratory rate, auscultate breath sounds, and monitor oxygen saturation.
- Be alert for a patient who was wheezing but suddenly stops wheezing and continues to show signs of respiratory distress. In this case, the absence of wheezing may be due to severe bronchial constriction that narrows the airways severely during inhalation and exhalation. As a result, so little air passes through the narrowed airways that no sound is made. This is a sign of imminent respiratory collapse; the patient needs ET intubation and mechanical ventilation. Reassure the patient and stay with him. Help him to relax as much as possible.
- Assess the patient's mental status for confusion, agitation, or lethargy.
- Assess the patient's heart rate and rhythm. Be alert for cardiac arrhythmias related to bronchodilator therapy or hypoxemia.
- Obtain ordered tests and report results promptly.
- Administer medications as ordered. I.V. fluids are commonly ordered to replace insensible fluid loss from hyperventilation.

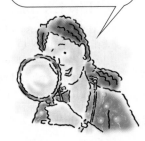

Watch closely for signs of imminent respiratory collapse.

- When the acute phase is over, position the patient for maximum comfort, usually in semi-Fowler's position. Encourage coughing to clear secretions. Offer emotional support and reassurance.

Quick quiz

1. When auscultating a patient's lungs, you hear crackles. These are caused by:
    A. secretions blocking the bronchial airways.
    B. collapsed or fluid-filled alveoli snapping open.
    C. a foreign body obstructing the trachea.
    D. consolidation.

Answer: B. Crackles are caused by alveoli opening and are usually associated with fluid in the alveolar space.

2. Which ABG analysis results would you expect to find in a patient with acute respiratory failure?
    A. pH 7.25, Pao_2 48, $Paco_2$ 55
    B. pH 7.40, Pao_2 82, $Paco_2$ 45
    C. pH 7.50, Pao_2 60, $Paco_2$ 30
    D. pH 7.30, Pao_2 85, $Paco_2$ 48

Answer: A. The patient with a Pao_2 less than 50, a decreased pH, and elevated $Paco_2$ is hypoxemic and in respiratory acidosis.

3. Which option isn't a method of weaning a patient from mechanical ventilation?
    A. Intermittent mandatory ventilation
    B. Pressure support ventilation
    C. Spontaneous breathing trials with T-piece
    D. Controlled mandatory ventilation

Answer: D. Controlled mandatory ventilation is used when the patient can't initiate spontaneous breaths, such as a patient paralyzed because of a spinal cord injury. It isn't an acceptable weaning method.

4. ET tubes have inflatable cuffs to:
    A. measure pressure on tracheal tissues.
    B. drain gastric contents.
    C. prevent backflow of oxygen.
    D. treat laryngeal edema.

Answer: C. ET tube cuffs prevent backflow of oxygen so that it's delivered fully to the lungs.

5.   A patient diagnosed with status asthmaticus who was previously wheezing suddenly stops wheezing and continues to show signs of respiratory distress. Your assessment findings would indicate that:
    A.   his condition is slowly improving.
    B.   he's in imminent danger of respiratory collapse.
    C.   he isn't as sick as you thought because he stopped wheezing.
    D.   you need more information because wheezing isn't a sensitive indicator of asthma.

Answer: B. Wheezing that stops suddenly when signs of respiratory distress continue indicates severe bronchial constriction with little air movement during inspiration and expiration. This is a dangerous event, requiring immediate intervention to prevent respiratory collapse.

6.   Which strategy is recommended to prevent ventilator-associated pneumonia?
    A.   Administering antibiotics
    B.   Elevating the head of the bed 30 to 45 degrees
    C.   Opening the ventilator circuit when removing condensate
    D.   Avoiding routine mouth care

Answer: B. A key prevention strategy for preventing ventilator-associated pneumonia is to elevate the head of the bed 30 to 45 degrees.

7.   A possible cause of a ventilator low-pressure alarm is:
    A.   condensation in the ventilator tubing.
    B.   patient coughing.
    C.   ET tube disconnected from ventilator.
    E.   secretions in the patient's airway.

Answer: C. If the ET tube becomes disconnected from the ventilator, a low-pressure alarm will sound.

Scoring

☆☆☆   If you answered all seven questions correctly, breathe a big sigh of relief. You re a respiratory mastermind!

☆☆   If you answered four questions correctly, don't wait to exhale. You're an inspiration!

☆   If you answered fewer than four questions correctly, don't panic— you aren't on the verge of expiration. Take a deep breath and dive back into the chapter.

Suggested References

Alspach, J. G. (Ed.). (2013). *Core curriculum for critical care nursing* (6th ed.). St. Louis, MO: Elsevier.

Hess, D. R. (2013). Noninvasive ventilation for acute respiratory failure. *Respiratory Care, 58*(6), 950–972.

McCance, K. L., & Huether, S. E. (Eds.). (2013). *Pathophysiology: The biologic basis for disease in adults and children* (7th ed.). St. Louis, MO: Elsevier.

Roberts, P. R., & Todd, S. R. (2012). *Comprehensive critical care: Adult.* Mt. Prospect, IL: Society of Critical Care Medicine.

Tulaimat, A., Gueret, R. M., Wisniewski, M. F., & Samuel, J. (2014). Association between rating of respiratory distress and vital signs, severity of illness, intubation, and mortality in acutely ill subjects. *Respiratory Care, 59*(9), 1338–1344.

Chapter 6

Gastrointestinal system

Just the facts

In this chapter, you'll learn:

◆ structure and function of the GI system

◆ assessment of the GI system

◆ diagnostic tests and treatments

◆ GI disorders and related nursing care.

Understanding the GI system

The GI system has two major components: the alimentary canal (also called the *GI tract*) and accessory organs of digestion.

GI function

The two major functions of the GI tract are:

1. digestion, or breaking down food and fluid into simple chemicals that can be absorbed into the bloodstream and transported through the body
2. elimination of wastes through excretion of stool.

GI failure

The GI system has a profound effect on a person's overall health. When a GI process malfunctions, the patient can experience problems ranging from loss of appetite to acid–base imbalance.

Alimentary canal

The alimentary canal is a hollow muscular tube that begins in the mouth and extends to the anus. It includes the pharynx, esophagus, stomach, and small and large intestines. (See *Structures of the GI system*.)

> Can someone please point me toward the Alimentary Canal? I think I took a wrong turn at the Canal Grande.

Structures of the GI system

The GI system includes the alimentary canal (pharynx, esophagus, stomach, and small and large intestines) and the accessory organs (liver, biliary duct system, and pancreas). These structures are illustrated below.

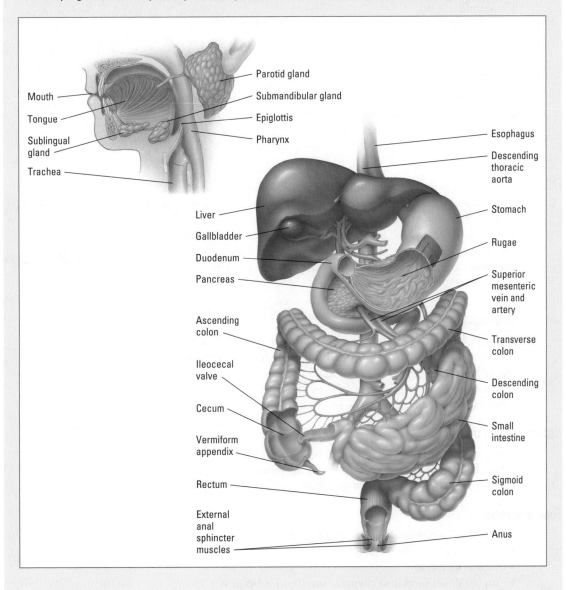

Mouth

Digestion begins in the mouth with chewing, salivating, and swallowing. The tongue provides a person's sense of taste. Saliva moistens food during chewing and is produced by three pairs of glands:
1. parotid
2. submandibular
3. sublingual.

Pharynx

The pharynx, or throat, is a cavity that extends from the oral cavity to the esophagus. The pharynx assists in swallowing by grasping food and propelling it toward the esophagus.

Esophagus

The esophagus is a muscular tube that connects the pharynx to the stomach at the cardiac orifice. The esophagus is posterior to the trachea, in the posterior mediastinum, and crosses through the diaphragm into the stomach. When food is swallowed, the cricopharyngeal sphincter—a sphincter at the upper border of the esophagus—relaxes for food to enter the esophagus. Peristalsis propels liquids and solids through the esophagus into the stomach.

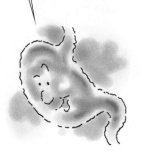

How perfect! Peristalsis propels liquids and solids through the esophagus into me!

Stomach

The stomach, a reservoir for food, is a collapsible, pouchlike structure in the left upper part of the abdominal cavity, just below the diaphragm. Its upper border is attached to the lower end of the esophagus. The lateral surface of the stomach is called the *greater curvature*; the medial surface, the *lesser curvature*.

Distinctive sphincters

The stomach contains two important sphincters:
1. the cardiac sphincter, which protects the entrance to the stomach
2. the pyloric sphincter, which guards the exit.

Food processor

The stomach has several major functions. It:
- serves as a temporary storage area for food
- begins digestion
- breaks down food into chyme, a semifluid substance
- moves the gastric contents into the small intestine
- produces intrinsic factor, which is necessary for absorption of vitamin B_{12}.

Small intestine

The small intestine is about 20′ (6 m) long and is named for its diameter, not its length. Nearly all digestion and nutrient absorption takes place in the small intestine.

There are three major divisions of the small intestine:
1. duodenum, the shortest (25 to 30 cm or 10″ to 12″) and most superior division
2. jejunum, (2.6 m or 8½′) the middle and longest segment
3. ileum (1 m or 3½′) the most inferior portion.

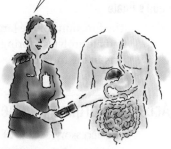

There's nothing small about the job of the small intestine. It does most of the digesting and absorbing!

Absorptive wall

The intestinal wall has several structural features that increase its absorptive surface area, including:
- plicae circulares, which are circular folds of the intestinal mucosa
- villi, which are fingerlike projections on the mucosa
- microvilli, which are tiny cytoplasmic projections on the surface of epithelial cells.

The small intestine also contains:
- intestinal crypts of Lieberkühn, which are simple glands lodged in the grooves separating villi. The functions of the crypts of Lieberkühn are to secrete inactivated pepsin, hydrochloric acid (to lower pH and activate pepsin), and mucus (to protect epithelial cells).
- Peyer's patches, which are collections of lymphatic tissue within the submucosa, which absorb viral and bacterial debris.
- Brunner's glands, which secrete mucus.

Small intestine functions, no small feat

The small intestine functions by:
- completing food digestion
- absorbing food molecules, water, and vitamins through its wall into the circulatory system, which then delivers them to cells throughout the body
- secreting hormones that control the secretion of bile, pancreatic juices, and intestinal juice.

Large intestine

The large intestine, or colon, has six segments:
1. The cecum, a saclike structure, makes up the first few inches. It's connected to the ileum of the small intestine by the ileocecal pouch.
2. The ascending colon rises on the right posterior abdominal wall and then turns sharply under the liver at the hepatic flexure.

3. The transverse colon is situated above the small intestine, passing horizontally across the abdomen and below the liver, stomach, and spleen. At the left colic flexure, it turns downward.
4. The descending colon starts near the spleen and extends down the left side of the abdomen into the pelvic cavity.
5. The sigmoid colon descends through the pelvic cavity, where it becomes the rectum.
6. The rectum, the last few inches of the large intestine, terminates at the anus.

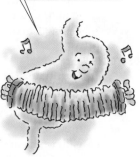

The large intestine, or colon, consists of six segments. And when they're all in tune, they play like a symphony.

Food's finale

The functions of the large intestine include absorbing excess water and electrolytes, storing food residue, and eliminating waste products in the form of feces.

Accessory organs of digestion

The accessory organs of the GI tract are the liver, gallbladder, and pancreas. They contribute hormones, enzymes, and bile, which are vital to digestion.

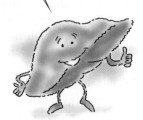

I may be considered an accessory, but my role is important.

Liver

The liver is located in the right upper quadrant under the diaphragm. It has four lobes:
1. left lobe
2. right lobe
3. caudate lobe (behind the right lobe)
4. quadrate lobe (behind the left lobe).

Liver's lobule

The liver's functional unit is called the *lobule*. It consists of hepatic cells, or hepatocytes, that encircle a central vein and radiate outward. Hepatocytes secrete bile and perform many metabolic, endocrine, and secretory functions.

Separating the hepatocytes' plates from each other are sinusoids, the liver's capillary system. Reticuloendothelial macrophages (Kupffer's cells) that line the sinusoids remove bacteria and toxins that enter the blood through the intestinal capillaries.

Liver at work

The liver's functions include:
*   metabolizing carbohydrates, fats, and proteins
*   detoxifying various endogenous and exogenous toxins in plasma
*   converting ammonia to urea for excretion

- synthesizing plasma proteins, nonessential amino acids, and lipoproteins
- storing essential nutrients, such as iron and vitamins A D, K, and B_{12}
- regulating blood glucose levels
- synthesizing and secreting bile.

Gallbladder

The gallbladder is a small, pear-shaped organ that lies halfway under the right lobe of the liver. It stores and concentrates bile produced by the liver and then releases bile into the common bile duct for delivery to the duodenum in response to the contraction and relaxation of the sphincter of Oddi.

Bile talk

Bile is a greenish liquid composed of water, cholesterol, bile salts, and phospholipids. It has several functions, including emulsifying (breaking down) fat and promoting intestinal absorption of fatty acids, cholesterol, and other lipids.

Pancreas

The pancreas lies horizontally in the abdomen behind the stomach. Its head and neck extend into the curve of the duodenum and its tail lies against the spleen. The pancreas performs exocrine and endocrine functions. (See *A look at the biliary tract*, page 438.)

Exocrine function and enzymes

The pancreas's exocrine function involves scattered cells that secrete more than 1,000 ml of digestive enzymes every day. Vagal stimulation and release of the hormones secretin and cholecystokinin control the rate and amount of pancreatic secretion.

Clustered lobules and lobes (acini) of enzyme-producing cells release their secretions into the pancreatic duct. The pancreatic duct runs the length of the pancreas and joins the bile duct from the gallbladder before entering the duodenum.

Endocrine function and hormones

The endocrine function of the pancreas involves the islets of Langerhans, located between the acinar cells. More than 1 million of these islets house two cell types:

1. beta cells, which secrete insulin to promote carbohydrate metabolism
2. alpha cells, which secrete glucagon, a hormone that stimulates glycogenolysis in the liver.

Insulin and glucagon flow directly into the blood. Blood glucose levels stimulate their release.

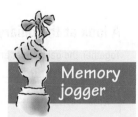

Memory jogger

To remember the difference between exocrine and endocrine, just remember **ex**ocrine refers to **ex**ternal. That leaves **en**docrine, which refers to **in**ternal.

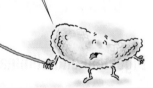

I'm a multitasking little organ! I perform exocrine and endocrine functions.

A look at the biliary tract

Together, the gallbladder and pancreas constitute the biliary tract. This illustration shows the parts of the biliary tract.

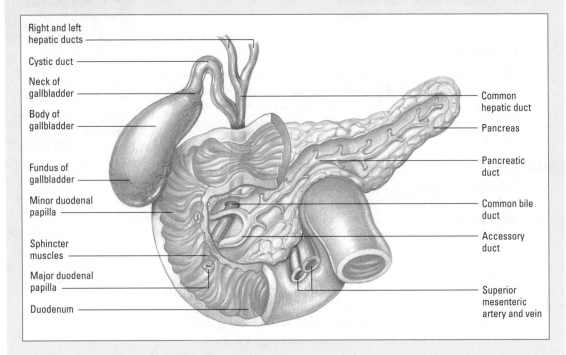

Right and left hepatic ducts

Cystic duct

Neck of gallbladder

Body of gallbladder

Fundus of gallbladder

Minor duodenal papilla

Sphincter muscles

Major duodenal papilla

Duodenum

Common hepatic duct

Pancreas

Pancreatic duct

Common bile duct

Accessory duct

Superior mesenteric artery and vein

Digestion and elimination

Digestion starts in the oral cavity, where chewing (mastication), salivating (the beginning of starch digestion), and swallowing (deglutition) all take place.

Down it goes!

When a person swallows, the hypopharyngeal sphincter in the upper esophagus relaxes, allowing food to enter the esophagus. In the esophagus, the glossopharyngeal nerve activates peristalsis, which moves the food down toward the stomach. As food passes through the esophagus, glands secrete mucus, which lubricates the food bolus.

Gotta get gastrin'

As the food bolus reaches the stomach, digestive juices (hydrochloric acid and pepsin) are secreted. When the food enters the stomach

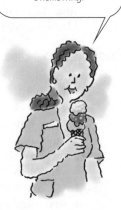

Yum! Digestion starts with chewing, salivation, and swallowing.

through the cardiac sphincter, the stomach wall stretches. This distention of the stomach wall stimulates the stomach to release gastrin.

Gastrin stimulates the stomach's motor functions and secretion of gastric juices by the gastric gland. These digestive secretions consist mainly of:

- pepsin
- hydrochloric acid
- intrinsic factor
- proteolytic enzymes.

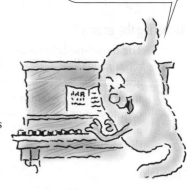

The digestive process takes some time. So sit back, relax, and enjoy the dinner show.

Not much for absorption

Little food absorption, except for alcohol, occurs in the stomach. Peristaltic contractions churn the food into tiny particles and mix it with gastric juices, forming chyme. Peristaltic waves move the chyme into the antrum of the stomach, where it backs up against the pyloric sphincter before being released into the duodenum.

Digestion and absorption powerhouse

The small intestine performs most of the work of digestion and absorption. Intestinal contractions and various digestive secretions break down carbohydrates, proteins, and fats, actions that enable the intestinal mucosa to absorb these nutrients into the bloodstream (along with water and electrolytes).

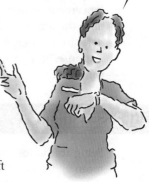

By the time chyme enters the large intestine, it's mostly indigestible.

Small to large

By the time chyme passes through the small intestine and enters the ascending colon of the large intestine, it has been reduced to mostly indigestible substances.

Journey through the large intestine

The food bolus begins its journey through the large intestine where the ileum and cecum join with the ileocecal pouch. Then the bolus moves up the ascending colon, past the right abdominal cavity, to the liver's lower border. It crosses horizontally below the liver and stomach by way of the transverse colon and descends through the left abdominal cavity to the iliac fossa through the descending colon.

From there, the bolus travels through the sigmoid colon to the lower midline of the abdominal cavity, then to the rectum, and finally to the anal canal. The anus opens to the exterior through two sphincters:

1. The internal sphincter contains thick, circular smooth muscle under autonomic control.
2. The external sphincter contains skeletal muscle under voluntary control.

All about the absorption

The large intestine produces no hormones or digestive enzymes; it continues the absorptive process. Through blood and lymph vessels in the submucosa, the proximal half of the large intestine absorbs all but about 100 ml of the remaining water in the colon. It also absorbs large amounts of sodium and chloride.

Harboring the enemy?

The large intestine harbors the bacteria *Escherichia coli*, *Enterobacter aerogenes*, *Clostridium perfringens*, and *Lactobacillus bifidus*. All of these bacteria aid in synthesizing vitamin K and breaking down cellulose into a usable carbohydrate. Bacterial action also produces flatus, which helps propel stool toward the rectum.

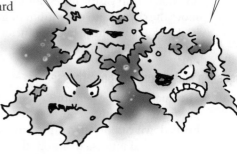

We're not all bad! Some bacteria help break down cellulose into a usable carbohydrate.

Yeah. Sometimes we make beautiful music together.

Lube job

In addition, the mucosa of the large intestine produces alkaline secretions. This alkaline mucus lubricates the intestinal walls and protects the mucosa from acidic bacterial action.

Elimination round

In the lower colon, long and relatively sluggish contractions cause propulsive waves. Normally occurring several times per day, these movements propel intestinal contents into the rectum and produce the urge to defecate. Defecation normally results from the defecation reflex, a sensory and parasympathetic nerve-mediated response, along with the voluntary relaxation of the external anal sphincter.

GI assessment

Being able to identify subtle changes in a patient's GI system can mean all the difference between effective and ineffective care. GI signs and symptoms can have many baffling causes. When your patient is critically ill, your GI assessment can be used to determine whether the patient's signs and symptoms are related to his current medical problem or indicate a new problem.

Unless the critically ill patient requires immediate stabilizing treatment, begin by taking a thorough patient history. Then probe further by conducting a thorough physical examination, using inspection, auscultation, palpation, and percussion.

History

In the health history, include information about the patient's chief complaint, medications used, family history, and social history. Conduct this part of the assessment as privately as possible because the patient may feel embarrassment when talking about GI functions.

Current health status

The patient with a GI problem usually complains of:
- pain
- heartburn
- nausea
- vomiting
- altered bowel habits.

To investigate these and other signs and symptoms, ask about the onset, duration, and severity of each. Also, inquire about the location of the pain, precipitating factors, alleviating factors, and associated symptoms. (See *Asking the right questions*, page 442.)

Previous health status

To determine if the patient's problem is new or recurring, ask about GI illnesses, such as an ulcer, gallbladder disease, inflammatory bowel disease, or GI bleeding. Also, ask if he has had abdominal surgery or trauma.

Further questions

Ask the patient additional questions, such as:
- Are you allergic to any foods or medications?
- Have you noticed a change in the color, amount, and appearance of your stool? Have you ever seen blood in your stool?
- Have you recently travelled abroad? (if reason for seeking care is diarrhea because diarrhea, hepatitis, and parasitic infections can result from ingesting contaminated food or water)
- How is your dental health? What kind of dental care have you received? (Poor dentition may impair the ability to chew and swallow food.)

Don't forget the drugs

Ask the patient if he's taking medication. Several drugs, including aspirin, sulfonamides, nonsteroidal anti-inflammatory drugs (NSAIDs), analgesics, and some antihypertensives, can cause nausea, vomiting, diarrhea, constipation, and other GI signs and symptoms. Be sure to ask about laxative use because habitual intake can cause constipation.

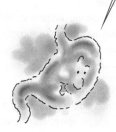

Your patient may complain of pain, heartburn, nausea, vomiting, or altered bowel habits. Be discreet when asking about these problems to avoid embarrassment.

Asking the right questions

When assessing a patient with GI-related signs and symptoms, be sure to ask the right questions. To establish a baseline for comparison, ask about the patient's current state of health, including questions about the onset, duration, quality, severity, and location of problems as well as precipitating factors, alleviating factors, and associated symptoms.

Onset

How did the problem start? Was it gradual or sudden and with or without previous symptoms? What was the patient doing when he noticed it? If he has diarrhea, has he been traveling? If so, when and where?

Duration

When did the problem start? Has the patient had the problem before? Has he had any abdominal surgery. If yes, when? If he's in pain, find out when the problem began. Is the pain continuous or intermittent?

Quality

Ask the patient to describe the problem. Has he ever had it before? Was it diagnosed? If he's in pain, find out whether the pain feels sharp, dull, aching, colicky (cramp-like), or burning.

Severity

Ask the patient to describe how much the problem bothers him—for example, have him rate it on a pain scale of 0 to 10. Does it keep him from his normal activities? Has it improved or worsened since he first noticed it? Does it wake him at night? If he's in pain, does he double over from it?

Location

Where does the patient feel the problem? Does it spread, radiate, or shift? Ask him to point to where he feels it the most.

Precipitating factors

Does anything seem to bring on the problem? What makes it worse? Does it occur at the same time each day or with certain positions? Does the patient notice it after eating or drinking certain foods or after certain activities?

Alleviating factors

Does anything relieve the problem? Does the patient take any prescribed or over-the-counter medications for relief? Has he tried anything else for relief?

Associated symptoms

What else bothers the patient when he has the problem? Has he had nausea, vomiting, dry heaves, diarrhea, constipation, bloating, or flatulence? Has he lost his appetite or lost or gained any weight? If so, how much? When was the patient's last bowel movement? Was it unusual? Has he seen blood in his vomitus or stool? Has his stool changed in size or color or included mucus? Ask the patient whether he can eat normally and hold down foods and liquids. Also, ask about alcohol consumption.

Family history

Because some GI disorders are hereditary, ask the patient whether anyone in his family has had a GI disorder. Disorders with a familial link include:

- ulcerative colitis
- colon cancer
- stomach ulcers
- diabetes
- alcoholism
- Crohn's disease.

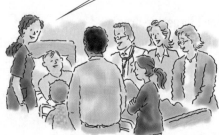

Family history can be important because some GI disorders can be hereditary.

Lifestyle patterns

Psychological and sociologic factors can profoundly affect health. To determine factors that may have contributed to your patient's problem, ask about his occupation, home life, financial situation, stress level, and recent life changes.

Be sure to ask about alcohol, recreational drug, herbal supplement, caffeine, and tobacco use as well as food consumption, exercise habits, and oral hygiene. Also ask about sleep patterns, such as hours of sleep and whether sleep is restful.

Cultural factors may affect a patient's dietary habits, so ask about any dietary restrictions the patient has such as following a vegetarian diet. Some patients may also have dietary restrictions due to a previous medical problem or procedure (i.e., bariatric surgery). Seek information regarding these as well.

Physical examination

A physical assessment begins by observing the patient's overall appearance and interactions. Physical examination of the GI system usually includes evaluation of the mouth, abdomen, liver, and rectum. Before beginning your examination, explain the techniques you'll be using and warn the patient that some procedures might be uncomfortable. Perform the examination in a private, quiet, warm, and well-lighted room.

Assessing the mouth

Use inspection and palpation to assess the oral cavity:
- First, inspect the patient's mouth and jaw for asymmetry and swelling. Check his bite, noting malocclusion from an overbite or underbite. If the patient has dentures, do they fit? Are they intact or broken? If the patient is intubated and mechanically ventilated, are the dentures still in place or removed?
- Inspect the inner and outer lips, teeth, and gums with a penlight. Note bleeding; gum ulcerations; cavity lesions; and missing, displaced, or broken teeth.
- Assess the tongue, checking for coating, tremors, swelling, and ulcerations. Note unusual breath odors.
- Finally, examine the pharynx, looking for uvular deviation, tonsillar abnormalities, lesions, plaques, and exudate.

Assessing the abdomen

When assessing the abdomen, perform the four basic steps in the following sequence: inspection, auscultation, percussion, and palpation. The GI system requires abdominal auscultation

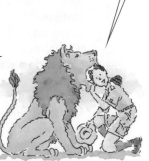

Begin your physical exam by assessing the oral cavity. Check out your patient's mouth, jaw, teeth, lips, gum, and tongue for starters.

before percussion and palpation because the latter can alter intestinal activity and bowel sounds.

Prepping for accuracy

To ensure an accurate assessment, before the examination:
- Drape the patient appropriately.
- Place a small pillow under the patient's knees to relax the abdominal muscles.
- Keep the room warm. Chilling can cause abdominal muscles to tense.
- Warm your hands and the stethoscope.
- Speak softly and encourage the patient to perform breathing exercises or use imagery during uncomfortable procedures.
- Assess painful areas last to avoid the patient becoming tense.

Abdominal inspection

Before inspecting the abdomen, mentally divide it into four quadrants. (See *Identifying abdominal landmarks*.)

Inspector General

Begin by performing a general inspection of the patient:
- Observe the skin, oral mucosa, nail beds, and sclera for jaundice or signs of anemia.
- Stand at the foot of the bed and observe the abdomen for symmetry, checking for bumps, bulges, or masses. A bulge may indicate bladder distention or hernia.
- Note the patient's abdominal shape and contour. The abdomen should be flat to rounded in people of average weight. A protruding abdomen may be caused by obesity, pregnancy, ascites, or abdominal distention. A slender person may have a slightly concave abdomen.
- Next, inspect the abdominal skin, which normally appears smooth and intact. Observe for discoloration, rashes, ecchymosis, or lesions. Striae, or stretch marks, can be caused by pregnancy, excessive weight gain, or ascites. New striae are pink or blue; old striae are silvery white. In patients with darker skin, striae may be dark brown. Note dilated veins. Record the length of any surgical scars on the abdomen and the stage of healing if warranted.
- Note abdominal movements and pulsations. Usually, waves of peristalsis aren't visible unless the patient is very thin, in which case they may be visible as slight wavelike motions. Marked visible rippling may indicate bowel obstruction; report it immediately. In a thin patient, pulsation of the aorta is visible in the epigastric area. Marked pulsations may occur with

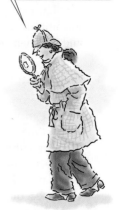

You'll need to rely on your keen assessment skills when performing a general inspection.

Identifying abdominal landmarks

To aid accurate abdominal assessment and documentation of findings, you can mentally divide the patient's abdomen into regions. Use the quadrant method—the easiest and most commonly used method—to divide the abdomen into four equal regions using two imaginary perpendicular lines crossing just above the umbilicus.

Right upper quadrant
- Liver and gallbladder
- Pylorus
- Duodenum
- Head of pancreas
- Hepatic flexure of colon
- Portions of ascending and transverse colon

Left upper quadrant
- Left liver lobe
- Stomach
- Body of pancreas
- Splenic flexure of colon
- Portions of transverse and descending colon

Right lower quadrant
- Cecum and appendix
- Portion of ascending colon
- Lower portion of right kidney
- Bladder (if distended)

Left lower quadrant
- Sigmoid colon
- Portion of descending colon
- Lower portion of left kidney
- Bladder (if distended)

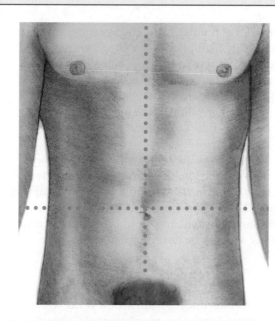

hypertension, aortic insufficiency, and other conditions causing widening pulse pressure.

Abdominal auscultation
Auscultation provides information about bowel motility and the underlying vessels and organs.

Follow the clock

Use a stethoscope to auscultate for bowel and vascular sounds. Lightly place the stethoscope diaphragm in the right lower quadrant, slightly below and to the right of the umbilicus. Auscultate in a clockwise fashion in each of the four quadrants, spending at least 2 minutes in each area. Note the character and quality of bowel sounds in each quadrant. In some cases, you may need to auscultate for 5 minutes before you hear sounds. Be sure to allow enough time to listen in each quadrant before you decide that bowel sounds are absent.

Auscultate for at least 2 minutes in each of the four abdominal quadrants.

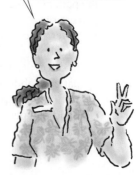

Tube tip

Before auscultating the abdomen of a patient with a nasogastric (NG) tube or another abdominal tube connected to suction, briefly clamp the tube or turn off the suction. Suction noises can obscure or mimic actual bowel sounds.

Sound class

Bowel sounds are classified as normal, hypoactive, or hyperactive:
- *Normal* bowel sounds are high-pitched, gurgling noises caused by air mixing with fluid during peristalsis. The noises vary in frequency, pitch, and intensity and occur irregularly from 5 to 34 times per minute. They're loudest before mealtimes. Borborygmus, or stomach growling, is the loud, gurgling, splashing sound heard over the large intestine as gas passes through it.
- *Hypoactive* bowel sounds are heard infrequently. They're associated with ileus, bowel obstruction, or peritonitis and indicate diminished peristalsis. Paralytic ileus, torsion of the bowel, or the use of opioids and other medications can decrease peristalsis.
- *Hyperactive* bowel sounds are loud, high-pitched, tinkling sounds that occur frequently and may be caused by diarrhea, constipation, or laxative use.

Sound off

Next, use the bell of the stethoscope to auscultate for vascular sounds. Normally, you should detect no vascular sounds. Note a bruit, venous hum, or friction rub. If you identify a bruit, don't proceed with palpation and percussion; if it's a new finding, notify the doctor. (See *Interpreting abnormal abdominal sounds*.)

Abdominal percussion
Use abdominal percussion to determine the size and location of abdominal organs and detect excessive accumulation of fluid and air. Begin percussion in the right lower quadrant and proceed clockwise, covering all four quadrants. Keep the approximate locations of the patient's organs in mind as you progress. Use direct or indirect percussion:
- Defer abdominal percussion if the patient exhibits abdominal guarding.
- In direct percussion, strike your hand or finger directly over the patient's abdomen.
- With indirect percussion, use the middle finger of your dominant hand or a percussion hammer to strike a finger resting on the patient's abdomen.

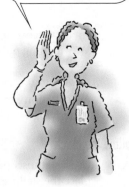

Listen for normal, hypoactive, or hyperactive bowel sounds.

Interpreting abnormal abdominal sounds

Sound and description	Location	Possible cause
Abnormal bowel sounds		
Hyperactive sounds (unrelated to hunger)	Any quadrant	Diarrhea, laxative use, or early intestinal obstruction
Hypoactive, then absent sounds	Any quadrant	Paralytic ileus or peritonitis
High-pitched tinkling sounds	Any quadrant	Intestinal fluid and air under tension in a dilated bowel
High-pitched rushing sounds coinciding with abdominal cramps	Any quadrant	Intestinal obstruction
Systolic bruits		
Vascular blowing sounds resembling cardiac murmurs	Over abdominal aorta	Partial arterial obstruction or turbulent blood flow
	Over renal artery	Renal artery stenosis
	Over iliac artery	Iliac artery obstruction
Venous hum		
Continuous, medium-pitched tone created by blood flow in a large engorged vascular organ such as the liver	Epigastric and umbilical regions	Increased collateral circulation between portal and systemic venous systems such as in cirrhosis
Friction rub		
Harsh, grating sound like two pieces of sandpaper rubbing together	Over liver and spleen	Inflammation of the peritoneal surface of liver such as from a tumor

Percussion precaution

Don't percuss the abdomen of a patient with an abdominal aortic aneurysm or a transplanted abdominal organ. Doing so can precipitate a rupture or organ rejection.

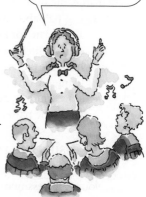

The degree of tympany you hear depends on the amount of air in the stomach and bowel.

Tympany and dullness

Normally, you should hear two sounds during percussion of the abdomen: tympany and dullness. When you percuss over hollow organs, such as an empty stomach or bowel, you should hear a clear, hollow sound like a drum beating. This sound, tympany, predominates because air is normally present in the stomach and bowel. The degree of tympany depends on the amount of air and gastric dilation.

When you percuss over solid organs, such as the liver, kidney, or feces-filled intestines, the sound changes to dullness. Note where percussed sounds change from tympany to dullness, which may indicate a solid mass or enlarged organ.

Abdominal palpation

Abdominal palpation includes light and deep touch to determine the size, shape, position, and tenderness of major abdominal organs and to detect masses and fluid accumulation. Palpate all four quadrants, leaving painful and tender areas for last.

Light palpation

Use light palpation to identify muscle resistance and tenderness as well as the location of some superficial organs. To do so, gently press your fingertips ½″ to ¾″ (1.5 to 2 cm) into the abdominal wall. Use the lightest touch possible because too much pressure blunts your sensitivity.

Deep palpation

Use deep palpation by pressing the fingertips of both hands about 1½″ (3.5 cm) into the abdominal wall. Move your hands in a slightly circular fashion so that the abdominal wall moves over the underlying structures.

Deep palpation may evoke rebound tenderness when you suddenly withdraw your fingertips, a possible sign of peritoneal inflammation. (See *Eliciting abdominal pain*.)

Assessing the liver

You can estimate the size and position of the liver through percussion and palpation.

Percussion discussion

Percussing the liver allows you to estimate its size. Hepatomegaly is commonly associated with hepatitis and other liver disease. Liver borders may be obscured and difficult to assess. (See *Percussing the liver*, page 450.)

Palpation problem

It's usually impossible to palpate the liver in an adult patient. If palpable, the liver border feels smooth and firm, with a rounded, regular edge. A palpable liver may indicate hepatomegaly.

To palpate for hepatomegaly:
- start at the lower right quadrant
- have the patient take a deep breath and hold it while you palpate using the tips of your fingers
- slowly move your hand up toward the costal margin and palpate while the patient exhales.

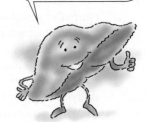

It's usually impossible to palpate the liver in an adult patient.

Assessing the rectum

If your patient is age 40 or older, a rectal examination may be part of your GI assessment. Explain the procedure to reassure the patient.

Eliciting abdominal pain

Rebound tenderness and the iliopsoas and obturator signs can indicate such conditions as appendicitis and peritonitis. You can elicit these signs of abdominal pain, as illustrated below.

Rebound tenderness

Help the patient into a supine position with his knees flexed to relax the abdominal muscles. Place your hands gently on the right lower quadrant at McBurney's point (located about midway between the umbilicus and the anterior superior iliac spine). Slowly and deeply dip your fingers into the area; then release the pressure in a quick, smooth motion. Pain on release—rebound tenderness—is a positive sign. The pain may radiate to the umbilicus.

Caution: To minimize the risk of rupturing an inflamed appendix, don't repeat this maneuver.

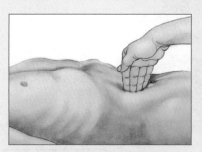
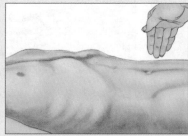

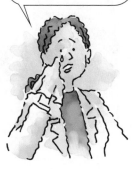

Eliciting pain . . . it gets me every time!

Iliopsoas sign

Help the patient into a supine position with his legs straight. Instruct him to raise his right leg upward as you exert slight pressure with your hand. Repeat the maneuver with the left leg. When testing either leg, increased abdominal pain is a positive result, indicating irritation of the psoas muscle.

Obturator sign

Help the patient into a supine position with his right leg flexed 90 degrees at the hip and knee. Hold the leg just above the knee and at the ankle; then rotate the leg laterally and medially. Pain in the hypogastric region is a positive sign, indicating irritation of the obturator muscle.

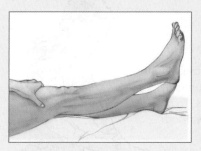
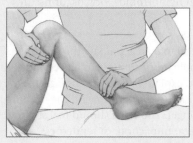

Percussing the liver

Begin percussing the abdomen along the right midclavicular line, starting below the level of the umbilicus. Move upward until the percussion notes change from tympany to dullness, usually at or slightly below the costal margin.

Then percuss downward along the right midclavicular line, starting above the nipple.

Move downward until percussion notes change from normal lung resonance to dullness, usually at the fifth to seventh intercostal space. Again, mark the point of change with a felt-tip pen. Estimate the liver size by measuring the distance between the two marks.

Anatomic landmarks for liver percussion

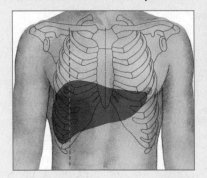

Hand position for liver percussion

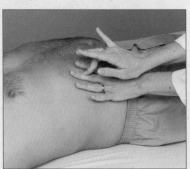

Perianal is primary

To perform a rectal examination, first inspect the perianal area following these steps:
- Put on gloves and spread the buttocks to expose the anus and surrounding tissue, checking for fissures, lesions, scars, inflammation, discharge, rectal prolapse, and external hemorrhoids.
- Ask the patient to strain as if he's having a bowel movement; this may reveal internal hemorrhoids, polyps, or fissures.

Rectum is next

After examining the perianal area, palpate the rectum:
- Apply a water-soluble lubricant to your gloved index finger. Tell the patient to relax and explain to him that he'll feel some pressure.
- Insert your finger into the rectum toward the umbilicus. To palpate, rotate your finger. The walls should feel soft and smooth without masses, fecal impaction, or tenderness.
- Remove your finger from the rectum and inspect the glove for stool, blood, or mucus. Test fecal material adhering to the glove for occult blood using a guaiac test.

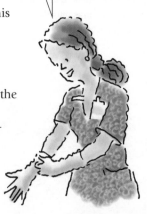

A rectal exam may be part of the GI assessment for a patient age 40 or older. Don't forget to lubricate your gloved finger before palpating the rectum.

Diagnostic tests

Many tests provide information used to guide your care of the patient with a GI problem. Even if you don't participate in testing, you should know why the test was ordered; what the results mean; and what your responsibilities are before, during, and after the test.

Diagnostic tests commonly ordered for patients with known or suspected GI disorders include endoscopy, laboratory tests, nuclear imaging scans, and radiographic tests.

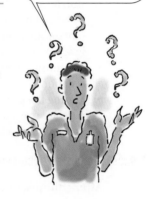

Know why a test was ordered; what the results mean; and what your responsibilities are before, during, and after testing.

Endoscopy

The practitioner can directly view hollow visceral linings by using a fiber-optic endoscope. This test is used to diagnose inflammatory, ulcerative, and infectious diseases; benign and malignant neoplasms; and other esophageal, gastric, and intestinal mucosal lesions. Endoscopy can also be used for therapeutic interventions or to obtain a biopsy.

Bedside or not

The endoscopic procedure is commonly done at the bedside in the critical care unit. However, if it's performed in the procedure suite, you may accompany an unstable patient who requires monitoring.

Colonoscopy

Colonoscopy, also referred to as *lower GI endoscopy*, is used to:
- diagnose inflammatory and ulcerative bowel disease
- pinpoint lower GI bleeding and treat if able
- detect and treat lower GI abnormalities, such as tumors, polyps, hemorrhoids, and abscesses.

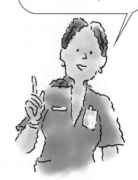

Remember, good bowel prep is important to ensure a successful colonoscopy.

Nursing considerations
- Explain the procedure and its purpose and tell the patient he'll receive I.V. premedication and conscious sedation for the procedure.
- Make sure that an informed consent form has been signed.
- Withhold all fluids and food for at least 6 to 8 hours before the test. If the patient has tube feedings running, obtain practitioner order to discontinue. Supplementation of I.V. fluids such as dextrose 5% may be warranted for glucose stability.
- Administer bowel preparation, as ordered, such as a clear liquid diet and bowel cleaning solution with electrolyte lavage. If the patient can't swallow or is unconscious, administer electrolyte lavage solution through a feeding tube or an NG tube.

- To decrease the risk of aspiration in a patient receiving electrolyte lavage solution through an NG tube, ensure proper tube placement and elevate the head of the bed or position the patient on his side. Have suction equipment available. (See *Increased risk in elderly patients.*)
- Advise the patient that he may feel the urge to defecate when the scope is inserted; encourage slow, deep breathing through the mouth, as appropriate.
- If the procedure is to be performed at the bedside, have necessary equipment for the procedure available, including emergency equipment, medications, and suction.
- Initiate an I.V. line if one isn't already in place for a patient who'll be receiving conscious sedation.
- Obtain the patient's baseline vital signs and oxygen saturation levels. Monitor cardiac rhythm.
- Administer medications, as ordered, such as midazolam for sedation. Provide supplemental oxygen, as ordered.
- During the procedure, monitor the patient's vital signs, airway patency, oxygen saturation, cardiac rhythm, skin color, abdominal distention, level of consciousness (LOC), and pain tolerance.

Assess, administer, document

After colonoscopy
- Assess your patient's vital signs and cardiopulmonary status, breath sounds, oxygen saturation, and LOC every 15 minutes for the first hour, every 30 minutes for the next hour, and then hourly until the patient stabilizes.
- Administer supplemental oxygen, as ordered and as indicated by oxygen saturation levels.
- Watch for adverse effects of sedation, such as respiratory depression, apnea, hypotension, excessive diaphoresis, bradycardia, and laryngospasm. Notify the practitioner if any occur.
- Assess the patient's stool for evidence of frank or occult bleeding.
- Monitor the patient for signs and symptoms of perforation, such as vomiting, severe abdominal pain, abdominal distention or rigidity, and fever. Notify the practitioner if any occur.
- Document the procedure, interventions, and assessment findings.

EGD

Esophagogastroduodenoscopy (EGD), also called *upper GI endoscopy*, is used to identify abnormalities of the esophagus, stomach, and small intestine, such as esophagitis, inflammatory bowel disease, Mallory-Weiss syndrome, bleeding lesions, tumors, gastritis, and polyps.

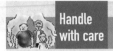

Handle with care

Increased risk in elderly patients

Elderly patients are at increased risk for experiencing adverse effects from the lavage solution, including nausea, vomiting, abdominal cramps, abdominal fullness, dizziness, and fluid and electrolyte imbalances. What's more, elderly patients may have difficulty ingesting the required amount of solution because of these adverse effects. Be sure to allow elderly patients ample time to ingest the solution.

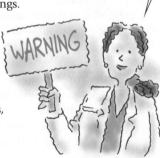

After colonoscopy, watch for any adverse effects of sedation and monitor for signs and symptoms of perforation. Report these problems immediately to the practitioner.

WARNING

Bypass the surgery

EGD eliminates the need for extensive exploratory surgery and can be used to detect small or surface lesions missed by radiography. It can also be used for sclerotherapy or to remove foreign bodies by suction (for small, soft objects) or electrocautery, snare, or forceps (for large, hard objects).

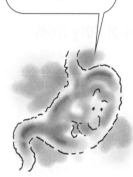

EGD is A-OK! It can even eliminate the need for extensive exploratory surgery.

Nursing considerations

Before EGD

- Explain the procedure and its purpose to the patient.
- Tell him the procedure takes about 30 minutes and that he'll receive I.V. premedication and anesthetic spray in his mouth and nose, followed by conscious sedation during the procedure.
- Restrict food and fluids for at least 6 to 12 hours before the test.
- If the patient is on anticoagulation, confer with the physician regarding timing of discontinuance prior to procedure to limit risk of bleeding.
- Make sure that an informed consent form has been signed.
- If the test is an emergency procedure, expect to insert an NG tube to aspirate contents and minimize the risk for aspiration.
- Make sure that the patient's dentures and eyeglasses are removed before the test.
- If the procedure is to be performed at the bedside, have the necessary equipment available for the procedure, including suction and emergency equipment (medications such as atropine, a monitor defibrillator, and endotracheal [ET] intubation equipment), and initiate an I.V. line if one isn't already in place.
- Monitor the patient before and throughout the procedure, including airway patency, vital signs, oxygen saturation, cardiac rhythm, abdominal distention, LOC, and pain tolerance.

After it's over

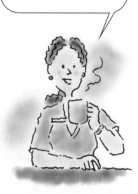

After endoscopy, withhold all food and fluids until your patient's gag reflex returns. I may just be able to squeeze in a second cup!

After EGD

- Monitor your patient's vital signs, oxygen saturation, cardiac rhythm, and LOC every 15 minutes for the first hour, every 30 minutes for the next hour, and then hourly until the patient stabilizes.
- Administer oxygen therapy, as ordered.
- Place the patient in a semi-Fowler's position (head of bed at 30 degrees) until sedation wears off.
- Withhold all food and fluids until your patient's gag reflex returns. After it returns, offer ice chips and sips of water, gradually increasing the patient's intake as tolerated and allowed.
- Observe for adverse effects of sedation, such as respiratory depression, apnea, hypotension, excessive diaphoresis, bradycardia, and laryngospasm. Notify the practitioner if any occur.

- Monitor the patient for signs and symptoms of perforation, such as difficulty swallowing, pain, fever, or bleeding as evidenced by black stools or bloody vomitus. Notify the practitioner if any occur.
- Document the procedure, interventions, and assessment findings.

Laboratory tests

Common laboratory tests used to diagnose GI disorders include studies of stool and peritoneal contents. Percutaneous liver biopsy may also be done.

Fecal studies

Normal stool appears brown and formed but soft. These abnormal findings may indicate a problem:
- Narrow, ribbonlike stool signals spastic or irritable bowel, partial bowel obstruction, or rectal obstruction.
- Constipation may be caused by diet or medications, especially narcotics.
- Diarrhea may indicate spastic bowel or viral infection.
- Mixed with blood and mucus, soft stool can signal bacterial infection; mixed with blood or pus, colitis.

In living color

- Yellow or green stool suggests severe, prolonged diarrhea; black stool suggests GI bleeding or intake of iron supplements or raw-to-rare meat. Tan or white stool shows hepatic duct or gallbladder-duct blockage, hepatitis, or cancer. Red stool may signal colon or rectal bleeding; however, drugs and foods can also cause this coloration.
- Most stool contains 10% to 20% fat. A higher fat content can turn stool pasty or greasy, a possible sign of intestinal malabsorption or pancreatic disease.

Nursing considerations
- Collect the stool specimen in a clean, dry container and immediately send it to the laboratory.
- Don't use stool that has been in contact with toilet bowl water or urine.
- Use commercial fecal occult blood slides as a simple method of testing for blood in stool. Follow package directions because certain medications and foods can interfere with test results.

Percutaneous liver biopsy

Percutaneous liver biopsy involves the needle aspiration of a core of liver tissue for histologic analysis. It's done under a local or general anesthetic. (See *Using a Menghini needle*.)

Last resort

Biopsy is used to detect hepatic disorders and cancer after ultrasonography, computed tomography (CT) scans, and radionuclide studies have failed or as an adjunct for definitive diagnosis. Because many patients with hepatic disorders have clotting defects, a clotting profile (prothrombin time [PT] and partial thromboplastin time)—along with blood type and crossmatching—should precede liver biopsy.

Nursing considerations

- Explain the procedure to the patient and tell him he'll be awake during the test and that the test may cause discomfort. Reassure him that a medication will be administered to help him relax.
- Restrict food and fluids for at least 4 hours before the test.
- Make sure the patient has signed an informed consent form.
- Check the patient's laboratory values, especially complete blood count (CBC), platelets, and clotting studies. Inform the practitioner of abnormal values.

Using a Menghini needle

In percutaneous liver biopsy, a Menghini needle attached to a 5-ml syringe containing normal saline solution is introduced through the chest wall and intercostal space (1). Negative pressure is created in the syringe. Then the needle is pushed rapidly into the liver (2) and pulled out of the body entirely (3) to obtain a tissue specimen.

1

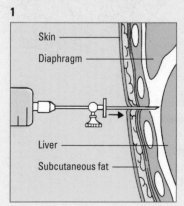

Skin

Diaphragm

Liver

Subcutaneous fat

2

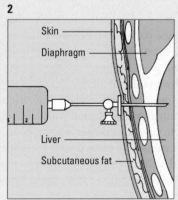

Skin

Diaphragm

Liver

Subcutaneous fat

3

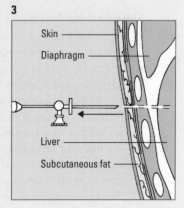

Skin

Diaphragm

Liver

Subcutaneous fat

Are we done yet?

After the procedure
- Watch the patient for bleeding and symptoms of bile peritonitis, including tenderness and rigidity around the biopsy site.
- Be alert for symptoms of pneumothorax, such as rising respiratory rate, decreased breath sounds, dyspnea, persistent shoulder pain, and pleuritic chest pain. Report these complications promptly.
- Apply a gauze dressing to the puncture site and reinforce or apply a pressure dressing if needed.
- Maintain the patient in a right side-lying position for several hours; the pressure enhances coagulation at the site.
- Monitor urine output for at least 24 hours and watch for hematuria, which may indicate bladder trauma.

Peritoneal fluid analysis

Peritoneal fluid analysis includes examination of gross appearance; erythrocyte and leukocyte counts; cytologic studies; microbiologic studies for bacteria and fungi; and determinations of protein, glucose, amylase, ammonia, and alkaline phosphatase levels.

Abdominal paracentesis

Abdominal paracentesis is a bedside procedure involving aspiration of fluid from the peritoneal space through a needle, trocar, or cannula inserted in the abdominal wall.

Paracentesis is used to:
- diagnose and treat massive ascites resistant to other therapy
- detect intra-abdominal bleeding after traumatic injury
- obtain a peritoneal fluid sample for laboratory analysis
- decrease intra-abdominal pressure and alleviate dyspnea.

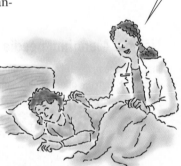

Aspiration of fluid from the peritoneal space is one procedure that can be easily done at the bedside, as long as the patient can sit up in bed.

Nursing considerations
- Explain the procedure to the patient. Make sure an informed consent form has been signed.
- Review the patient's coagulation studies.
- Have the patient empty his bladder if alert.
- Record the patient's baseline vital signs, weight, and abdominal girth. Indicate the abdominal area measured with a felt-tipped marking pen for consistency in practitioner assessments.
- The trocar or introducer cannula is inserted with the patient supine in the left lateral decubitus or semi-Fowler's position. After cannula insertion, assist the patient to sit up in bed if able. (See *Positioning for abdominal paracentesis*.)
- Remind the patient to remain as still as possible during the procedure.

Positioning for abdominal paracentesis

When positioning a patient to facilitate drainage after abdominal paracentesis, help him sit up in bed or allow him to sit on the edge of the bed with additional support for his back and arms if physical condition warrants.

In this position, gravity causes fluid to accumulate in the lower abdominal cavity. The internal organs provide counter resistance and pressure to aid fluid flow.

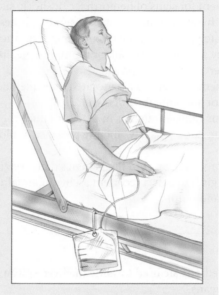

- Immediately before the procedure, participate in a "time-out" to ensure it's the correct patient, correct procedure, and correct site marking.
- During the procedure, monitor the patient's vital signs, oxygen saturation, and cardiac rhythm every 15 minutes and observe for tachycardia, hypotension, dizziness, pallor, diaphoresis, and increased anxiety, especially if more than 1,500 ml of peritoneal fluid is aspirated at one time.
- If the patient shows signs of hypovolemic shock, slow the drainage rate by raising the collection container vertically so it's closer to the height of the needle, trocar, or cannula. Stop the drainage if necessary. Limit aspirated fluid to between 1,500 and 2,000 ml.
- After the doctor removes the needle, trocar, or cannula and, if necessary, sutures the incision, apply a dry sterile pressure dressing.
- If the catheter is to remain, assure catheter is intact, sterile technique with dressing changes is performed, and specific time frames/fluid limits to drain the abdominal cavity must be ordered.

Let the monitoring begin

After the procedure
- Monitor the patient's vital signs, oxygen saturation, and cardiac rhythm, and check the dressing for drainage every 15 minutes for

the first hour, every 30 minutes for the next 2 hours, every hour for 4 hours, and then every 4 hours for 24 hours.

- Observe the patient for signs of hemorrhage or shock, such as hypotension, tachycardia, pallor, and excessive diaphoresis. These signs may indicate puncture of the inferior epigastric artery, hematoma of the anterior cecal wall, or rupture of the iliac vein or bladder. Observe for hematuria.
- Observe the patient for signs of a perforated intestine, such as increasing pain or abdominal tenderness.
- If the paracentesis catheter remains in place, monitor the fluid for volume, color, odor, viscosity, and the presence of blood or fecal matter.
- Document the procedure; record the patient's daily weight and abdominal girth to detect recurrent ascites; maintain accurate intake and output.

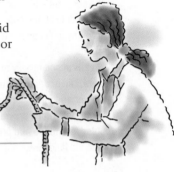

Don't forget to measure the patient's abdominal girth to check for recurrent ascites.

Nuclear imaging

Nuclear imaging methods are used to study the liver, spleen, and other abdominal organs.

Hepatobiliary scan

In a hepatobiliary scan, a scanner or gamma camera records the distribution of radioactivity within the liver and spleen after I.V. injection of a radioactive colloid. Kupffer's cells in the liver take up most of this colloid, whereas smaller amounts lodge in the spleen and bone marrow.

Ultrasonography, CT or gallium scanning, or biopsy is used to confirm the clues revealed by liver–spleen scanning.

Detective device

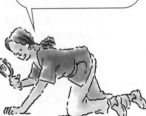

By registering the extent of this absorption, the imaging device aids in the diagnosis of common bile duct obstruction, acute and chronic cholecystitis, bile leaks, biliary atresia, and liver function. Because the test demonstrates disease nonspecifically (as a cold spot, which is an area that fails to take up the colloid), test results usually require confirmation by ultrasonography, CT or gallium scan, or biopsy.

Nursing considerations

- Describe the test to the patient and explain that it's used to examine the liver and spleen through pictures taken with a special scanner or camera.
- Tell the patient he'll receive an injection of a radioactive substance (technetium-99m sulfide) through an I.V. line in his hand or arm to allow better visualization of the liver and spleen.
- Instruct the patient to immediately report adverse reactions, such as flushing, fever, light-headedness, or difficulty breathing.

Magnetic resonance imaging

Magnetic resonance imaging (MRI) is used to examine the liver and abdominal organs. It's useful in evaluating liver disease by characterizing tumors, masses, or cysts found on other noninvasive studies. An image is generated by energizing protons in a strong magnetic field. Radio waves emitted as protons return to their former equilibrium and are recorded. No ionizing radiation is transmitted during the scan.

MRI mire

Disadvantages of MRI include the closed tubelike space required for the scan. Newer MRI centers offer a less confining "open-MRI" scan. In addition, the test can't be performed on patients with implanted metal prostheses or devices.

Nursing considerations

- Explain the procedure to the patient and stress the need to remove metal objects, such as jewelry, including piercings, before the procedure.
- Explain to the patient that he must lie still for 1 to 1½ hours for the procedure.
- Generally, you'll accompany the patient to the MRI suite. If he becomes claustrophobic during the test, administer mild sedation, as ordered.
- If the patient is unstable, make sure that an I.V. line without metal components is in place and that all equipment is compatible with MRI imaging. Monitor the patient's oxygen saturation, cardiac rhythm, and respiratory status during the test.

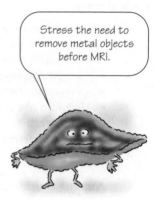

Stress the need to remove metal objects before MRI.

Radiographic tests

Radiographic tests include abdominal X-rays, various contrast media studies, and CT scans.

Abdominal X-rays

An abdominal X-ray, also called *flat plate of the abdomen* or *kidney-ureter-bladder radiography*, is used to detect and evaluate tumors, kidney stones, abnormal gas collection, and other abdominal disorders. The test consists of two plates: one taken with the patient supine and the other taken while he stands, if he is able to.

Reading the rays

On X-ray, air appears black, fat appears gray, and bone appears white. Although a routine X-ray doesn't reveal most abdominal organs, it does show the contrast between air and fluid. For example, intestinal blockage traps large amounts of detectable fluids and air inside organs. When an intestinal wall tears, air leaks into the abdomen and becomes visible on X-ray.

Nursing considerations
- Explain the procedure to the patient. Radiography requires no special pretest or posttest care. In the critical care unit, it's usually done at the bedside using portable X-ray equipment.

CT scan
In CT scanning, a computer translates multiple X-ray beams into three-dimensional oscilloscope images of the patient's biliary tract, liver, and pancreas.

Scads of scans
CT scanning is used to:
- evaluate for fluid or air collections or bleeding
- distinguish between obstructive and nonobstructive jaundice
- identify abscesses, cysts, hematomas, tumors, and pseudocysts
- evaluate the cause of weight loss and look for occult malignancy
- diagnose and evaluate pancreatitis.

The test can be done with or without a contrast medium, but contrast is preferred unless the patient is allergic to contrast media or concern for renal impact is warranted.

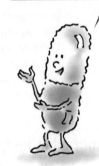

A pretest prep kit may be necessary if the patient requires a contrast medium but is allergic to iodine, shellfish, or dye.

Nursing considerations
- Explain the procedure to the patient and tell him that he should lie still, relax, and breathe normally during the test. Explain that if the practitioner orders an I.V. contrast medium, he may experience discomfort from the needle puncture and a localized feeling of warmth on injection.
- Restrict food and fluids after midnight before the test but continue any drug regimen as ordered.
- Confirm if the patient has an allergy to iodine or shellfish. If an allergy is identified, the physician will order steroids such as Solu-Medrol or prednisone and antihistamine (Benadryl) to reduce the risk of a reaction to the dye. Report immediately any adverse reactions, such as nausea, vomiting, dizziness, headache, urticaria, and respiratory distress.
- If the patient is on nothing-by-mouth status, increase the I.V. fluid rate as ordered after the procedure to flush the contrast medium from his system. Monitor serum creatinine and blood urea nitrogen (BUN) levels for signs of acute kidney injury, which may be caused by the contrast medium.

Treatments

GI dysfunctions present many treatment challenges because they stem from various mechanisms occurring separately or simultaneously, including tumors, hyperactivity and hypoactivity, malabsorption, infection and inflammation, vascular disorders, intestinal obstruction, and degenerative disease. Treatment options include drug therapy, surgery, GI intubation, and nutritional support.

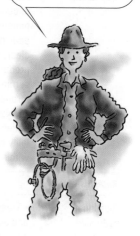

GI dysfunctions stem from various mechanisms occurring separately or simultaneously, making treatment tricky. Are you up to the challenge?

Drug therapy

Drug therapy may be used for such disorders as acute GI bleeding, peptic ulcer disease, and hepatic failure. Some of the most commonly used drugs in critical care include ammonia detoxicants, antacids, antidiuretic hormone, antiemetics, histamine-2 (H_2) receptor antagonists, and proton pump inhibitors.

How fast?

Some of these drugs, such as antacids and antiemetics, provide relief immediately. Other drugs, such as ammonia detoxicants and H_2-receptor antagonists, may take several days or longer to alleviate the problem. (See *Common GI drugs*, page 462.)

Surgery

Surgery may be used to treat the patient with massive bleeding who hasn't responded to medical treatments, such as gastric lavage or sclerotherapy. Be ready to provide special postoperative support for your patient after GI surgery because he may have to make permanent and usually difficult lifestyle changes. Two surgical procedures for GI disorders are liver transplantation and LeVeen shunt insertion.

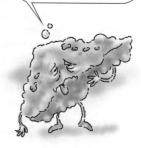

A liver transplant may be the last and best hope for a patient with a life-threatening liver disorder.

Liver transplantation

For a patient with a life-threatening liver disorder who doesn't respond to other treatment, a liver transplant may be the best hope. Candidates include patients with:
* congenital biliary abnormalities
* chronic hepatitis
* inborn errors of metabolism
* end-stage liver disease.
  Transplant candidates are placed on the transplant waiting list.

(Text continues on page 464.)

Common GI drugs

Drugs	Indications	Adverse reactions	Practice pointers
Ammonia detoxicant			
Lactulose (Cephulac)	• Prevention and treatment of portosystemic encephalopathy in patients with severe hepatic disease (increasing clearance of nitrogenous products and decreasing serum ammonia levels through laxative effects) • Laxative to treat constipation due to hyperosmolality and water retention within the colon	Abdominal cramps, diarrhea, flatulence, belching	• After administration through an NG tube, flush tube with water. • For administration by retention enema, instruct the patient to retain drug for 30 to 60 minutes. • Be aware that neomycin and other antibiotics may decrease effectiveness. • Monitor the patient's serum ammonia levels while receiving the drug. • Use for the treatment and prevention of hepatic encephalopathy. Titrate the dose to 2 to 3 soft stools per day.
Antacids			
Aluminum hydroxide (Amphojel)	• Treatment of heartburn and acid indigestion, and adjunct therapy for peptic ulcer disease Binds phosphates in the GI tract in hyperphosphatemia	Constipation, intestinal obstruction, hypophosphatemia	• Monitor phosphorus levels. • Use cautiously in patients with renal disease. • Don't administer within 1 to 2 hours of other oral medications. • After administration through an NG tube, flush tube with water.
Calcium carbonate (Tums)	• Treatment of heartburn and acid indigestion and adjunct therapy for peptic ulcer disease • Calcium supplement	Nausea, vomiting, hypercalcemia (with excessive use), renal calculi	• Use cautiously in patients with renal disease, cardiac disease, or sarcoidosis. • Monitor patients for hypercalcemia. • Don't administer within 1 to 2 hours of other oral medications.
Antidiuretic hormone			
Vasopressin (Pitressin)	• Injection administered I.V. or intra-arterially into the superior mesenteric artery during angiography or endoscopy. Used as treatment in acute, massive GI hemorrhage (such as peptic ulcer disease, ruptured esophageal varices, and Mallory-Weiss syndrome)	Angina, cardiac arrhythmias, cardiac arrest, water intoxication, seizures, bronchospasms, anaphylaxis, tremors, sweating, angioedema, myocardial ischemia	• Be aware that intra-arterial infusion requires angiographic catheter placement. • Monitor intake and output closely. • Monitor for water intoxication (drowsiness, headache, confusion, anuria). • Monitor cardiac rhythm. • Use cautiously in patients with coronary artery disease, heart failure, renal disease, asthma, or a seizure disorder. • Keep in mind that use is contraindicated in patients with chronic nephritis. • Use cautiously in elderly, preoperative, or postoperative patients.

Common GI drugs

Drugs	Indications	Adverse reactions	Practice pointers
Antiemetics			
Dolasetron (Anzemet) Ondansetron (Zofran) Aprepitant (Emend) Granisetron (Kytril)	• Prevention and treatment of postoperative nausea and vomiting and in conjunction with cancer chemotherapy	Diarrhea, liver test abnormalities, pruritus, headache, tachycardias, myalgia, anorexia, fatigue	• Monitor cardiac rhythm. • They're contraindicated in patients with prolonged QT intervals or with congenital QT syndrome. • Monitor liver function. • Correct hypokalemia and hypomagnesemia before administering.
Metoclopramide (Reglan)	• Prevention and treatment of postoperative nausea and vomiting and in conjunction with cancer chemotherapy • Treatment of delayed gastric emptying secondary to diabetic gastroparesis	Restlessness, anxiety, suicidal ideation, seizures, bradycardia, transient hypertension, extrapyramidal reactions, heart failure, drowsiness	• It's contraindicated in patients with GI hemorrhage or perforation and patients with seizure disorders or adrenal gland tumor. • Monitor the patient for onset of extrapyramidal reactions.
Histamine-2 receptor antagonists			
Famotidine (Pepcid) Ranitidine (Zantac)	• Treatment of duodenal and gastric ulcers, gastroesophageal reflux disease (GERD), and Zollinger-Ellison syndrome • Prevention of gastric stress ulcers • Treatment of duodenal and gastric ulcers, GERD, and Zollinger-Ellison syndrome • Prevention of gastric stress ulcers	Headache, palpitations, diarrhea, constipation, malaise, blurred vision, jaundice, leukopenia, angioedema, thrombocytopenia	• Be aware that the drug may cause irritation at the I.V. site. Dilute with a compatible solution before injecting. • After administration through an NG tube, flush tube with water. • Keep in mind that patients with renal insufficiency may need a decreased dose. • It may cause seizures, bronchospasm, or thrombocytopenia. • Because antacids decrease ranitidine absorption, give 1 hour apart. • Use cautiously in patients with renal disease. • Monitor renal and liver tests. • It may cause blood dyscrasias.

(continued)

Common GI drugs *(continued)*

Drugs	Indications	Adverse reactions	Practice pointers
Proton pump inhibitors			
Lansoprazole (Prevacid) Omeprazole (Prilosec) Pantoprazole (Protonix) Esomeprazole (Nexium)	• Treatment of duodenal and gastric ulcers, erosive esophagitis, GERD, Zollinger-Ellison syndrome, and eradication of *Helicobacter pylori* • Prophylaxis for gastric stress ulcer (in critically ill patients)	Diarrhea, abdominal pain, nausea, constipation, chest pain, dizziness, hyperglycemia, headaches	• Use cautiously in patients with severe liver disease. • Monitor liver function values and blood glucose levels.
Synthetic octapeptide			
Octreotide acetate (Sandostatin)	• Treatment for variceal bleeding, reduces portal blood flow by vasoconstriction of the splanchnic vessels	Dizziness, fatigue, headache, light-headedness, conduction abnormalities, edema, nausea, diarrhea, blurred vision, gallbladder abnormalities, pancreatitis, hypoglycemia, hyperglycemia, pain at injection site, suppression of growth hormone, gastroenterohepatic peptides	• Keep in mind this is contraindicated in patients hypersensitive to drug or its components. • Monitor baseline thyroid function tests. • Monitor IGF-1 (somatomedin C) levels every 2 weeks. Dosage adjustments may be made based on this level. • Monitor patients for gallbladder disease. • Monitor patients for signs and symptoms of glucose imbalance. • Monitor fluid and electrolyte balance.

The waiting list

A patient's position on the waiting list is determined by the model for end-stage liver disease (MELD) score. To provide organs in an efficient and fair way, the United Network for Organ Sharing (UNOS) uses the MELD score for transplant patient selection. The transplantation community also uses the MELD score to gauge the severity of liver disease in patient care management. (See *Calculating a MELD score.*)

Nursing considerations

When caring for a patient undergoing a liver transplantation, concentrate on preparing the patient and his family physically and emotionally for the procedure, including instructing the patient about the procedure and events after. Also, take steps to prevent

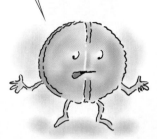

I'll do my best to help fight infection and immune reactions, but you gotta know transplants are serious procedures.

Calculating a MELD score

The model for end-stage liver disease (MELD) uses the patient's laboratory values for serum bilirubin, serum creatinine, and the international normalized ratio (INR). It's calculated according to the following formula:

MELD = 3.78 [estimated log of serum bilirubin (mg/dl)]
      + 11.2 [estimated log of INR]
      + 9.57 [estimated log of serum creatinine (mg/dl)]
      + 6.43

UNOS has made the following modifications to the score:
- If the patient has been dialyzed within the last 7 days, then the value for serum creatinine used should be 4.0.
- Any value less than 1 is given a value of 1. For example, if bilirubin is 0.8, use a value of 1.0.

In interpreting the MELD score in hospitalized patients, the 3-month mortality per MELD score is:
- 40 or more: 71.3% mortality
- 30 to 39: 52.6% mortality
- 20 to 29: 19.6% mortality
- 10 to 19: 6.0% mortality
- less than 9: 1.9% mortality.

Currently, the national average MELD score for a patient undergoing a liver transplant is 20.

postoperative complications. (See *Managing liver transplantation complications*, page 466.)

Before it begins

Before liver transplantation
- Instruct the patient and his family about the transplant, necessary diagnostic tests, immunosuppressant medications, and rejection risk. This is usually done in collaboration with the physician and transplant nurse coordinator.
- Review information about the equipment and procedures, such as cardiac monitoring, ET tube, NG tube, abdominal drainage tubes, indwelling urinary catheter, and arterial lines. Reassure the patient that discomfort should be minimal and that the equipment will be removed as soon as possible.
- Administer ordered medications such as immunosuppressant agents.
- Review incentive spirometry and range-of-motion (ROM) exercises with the patient.

Managing liver transplantation complications

Check this table to find possible complications of liver transplantation and assessment and nursing interventions for each complication.

Complication	Assessment and intervention
Hemorrhage and hypovolemic shock	• Assess the patient's vital signs and other indicators of fluid volume hourly and note trends indicating hypovolemia; hypotension; weak, rapid, irregular pulse; oliguria; decreased LOC; and signs of peripheral vasoconstriction. • Monitor the patient's hematocrit and hemoglobin levels daily. • Maintain patency of all I.V. lines and reserve 2 units of blood in case the patient needs a transfusion.
Vascular obstruction	• Be alert for signs and symptoms of acute vascular obstruction in the right upper quadrant—cramping pain or tenderness, nausea, and vomiting. Notify the practitioner immediately if any occur. • As ordered, prepare for emergency thrombectomy. Maintain I.V. infusions, check and document the patient's vital signs, and maintain airway patency.
Wound infection or abscess	• Assess the incision site daily and report any inflammation, tenderness, drainage, or other signs and symptoms of infection. • Change the dressing daily or as needed. • Note and report any signs or symptoms of peritonitis or abscess, including fever, chills, leukocytosis (or leukopenia with bands), and abdominal pain, tenderness, and rigidity. • Take the patient's temperature every 4 hours. • Collect abdominal drainage for culture and sensitivity studies. Document the color, amount, odor, and consistency of drainage. • Assess the patient for signs of infection in other areas, such as the urinary tract, respiratory system, and skin. Document and report any signs of infection.
Pulmonary insufficiency or failure	• Maintain ventilation at prescribed levels. • Monitor the patient's arterial blood gas levels and change ventilator settings as ordered. • Auscultate for abnormal breath sounds every 2 to 4 hours. • Suction the patient as needed. • If extubated, provide incentive spirometry to limit atelectasis and pneumonia risk. • Encourage cough and deep breathing as tolerated.
Effects of immunosuppressant therapy	• Note any signs or symptoms of opportunistic infection, including fever, tachycardia, chills, leukocytosis, leukopenia, and diaphoresis. • Maintain the patient on protective isolation as ordered. • Report adverse reactions to drugs. • Check the patient's weight daily. • Limit the patient's contact with people who are sick. • Educate the patient and his family about the need for hand hygiene.
Hepatic failure	• Monitor NG tube drainage for upper GI bleeding. • Frequently assess the patient's neurovascular status. • Note development of peripheral edema and ascites. • Monitor the patient's renal function by checking urine output, BUN levels, and serum creatinine and potassium levels. Monitor serum amylase levels daily.

- Make sure that an informed consent form has been signed.
- Instruct family members in measures to control infection and minimize rejection after transplantation and advise them to have all their immunizations up to date.
- Provide emotional support to the patient and his family during the pretransplant waiting time, which can be lengthy (weeks to months).

Posttransplant procedures

After liver transplantation
- Assess the patient's cardiopulmonary and hemodynamic status, including vital signs, oxygen saturation, and cardiac rhythm, at least every 15 minutes in the immediate postoperative period and then hourly or as indicated by his condition.
- Monitor the patient's temperature frequently, at least every hour initially and then every 2 to 4 hours. He may be hypothermic in the initial postoperative phase, and it's important to reestablish normal body temperature. Later in the postoperative phase, monitor the patient for fever and signs of infection. (See *What does fever mean?*)
- Monitor laboratory tests, especially liver enzymes, bilirubin, electrolytes, coagulation studies, and CBC.
- Assess insertion sites for indications of bleeding. Assess the incision site closely for oozing or active bleeding. If the patient has an NG tube, assess drainage color and amount at least every 2 hours.
- Institute strict infection control precautions.
- Administer prophylactic antibiotics and postoperative drugs, such as corticosteroids and immunosuppressants, as ordered.
- Assist with extubation as soon as possible (usually within 4 to 6 hours) and administer supplemental oxygen as needed. Encourage coughing, deep breathing, and incentive spirometry.
- Monitor the patient's intake and output at least hourly and notify the practitioner if urine output is less than 30 ml/hour. Maintain fluids at 2,000 to 3,000 ml/day, or as ordered, to prevent fluid overload.
- Maintain the patient on nothing-by-mouth status with NG decompression and attach the NG tube to low intermittent suction until bowel sounds return.
- Change the patient's position at least every 2 hours, getting him out of bed and to the chair within 24 hours if his condition is stable.
- Continually assess the patient for signs and symptoms of acute rejection, such as malaise, fever, graft enlargement, and diminished graft function (typically 7 to 14 days after the transplant).

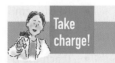

Take charge!

What does fever mean?

A sudden onset of high fever and an increase in liver enzymes suggest hepatic artery thrombosis. If your patient exhibits a fever and infection is suspected, be ready to obtain cultures of all body fluids, X-rays of the chest and abdomen, and a Doppler ultrasound of the hepatic vessels.

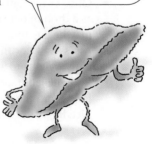

Stick with it. Continually assess the patient for signs and symptoms of acute rejection.

- To ease emotional stress, plan care to allow rest and provide as much privacy as possible. Allow family members to visit and comfort the patient as much as possible.
- Teach the patient and his family about danger signs and symptoms and the need to report these immediately. This typically occurs prior to the transplant surgery, but education continues well into the postoperative period.

Transjugular intrahepatic portosystemic shunt

The transjugular intrahepatic portosystemic shunt (TIPS) procedure creates an artificial path for the blood traveling from the intestines, through the liver, and back to the heart. This reduces portal vein pressure and the hypertension complications of recurrent variceal bleeding and ascites. (See *How the TIPS procedure works*.)

Who's the candidate?

TIPS is an effective therapeutic measure to reduce portal hypertension. The TIPS procedure provides a salvage therapy for those patients who have failed medical treatment and may be a bridge for those patients awaiting transplant.

Patients who may be candidates for the TIPS procedure include:
- patients who have experienced two or more variceal bleeds
- patients whose bleeding hasn't been controlled with endoscopy (band ligation and sclerotherapy)
- patients whose bleeding isn't controlled by medication (vasopressin, octreotide, and beta-adrenergic blocker)
- patients with variceal bleeding or refractory ascites who need a bridge to transplantation
- patients whose transplant has failed and are awaiting retransplantation.

Nursing considerations

A patient with a TIPS procedure needs special care and continuous monitoring:
- Assess the patient's vital signs, physical condition, and cognitive status.
- Observe the patient for signs and symptoms of hemorrhage (such as a drop in hematocrit) and for a spike in temperature, which may be due to a bile leak or developing bacteremia.
- Assess and document intake and output, abdominal girth, and daily weights to assess fluid status.
- Evaluate laboratory studies, such as serum ammonia, electrolyte levels, and coagulation studies for indications of encephalopathy, bleeding, and ascites, which would suggest shunt occlusion.

How the TIPS procedure works

A TIPS is used in patients with cirrhosis, where the scar tissue within the liver causes partial blockage of the blood flow through the liver from the portal vein to the hepatic vein. The blockage increases the pressure in the portal vein, which is called *portal hypertension*. This increase in pressure causes the blood to flow backward from the liver into the veins of the spleen, stomach, lower esophagus, and intestines, causing enlarged vessels, bleeding, and the accumulation of fluid in the chest or abdomen.

Because blood from the GI tract is shunted around the liver and back into the systemic circulation, there's an increase in circulating toxins (ammonia and bacteria) that increases the patient's risk for developing hepatic encephalopathy.

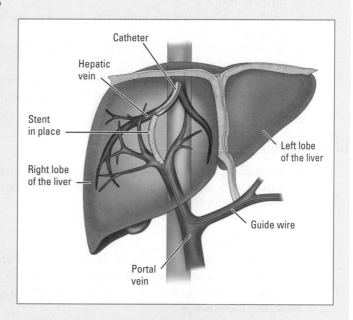

Shunt operation

TIPS is a nonsurgical method of placing a portosystemic shunt. The shunt is passed down the jugular vein and is inserted between the portal and hepatic veins within the liver.

Interventional radiologists use image guidance to make a tunnel through the liver to connect the portal vein to one of the hepatic veins (three veins that carry blood away from the liver back to the heart). A stent is then placed in this tunnel to keep the pathway open, allowing some of the blood that would ordinarily pass through the liver to bypass the liver entirely, reducing bleeding and high blood pressure in the portal vein.

- Observe the patient's cognitive status for signs and symptoms of encephalopathy (such as drowsiness and confusion to coma), which may occur as a result of the shunted blood bypassing the liver and being sent into the systemic circulation without being detoxified by the liver.
- Be alert for heart failure, which may result from increased blood volume being shunted to the heart.

When at home

- Teach the patient and his family about the treatment plan, including the need to avoid all alcohol intake; adhere to a low-sodium, low-protein diet; and to take all prescribed medication.

- Encourage the patient to check with his doctor before taking new medications.
- Teach the patient and his family that the patient needs to be weighed every day.
- Teach the patient and his family to report signs of complications to the doctor promptly.
- Instruct the patient's family to observe for changes in cognitive and emotional status, which need to be reported promptly.

GI intubation

Nasoenteric, NG, and other specialized tubes may be used in treating the patient with acute intestinal obstruction, bleeding, esophageal varices, or another GI dysfunction.

Gastric lavage

Gastric lavage is an emergency treatment for the patient with GI hemorrhage caused by peptic ulcer disease or ruptured esophageal or gastric varices and as emergency treatment for some drug overdoses.

It involves esophageal intubation with a large-bore, single- or double-lumen tube; instillation of irrigating fluid; and aspiration of gastric contents. In some cases, a vasoconstrictor, such as epinephrine, may be added to the irrigating fluid to enhance this action. (See *Types of NG tubes*.)

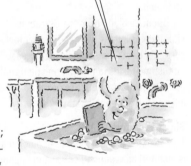

Just what I needed—a good washing. And it's not even Saturday night! Gastric lavage, take me away!

Rarities

Complications are rare and include:
- vomiting and aspiration
- fluid overload
- electrolyte imbalance or metabolic acidosis
- bradycardia.

Nursing considerations
- Explain the procedure to the patient.
- Determine the length of the tube for insertion. (See *Measuring NG tube length*, page 472.)
- Lubricate the end of the tube with a water-soluble lubricant and insert it into the patient's mouth or nostrils, as ordered. Advance the tube through the pharynx and esophagus and into the stomach.
- Check the tube for placement by attaching a piston or bulb syringe and aspirating the contents. Gastric aspirate is acidic, with a pH ranging from 0 to 4. An alkaline pH of 7 or greater indicates that the tube is in the respiratory tract.

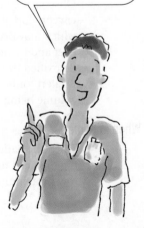

Don't guess how long your patient's NG tube should be. Measure carefully before beginning the insertion process.

Types of NG tubes

There are two common types of NG tubes: Levin and Salem sump. The practitioner will usually decide which tube to use.

Levin tube

The Levin tube is a rubber or plastic tube with a single lumen, 42″ to 50″ (106.7 to 127 cm) long, with holes at the tip and along the side.

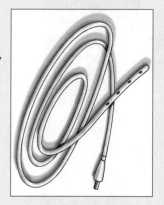

Salem sump tube

The Salem sump tube is a double-lumen tube made of clear plastic. It's used more commonly than the Levin tube because it causes less gastric mucosal irritation. It has a colored sump port (pigtail) that allows atmospheric air to enter the patient's stomach;

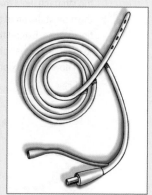

therefore, the tube floats freely and doesn't adhere to or damage gastric mucosa. The larger port of this 48″ (121.9 cm) tube serves as the main suction conduit. The tube has openings at 45, 55, 65, and 75 cm as well as a radiopaque line to verify placement.

- When the tube is in place, lower the head of the bed to 15 degrees and reposition the patient on his left side, if possible.
- Fill the syringe with 30 to 50 ml of irrigating solution—usually isotonic normal saline, which limits sodium removal—and begin instillation. Instill about 250 ml of fluid, wait 30 seconds, and then begin to withdraw the fluid into the syringe. If you can't withdraw any fluid, allow the tube to drain into an emesis basin.
- If the practitioner orders a vasoconstrictor to be added to the irrigating fluid, wait for the prescribed period before withdrawing fluid to allow absorption of the drug into the gastric mucosa.
- Carefully measure and record fluid return. If the volume of fluid return doesn't at least equal the amount of fluid instilled, abdominal distention and vomiting result.
- Continue lavage until return fluid is clear or as ordered. Remove the tube or secure it, as ordered. If appropriate, send lavage specimens to the laboratory for toxicology studies and gastric contents for pH and guaiac studies.
- Never leave the patient alone during gastric lavage.

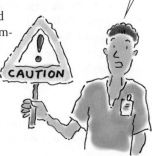

Never leave the patient alone during gastric lavage.

CAUTION

Measuring NG tube length

To determine how long the NG tube must be to reach the stomach, hold the end of the tube at the tip of the patient's nose. Extend the tube to the patient's earlobe and then down to the xiphoid process.

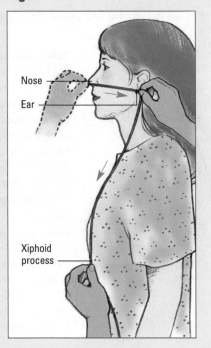

Nose

Ear

Xiphoid process

- Monitor the patient's cardiac rhythm and observe for possible complications, such as bradycardia, hypovolemia, vomiting, and aspiration.
- Monitor the patient's vital signs and oxygen saturation every 30 minutes until his condition stabilizes.
- Document the procedure and interventions.

Multilumen esophageal tube placement

In esophagogastric tamponade, an emergency treatment, a multilumen esophageal tube is inserted to control esophageal or gastric hemorrhage resulting from ruptured varices. It's usually a tentative measure until sclerotherapy can be done. (See *Comparing esophageal tubes.*)

Up, up, and away

The tube is inserted through a nostril, or sometimes the mouth, and then passed into the stomach. The tube's esophageal and

Comparing esophageal tubes

Types of esophageal tubes include the Linton tube, the Minnesota esophagogastric tamponade tube, and the Sengstaken-Blakemore tube.

Linton tube

The Linton tube, a three-lumen, single-balloon device, has ports for esophageal and gastric aspiration. Because the tube doesn't have an esophageal balloon, it isn't used to control bleeding in patients with esophageal varices but can be used for gastric bleeding.

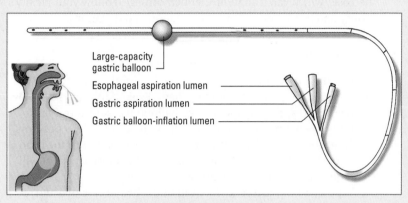

Large-capacity gastric balloon
Esophageal aspiration lumen
Gastric aspiration lumen
Gastric balloon-inflation lumen

Minnesota esophagogastric tamponade tube

The Minnesota esopha-gogastric tamponade tube has four lumens and two balloons. It has pressure-monitoring ports for both balloons. It can be used to control bleeding in patients with esophageal or gastric bleeding.

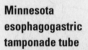
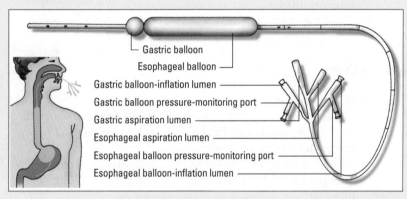

Gastric balloon
Esophageal balloon
Gastric balloon-inflation lumen
Gastric balloon pressure-monitoring port
Gastric aspiration lumen
Esophageal aspiration lumen
Esophageal balloon pressure-monitoring port
Esophageal balloon-inflation lumen

Sengstaken-Blakemore tube

The Sengstaken-Blakemore tube, a three-lumen device with esophageal and gastric balloons, has a gastric aspiration port that allows drainage from below the gastric balloon and is also used to instill medication.

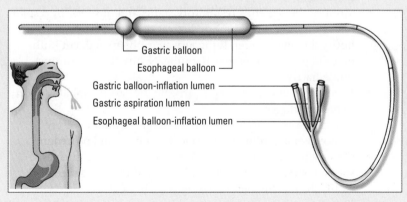

Gastric balloon
Esophageal balloon
Gastric balloon-inflation lumen
Gastric aspiration lumen
Esophageal balloon-inflation lumen

gastric balloons are inflated to exert pressure on the varices to stop bleeding, while a lumen allows esophageal and gastric contents to be aspirated.

Balloon inflation for longer than 48 hours may cause pressure necrosis, which can lead to further hemorrhage. Follow your facility's policy and procedure for balloon inflation and deflation.

Nursing considerations

Before the procedure
- Describe the procedure to the patient. Explain that a helmet may be used to apply traction to keep balloon pressure at the gastro-esophageal junction. Place the patient in semi-Fowler's position. (If unconscious, place the patient on his left side, with the head of the bed elevated to 15 degrees.) An unresponsive patient will require ET intubation for airway protection.
- Tape a pair of scissors to the head of the bed in case of acute respiratory distress.
- Check tube balloons for air leaks and patency before insertion.
- Never leave the patient alone during tamponade.

The pressure's on

After the procedure
- Closely monitor the patient's condition and lumen pressure. If the pressure changes or decreases, check for bleeding and notify the practitioner immediately.
- Monitor the patient's cardiac rhythm, vital signs, and oxygen saturation every 30 to 60 minutes. A change may indicate new bleeding.
- Monitor the patient's respiratory status and observe for respiratory distress. If respiratory distress develops, have someone notify the practitioner. If the airway is obstructed, cut both balloon ports and remove the tube. Notify the practitioner immediately.
- Maintain suction on the ports. Irrigate the gastric aspiration port to prevent clogging.
- Deflate the esophageal balloon for about 30 minutes every 12 hours or according to your facility's policy and procedure.
- Observe the patient for signs of esophageal rupture, such as shock, increased respiratory difficulty, and increased bleeding. Notify the practitioner if such signs are present.
- Keep the patient warm, comfortable, and as still as possible.
- When bleeding has been controlled, assist with tube removal.

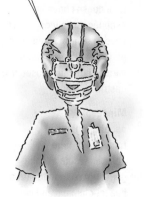

A helmet may be used to keep balloon pressure at the gastroesophageal junction.

Nasoenteric decompression tube

The nasoenteric decompression tube is used to aspirate intestinal contents for analysis and to correct intestinal obstruction. It's inserted nasally and advanced beyond the stomach into the intestinal tract. The tube may also prevent nausea, vomiting, and abdominal distention after GI surgery.

Safe passage

A balloon or rubber bag at one end of the tube holds air or water to stimulate peristalsis and aid the tube's passage through the pylorus and into the intestinal tract. (See *Common types of nasoenteric decompression tubes*.)

Nursing considerations

The patient with a nasoenteric decompression tube needs special care and continuous monitoring to:
- ensure tube patency
- maintain suction and bowel decompression
- detect such complications as fluid–electrolyte imbalance.

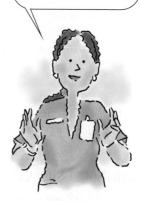

Nasoenteric decompression requires your close attention to ensure tube patency and maintain suction and bowel decompression.

Common types of nasoenteric decompression tubes

The type of nasoenteric decompression tube chosen for your patient will depend on the size of the patient and his nostrils, the estimated duration of intubation, and the reason for the procedure. For example, to remove viscous material from the patient's intestinal tract, the doctor may select a tube with a wide bore and a single lumen.

Whichever tube you use, you'll need to provide good mouth care and check the patient's nostrils often for signs of irritation. If you see any signs of irritation, retape the tube so that it doesn't cause tension, and then lubricate the nostril. Or, you can check with the doctor to see if the tube can be inserted through the other nostril.

Most tubes are impregnated with a radiopaque mark so that placement can be confirmed easily by X-ray or other imaging technique.

Tubes such as the preweighted Andersen Miller-Abbot type intestinal tube (shown on the right) have a tungsten-weighted inflatable latex balloon tip designed for temporary management of mechanical obstruction in the small or large intestines.

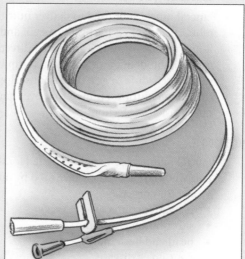

Dealing with obstruction

If your patient's tube appears to be obstructed, follow your facility's policy and procedure and notify the practitioner if you're unable to restore patency. He may order measures, such as those described here, to restore patency quickly and efficiently:

- First, disconnect the tube from suction and irrigate with normal saline solution. Use gravity flow to help clear the obstruction unless otherwise ordered.
- If irrigation doesn't reestablish patency, the tube may be obstructed by its position against the gastric mucosa. Tug slightly on the tube to move it away from the mucosa.
- If gently tugging doesn't work, the tube may be kinked and need additional manipulation. However, don't reposition or irrigate a tube in a patient who had GI surgery, in one who had the tube inserted during surgery (because this may disturb new sutures), or in a patient who was difficult to intubate.

Nutritional support

A patient with a GI problem who can't eat or otherwise ingest enough food may require enteral or parenteral nutrition.

Enteral nutrition

Enteral nutrition is used to deliver nutrients to the GI tract using a tube. The upper GI tract is bypassed, and pureed food or a special liquid enteral formula is delivered directly into the stomach (gastric gavage), duodenum, or jejunum. It can be administered on an intermittent schedule or as a continuous, slow infusion.

Enteral nutrition is preferred over parenteral because of the reduced risk for infection.

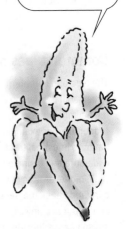

A blender? I can do a blender. But what does a puree involve?

Who needs it?

Enteral nutrition delivery is indicated for the patient with a functional GI tract who can't adequately take food by mouth, such as a patient with:

- Crohn's disease
- ulcerative colitis
- short-bowel syndrome
- head and neck injuries
- neurologic disease
- stroke
- oral cancers
- a psychiatric disorder
- an ET intubation device.

Who can't have it?

Tube feeding is contraindicated in the patient with suspected intestinal obstruction, acute pancreatitis, or absent bowel sounds.

Nursing considerations

Before the procedure

- Explain the procedure to the patient and obtain the necessary formula and equipment.
- Assess the patient's abdomen for bowel sounds and distention. Check placement of the feeding tube to ensure it hasn't slipped out since the last feeding. Never give a tube feeding until you're sure the tube is properly positioned in the patient's stomach. Administering a feeding through a misplaced tube can lead to aspiration.
- Check tube location at 4-hour intervals after feeding is started. Air bolus techniques are unreliable for identifying tube location. If unsure, obtain an X-ray to confirm tube position.
- Check for gastric residual to assess gastric emptying; aspirate and measure gastric residual contents. Follow your facility's policy regarding withholding feedings. Reinstill any aspirate obtained.
- When delivering the feeding, elevate the bed to semi-Fowler's or high Fowler's position to prevent aspiration and promote digestion.
- Irrigate the tube, administer the feeding as ordered, and then flush the tube again if intermittent use.
- If continuous feedings are ordered, provide by infusion pump, collaborate with nutrition support and the physician to identify free water support needs, usually every 4 hours a 30-ml bolus may be ordered.

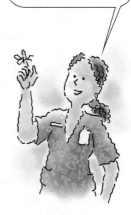

Remember . . . never give a tube feeding until you're sure the tube is properly positioned in the patient's stomach.

After lunch

After the procedure

- Record the amount of ingested formula. Note the patient's tolerance of tube feeding.
- Weigh the patient daily and monitor ordered laboratory tests.
- Provide meticulous mouth and tube care.

Parenteral nutrition

When a patient can't meet his nutritional needs by oral or enteral feedings, he may require I.V. nutritional support, or *parenteral nutrition*.

Who needs it?

The patient's diagnosis, history, and prognosis are used to determine the need for parenteral nutrition. Generally, this treatment is

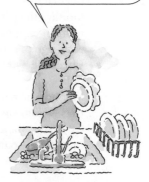

At least with enteral feedings there are no dishes to do—and no dishpan hands!

prescribed for any patient who can't absorb nutrients through the GI tract for more than 10 days.

More specific indications include:
- debilitating illness lasting longer than 2 weeks
- loss of 10% or more of pre-illness weight
- serum albumin level below 3.5 g/dl
- excessive nitrogen loss from wound infection, fistulas, or abscesses
- renal or hepatic failure
- severe pancreatitis
- severe burns
- nonfunctioning GI tract for 5 to 7 days in a severely catabolic patient.

Delivery route

Parenteral nutrition may be given through a peripheral or central venous (CV) line. Depending on the solution, parenteral nutrition boosts the patient's calorie intake or surpasses his calorie requirements. There are two types of parenteral nutrition:
- *Total parenteral nutrition (TPN)* refers to any nutrient solution, including lipids, given through a CV line.
- *Peripheral parenteral nutrition (PPN)* is delivered through a peripheral line. PPN is used to supply the patient's full calorie needs while avoiding the risks that accompany a CV line. (See *Types of parenteral nutrition*, pages 480 and 481.)

Nursing considerations
- Explain the procedure to the patient.
- Be sure to check the solution against the practitioner's order for correct patient name, expiration date, and formula components.
- Throughout the procedure, maintain strict sterile technique.
- Follow your facility's policy and procedure and administer using an infusion pump with the pump tubing and micron filter. Infuse at a constant rate without interruption to avoid blood glucose fluctuations.

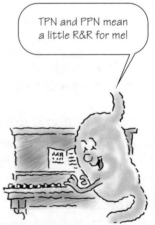

TPN and PPN mean a little R&R for me!

- Monitor the patient's vital signs at least every 2 to 4 hours, or more often if necessary. Watch him for increased temperature, an early sign of catheter sepsis.
- Check the patient's blood glucose level according to your facility's policy.
- Monitor the patient's intake and output and routine laboratory tests (serum electrolytes, calcium, BUN, creatinine, magnesium, CBC, and albumin).
- Monitor the patient's liver and kidney function.
- Weigh the patient daily.

- Change the dressing according to your facility's policy. Monitor the catheter site for swelling, which may indicate infiltration.
- Change the solution, tubing, and filter every 24 hours or according to your facility's policy.
- When discontinuing parenteral nutrition, decrease the infusion rate slowly, depending on the patient's current glucose intake, to minimize the risk for hyperinsulinemia and resulting hypoglycemia.

Monitor the catheter site for swelling, which may indicate infiltration or infection.

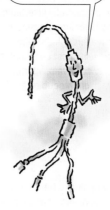

Gastrointestinal system disorders

Abdominal disorders commonly encountered in a critical care unit include acute GI bleeding, acute pancreatitis, bowel infarction, cirrhosis, hepatic failure and encephalopathy, and intra-abdominal hypertension.

Acute GI bleeding

GI bleeding can occur anywhere along the GI tract. Although GI bleeding stops spontaneously in most patients, acute bleeding accounts for significant morbidity and mortality.

Maybe multiple morbidities

GI bleeding is the most common cause for admission to an intensive care unit (ICU) in the United States. Twenty-five percent of critical care patients will develop GI bleeding during hospitalization. Additionally, they may have underlying comorbidities that contribute to the risk of upper GI bleeding, such as:

Many critical care patients have upper GI bleeding or conditions that place them at higher risk for bleeding.

- recent major surgery
- history of myocardial infarction (MI) and treatment with thrombolytic therapy
- renal failure
- history of chronic liver damage secondary to alcohol abuse or hepatitis
- history of radiation therapy
- chronic pain condition, such as arthritis, requiring treatment with NSAIDs.

What causes it?

Upper GI bleeding includes bleeding in the esophagus, stomach, and duodenum. Bleeding below the Treitz ligament is considered lower GI bleeding; the most common site is in the colon.

Types of parenteral nutrition

Type	Solution components per liter	Uses
Total parenteral nutrition by central venous (CV) catheter or peripherally inserted central catheter into the superior vena cava through the infraclavicular vein (most common), supraclavicular vein, internal jugular vein, or antecubital fossa	• $D_{15}W$ to $D_{25}W$ (1 L dextrose 25% = 850 nonprotein calories) • Crystalline amino acids 2.5% to 8.5% • Electrolytes, vitamins, trace elements, and insulin, as ordered • Lipid emulsion 10% to 20% (usually infused as a separate solution)	• Used for long-term (2 weeks or more) feedings • Meets substantial caloric and nutrient needs • Provides calories; restores nitrogen balance; and replaces essential vitamins, electrolytes, minerals, and trace elements • Promotes tissue synthesis, wound healing, and normal metabolic function • Allows bowel rest and healing; reduces activity in the gallbladder, pancreas, and small intestine • Improves tolerance of surgery
Peripheral parenteral nutrition by peripheral catheter	• D_5W to $D_{10}W$ • Crystalline amino acids 2.5% to 5% • Electrolytes, minerals, vitamins, and trace elements, as ordered • Lipid emulsion 10% or 20% (1 L dextrose 10% and amino acids 3.5% infused at the same time as 1 L of lipid emulsion = 1,440 nonprotein calories) • Heparin or hydrocortisone, as ordered	• Used for short-term (2 weeks or less) feedings • Provides up to 2,000 calories/day • Maintains adequate nutritional status in a patient who can tolerate relatively high fluid volume, one who usually resumes bowel function and oral feedings after a few days, and one susceptible to infections associated with the CV catheter

Upper causes

The causes of upper GI bleeding include:
• peptic ulcer disease
• rupture of esophageal varices
• esophagitis
• Mallory-Weiss tear
• erosive gastritis
• arteriovenous malformations.

Lower causes

The most common causes of lower GI bleeding include:
• diverticulitis
• polyps
• hemorrhoids

Special considerations	Uses
Basic solution	*I.V. lipid emulsion*
• Nutritionally complete	• Given by way of CV line
• Requires minor surgical procedure for CV line insertion	• May not be used effectively in a severely stressed patient (especially a patient with burns)
• Highly hypertonic solution	• May interfere with immune mechanisms; in a patient suffering from respiratory compromise, reduces carbon dioxide buildup
• May cause pneumothorax (typically during catheter insertion), phlebitis, thrombus formation, air embolus, infection, sepsis, and metabolic complications (glucose intolerance, electrolyte imbalance, essential fatty acid deficiency)	
• Must be delivered in a vein with high blood flow rate (the subclavian is preferred) because glucose content may be increased beyond the level a peripheral vein can handle (commonly six times more concentrated than blood)	
Basic solution	*I.V. lipid emulsion*
• Nutritionally complete for a short time	• As effective as dextrose for calorie source
• Can't be used in a nutritionally depleted patient	• Diminishes phlebitis if infused at the same time as basic nutrient solution
• Can't be used in a volume-restricted patient	• Reduces carbon dioxide buildup when pulmonary compromise is present
• Doesn't cause weight gain	• Irritates vein in long-term use
• Avoids insertion and care of a CV line but requires adequate venous access site; must be changed every 72 hours	
• May cause phlebitis and increases risk of metabolic complications	
• Less chance of metabolic complications than with CV line	
• To avoid venous sclerosis, must contain no more than 10% dextrose, so patient must tolerate large fluid volume to meet nutritional needs	

- neoplasm
- angiodysplasias
- Crohn's disease
- ulcerative colitis
- colitis.

How it happens

The patient experiences a loss of circulating blood volume, regardless of the cause of bleeding.

What happens

Because the arterial blood supply near the stomach and esophagus is extensive, bleeding can lead to a rapid loss of large amounts of blood, subsequent hypovolemia, and shock. Here's what else happens:

- Loss of circulating blood volume leads to a decreased venous return.
- Cardiac output and blood pressure decrease, causing poor tissue perfusion. In response, the body compensates by shifting interstitial fluid to the intravascular space.
- The sympathetic nervous system is stimulated, resulting in vasoconstriction and increased heart rate.
- The renin-angiotensin-aldosterone system is activated, leading to fluid retention and increasing blood pressure.
- If blood loss continues, cardiac output further decreases, leading to cellular hypoxia. Eventually, all organs fail due to hypoperfusion.

What to look for

Because GI bleeding can occur anywhere along the GI tract, assessment is crucial in determining the amount and possible location of bleeding.

Source signs

The appearance of blood in tube drainage, vomitus, and stool indicates the source of GI bleeding:

- Hematemesis—bright red blood in NG tube drainage or vomitus—typically indicates an upper GI source. However, if the blood has spent time in the stomach where it was exposed to gastric acid, the drainage or vomitus resembles coffee grounds.
- Hematochezia—bright red blood from the rectum—typically indicates a lower GI source of bleeding. It may also suggest an upper GI source if the transit time through the bowel was rapid.
- Melena—black, tarry, and sticky stool—usually indicates an upper GI bleeding source. However, it can result from bleeding in the small bowel or proximal colon.

Signs and symptoms

Typically, the patient exhibits signs and symptoms based on the amount and rate of bleeding. With acute GI bleeding and blood loss greater than 30% of the person's blood volume, he exhibits signs and symptoms of hypovolemic shock, including:

- cool, clammy skin
- pallor
- restlessness
- apprehension
- tachycardia
- diaphoresis

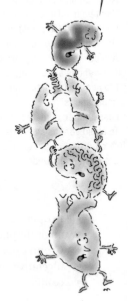

With continued bleeding, all organs eventually fail due to hypoperfusion.

- hypotension (mean arterial pressure [MAP] <60 mm Hg)
- syncope
- oliguria
- electrocardiogram (ECG) changes.

What tests tell you

These findings help diagnose acute GI bleeding:
- Upper GI endoscopy reveals the source of esophageal or gastric bleeding.
- The 12-lead ECG may reveal evidence of cardiac ischemia secondary to hypoperfusion.
- Abdominal X-ray may indicate air under the diaphragm, suggesting ulcer perforation.
- Angiography may aid in visualizing the bleeding site and may also be used to embolize a bleeding vessel.
- Coagulation studies may be prolonged, especially if the patient has liver disease.
- Mesenteric angiography can help locate the site of the bleeding.
- CBC reveals the amount of blood loss, but changes may not be seen for 4 to 6 hours.
- Arterial blood gas (ABG) analysis can indicate metabolic acidosis from hemorrhage and possible hypoxemia.

How it's treated

Treatment goals include stopping the bleeding and providing fluid replacement while maintaining the patient's hemodynamic stability. Treatment may include:
- fluid volume replacement with crystalloid solutions initially, followed by colloids and blood component therapy
- respiratory support
- gastric intubation with gastric lavage (unless the patient has esophageal varices) and gastric pH monitoring
- drug therapy, such as antacids, H_2-receptor antagonists, and proton pump inhibitors
- endoscopic or surgical repair of bleeding sites.

What to do

- Type and crossmatch at least 2 units of blood.
- Start at least two large-bore I.V. lines (16G or 18G preferred). Assess the patient for blood loss and begin fluid replacement therapy as ordered, initially delivering crystalloid solutions, such as normal saline or lactated Ringer's solution, followed by blood component products.

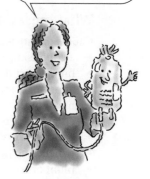

Treatment for GI bleeding may include fluid volume replacement with crystalloid solutions initially, followed by colloids and blood component therapy.

- Ensure your patient's patent airway. Monitor cardiac and respiratory status and assess LOC at least every 15 minutes until he stabilizes and then every 2 to 4 hours, as indicated by his status. Assist with insertion of hemodynamic monitoring devices and assess hemodynamic parameters.
- Administer supplemental oxygen as ordered. Monitor oxygen saturation levels.
- Position the patient with the head of the bed raised to at least 30 degrees to minimize the risk of aspiration.
- Monitor the patient's skin color and capillary refill for signs of hypovolemic shock.
- Obtain serial hemoglobin (Hb) levels and hematocrit (HCT). Administer albumin or blood as ordered.
- Monitor the patient's intake and output closely, including all losses from the GI tract. Check all stools and gastric drainage for occult blood.
- Assist with or insert an NG tube and perform lavage using room temperature saline to clear blood and clots from the stomach.
- Assess the patient's abdomen for bowel sounds and gastric pH, as ordered. Expect to resume enteral or oral feedings after bowel function returns and there's no evidence of further bleeding.
- Provide appropriate emotional support to the patient.
- Prepare the patient for endoscopic repair or surgery, if indicated.

Acute pancreatitis

Pancreatitis, inflammation of the pancreas, occurs in acute and chronic forms and may be due to edema, necrosis, or hemorrhage. In men, this disease is commonly associated with alcoholism, trauma, or peptic ulcer; in women, with biliary tract disease.

> Pancreatitis occurs in acute and chronic forms. It may be caused by edema, necrosis, or hemorrhage.

What causes it

Causes of pancreatitis may include:
- alcoholism (most common)
- biliary tract disease
- abnormal organ structure
- metabolic or endocrine disorders, such as high cholesterol levels and hyperparathyroidism
- pancreatic cysts or tumors
- penetrating peptic ulcers
- blunt or surgical trauma
- drugs, such as corticosteroids, sulfonamides, thiazides, procainamide, and tetracycline
- infection
- hereditary factors.

How it happens

Acute pancreatitis occurs in two forms:
1. edematous (interstitial) pancreatitis, which causes fluid accumulation and swelling (accounts for 80% of the cases)
2. necrotizing pancreatitis, which causes cell death and tissue damage (accounts for 20% of the cases).

Damage and destruction

The inflammation that occurs with both types of pancreatitis is caused by premature activation of enzymes, which leads to tissue damage. If pancreatitis damages the islets of Langerhans, diabetes mellitus may result. Sudden severe pancreatitis causes massive hemorrhage and total destruction of the pancreas, manifested as diabetic acidosis, shock, or coma.

Association affects outcome

The prognosis is good for a patient with pancreatitis associated with biliary tract disease but poor when associated with alcoholism. Mortality is as high as 60% when pancreatitis is associated with necrosis and hemorrhage.

Rating mortality

The severity of pancreatitis is predicted using Ranson's criteria. If the patient meets fewer than three of the criteria, the mortality rate is less than 1%. When three or four of the criteria are met, the mortality rate increases to 15% to 20%. With five or six criteria, the mortality rate is 40%. (See *Ranson's criteria*, page 486.)

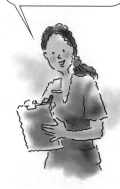

The prognosis is good when pancreatitis is associated with biliary tract disease but poor when associated with alcoholism.

What to look for

Commonly, the patient describes sudden onset of intense epigastric pain centered close to the umbilicus and radiating to the back. He typically reports that the pain is aggravated by:
- eating fatty foods
- consuming alcohol
- lying in a recumbent position.

Take notes

During the physical examination, you may note:
- persistent vomiting (in a severe attack) from hypermotility or paralytic ileus
- abdominal distention (in a severe attack) from bowel hypermotility and fluid accumulation in the peritoneal cavity
- diminished bowel activity (in a severe attack), suggesting altered motility secondary to peritonitis
- crackles at lung bases (in a severe attack) secondary to heart failure

Ranson's criteria

The severity of your patient's acute pancreatitis is determined by the existence of certain characteristics. The more criteria met by the patient, the more severe the episode of pancreatitis and, therefore, the greater the risk of mortality.

On admission

Admission criteria include:
- age older than 55
- white blood cell (WBC) count greater than 16,000/μl
- serum glucose greater than 200 mg/dl
- lactate dehydrogenase greater than 350 International Units/L
- aspartate aminotransferase greater than 250 units/L.

After admission

During the first 48 hours after admission, criteria include:
- 10% decrease in HCT
- BUN increase greater than 5 mg/dl
- serum calcium less than 8 mg/dl
- base deficit greater than 4 mEq/L
- partial pressure of arterial oxygen less than 60 mm Hg
- estimated fluid sequestration greater than 6 L.

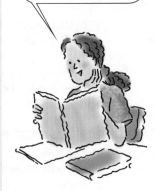

The more criteria your patient meets, the more severe his pancreatitis is . . . and, unfortunately, the greater his risk of mortality.

- steatorrhea (foul-smelling, bulky, pale stools)
- Chvostek's or Trousseau's sign (if the patient has hypocalcemia)
- jaundice
- ascites
- tachycardia
- low-grade fever
- diaphoresis
- Greg-Turner's sign (flank ecchymosis due to blood in the retroperitoneal space)
- Cullen's sign (ecchymosis surrounding the umbilicus due to blood in the peritoneum)
- restlessness related to pain
- decreased pulmonary artery pressure and cardiac output due to hemorrhage or dehydration; elevated cardiac output and decreased systemic vascular resistance if systemic inflammation or sepsis is present.

What tests tell you

These findings help diagnose acute pancreatitis:
- Serum amylase and lipase levels are elevated three to five times normal. Lipase remains elevated longer and thus is useful for delayed presentations/diagnosis.
- Urine amylase is increased for 1 to 2 weeks.

- WBC count is elevated, Hb and HCT are decreased with hemorrhage and increased with dehydration, coagulation is decreased.
- Serum calcium level may be decreased.
- Serum potassium level is decreased.
- C-reactive protein is present in blood.
- Serum bilirubin levels, aspartate aminotransferase, alanine aminotransferase, lactate dehydrogenase (LD), and alkaline phosphatase are elevated.
- Abdominal and chest X-rays show pleural effusions and bowel dilation and ileus.
- CT scan, and MRI, show an enlarged pancreas with fluid collection, cysts, abscess, masses, and pseudocysts.
- Abdominal ultrasound is effective to evaluate for biliary tree patency, gallstones, or ductal dilatation.
- ECG may reveal ST-segment depression and T-wave inversion.
- Peritoneal lavage possibly positive for blood (in hemorrhagic pancreatitis).

How it's treated

Treatment for the patient with acute pancreatitis may include:
- fluid and electrolyte replacement to treat shock
- blood transfusions as necessary for hemorrhage
- pain management
- withholding food and fluids to rest the pancreas
- NG tube suctioning to decompress the stomach and limit stimulation of secretin
- drugs, such as analgesics, antacids, H_2-receptor antagonists, antibiotics, anticholinergics, and insulin
- peritoneal lavage: removes toxins that may have leaked into the peritoneal fluid
- surgical drainage for a pancreatic abscess or pseudocyst
- laparotomy (if biliary tract obstruction causes acute pancreatitis) to remove the obstruction.

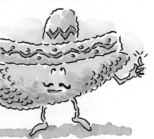

Treatment for pancreatitis may include I.V. fluids, drugs, and peritoneal lavage—and withholding food and fluid so I can take a siesta.

What to do

- Ensure a patent airway and assess the patient's respiratory status at least every hour or more often. Assess oxygen saturation levels and breath sounds for adventitious or diminished breath sounds.
- Closely monitor the patient's cardiac and hemodynamic status at least every hour or more often, as ordered.
- Place the patient in a comfortable position that maximizes air exchange, such as semi-Fowler's or high Fowler's.
- Allow for periods of rest and activity.

- If the patient develops acute respiratory distress syndrome, anticipate the need for additional therapies, such as mechanical ventilation or prone positioning.

Chemistry 101

- Initiate I.V. fluid replacement therapy. Monitor serum laboratory values (hematology, coagulation, and chemistry) for changes.
- Be especially alert for signs and symptoms of hypokalemia (hypotension, muscle weakness, apathy, confusion, and cardiac arrhythmias), hypomagnesemia (hypotension, tachycardia, confusion, tremors, twitching, tetany, and hallucinations), and hypocalcemia (positive Chvostek's and Trousseau's signs, seizures, and prolonged QT interval on ECG). Have emergency equipment readily available.
- Monitor the patient's intake and output closely and notify the practitioner if urine output is less than 0.5 ml/kg/hour. Weigh the patient daily.
- Monitor the patient's neurologic status, noting confusion or lethargy.
- Maintain your patient in a normothermic state to reduce the body's demand for oxygen.
- Assess the patient's pain level and administer analgesics, as ordered.
- Administer antibiotics, as ordered, and monitor serum peak and trough levels, as appropriate.
- Withhold all oral fluids and food to prevent stimulation of pancreatic enzymes.
- Insert an NG tube as ordered. Check placement at least every 4 hours. Irrigate with normal saline solution for patency. Monitor drainage for frank bleeding. Monitor vomitus and stool for bleeding.
- Assess the patient's abdomen for distention and bowel sounds; measure his abdominal girth.
- Administer parenteral nutrition therapy, as ordered. Monitor for hyperglycemia related to the therapy as well as injured pancreas. Administer insulin as ordered.
- When bowel sounds become active, anticipate switching to enteral or oral feedings.
- Perform ROM exercises to maintain joint mobility.
- Perform meticulous skin care.

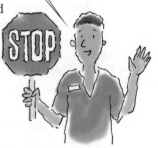

Hold it! Withhold all oral fluids and food to prevent stimulation of pancreatic enzymes.

Offer a shoulder

- Provide emotional support to the patient.
- Prepare the patient for surgery if indicated.

Bowel infarction

Bowel infarction is a decreased blood flow to the major mesenteric vessels. It leads to vasoconstriction and vasospasm of the bowel and contracted bowel with mucosal ulceration.

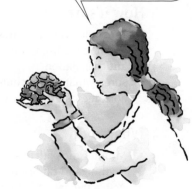

Just how slow can the blood flow in an infarcted bowel? I wonder.

What causes it

Bowel infarction can be caused by:
- thrombosis after an MI
- cholesterol plaques in the aorta that become dislodged
- emboli in patients with endocarditis or atrial fibrillation
- arteriosclerosis
- cirrhosis of the liver
- hypercoagulation as seen in polycythemia or after splenectomy
- reduced perfusion from heart failure or shock.

How it happens

Here's what happens with bowel infarction:
- Decreased blood flow to the mesenteric vessels leads to spasms.
- When the spasms subside, the muscles of the bowel are fatigued and unable to receive essential oxygen and nutrients.
- The bowel becomes edematous and cyanotic, and necrosis can occur.
- As pressure in the lumens of the bowel increases, perforation can occur, leading to peritonitis or abscess formation.

What to look for

Look for signs and symptoms that may occur with bowel infarction, including:
- acute abdominal pain
- vomiting
- bloody diarrhea
- weight loss
- abdominal distention with tenderness and guarding
- absent or hypoactive bowel sounds
- signs and symptoms of shock
- fever.

Abdominal distention with tenderness and guarding may indicate bowel infarction. Ow, that hurts!

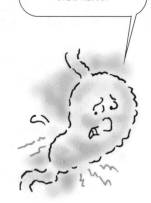

What tests tell you

These test results may help diagnose bowel infarction:
- Abdominal X-rays reveal dilated loops of bowel.
- Barium studies show the infarction location.
- Angiography reveals the infarction location.

- Fecal occult blood test is positive for blood.
- CT scan may reveal the area of infarction.
- Serum phosphate, HCT, and serum osmolality levels are elevated.
- Sigmoidoscopy reveals an ischemic bowel.

How it's treated

Treatment for your patient with bowel infarction may include:
- vasodilators for perfusion and pain relief
- anticoagulation
- surgery that may include endarterectomy, thrombectomy, and aortomesenteric bypass grafting.

What to do

- Monitor the patient's vital signs, oxygen saturation, cardiac rhythm, and cardiopulmonary status.
- Assess the patient's abdomen for bowel sounds at least every 2 to 4 hours per facility policy and monitor his abdominal girth and weight daily.
- Monitor skin temperature and capillary refill.
- Administer fluid replacement as ordered.
- Administer vasoactive agents such as dopamine, as ordered.
- Prepare the patient for surgical repair, as indicated.
- Monitor the patient's intake and output.
- Administer analgesics and antibiotics, as ordered.
- Observe electrolyte and glucose levels for imbalances.
- Provide nutritional support as ordered.

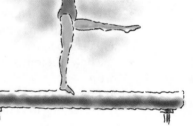

Monitor your patient's electrolyte and glucose levels for imbalances.

Cirrhosis

Cirrhosis is a chronic disorder marked by diffuse destruction and fibrotic regeneration of hepatic cells. As necrotic tissue yields to fibrosis, this disease damages liver tissue and normal vasculature, impairs blood and lymph flow, and ultimately causes hepatic insufficiency.

What causes it

There are several types of cirrhosis, including:
- portal (Laënnec's), caused by malnutrition and chronic alcohol ingestion
- biliary, caused by bile duct disease that suppresses bile flow
- postnecrotic, caused by various types of hepatitis
- pigment, caused by hemochromatosis
- cardiac, caused by liver damage from right-sided heart failure.

How it happens

Cirrhosis is characterized by irreversible chronic injury of the liver, extensive fibrosis, and nodular tissue growth. The changes result from liver cell death (hepatocyte necrosis), collapse of the liver's supporting structure (the reticulin network), distortion of the vascular bed, and nodular regeneration of remaining liver tissue.

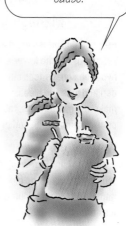

Your patient may have one of several types of cirrhosis, including portal, biliary, postnecrotic, pigment, and cardiac.

What to look for

Assess your patient for these signs and symptoms, which are the same regardless of the cause:

- *GI*—anorexia, indigestion, nausea and vomiting, constipation or diarrhea, dull abdominal ache, clay-colored stools
- *respiratory*—pleural effusion, limited thoracic expansion
- *central nervous system (CNS)*—lethargy, mental changes, slurred speech, asterixis
- *hematologic*—bleeding tendencies, anemia
- *endocrine*—testicular atrophy, menstrual irregularities, loss of chest and axillary hair
- *skin*—severe pruritus, extreme dryness, poor tissue turgor, abnormal pigmentation, spider angiomas, purpura
- *hepatic*—jaundice, hepatomegaly, ascites, edema of the legs
- *miscellaneous*—musty breath, muscle atrophy, palpable liver or spleen, tachycardia.

The signs and symptoms of cirrhosis affect all body systems and are the same regardless of the cause.

What tests tell you

These findings help diagnose cirrhosis:

- Liver biopsy is the gold standard to diagnose cirrhosis.
- Liver scan shows abnormal thickening and a liver mass.

These help, too

Other helpful tests include:

- cholecystography and cholangiography to visualize the gallbladder and biliary duct system
- percutaneous transhepatic cholangiography to visualize the portal venous system
- WBC count, HCT and Hb, albumin, serum electrolyte, and cholinesterase levels (all decreased)
- serum ammonia, total bilirubin, PT, international normalized ratio, and LD levels (all increased).

How it's treated

Treatment for your patient with cirrhosis may include:

- high-calorie and moderate- to high-protein diet; restricted protein if hepatic encephalopathy develops
- sodium restricted to 200 to 500 mg per day; fluids to 1,000 to 1,500 ml per day
- possible enteral or parenteral feeding if the patient's condition continues to deteriorate
- drug therapy (requires special caution because the cirrhotic liver can't detoxify harmful substances efficiently; sedatives avoided or prescribed with great care)
- paracentesis and salt-poor albumin infusions to relieve ascites
- surgery (ligation of varices, splenectomy, esophagogastric resection, or liver transplantation).

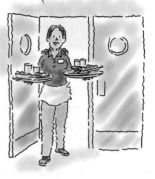

Treatment for cirrhosis includes following a special diet and fluid regimen and possible enteral or parenteral feedings if the patient's condition deteriorates.

What to do

A patient with cirrhosis is generally admitted to the critical care unit because of a complication of cirrhosis, such as hepatic failure or bleeding esophageal varices (See *Managing bleeding from esophageal varices.*)

- Monitor the patient's vital signs, oxygen saturation, cardiac rhythm, and cardiopulmonary status.

Take charge!

Managing bleeding from esophageal varices

Esophageal varices are dilated, tortuous veins in the submucosa of the lower esophagus resulting from portal hypertension. Varices can go undetected and result in sudden and massive bleeding. Such varices commonly cause massive hematemesis, requiring emergency treatment to control hemorrhage and prevent hypovolemic shock.

What to do

- Vasopressin (Pitressin) infused into the superior mesenteric artery may stop bleeding temporarily. Vasopressin infused by I.V. drip diluted with dextrose 5% in water is less effective.
- Octreotide (Sandostatin) infused by I.V. bolus causes splanchnic vasoconstriction and decreases portal inflow.
- Sclerotherapy is done by endoscopy to cause fibrosis and obliteration of the varices.

- A Minnesota or Sengstaken-Blakemore tube is used to control hemorrhage by applying pressure on the bleeding site.
- Saline lavage through the tube is used to control bleeding.
- Fresh blood and frozen plasma are given to replace clotting factors.
- Lactulose (Cephulac) is administered to promote elimination of old blood from the GI tract and to combat excessive production and accumulation of ammonia, which contributes to encephalopathy.
- Surgical bypass procedures include portosystemic anastomosis, and splenorenal, portacaval, or mesocaval shunt insertion.
- Nonsurgical bypass procedures such as TIPS.

- Observe the patient closely for signs of behavioral or personality changes. Report increasing stupor, lethargy, hallucinations, or neuromuscular dysfunction. Watch for asterixis, a sign of developing hepatic encephalopathy.
- Assess the patient for fluid retention, weigh and measure his abdominal girth daily, and inspect his ankles and sacrum for dependent edema.
- Accurately record the patient's intake and output.

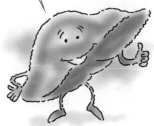

Watch the patient with cirrhosis closely for signs of behavioral or personality changes.

Hepatic failure and encephalopathy

Hepatic failure is the possible end result of any liver disease. When the liver fails, a complex syndrome involving impairment of many organs and body functions ensues. Failure can be caused by hepatitis, cirrhosis, or liver cancer. (See *Viral hepatitis from A to E—plus G*, page 494.)

Ammonia coma

Hepatic encephalopathy, also called *hepatic coma*, is a neurologic syndrome that develops as a manifestation of hepatic failure. It usually reflects ammonia intoxication of the brain.

What causes it

Hepatic encephalopathy is the result of increasing blood ammonia levels from:
- improper shunting of blood from portal hypertension or from surgically created portosystemic shunts
- excessive protein intake
- sepsis
- excessive accumulation of nitrogenous body wastes (caused by constipation or GI bleeding)
- bacterial action on protein and urea to form ammonia
- drugs (sedatives, analgesics, and diuretics)
- dehydration
- hypokalemia, which increases ammonia production in the kidneys.

How it happens

Hepatic encephalopathy—a set of CNS disorders—results when the liver can no longer detoxify the blood. Liver dysfunction and collateral vessels that shunt blood around the liver to the systemic circulation permit toxins absorbed from the GI tract to circulate freely to the brain.

Viral hepatitis from A to E—plus G

Use this table to compare the features of various types of viral hepatitis characterized to date. Other types are emerging.

Feature	Hepatitis A	Hepatitis B	Hepatitis C	Hepatitis D	Hepatitis E	Hepatitis G
Incubation	15 to 45 days	30 to 180 days	15 to 160 days	14 to 64 days	14 to 60 days	14 to 42 days
Onset	Acute	Insidious	Insidious	Acute	Acute	Presumed insidious
Age-group commonly affected	Children, young adults	Any age	More common in adults	Any age	Ages 20 to 40	Any age, primarily adults
Transmission	Fecal-oral, sexual (especially oral-anal contact), non-percutaneous (sexual, maternal-neonatal), percutaneous (rare)	Blood-borne; parenteral route, sexual, maternal-neonatal; virus is shed in all body fluids	Blood-borne; parenteral route, sexual	Parenteral route; most people infected with hepatitis D are also infected with hepatitis B	Primarily fecal-oral	Blood-borne; similar to hepatitis B and C
Severity	Mild	Commonly severe	Moderate	Can be severe and lead to fulminant hepatitis	Highly virulent with common progression to fulminant hepatitis and hepatic failure, especially in pregnant patients	Moderate
Prognosis	Generally good	Worsens with age and debility	Moderate	Fair, worsens in chronic cases; can lead to chronic hepatitis D and chronic liver disease	Good unless pregnant	Generally good; no current treatment recommendations
Progression to chronicity	None	Occasional	10% to 50% of cases	Occasional	None	Not known; no association with chronic liver disease

Ammonia's role

Ammonia is one of the main toxins causing hepatic encephalopathy. Ammonia is a by-product of protein metabolism. The liver transforms ammonia to urea, which the kidneys excrete. When the liver fails to do this, ammonia levels increase and ammonia is delivered to the brain.

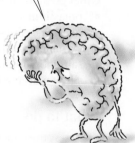

When the liver can't transform ammonia to urea, ammonia is delivered to the brain.

What to look for

Signs and symptoms vary, depending on the severity of neurologic involvement.

The disorder progresses through these four stages, with symptoms that can fluctuate from one stage to another:
1. prodromal stage—slight personality changes (disorientation, forgetfulness, and slurred speech), changes in sleep patterns, and a slight tremor
2. impending stage—tremor progresses to asterixis (the hallmark of hepatic encephalopathy), characterized by quick irregular extensions and flexions of the wrists and fingers, lethargy, aberrant behavior, confusion, and apraxia
3. stuporous stage—hyperventilation with stupor; noisy and abusive patient when stimulated; severe confusion; hyperactive deep tendon reflexes
4. comatose stage—includes a positive Babinski's sign; coma; abnormal posturing; and a musty, sweet breath odor.

What tests tell you

These findings help diagnose hepatic encephalopathy:
- Liver function tests are elevated.
- Serum albumin level is decreased and BUN and blood glucose levels are increased.
- Serum electrolyte levels reveal hypokalemia and hyponatremia.
- Bilirubin and ammonia levels are elevated.
- Coagulation studies are prolonged.
- EEG is commonly abnormal but with nonspecific changes.

How it's treated

Treatment goals for the patient with hepatic failure are correcting the underlying cause and reducing blood ammonia levels. Treatment measures include:
- administration of neomycin or metronidazole to destroy intestinal bacteria that breaks down protein into ammonia
- sorbitol-induced catharsis to produce osmotic diarrhea
- continuous aspiration of blood from the stomach

- reduction of dietary protein to 20 to 40 g daily.
- lactulose administration to decrease colonic pH to prevent absorption of ammonia and reduce blood ammonia levels.

But wait, there's more

Other possible treatments include:
- potassium supplements
- hemodialysis to temporarily clear toxic blood
- exchange transfusions
- salt-poor albumin to maintain fluid and electrolyte balance
- shunt placement or paracentesis if ascites is a problem.

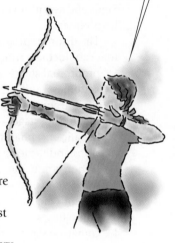

Aim for the treatment targets: correcting the underlying cause and reducing your patient's blood ammonia levels.

What to do

- Assess the patient's airway and respiratory status frequently, at least every 1 to 2 hours. Maintain a patent airway and position the patient with the head of the bed elevated.
- Monitor the patient's oxygen saturation levels.
- Assess the patient's neurologic status to establish a baseline and report any changes. Reorient the patient as necessary. Assure patient safety measures are in place.
- Monitor the patient's cardiac status and vital signs often, at least every hour.
- Assess the patient's hemodynamic parameters closely, at least every hour. Monitor for indications of fluid volume deficit or excess.
- Assess the patient's urinary output hourly. Notify the practitioner if output is less than 0.5 ml/kg/hour.
- Measure the patient's abdominal girth and weight daily.
- Assess the patient for signs and symptoms of fluid excess, including peripheral edema, jugular vein distention, tachypnea, and crackles that don't clear with coughing.
- Monitor laboratory studies, such as renal function, liver enzymes, serum ammonia, serum albumin, total protein, coagulation studies, and serum electrolytes.
- Monitor the patient's nutritional intake and maintain calorie count.
- Check capillary blood glucose levels every 4 hours or as ordered and assess for signs and symptoms of hyperglycemia and hypoglycemia.
- Institute bleeding precautions and monitor the patient for signs and symptoms of bleeding.
- Administer prescribed medications. Check with the practitioner to adjust the dose of lactulose to allow for 2 to 3 semiformed stools per day.
- Assist with paracentesis as indicated.
- Begin emergency treatment to control bleeding if variceal rupture occurs.
- Provide supportive care to the patient and his family.

Intra-abdominal hypertension

Intra-abdominal hypertension, the elevation of intra-abdominal pressure, commonly occurs in the critical care unit and affects medical patients just as often as it does trauma and surgical patients. If untreated, intra-abdominal hypertension can lead to abdominal compartment syndrome, a medical emergency that accounts for significant morbidity and mortality in critically ill patients.

Clear-cut measures

Intra-abdominal hypertension is defined as sustained or repeated pathologic elevation of intra-abdominal pressure (IAP) of 12 mm Hg or greater. The World Society on Abdominal Compartment Syndrome has identified four grades of severity of intra-abdominal hypertension:
1. Grade I—IAP between 12 and 15 mm Hg
2. Grade II—IAP between 16 and 20 mm Hg
3. Grade III—IAP between 21 and 25 mm Hg
4. Grade IV—IAP greater than 25 mm Hg.

Organ breakdown

According to the World Society, abdominal compartment syndrome is organ dysfunction that occurs as the end-stage complication of untreated intra-abdominal hypertension. This complication affects the mesenteric, hepatic, and intestinal arterial systems and can diminish blood flow to various intra-abdominal organs.

> Abdominal compartment syndrome, the end-stage complication of untreated intra-abdominal hypertension, can diminish blood flow to various intra-abdominal organs.

What causes it

Both intra-abdominal hypertension and abdominal compartment syndrome result from capillary endothelial damage and widespread interstitial edema in the body, including the bowel and mesentery. Many medical and surgical patients requiring care in the critical care unit have these conditions. The incidence of intra-abdominal hypertension in high-risk critical care unit patients is 5% to 50%.

Common conditions

Intra-abdominal hypertension has several etiologies but can be categorized into three main factors which relate to alterations in intra-abdominal pressure. These are:
1. decreased abdominal wall compliance
2. capillary leakage or fluid resuscitation
3. increased intraluminal contents.
    Intra-abdominal hypertension is especially prevalent in patients with systemic inflammatory response syndrome and sepsis. Other causes include:
* abdominal trauma
* GI hemorrhage

- pancreatitis
- pelvic fracture
- ruptured aortic aneurysm
- burns (large areas, full-thickness)
- shock
- aggressive fluid resuscitation
- cirrhosis
- peritonitis
- post-abdominal surgery
- morbid obesity.

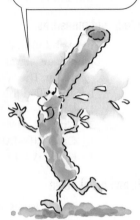

Sorry . . . it's my fault! My lining sprung a leak, and now I'm dripping all over the intra-abdominal compartment. I could use a bucket—quick!

How it happens

Interstitial edema in the bowel and mesentery as a result of capillary endothelial damage is the primary pathophysiologic cause of intra-abdominal hypertension and abdominal compartment syndrome. Although an initial event triggers the capillary damage, the release of proinflammatory cytokines in response to this insult also contributes to the widespread endothelial damage that occurs.

Leaks and stretching

As a result of "leaky" capillaries, several liters of interstitial fluid can accumulate in the intra-abdominal compartment. The abdominal wall and fascia slowly stretch as this fluid accumulates. Overstretching of the abdominal tissues quickly leads to decreased abdominal compliance, which results in elevated intra-abdominal pressure. Sustained elevation of intra-abdominal pressure has significant adverse effects on organ perfusion throughout the body.

Body system effects

Pathophysiologic changes associated with intra-abdominal hypertension and abdominal compartment syndrome produce these body system effects:

- *GI*—Elevated pressure in the abdominal cavity leads to abdominal distention and compression on the mesenteric, hepatic, and intestinal vessels. Capillary blood flow within the abdomen becomes completely obstructed if the intra-abdominal pressure rises to the point that it equals that of the capillary bed (15 to 25 mm Hg). Obstruction of capillary blood flow results in decreased venous flow, venous congestion, worsening ischemia, and eventually, bowel necrosis. In addition, decreased portal blood flow results in visceral edema within the portal system, further aggravating the rise in intra-abdominal pressure.
- *Cardiovascular*—Compression of the vena cava and portal vein results in decreased venous return to the heart (decreased preload), resulting in decreased cardiac output. Intrathoracic pressure rises as

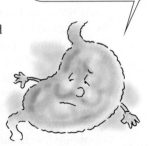

It's hard to believe that a little extra fluid in the gut can wreak so much havoc on the body.

the intra-abdominal pressure increases, causing a reduction in cardiac compliance and severe diastolic dysfunction. Increased systemic afterload also occurs as the body responds to the drop in cardiac output by promoting vasoconstriction. This vasoconstriction, along with the low cardiac output, leads to further cardiac decompensation.

- *Pulmonary*—As intrathoracic pressure rises due to increased intra-abdominal pressure, the diaphragm is pushed cephalad (upward into the chest), resulting in respiratory compromise. In an effort to maintain an adequate tidal volume, peak pressures rise (increased pulmonary vascular resistance) as the ventilator drives air into the lungs. If these pressures continue to go unchecked, barotrauma can result quickly, leading to hypercapnia (elevated carbon dioxide) and hypoxia. Decreased cardiac output in combination with increased pulmonary vascular resistance can trigger the release of inflammatory mediators from the gut, resulting in pulmonary capillary damage, pulmonary interstitial edema, and a syndrome that closely mirrors acute respiratory distress syndrome.
- *Renal*—Direct pressure on the renal parenchyma (especially the renal capsule) and renal veins leads to edema of the kidneys. At the same time, decreased cardiac output and aortic compression compromise renal perfusion. Consequently, glomerular filtration decreases, leading to decreased urine output and possible renal insufficiency and failure.
- *CNS*—Venous return to the chest is hampered by increased intrathoracic pressure caused by intra-abdominal hypertension. This decrease in venous return results in venous congestion of the arms and neck. Elevations in intracranial pressure occur as the congestion progresses up through the internal jugular vein into the cranial vault.

What to look for

Intra-abdominal hypertension and abdominal compartment syndrome produce significant adverse systemic and hemodynamic effects. Assess the patient for these signs and symptoms:
- tense abdominal wall
- increased abdominal girth (round belly sign characterized by abdominal distention with increased ratio of anteroposterior-to-transverse diameter)
- abdominal tenderness
- shallow respirations
- oliguria or anuria
- tachycardia
- hypotension
- hypercapnia

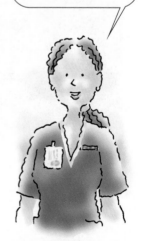

Assess the abdomen for tenseness, tenderness, and increased girth. And don't forget to check for a positive round belly sign.

- hypoxia
- decreased cardiac output and index
- increased central venous pressure (CVP)
- increased pulmonary artery wedge pressure
- increased pulmonary artery pressure
- increased intra-abdominal pressure (via urinary bladder catheter).

What tests tell you

The gold standard for diagnosing intra-abdominal hypertension is measurement of the intra-abdominal pressure. (See *Measuring intra-abdominal pressure.*)

Measuring intra-abdominal pressure

You can perform intra-abdominal pressure monitoring through direct or indirect means. The direct method is preferred for intra-abdominal pressure monitoring and involves inserting an indwelling urinary catheter into the patient's bladder. The bladder will reflect intra-abdominal pressure when it has a volume of 100 ml or less.

Insert a needle into the catheter sample port of the indwelling catheter. Then attach the needle to pressure tubing and a transducer, which allows you to view the intra-abdominal pressure on a monitor. The photo below shows a completed intra-abdominal pressure set-up.

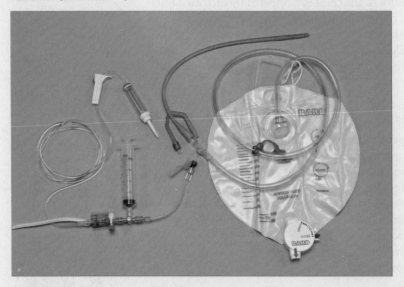

Off the gold standard

Other diagnostic findings include:

- elevated BUN and creatinine
- ABG levels that indicate hypoxia and high partial pressure of arterial carbon dioxide levels.

How it's treated

Intra-abdominal hypertension detected early is amenable to nonsurgical intervention. Treatment goals include reducing intra-abdominal pressure and improving perfusion to the affected organs. Specific treatments may include:

- diuretics to reduce interstitial edema
- possible fluid restriction
- I.V. albumin to maintain CVP between 8 and 12 mm Hg
- inotropic support with vasopressors to improve cardiac output and tissue perfusion
- continuous renal replacement therapy for fluid removal and management
- mechanical ventilation to maintain adequate gas exchange
- NG suctioning to remove excess air and fluid from intestinal lumen
- possible bowel purging using cathartics, enemas, or rectal tubes
- surgical decompression (medical management is preferred).

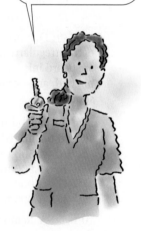

The key to success is reducing intra-abdominal pressure and improving perfusion to the affected organs.

What to do

- Administer I.V. fluids to help minimize abdominal ischemia.
- Administer oxygen to help maximize tissue perfusion.
- Be prepared to provide mechanical ventilation if the patient begins to experience respiratory distress.
- Administer sedation and analgesics to help decrease tissue oxygenation needs. In some cases, the practitioner may order a neuromuscular blocker for the patient.
- Be prepared to assist with paracentesis.
- Monitor intra-abdominal pressures at least every 2 hours, or according to your facility's policy.
- Maintain NG suctioning to remove all air and fluid from the intestinal tract.
- If the patient needs surgical decompression, prepare the patient for surgery.
- Provide emotional support to the patient and his family.

Quick quiz

1. The stomach's major functions include all of these actions except:
- A. moving the gastric contents into the small intestine.
- B. completing digestion.
- C. serving as a temporary storage area for food.
- D. breaking down food into chyme.

Answer: B. The stomach doesn't complete the digestion process. It begins the digestion process by being a temporary storage area for food where it begins to break down into chyme before being moved into the small intestine.

2. Bowel sounds that are high-pitched and gurgling and occur 10 times per minute are classified as:
- A. hypoactive.
- B. hyperactive.
- C. dull.
- D. normal.

Answer: D. Normal bowel sounds are high-pitched and gurgling and occur irregularly from 5 to 34 times per minute. Hypoactive sounds are heard infrequently. Hyperactive bowel sounds are loud, high-pitched, and occur frequently. There's no such thing as dull bowel sounds.

3. During abdominal paracentesis, the aspirated fluid amount should be limited to:
- A. 1,500 to 2,000 ml.
- B. 2,000 to 3,000 ml.
- C. 1,000 to 2,000 ml.
- D. 1,000 to 1,500 ml.

Answer: A. Removing more than 1,500 to 2,000 ml of peritoneal fluid at one time may lead to hypovolemic shock.

4. What symptom would make a patient a candidate for enteral nutrition?
- A. Acute pancreatitis
- B. Ulcerative colitis
- C. Absent bowel sounds
- D. Bowel obstruction

Answer: B. Ulcerative colitis is an indication for the use of enteral nutrition. All of the other conditions are indications for parenteral nutrition.

5. Which of the following feeding methods is the preferred choice for critically ill adult patients?
    A. Duodenal tube
    B. Enteral nutrition
    C. Total parenteral nutrition
    D. Peripheral parenteral nutrition

Answer: A. The duodenal tube is preferred due to long-term use potential and decreased risk of aspiration.

Scoring

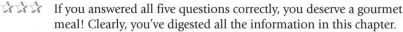

If you answered all five questions correctly, you deserve a gourmet meal! Clearly, you've digested all the information in this chapter.

If you answered four questions correctly, read up and try again! Your hunger for GI information makes it easy to swallow.

If you answered fewer than four questions correctly, you may be fact-starved. Chew over the chapter and then take the test again.

Suggested References

American Association of Critical Care Nurses. (2010). *AACN PracticeAlert: Verification of feeding tube placement*. Retrieved from http://www.aacn.org/wd/practice /content/feeding-tube-practice-alert.pcms?menu=practice

Castello, H., Schoch, L., & Grogan, T. (2013). Acute liver failure in an obstetric patient: Challenge of critical care for 1 patient with 2 subspecialty needs. *Critical Care Nurse, 33*(1), 48–56.

Gallagher, J. (2007). Ask the experts: Intra-abdominal pressure monitoring via indwelling urinary catheter. *Critical Care Nurse, 27*(5), 64–70.

Hunt, L., Frost, S. A., Hillman, K., Newton, P. J., & Davidson, P. M. (2014). Management of intra-abdominal hypertension and abdominal compartment syndrome: A review. *Journal of Trauma Management & Outcomes, 8*(1), 2.

Kramer, C., & Jeffery, A. (2014). Pancreatitis in children. *Critical Care Nurse, 34*(4), 43–52.

Morton, P. G., Fontaine, D., Hudak, C. M., & Gallo, B. M. (Eds.). (2005). *Critical care nursing: A holistic approach* (8th ed.). Philadelphia, PA: Lippincott Williams & Wilkins.

Perrin, K. O. (2009). *Understanding the essentials of critical care nursing*. Upper Saddle River, NJ: Pearson/Prentice Hall.

Chapter 7

Renal system

Just the facts

In this chapter, you'll learn:

♦ structure and function of the renal system

♦ assessment of the renal system

♦ diagnostic tests and treatments

♦ common renal disorders and related nursing care.

Understanding the renal system

The renal system is the body's water treatment plant. Its job is to collect waste products and expel them as urine. The structures of the renal system include:

- kidneys
- ureters
- bladder
- urethra.

Kidney sitting

The kidneys are located on each side of the abdomen near the lower back. These compact organs contain a filtration system that processes about 45 gallons of fluid each day. The by-product of this process is urine, which contains water and waste products. (See *A close look at a kidney*.)

It's all downhill from there

After it's produced by the kidneys, urine passes through the urinary system and is expelled from the body. The other structures of the system, extending downward from the kidneys, include the:

- ureters—two 16″ to 18″ (40.5- to 45.5-cm) muscular tubes that contract rhythmically (peristalsis) to transport urine from each kidney to the bladder
- urinary bladder—a sac with muscular walls that collects and holds urine (300 to 500 ml) expelled from the ureters every few seconds

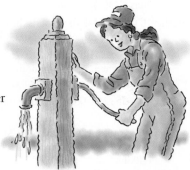

The renal system is the body's water treatment plant; it collects waste products and expels them as urine.

A close look at a kidney

Illustrated below is a kidney along with an enlargement of a nephron, the kidney's functional unit.

Kidney keys

Major structures of the kidney include:
• medulla—inner portion of the kidney, made up of renal pyramids and tubular structures
• renal artery—supplies blood to the kidney
• renal pyramid—channels output to the renal pelvis for excretion
• renal calyx—channels formed urine from the renal pyramids to the renal pelvis
• renal vein—about 99% of filtered blood is circulated through the renal vein back to the general circulation; the remaining 1%, which contains waste products, undergoes further processing in the kidney
• renal pelvis—after blood that contains waste products is processed in the kidney, formed urine is channeled to the renal pelvis
• ureter—a tube that terminates in the urethra; urine enters the urethra for excretion
• cortex—outer layer of the kidney.

Note the nephron

The nephron is the functional and structural unit of the kidney. Each kidney contains about 1 million nephrons. Their two main activities are selective resorption and secretion of ions and mechanical filtration of fluids, wastes, electrolytes, and acids and bases.

Components of the nephron include:
• glomerulus—a network of twisted capillaries that acts as a filter for the passage of protein-free and red blood cell (RBC)–free filtrate to the proximal convoluted tubules
• Bowman's capsule—the structure that contains the glomerulus and acts as a filter for urine
• proximal convoluted tubule—the site of resorption of glucose, amino acids, metabolites, and electrolytes from filtrate; resorbed substances then return to the circulation
• loop of Henle—a U-shaped nephron tubule located in the medulla and extending from the proximal convoluted tubule to the distal convoluted tubule; the site for further concentration of filtrate through resorption
• distal convoluted tubule—the site from which filtrate enters the collecting tubule
• collecting tubule—the structure that releases urine.

Kidney

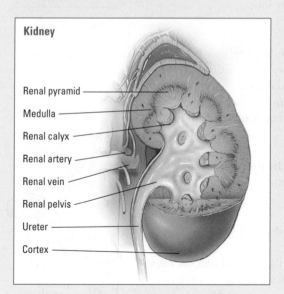

Renal pyramid
Medulla
Renal calyx
Renal artery
Renal vein
Renal pelvis
Ureter
Cortex

Nephron

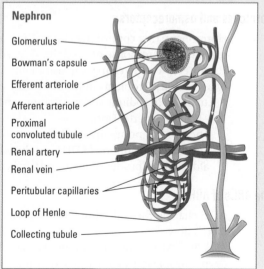

Glomerulus
Bowman's capsule
Efferent arteriole
Afferent arteriole
Proximal convoluted tubule
Renal artery
Renal vein
Peritubular capillaries
Loop of Henle
Collecting tubule

- urethra—a narrow passageway (surrounded by the prostate gland in men) from the bladder to the outside of the body through which urine is excreted.

That isn't all

The renal system is a major regulatory system as well. Its roles include:
- maintaining fluid and electrolyte balance
- maintaining acid–base balance
- detoxifying the blood and eliminating wastes
- regulating blood pressure
- aiding RBC production.

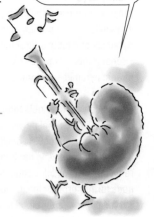

I'm a major player in a major regulatory system. Doo-wah-doo, Daddio.

Fluid and electrolyte balance

The kidneys maintain fluid and electrolyte balance in the body by regulating the amount and makeup of the fluid inside and around the cells.

Exchange interchange

The kidneys maintain the volume and composition of extracellular and, to a lesser extent, intracellular fluid. They do so by continuously exchanging water and solutes across their cell membranes. The solutes include electrolytes such as hydrogen, sodium, potassium, chloride, bicarbonate, sulfate, and phosphate ions.

Hormones and osmoreceptors

Hormones partly control the kidneys' role in fluid balance by regulating the response of specialized sensory nerve endings (osmoreceptors) to changes in osmolality (the ionic concentration of a solution). Problems in hormone concentration can cause fluctuations in sodium and potassium concentrations that, in turn, may lead to hypertension.

The two hormones involved are:
1. antidiuretic hormone (ADH), produced by the pituitary gland
2. aldosterone, produced by the adrenal cortex.

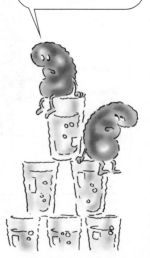

Two hormones—ADH and aldosterone—are involved in fluid balance.

The ABCs of ADH

ADH changes the collecting tubules' permeability to water. Here's how:
- When ADH concentration in plasma is high, the tubules are most permeable to water. This condition creates a highly concentrated but small volume of urine.
- When ADH concentration is low, the tubules are less permeable to water. This situation creates a larger volume of less concentrated urine.

Age and ADH

As a person ages, tubular resorption and renal concentrating ability decline because the size and number of functioning nephrons decrease.

All about aldosterone and sodium

Aldosterone regulates water resorption by the distal tubules and changes urine concentration by increasing sodium resorption. Here's how:

- A high plasma aldosterone concentration increases sodium and water resorption by the tubules and decreases sodium and water excretion in the urine.
- A low plasma aldosterone concentration promotes sodium and water excretion.

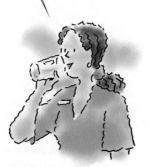

Aldosterone regulates water resorption and changes urine concentration by increasing sodium resorption.

Aldosterone and potassium

Aldosterone also helps control the secretion of potassium by the distal tubules. A high aldosterone concentration increases the excretion of potassium. Other factors that affect potassium secretion include:

- amount of potassium ingested
- number of hydrogen ions secreted
- potassium levels in the cells
- amount of sodium in the distal tubule
- glomerular filtration rate (GFR), which is the rate at which plasma is filtered as it flows through the glomerular capillary filtration membrane.

Going against the current

The kidneys concentrate urine through the countercurrent exchange system. In this system, fluid flows in opposite directions through parallel tubes, up and down parallel sides of the loops of Henle. A concentration gradient causes fluid exchange; the longer the loop, the greater the concentration gradient.

Acid–base balance

To regulate acid–base balance, the kidneys:

- secrete hydrogen ions
- resorb sodium and bicarbonate ions
- acidify phosphate salts
- produce ammonia.

Earning a PhD in pH balance

All of these regulating activities keep the blood at its normal pH of 7.35 to 7.45. Acidosis occurs when the pH falls below 7.35, and alkalosis occurs when the pH rises above 7.45.

Detoxification and waste elimination

The kidneys collect and eliminate wastes from the body in a three-step process:

1. *glomerular filtration*, in which the kidney's blood vessels, or glomeruli, filter blood flowing through them
2. *tubular resorption*, in which the tubules (minute canals that make up the kidney) resorb the filtered fluid
3. *tubular secretion*, in which the filtered substance is then released by the tubules.

Clear the way

Clearance is the complete removal of a substance from the blood. It's commonly described as the amount of blood that can be cleared in a specific time. For example, creatinine clearance is the volume of blood in milliliters that the kidneys can clear of creatinine in 1 minute.

Some substances are filtered out of the blood by the glomeruli. Dissolved substances that remain in the fluid may be resorbed by the renal tubular cells. (See *Understanding GFR.*)

Nephron compensation

In a patient whose kidneys have atrophied from disease, healthy nephrons (the filtering units of the kidney) enlarge to compensate. As nephron damage progresses, the enlargement no longer adequately compensates, and the patient's GFR slows. (See *Age-related renal changes.*)

Tubular transport-ability

The amount of a substance that's resorbed or secreted depends on the substance's maximum tubular transport capacity, or the maximum amount of a substance that can be resorbed or secreted in 1 minute without saturating the renal system.

For example, in diabetes mellitus, excess glucose in the blood overwhelms the renal tubules and causes glucose to appear in the urine (glycosuria). In other cases, when glomeruli are damaged, protein appears in the urine (proteinuria) because the large protein molecules pass into the urine instead of being resorbed.

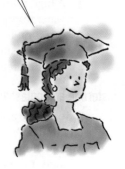

Normal blood pH has a narrow range. Acidosis occurs when pH falls below 7.35, and alkalosis occurs when pH rises above 7.45. PhDs need a different kind of grading system.

Understanding GFR

GFR is the rate at which the glomeruli filter blood. A normal GFR is about 120 ml/minute. GFR depends on:
- permeability of capillary walls
- vascular pressure
- filtration pressure.

GFR and clearance

Clearance is the complete removal of a substance from the blood. The most accurate measure of glomerular filtration is creatinine clearance because creatinine is filtered by the glomeruli but not resorbed by the tubules.

Equal to, greater than, or less than

Here's more about how the GFR affects clearance measurements for a substance in the blood:
- If the tubules neither resorb nor secrete the substance—as happens with creatinine—clearance is equal to the GFR.
- If the tubules resorb the substance, clearance is less than the GFR.
- If the tubules secrete the substance, clearance exceeds the GFR.
- If the tubules resorb and secrete the substance, clearance may be less than, equal to, or greater than the GFR.

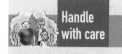

Handle with care

Age-related renal changes

By age 70, a person's blood urea nitrogen levels increase by 21%. Other age-related changes that affect renal function include:
- diminished kidney size
- impaired renal clearance of drugs
- reduced bladder size and capacity
- decreased renal response to sodium intake.

Blood pressure regulation

High blood pressure (hypertension) can damage blood vessels as well as cause hardening of the kidneys (nephrosclerosis), a leading cause of chronic renal failure.

Hypertension regulation

Hypertension can stem from renin-angiotensin hyperactivity (as well as from fluid and electrolyte imbalance). The kidneys aid blood pressure regulation by producing and secreting the enzyme renin in response to an actual or perceived decline in extracellular fluid volume. Renin, in turn, forms angiotensin I, which is converted to the more potent angiotensin II.

Pressure promotion

Angiotensin II increases low arterial blood pressure levels by:
- increasing peripheral vasoconstriction
- stimulating aldosterone secretion.

The increase in aldosterone promotes the resorption of sodium and water to correct the fluid deficit and inadequate blood flow (renal ischemia).

Simply put, the kidneys secrete renin, which forms angiotensin I, which is converted to angiotensin II.

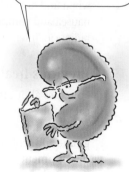

RBC production

Erythropoietin is a hormone that prompts the bone marrow to increase RBC production (erythropoiesis).

Vitamin D and calcium formation

The kidneys secrete erythropoietin when the oxygen supply in blood for tissues drops. They also produce active vitamin D and help regulate calcium balance and bone metabolism. Loss of renal function results in chronic anemia and insufficient calcium levels (hypocalcemia) because of a decrease in erythropoietin.

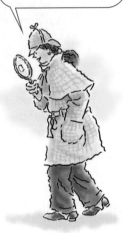

Collect clues from the patient's health history to find out about the cause and severity of his renal condition.

Renal assessment

Begin the renal assessment by collecting a patient health history. Next, conduct a thorough physical examination.

History

Collect a thorough health history to gain the information you need to find the cause and severity of the patient's renal disease. The health history includes information about the patient's current and previous illnesses and treatments as well as medication and family and lifestyle factors.

Current health status

Find out how the patient's symptoms developed and progressed. Ask how long he has had the problem, how it affects his daily routine, and when and how it began. Ask about related signs and symptoms, such as nausea and vomiting. If your patient has any pain, ask about its location, radiation, intensity, duration, and what precipitates or relieves it.

Previous health status

For clues about the patient's current condition, explore his past medical problems. Certain systemic diseases, such as diabetes mellitus, systemic lupus erythematosus, hypertension, sickle cell anemia, acute glomerulonephritis, and acute pyelonephritis, may contribute to the development of acute renal failure.

Ask the patient whether he has a history of renal disease or has ever had a kidney or bladder tumor. Find out what treatments he received and the treatment outcomes. Ask about any traumatic injuries, surgery, or conditions that required hospitalization or any recent diagnostic test that involved the use of a contrast medium.

Drug check

Ask your patient if he's now taking any medications and what they are. Ask if he has any known allergies to foods or medications.

Many drugs are eliminated by the kidneys, so the patient with compromised kidney function, such as chronic renal failure, may need to avoid certain drugs or receive reduced dosages to prevent further renal problems. Drugs that may require a reduced dosage include angiotensin-converting enzyme inhibitors, ciprofloxacin (Cipro), digoxin (Lanoxin), histamine-2 receptor antagonists, penicillins, nonsteroidal anti-inflammatory drugs (NSAIDs) including cyclo-oxygenase type 2 inhibitors (COX-2), and sulfonamides.

Examples of drugs that impose a risk of nephrotoxicity include aminoglycosides (such as gentamicin [Garamycin], neomycin [Mycifradin], and tobramycin), cisplatin (Platinol-AQ), and lithium carbonate (Eskalith).

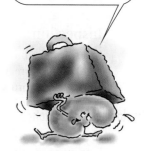

I need to stay in shape. Many drugs are eliminated by the kidneys.

Family history

Because some renal disorders are hereditary, ask the patient whether anyone in his family has a history of renal disease. Polycystic kidney disease is one example of an inherited disorder that can lead to renal failure.

Lifestyle patterns

Psychological and sociologic factors can affect the patient's health.

To determine how such factors may have contributed to your patient's current problem, ask about his:

- home life
- stress level
- occupation.

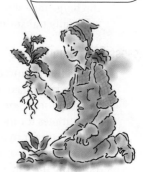

Environmental agents—including pesticides—that could cause kidney problems might be found in the patient's home or workplace.

At work and play

Ask your patient about possible exposure at work or home to agents that may be nephrotoxic, such as cleaning products, pesticides, lead, and mercury. Also ask about his alcohol, tobacco, caffeine, and drug use as well as his dietary habits, cultural practices that affect diet, and dietary restrictions, such as a vegetarian or low-potassium diet.

Physical examination

Proceed in an orderly way with the physical examination of your patient's renal system using inspection, auscultation, percussion, and palpation.

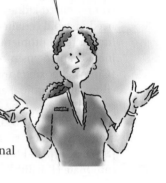

Compare the left and right sides of the abdomen and note asymmetrical areas.

Inspection

In a normal adult, the abdomen is smooth, flat or scaphoid (concave), and symmetrical. Abdominal skin should be free from scars, lesions, bruises, and discoloration.

Disclosing dysfunction

Inspect your patient's abdomen for gross enlargements or fullness by comparing the left and right sides, noting asymmetrical areas. Extremely prominent veins may accompany other vascular signs associated with renal dysfunction, such as hypertension or renal artery bruits.

Distention, skin tightness and glistening, and striae (streaks or linear scars caused by rapidly developing skin tension) may signal fluid retention. If you suspect ascites, perform the fluid wave test. Ascites may suggest nephrotic syndrome.

Urethral meatus inspection

Urethral meatus inspection may reveal several abnormalities. In a male patient, a meatus deviating from the normal central location may represent a congenital defect. In any patient, inflammation and discharge may signal urethral infection. Ulceration usually indicates a sexually transmitted disease.

Assess fluid volume status

Assess fluid volume status by observing for jugular vein distention and peripheral edema, periorbital edema, and sacral edema. Check the skin for turgor and mobility. Inspect the tongue and mucous membranes for moisture.

Skin turgor may be an unreliable sign of hydration in older people because of reduced subcutaneous tissue. Check turgor by pinching the subcutaneous tissue at the forehead or over the xiphoid process and watching for a quick return to baseline.

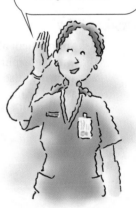

Listen up! Systolic bruits and other unusual sounds can be signs of trouble.

Auscultation

Auscultate the renal arteries in the left and right upper abdominal quadrants by pressing the stethoscope bell lightly against the abdomen and instructing the patient to exhale deeply. Begin auscultating at the midline and work to the left. Then return to the midline and work to the right.

Whoosh

Systolic bruits (whooshing sounds) or other unusual sounds are potentially significant abnormalities. For example, in a patient with hypertension, systolic bruits suggest renal artery stenosis.

Tube talk

Before auscultating the abdomen of a critically ill patient with a nasogastric (NG) tube or another abdominal tube connected to suction, briefly clamp the tube or turn off the suction. Suction noises can obscure or mimic abdominal sounds.

Percussion

After auscultating the renal arteries, percuss the patient's kidneys to detect tenderness or pain and percuss the bladder to evaluate its position and contents.

Percuss the kidneys to detect tenderness or pain. Percuss the bladder to evaluate its position and contents.

How to

To percuss over the kidneys, have the patient sit up. Place your nondominant hand on the patient's back at the costovertebral angle of the 12th rib. Strike that hand with the ulnar surface of your other fist. Use just enough force to cause a painless but perceptible thud.

Percussing problems

Abnormal kidney percussion findings include tenderness and pain, suggesting glomerulonephritis or glomerulonephrosis. A dull sound heard on percussion in a patient who has just urinated may indicate urine retention, reflecting bladder dysfunction or infection.

In an elderly patient, you may be able to palpate both kidneys because of decreased muscle tone and elasticity.

Palpation

Palpate the kidneys and bladder to detect lumps, masses, or tenderness. (See *Palpating the renal organs*, page 514.) To achieve optimal results, ask the patient to relax the abdomen by taking deep breaths through the mouth.

Peek-a-boo

Because the kidneys lie behind other organs and are protected by muscle, they normally aren't palpable unless they're enlarged. However, in a thin patient,

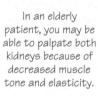

Palpating the renal organs

In the normal adult, the kidneys usually can't be palpated because of their location deep in the abdomen. However, they may be palpable in a thin patient or in one with reduced abdominal muscle mass. (Because the right kidney is slightly lower than the left, it may be easier to palpate.) Both kidneys descend with deep inhalation. An adult's bladder may not be palpable, either. If palpable, the bladder normally feels firm and relatively smooth. Using bimanual palpation, begin on the patient's right side and proceed with palpating the renal organs as outlined below.

Kidney palpation

1. Help the patient to a supine position and expose the abdomen from the xiphoid process to the symphysis pubis. Standing at the right side, place your left hand under the back, midway between the lower costal margin and the iliac crest, as shown below.

2. Next, place your right hand on the patient's abdomen directly above your left hand. Angle this hand slightly toward the costal margin. To palpate the right lower edge of the right kidney, press your right fingertips about 1½" (3.8 cm) above the right iliac crest at the midinguinal line; press your left fingertips upward into the right costovertebral angle.

3. Instruct the patient to inhale deeply so that the lower portion of the right kidney can move down between your hands. If it does, note the shape and size of the kidney. Normally, it feels smooth, solid, and firm, yet elastic. Ask the patient if palpation causes tenderness. Avoid using excessive pressure to palpate the kidney because this may cause intense pain.

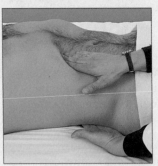

4. To assess the left kidney, move to the patient's left side and

position your hands, as described in the preceding figure, but position your right hand 2" (5 cm) above the left iliac crest. Then apply pressure with both hands as the patient inhales. If the left kidney can be palpated, compare it with the right kidney; it should be the same size.

Bladder palpation

Before palpating the bladder, make sure the patient has voided. Then locate the edge of the bladder by pressing deeply in the midline about 1" to 2" (2.5 to 5 cm) above the symphysis pubis. As the bladder is palpated, note its size and location and check for lumps, masses, and tenderness. The bladder normally feels firm and relatively smooth. During deep palpation, the patient may report the urge to urinate—a normal response.

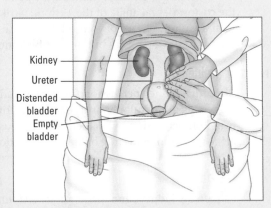

Kidney
Ureter
Distended bladder
Empty bladder

you may be able to feel the lower end of the right kidney as a smooth round mass that drops on inspiration. In an elderly patient, you may be able to palpate both kidneys because of decreased muscle tone and elasticity.

Finding fault

On palpation, a lump, mass, or tenderness may indicate a tumor or cyst. A soft kidney may reflect chronic renal disease; a tender kidney, acute infection. Unequal kidney size may reflect hydronephrosis, a cyst, a tumor, or another disorder. Bilateral enlargement suggests polycystic kidney disease.

Abnormal bladder palpation findings include a lump or mass, possibly signaling a tumor or cyst, and tenderness, which may stem from infection. (See *Interpreting renal findings*, page 516.)

Calcium culprit

When your patient complains of muscle spasms and paresthesia in his limbs, check for signs of calcium deficiency. (See *Checking for hypocalcemia*, page 517.)

Diagnostic tests

Diagnostic tests commonly ordered for a patient with known or suspected renal disease may include blood studies, kidney-ureter-bladder (KUB) radiography, kidney computed tomography (CT) scan, renal angiography, renal ultrasound, and urine studies.

Blood studies

Blood studies used to diagnose and evaluate kidney function include:
- complete blood count (CBC) to evaluate white blood cells (WBCs), RBCs, hemoglobin (Hb), and hematocrit (HCT)
- blood urea nitrogen (BUN) testing
- electrolyte measurements to evaluate calcium, phosphorus, chloride, potassium, and sodium levels
- serum creatinine, serum osmolality, serum protein, uric acid, creatinine clearance, and urea clearance measurements. (See *Interpreting blood studies in renal disease*, page 518, and *Calculating GFRs*, page 519.)

KUB radiography

KUB radiography, consisting of plain, contrast-free X-rays, shows kidney size, position, and structure. It can also reveal calculi and other lesions. Before performing a renal biopsy, the doctor may use this test to determine kidney placement. For diagnostic purposes, however, the KUB study provides limited information.

Interpreting renal findings

After completing your assessment, you're ready to form a diagnostic impression of the patient's condition. Check this table to find groupings of significant signs and symptoms, related findings you may discover during the health history and physical assessment, and the possible cause indicated by a cluster of these findings.

Key signs and symptoms	Related findings		Possible cause
• Oliguria, possibly progressing to anuria • Hematuria or coffee-colored urine • Smoky urine	• Poststreptococcal throat or skin infection • Systemic lupus erythematosus, vasculitis, or scleroderma • Pregnancy	• Elevated blood pressure • Periorbital edema progressing to dependent edema • Ascites • Pleural effusion	Acute glomerulonephritis
• Oliguria • Dark, smoky urine • Anorexia and vomiting	• Crush injury or illness associated with shock such as burns • Muscle necrosis • Exposure to nephrotoxic agent such as lead • Excretory urography using dye injection	• Recent aminoglycoside therapy • Oliguria progressing to anuria • Dyspnea • Bibasilar crackles • Dependent edema	Acute tubular necrosis
• Proteinuria, hematuria, vomiting, and pruritus (patient may be asymptomatic until advanced disease stage)	• Primary renal disorder, such as membranoproliferative glomerulonephritis and focal segmental glomerulosclerosis	• Elevated blood pressure • Ascites and dependent edema • Dyspnea • Bibasilar crackles	Chronic glomerulonephritis
• Urinary frequency and urgency • Burning sensation on urination • Nocturia, cloudy hematuria, and dysuria • Lower back or flank pain	• Female patient • Recurrent urinary tract infection (UTI) • Recent chemotherapy or systemic antibiotic therapy	• Recent vigorous sexual activity • Suprapubic pain on palpation • Fever and chills • Inflamed perineal area	Cystitis
• Severe radiating pain from costovertebral angle to flank and suprapubic region and from external genitalia • Nausea and vomiting • Hematuria	• Strenuous physical activity in hot environment • Previous renal calculi • Recent kidney infection	• Fever and chills • Poor skin turgor, concentrated urine, and dry mucous membranes	Nephrolithiasis

Checking for hypocalcemia

Two signs that indicate tetany associated with hypocalcemia are Chvostek's and Trousseau's signs. To elicit these signs, follow the procedures described here. If you detect them, notify the practitioner immediately.

While conducting these tests, watch the patient for laryngospasm, monitor his cardiac status, and have resuscitation equipment nearby. Keep in mind the discomfort these tests typically cause.

Chvostek's sign

To elicit this sign, tap the patient's facial nerve just in front of the earlobe and below the zygomatic arch or between the zygomatic arch and the corner of the mouth, as shown below.

A positive response (indicating latent tetany) ranges from simple mouth-corner twitching to twitching of all facial muscles on the side tested. Simple twitching may be normal in some patients. However, a more pronounced response usually confirms Chvostek's sign.

Trousseau's sign

In this test, occlude the brachial artery by inflating a blood pressure cuff on the patient's upper arm to a level between diastolic and systolic blood pressure. Maintain this inflation for 3 minutes while observing the patient for Trousseau's sign, or carpal spasm (shown below).

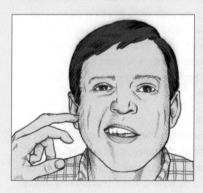

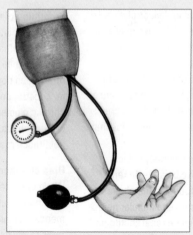

Interpreting blood studies in renal disease

Here's how you may interpret the results of blood studies used in diagnosing renal disease.

Complete blood count

An increased WBC count may indicate UTI, peritonitis (in peritoneal dialysis patients), or kidney transplantation infection and rejection.

RBC count, Hb level, and HCT decrease in a patient with chronic renal insufficiency resulting from decreased erythropoietin production by the kidneys. HCT also provides an index of fluid balance because it indicates the percentage of RBCs in the blood.

Blood urea nitrogen

Increased BUN levels may indicate glomerulonephritis, extensive pyogenic infection, oliguria (from mercuric chloride poisoning or posttraumatic renal insufficiency), tubular obstruction, or other obstructive uropathies. Because nonrenal conditions can cause BUN levels to increase, interpret BUN levels in conjunction with serum creatinine levels.

Electrolytes

Because the kidneys regulate fluid and electrolyte balance, a critically ill patient with renal disease may experience significant serum electrolyte imbalances. The most commonly measured electrolytes are:

• *calcium and phosphorus*—Calcium and phosphorus levels have an inverse relationship; when one increases, the other decreases. In renal failure, the kidneys aren't able to excrete phosphorus, resulting in hyperphosphatemia and hypocalcemia.

• *chloride*—Chloride levels relate inversely to bicarbonate levels, reflecting acid–base balance. In renal disease, elevated chloride levels suggest metabolic acidosis. Hyperchloremia occurs in renal tubular necrosis, severe dehydration, and complete renal shutdown. Hypochloremia may occur with pyelonephritis.

• *potassium*—Hyperkalemia occurs with renal insufficiency or acidosis. In renal shutdown, potassium may rapidly increase to life-threatening levels. Hypokalemia may reflect renal tubular disease.

• *sodium*—Sodium helps the kidneys regulate body fluid. Renal disease may result in the loss of sodium through the kidneys.

Serum creatinine

Serum creatinine level reflects the GFR. Renal damage is indicated more accurately by increases in serum creatinine than by BUN level.

Serum osmolality

An increase in serum osmolality with a simultaneous decrease in urine osmolality indicates diminished distal tubule responsiveness to circulating ADH.

Serum proteins

Levels of the serum protein albumin may decline sharply from loss in the urine during nephritis or nephrosis, which in turn causes edema. Nephrosis may also cause total serum protein levels to decrease.

Uric acid

Because uric acid clears from the body by glomerular filtration and tubular secretion, elevated levels may indicate impaired renal function; below-normal levels may indicate defective tubular absorption.

Creatinine clearance

Creatinine clearance indicates GFR. Typically, high creatinine clearance rates have little diagnostic value. Low creatinine clearance rates may indicate reduced renal blood flow (associated with shock or renal artery obstruction), acute tubular necrosis, acute or chronic glomerulonephritis, advanced bilateral chronic pyelonephritis, advanced bilateral renal lesions, or nephrosclerosis.

Urea clearance

While urea clearance is a less reliable measurement of GFR than creatinine clearance, it still provides a good measure of overall renal function. High urea clearance rates rarely have diagnostic value. Low urea clearance rates may reflect decreased renal blood flow, acute or chronic glomerulonephritis, advanced bilateral chronic pyelonephritis, acute tubular necrosis, nephrosclerosis, advanced bilateral renal lesions, bilateral ureteral obstruction, or dehydration.

Calculating GFRs

The National Institutes of Health has formed the National Kidney Disease Education Program (NKDEP) to help decrease the incidence of chronic renal disease progressing to renal failure. One of the first goals of the NKDEP was to encourage the use of the estimated GFR using the Modification of Diet in Renal Disease (MDRD) equation. The MDRD equation factors in serum creatinine values, age, gender, and race.

If the GFR is less than 60 over a 3-month period, it suggests chronic renal disease. A GFR less than 15 indicates renal failure.

$$GFR = 186 \times (P_{cr})^{-1.154} \times (Age)^{-0.203} \times (0.742 \text{ if female})$$

If the patient is African-American, multiply the result by 1.21 because African-Americans tend to have more muscle mass than other races.

P_{cr} = serum creatinine value

Nursing considerations
- KUB radiography requires no special pretest or posttest care. It's commonly a portable X-ray test performed at the bedside in the critical care unit.
- Explain the procedure to the patient.

Kidney CT scan

A CT scan of the kidney would be performed to evaluate for trauma or to assess for tumors, lesions, or other disease such as polycystic kidney disease or abscesses. Contrast dye may be used.

Nursing considerations
- If contrast dye is not used, then no preparation is needed.
- Explain the procedure to the patient and confirm that he isn't allergic to iodine or shellfish. A patient with these allergies may have an adverse reaction to the contrast medium. If he has a seafood or dye allergy, a pretest preparation kit with prednisone (Deltasone) and diphenhydramine (Benadryl) may be given.
- Report adverse reactions, such as nausea, vomiting, dizziness, headache, and urticaria.
- Depending on the patient's renal status, the practitioner may order increased fluids after the procedure or an increased rate of I.V. fluid infusion to flush the contrast medium out of the patient's system.
- The practitioner may also order N-acetylcysteine (Mucomyst) to help limit the damage done to the renal tissues by the contrast medium.

- After the procedure, check the patient's serum creatinine and BUN levels to evaluate renal function (contrast media can cause acute renal failure).

Renal angiography

Renal angiography is used to visualize the arterial tree, capillaries, and venous drainage of the kidneys. The test involves the use of a contrast medium injected under fluoroscopy into a catheter in the femoral artery or vein.

Angiography of arteries

Renal arteriography (angiography of the arteries) may reveal:
- abnormal renal blood flow
- hypervascular renal tumors
- renal cysts
- renal artery stenosis
- renal artery aneurysms and arteriovenous (AV) fistulas
- pyelonephritis
- renal abscesses or inflammatory masses
- renal infarction
- renal trauma.

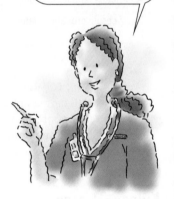

Renal arteriography may reveal disorders such as these.

Nursing considerations
- Explain the procedure to the patient and confirm that he isn't allergic to iodine or shellfish. A patient with these allergies may have an adverse reaction to the contrast medium. If he has a seafood or dye allergy, a pretest preparation kit with prednisone (Deltasone) and diphenhydramine (Benadryl) may be given.
- Preprocedure testing should include evaluation of renal function (serum creatinine and BUN) and potential risk of bleeding (prothrombin time, partial thromboplastin time, and platelet count). Notify the practitioner if results are abnormal.
- Report adverse reactions, such as nausea, vomiting, dizziness, headache, and urticaria.
- Depending on the patient's renal status, the practitioner may order increased fluids after the procedure or an increased rate of I.V. fluid infusion to flush the contrast medium out of the patient's system.
- The practitioner may also order N-acetylcysteine (Mucomyst) to help limit the damage done to the renal tissues by the contrast medium.
- After the procedure, check the patient's serum creatinine and BUN levels to evaluate renal function (contrast media can cause acute renal failure).

Renal ultrasound

Renal ultrasound is used to visualize kidney size, shape, and placement. Renal ultrasound may reveal:
- hydronephrosis
- tumors
- cysts
- abscess
- trauma.

Nursing considerations
- Explain the procedure to the patient.
- No pretest preparation is needed.
- The test may be done at the bedside if the patient is unstable.

Urine studies

Urine studies, such as urinalysis and urine osmolality, can indicate acute renal failure, renal trauma, and other disorders. Urinalysis can indicate renal or systemic disorders, warranting further investigation. A random urine specimen is used, preferably the first-voided morning specimen. (See *What urinalysis findings mean*, page 522.)

Urine osmolality is used to evaluate the diluting and concentrating ability of the kidneys and varies greatly with diet and hydration status. The ability to concentrate urine is one of the first functions lost in renal failure.

Nursing considerations
- Before urinalysis, collect a random urine specimen from the indwelling urinary catheter or, preferably, the first-voided morning specimen. Send the specimen to the laboratory immediately.
- For urine osmolality testing, collect a random urine sample, preferably the first-voided morning specimen.

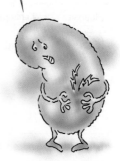

A renal disorder can affect every body system of a critically ill patient. It may be fatal without effective treatment.

Treatments

Renal disorders can adversely affect virtually every body system in a critically ill patient and may be fatal without effective treatment. Drug therapy is a treatment option in some cases, and others require dialysis of some kind.

What urinalysis findings mean

Test	Normal values or findings	Abnormal findings	Possible causes of abnormal findings
Color and odor	• Straw color	Clear to black	Dietary changes; use of certain drugs; metabolic, inflammatory, or infectious disease
	• Slightly aromatic odor	Fruity odor	Diabetes mellitus, starvation, dehydration
	• Clear appearance	Turbid appearance	Renal infection
Specific gravity	• Between 1.005 and 1.030, with slight variations from one specimen to the next	Below-normal specific gravity	Diabetes insipidus, glomerulonephritis, pyelonephritis, acute renal failure, alkalosis
		Above-normal specific gravity	Dehydration, nephrosis
		Fixed specific gravity	Severe renal damage
pH	• Between 4.5 and 8.0	Alkaline pH (above 8.0)	Fanconi's syndrome (chronic renal disease), UTI, metabolic or respiratory alkalosis
		Acidic pH (below 4.5)	Renal tuberculosis, phenylketonuria, acidosis
Protein	• No protein	Proteinuria	Renal disease (such as glomerulosclerosis, acute or chronic glomerulonephritis, nephrolithiasis, polycystic kidney disease, and acute or chronic renal failure)
Ketones	• No ketones	Ketonuria	Diabetes mellitus, starvation, conditions causing acutely increased metabolic demands and decreased food intake (such as vomiting and diarrhea)
Glucose	• No glucose	Glycosuria	Diabetes mellitus
RBCs	• 0 to 3 RBCs per high-power field	Numerous RBCs	UTI, obstruction, inflammation, trauma, or tumor; glomerulonephritis; renal hypertension; lupus nephritis; renal tuberculosis; renal vein thrombosis; hydronephrosis; pyelonephritis; parasitic bladder infection; polyarteritis nodosa; hemorrhagic disorder
Epithelial cells	• Few epithelial cells	Excessive epithelial cells	Renal tubular degeneration

What urinalysis findings mean *(continued)*

Test	Normal values or findings	Abnormal findings	Possible causes of abnormal findings
WBCs	• 0 to 4 WBCs per high-power field	Numerous WBCs	Urinary tract inflammation, especially cystitis or pyelonephritis
		Numerous WBCs and WBC casts	Renal infection (such as acute pyelonephritis and glomerulonephritis, nephrotic syndrome, pyogenic infection, and lupus nephritis)
Casts	• No casts (except occasional hyaline casts)	Excessive casts	Renal disease
		Excessive hyaline casts	Renal parenchymal disease, inflammation, glomerular capillary membrane trauma
		Epithelial casts	Renal tubular damage, nephrosis, eclampsia, chronic lead intoxication
		Fatty, waxy casts	Nephrotic syndrome, chronic renal disease, diabetes mellitus
		RBC casts	Renal parenchymal disease (especially glomerulonephritis), renal infarction, subacute bacterial endocarditis, sickle cell anemia, blood dyscrasias, malignant hypertension, collagen disease
Crystals	• Some crystals	Numerous calcium oxalate crystals	Hypercalcemia
		Cystine crystals (cystinuria)	Inborn metabolic error
Yeast cells	• No yeast crystals	Yeast cells in sediment	External genitalia contamination, vaginitis, urethritis, prostatovesiculitis
Parasites	• No parasites	Parasites in sediment	External genitalia contamination
Creatinine clearance	• Males (age 20): 90 mg/minute/1.73 m² of body surface • Females (age 20): 84 ml/minute/1.73 m² of body surface • Older patients: normally decreased concentrations (by 6 ml/minute/decade)	Above-normal creatinine clearance	Little diagnostic significance
		Below-normal creatinine clearance	Reduced renal blood flow (associated with shock or renal artery obstruction), acute tubular necrosis, acute or chronic glomerulonephritis, advanced bilateral renal lesions (as in polycystic kidney disease, renal tuberculosis, and cancer), nephrosclerosis, heart failure, severe dehydration

Drug therapy

Drug therapy for renal disorders includes such agents as alkalinizing agents, diuretics, and sulfonate cation-exchange resins to correct hyperkalemia. (See *Commonly used drugs for renal disorders.*)

Ideally, drug therapy should be effective without impairing renal function. Drugs excreted mainly by the kidneys may require dosage adjustments to prevent nephrotoxicity.

Dialysis

A critically ill patient with a renal disorder may need dialysis treatments to remove toxic waste and excess fluid from the body. Depending on the patient's condition, hemodialysis or peritoneal dialysis may be used. In addition, a hemodynamically unstable patient may be treated with continuous renal replacement therapy (CRRT).

Continuous renal replacement therapy

CRRT is used to treat a patient with acute renal failure. Unlike the more traditional intermittent hemodialysis (IHD), CRRT is administered around the clock, providing the patient with continuous therapy without the destabilizing hemodynamic and electrolytic changes of IHD.

CRRT for whom?

CRRT is used for a patient who can't tolerate traditional hemodialysis, such as one with hypotension. Also, a patient who has had abdominal surgery and can't receive peritoneal dialysis because of an overwhelming risk of infection is a candidate for CRRT. (See *Understanding CRRT*, page 526.)

CRRT ABCs

CRRT techniques vary in complexity:
* Slow continuous ultrafiltration (SCUF) uses AV access and the patient's blood pressure to circulate blood through a hemofilter. Because the goal of this therapy is fluid removal, the patient doesn't receive any replacement fluids.
* Continuous venovenous hemofiltration (CVVH) combines fluid removal with a venous blood pump. A double-lumen catheter provides access to a vein, and a pump moves blood through the hemofilter.
* In continuous venovenous hemodialysis (CVVH-D), a vein provides the access while a pump is used to move dialysate solution across the hemofilter concurrent with blood flow.

Nursing considerations
* If the patient is undergoing CRRT for the first time, explain its purpose and what to expect during treatment.

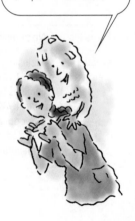

Because the goal of SCUF therapy is fluid removal, don't administer replacement fluids.

Commonly used drugs for renal disorders

Drugs	Indications	Adverse reactions	Practice pointers
Alkalinizing agent			
Sodium bicarbonate	To correct metabolic acidosis in patients with renal failure	Metabolic alkalosis, hypernatremia, local pain and irritation at the injection site, hypokalemia	• Use with caution in patients with heart failure or renal insufficiency and patients receiving corticosteroids. • Assess the patient's cardiopulmonary status. • Monitor the patient for metabolic alkalosis and electrolyte imbalance, especially hypocalcemia and hypokalemia. • Monitor the I.V. site for irritation and infiltration. (Extravasation may cause tissue damage and necrosis.)
Loop diuretics			
Bumetanide (Bumex) Furosemide (Lasix) Torsemide (Demadex)	To inhibit sodium resorption in the renal tubule, promote diuresis, and manage edema.	Dizziness, muscle cramps, hypotension, headache, fluid and electrolyte imbalance (hypokalemia, hypochloremia, and hyponatremia), electrocardiogram (ECG) changes, chest pain, renal failure	• Monitor the patient for fluid and electrolyte imbalance. • Monitor the patient for cardiac arrhythmias, especially ventricular. • Avoid using in the patient with sulfonamide hypersensitivity. • Use is contraindicated in anuria. • Be aware that ototoxicity may result with rapid I.V. administration of high dosages. • Carefully monitor the patient's intake and output.
Sulfonate cation-exchange resin			
Sodium polystyrene sulfonate (Kayexalate)	To correct hyperkalemia	GI irritation, anorexia, nausea, vomiting, constipation, hypokalemia, hypocalcemia, diarrhea	• Monitor the patient for electrolyte imbalance, hypokalemia, and hypocalcemia. • Monitor the patient for ECG changes (flat, inverted T wave and prominent U wave) and ventricular arrhythmias. • For oral administration, mix resin with water or sorbitol—never orange juice because of high potassium content. • Monitor elderly patients for constipation and fecal impaction. • Use cautiously in patients who require sodium restriction, such as those with heart failure or hypertension, to prevent the risk of sodium overload.

Understanding CRRT

CRRT filters toxic wastes from a patient's blood and may include a replacement solution. It's used to correct fluid overload that doesn't respond to diuretics and to treat critically ill patients who have acute renal failure, can't tolerate hemodialysis, or have some electrolyte and acid–base disturbances.

Hemofilter how-to

All CRRT equipment is located at the patient's bedside. The procedure doesn't require the immediate supervision of a dialysis nurse. The patient's blood may be accessed by catheter, internal AV graft, or AV shunt. The hemofilter is made up of hollow fiber capillaries that filter blood at a rate of about 150 to 300 ml per minute, driven by the patient's arterial blood pressure in continuous AV hemofiltration or by a blood pump in CVVH. Because the amount of fluid removed is greater than the patient's intake, the patient gradually loses fluid (12 to 15 L per day).

- Prime the hemofilter and tubing according to the manufacturer's instructions. (See *Setup for CVVH.*)
- Assist with catheter insertion, if necessary, using strict sterile technique.
- If ordered, flush the catheters with a heparin flush solution to prevent clotting.

Get dressed

- Apply occlusive dressings to the insertion sites and mark the dressings with the date and time.
- Before treatment, weigh the patient, take baseline vital signs, and make sure all necessary laboratory studies have been done (usually electrolyte levels, coagulation factors, CBC, BUN, and creatinine studies).
- Monitor the patient's vital signs and oxygen saturation.
- If a pulmonary artery (PA) catheter has been placed, assess the patient's hemodynamic parameters, including central venous pressure (CVP), pulmonary artery pressure (PAP), and pulmonary artery wedge pressure (PAWP).
- Be alert for indications of hypovolemia (such as decreasing blood pressure and decreases in PAP, CVP, and PAWP) from too rapid removal of ultrafiltrate or hypervolemia due to excessive fluid replacement with a decrease in ultrafiltrate.

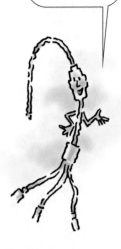

Flush the catheters with a heparin flush solution to prevent clotting.

Setup for CVVH

CRRT is typically performed using CVVH. For this technique, the doctor inserts a special double-lumen catheter into a large vein, commonly the subclavian, femoral, or internal jugular vein. Because the catheter is in a vein, an external pump is used to move blood through the system. The patient's venous blood moves through the "arterial" lumen to the pump, which then pushes the blood through the catheter to the hemofilter. Here, water and toxic solutes (ultrafiltrate) are removed from the patient's blood and drain into a collection device. Blood cells aren't removed because they are too large to pass through the filter. As the blood exits the hemofilter, it's then pumped through the "venous" lumen back to the patient.

Several components of the pump provide safety mechanisms. Pressure monitors on the pump maintain the flow of blood through the circuit at a constant rate. An air detector traps air bubbles before the blood returns to the patient. A venous trap collects blood clots that may be in the blood. A blood leak detector signals when blood is found in the dialysate; a venous clamp operates if air is detected in the circuit or if there's disconnection in the blood line.

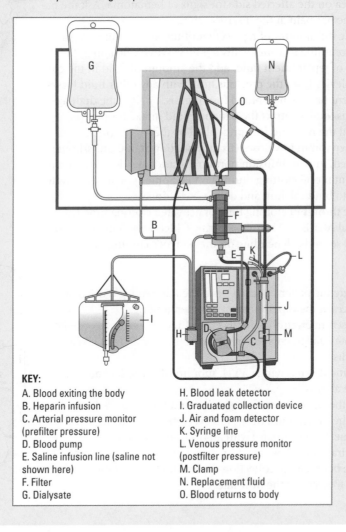

KEY:

A. Blood exiting the body
B. Heparin infusion
C. Arterial pressure monitor (prefilter pressure)
D. Blood pump
E. Saline infusion line (saline not shown here)
F. Filter
G. Dialysate

H. Blood leak detector
I. Graduated collection device
J. Air and foam detector
K. Syringe line
L. Venous pressure monitor (postfilter pressure)
M. Clamp
N. Replacement fluid
O. Blood returns to body

- Provide continuous cardiac monitoring because arrhythmias can occur with electrolyte imbalances.
- Monitor the patient's weight and vital signs frequently.

Color is key

- Inspect the ultrafiltrate during the procedure. It should remain clear yellow, with no gross blood.
- Pink-tinged or bloody ultrafiltrate may signal a membrane leak in the hemofilter, which permits bacterial contamination. With a CVVH system, look for the blood leak detector to signal this. If a leak occurs, notify the doctor so the hemofilter can be replaced.
- Assess the leg used for vascular access for signs of obstructed blood flow, such as coolness, pallor, and weak pulse. Check the groin area on the affected side for signs of hematoma. Ask the patient if he has pain at the insertion sites.
- Calculate the amount of replacement fluid every hour or as ordered, according to your facility's policy. When calculating the amount of replacement fluid, add the amount of fluid in the collection device from the previous hour with any other fluid losses the patient has, such as blood loss, emesis, or NG tube drainage. From this total, subtract the patient's fluid intake for the past hour and the net fluid loss prescribed by the practitioner.
- Infuse heparin in low doses (usually starting at 500 units/hour), as ordered, into an infusion port on the arterial side of the setup to prevent blood clotting during CVVH. Some systems use citrate instead to bind calcium and decrease clotting.
- Measure thrombin clotting time or activated clotting time (ACT). A normal ACT is 100 seconds; during CRRT, keep it between 100 and 300 seconds, depending on the patient's clotting times.

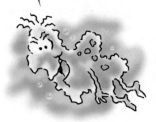

I'm in! A membrane leak in the hemofilter could permit bacterial contamination.

No bending allowed

- Make sure the patient doesn't bend the affected leg more than 30 degrees at the hip to prevent catheter kinking.
- Obtain serum electrolyte levels every 4 to 6 hours or as ordered; anticipate adjustments in replacement fluid or dialysate based on the results.
- If the patient is receiving CVVH, monitor the arterial and venous pressure alarms.
- Inspect the site dressing for infection and bleeding. Perform skin care at the catheter insertion sites every 48 hours, using sterile technique. Cover the sites with an occlusive dressing.
- If the ultrafiltrate flow rate decreases, raise the bed to increase the distance between the collection device and the hemofilter. Lower the bed to decrease the flow rate.

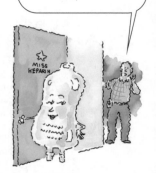

Five minutes to curtain call, Miss Heparin.

- Clamping the ultrafiltrate line is contraindicated with some types of hemofilters because pressure may build up in the filter, clotting it and collapsing the blood compartment.
- Record the time the treatment begins, fluid balance figures, vital signs, weight, times of dressing changes, complications, medications given, and the patient's tolerance of the procedure. Document patient assessment parameters when the treatment course has ended.

Hemodialysis

Hemodialysis is used to remove toxic wastes and other impurities from the blood of a patient with renal failure. It's also used to restore or maintain acid–base and electrolyte balance and prevent the complications associated with uremia. To do so, this method extracts the by-products of protein metabolism—notably urea and uric acid—as well as creatinine and excess water from the patient's blood.

Blood, out and back

During hemodialysis, the patient's blood is removed from the body through a surgically created access site, pumped through a dialyzing unit to remove toxins, and then returned to the body.

Osmosis, diffusion, and filtration

The extracorporeal dialyzer works through a combination of osmosis, diffusion, and filtration. (See *How hemodialysis works*, page 530.)

Acute use or long-term therapy

Hemodialysis can be done in an emergency in acute renal failure or as regular long-term therapy in end-stage renal disease. In chronic renal failure, the frequency and duration of treatments depend on the patient's condition; up to several treatments per week, each lasting 3 to 4 hours, may be required. Rarely, hemodialysis is done to treat acute poisoning or drug overdose.

Specially trained nurses usually perform the procedure in a hemodialysis unit; in the critically ill patient, it's performed at the bedside using portable equipment.

Nursing considerations

- If the patient is undergoing hemodialysis for the first time, explain its purpose and what to expect during and after treatment. Explain that he'll first undergo a procedure to create a vascular access. (See *Hemodialysis access sites*, page 531.)

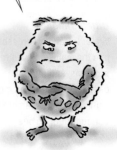

Here's how hemodialysis works: Blood is removed from the body, toxins are removed, and then the blood is returned to the body.

How hemodialysis works

In hemodialysis, blood flows from the patient to an external dialyzer (or artificial kidney) through an arterial access site.

Inside the dialyzer

Inside the dialyzer, blood and dialysate flow countercurrently, divided by a semipermeable membrane. The composition of the dialysate resembles normal extracellular fluid. The blood contains an excess of specific solutes (such as metabolic waste products and electrolytes), and the dialysate contains electrolytes that may be at abnormal levels in the patient's bloodstream. The dialysate's electrolyte composition can be modified to raise or lower electrolyte levels, depending on the patient's needs.

Diffusion

Excretory function and electrolyte homeostasis are achieved by diffusion—the movement of molecules across the dialyzer's semipermeable membrane—from an area of higher solute concentration to an area of lower concentration.

Ultrafiltration

Water (a solvent) crosses the membrane from the blood into the dialysate by ultrafiltration. Excess water, waste products, and other metabolites are removed through osmotic pressure, the movement of water across the semipermeable membrane from an area of lesser solute concentration to one of greater solute concentration, and

hydrostatic pressure, which forces water from the blood compartment into the dialysate compartment.

After it's cleaned of impurities and excess water, the blood returns to the body through a venous site.

Three systems

Three system types are used to deliver dialysate:
1. The proportioning system—the most common type—mixes concentrate with water to form dialysate, which then circulates through the dialyzer and goes down a drain after a single pass, followed by fresh dialysate.
2. The batch system uses a reservoir for circulating dialysate.
3. The regenerative system uses sorbents to purify and regenerate recirculating dialysate.

Hollow-filter dialyzer

The hollow-filter dialyzer contains fine capillaries with a semipermeable membrane enclosed in a plastic chamber. Blood flows through these capillaries as the system pumps dialysate in the opposite direction on the outside of the capillaries.

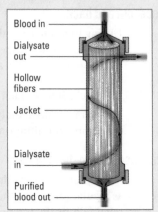

Blood in

Dialysate out

Hollow fibers

Jacket

Dialysate in

Purified blood out

Access obtained

After vascular access
- Weigh the patient, take his vital signs, and assess breath and heart sounds. Check for edema and jugular vein distention.
- Use good hand-washing technique and wear protective eyewear, gown, and gloves during the hemodialysis procedure.
- Discard (don't recap) all needles used in the procedure in designated containers.
- Assess the vascular access site for the presence of a bruit and thrill and keep the vascular access site well-supported and resting on a sterile drape or sterile barrier shield.

Hemodialysis access sites

Hemodialysis requires vascular access through a subclavian or femoral vein or an AV fistula or graft. The site and type of access used depend on the expected duration of dialysis, the surgeon's preference, and the patient's condition.

Subclavian vein catheterization

Using the Seldinger technique, the doctor or surgeon inserts an introducer needle into the subclavian vein. He then inserts a guide wire through the introducer needle and removes the needle. Using the guide wire, he then threads a 5" to 12" (12.5 to 30.5 cm) plastic or Teflon catheter with a Y-hub into the patient's vein.

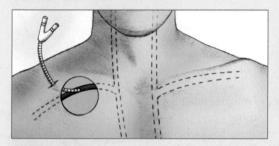

Femoral vein catheterization

Using the Seldinger technique, the doctor or surgeon inserts an introducer needle into the right or left femoral vein. He then inserts a guide wire through the introducer needle and removes the needle. Using the guide wire, he then threads a 5" to 12" plastic or Teflon catheter with a Y-hub or two catheters—one for inflow and another, placed about $1/2$" (1.3 cm) distal to the first, for outflow.

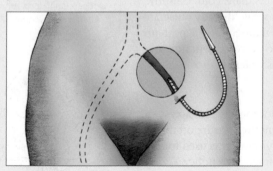

AV fistula

To create an AV fistula, the surgeon makes an incision in the patient's wrist or lower forearm, then a small incision in the side of an artery and another in the side of a vein. He then sutures the edges of the incisions together to make a common opening approximately 1" to 3" (2.5 to 7.5 cm) long.

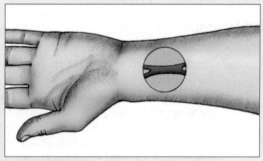

AV graft

To create a graft, the surgeon makes an incision in the patient's forearm, upper arm, or thigh. He then tunnels a natural or synthetic graft under the skin and sutures the distal end to an artery and the proximal end to a vein.

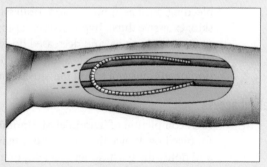

- As ordered, prepare the hemodialysis equipment. Follow the manufacturer's and your facility's protocols and maintain strict sterile technique to prevent the introduction of pathogens into the patient's bloodstream during treatment.
- Check and record the patient's vital signs every 30 minutes or according to your facility's policy, during treatment to detect possible complications. Fever may point to infection from pathogens in the dialysate or equipment; give an antipyretic, an antibiotic, or both, as ordered. Hypotension may indicate hypovolemia or a drop in HCT; give blood or fluid supplements I.V., as ordered. Rapid respirations may signal hypoxemia or fluid overload. Assess breath sounds and oxygen saturation and give supplemental oxygen, as ordered.

> Assess your patient for headache and other problems caused by rapid fluid removal and electrolyte changes.

He's got rhythm

- Monitor the patient's cardiac rhythm for arrhythmias that may result from electrolyte and pH changes in the blood due to hemodialysis.
- Periodically check the dialyzer blood lines to make sure all connections are secure. Monitor the lines for clotting.
- Assess the patient for headache, muscle twitching, backache, nausea or vomiting, and seizures, which may indicate disequilibrium syndrome caused by rapid fluid removal and electrolyte changes.
- If disequilibrium syndrome occurs, notify the practitioner immediately; he may reduce the blood flow rate or stop dialysis. Muscle cramps may also result from rapid fluid and electrolyte shifts. As ordered, relieve cramps by injecting normal saline solution into the venous return line.
- Observe the patient carefully for signs and symptoms of internal bleeding, such as apprehension; restlessness; pale, cold, clammy skin; excessive thirst; hypotension; rapid, weak, thready pulse; increased respirations; and decreased body temperature. Report any of these signs immediately and prepare to decrease heparinization or administer a blood transfusion, as ordered.

> Make sure the arm used for vascular access isn't used for another procedure.

Patient access

- After completion of hemodialysis, monitor the vascular access site for bleeding. If bleeding is excessive, maintain pressure on the site and notify the practitioner. If a temporary catheter is used for dialysis, flush the catheter according to your facility's policy.
- Make sure that the arm used for vascular access isn't used for another procedure, including I.V. line insertion, blood pressure monitoring, and venipuncture.

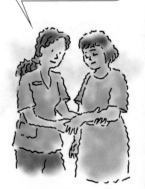

- Assess circulation at the access site by auscultating for the presence of bruits and palpating for thrills. Lack of bruits at a vascular access site for dialysis may indicate a blood clot, requiring immediate surgical attention.
- Keep an accurate record of the patient's food and fluid intake and encourage him to comply with prescribed restrictions, such as increased calorie intake; decreased fluid intake; and limited protein, potassium, and sodium intake.

Peritoneal dialysis

Like hemodialysis, peritoneal dialysis is used to remove toxins from the blood of a patient with acute or chronic renal failure who doesn't respond to other treatments. Unlike hemodialysis, peritoneal dialysis uses the patient's peritoneal membrane as a semipermeable dialyzing membrane.

How it's done

In peritoneal dialysis, the dialysate (the solution instilled into the peritoneal cavity by catheter) draws waste products, excess fluid, and electrolytes from the blood across the semipermeable peritoneal membrane. (See *Principles of peritoneal dialysis*, page 534.) After a prescribed period, the dialysate is drained from the peritoneal cavity, removing impurities with it. The dialysis procedure is then repeated, using a new dialysate each time, until waste removal is complete and fluid, electrolyte, and acid–base balance has been restored.

With special preparation, the critical care nurse may perform peritoneal dialysis using an automatic or semiautomatic cycle machine.

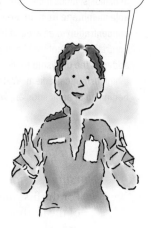

Peritonitis results when bacteria enter the peritoneal cavity through the catheter or insertion site.

Upside

Peritoneal dialysis has several advantages over hemodialysis—it's simpler, less costly, and less stressful. Also, it's nearly as effective as hemodialysis while posing fewer risks.

Downside

Even so, peritoneal dialysis can cause severe complications. The most serious one, peritonitis, results from bacteria entering the peritoneal cavity through the catheter or the insertion site. In addition to causing infection, peritonitis can scar the peritoneum, causing thickening of the membrane and preventing its use as a dialyzing membrane.

Other complications include catheter obstruction from clots, lodging against the abdominal wall, or kinking; hypotension; and hypovolemia from excessive plasma fluid removal.

Principles of peritoneal dialysis

Peritoneal dialysis works through a combination of diffusion and osmosis.

Diffusion

In diffusion, particles move through a semipermeable membrane from an area of high solute concentration to an area of low solute concentration. In peritoneal dialysis, the water-based dialysate being infused contains glucose, sodium chloride, calcium, magnesium, acetate or lactate, and no waste products. Therefore, waste products and excess electrolytes in the blood cross through the semipermeable peritoneal membrane into the dialysate. Removing the waste-filled dialysate and replacing it with fresh solution keeps the waste concentration low and encourages further diffusion.

Osmosis

In osmosis, fluids move through a semipermeable membrane from an area of low solute concentration to an area of high solute concentration. In peritoneal dialysis, dextrose is added to the dialysate to give it a higher solute concentration than the blood, creating a high osmotic gradient. Water migrates from the blood through the membrane at the beginning of each infusion, when the osmotic gradient is highest.

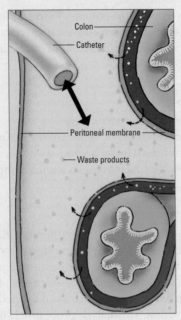

Colon

Catheter

Peritoneal membrane

Waste products

Nursing considerations

- For the first-time peritoneal dialysis patient, explain the purpose of the treatment and what he can expect during and after the procedure.
- Explain that the doctor first inserts a catheter into the abdomen to allow instillation of dialysate. (See *Comparing peritoneal dialysis catheters.*)
- Before catheter insertion, take and record the patient's baseline vital signs and weight.
- Ask the patient to urinate to reduce the risk of bladder perforation and increase comfort during catheter insertion. If he can't

Comparing peritoneal dialysis catheters

The first step in any type of peritoneal dialysis is the insertion of a catheter to allow instillation of dialyzing solution. The doctor may insert a Tenckhoff, Swan neck, or Toronto-Western Hospital (TWH) catheter.

Tenckhoff catheter

To implant a Tenckhoff catheter, the doctor inserts the first 6³/₄" (17.1 cm) of the catheter into the patient's abdomen. The next 2³/₄" (7-cm) segment, which may have a Dacron cuff at one or both ends, is imbedded subcutaneously. Within a few days after insertion, the patient's tissues grow around the cuffs, forming a tight barrier against bacterial infiltration. The remaining 3⁷/₈" (9.8 cm) of the catheter extends outside of the abdomen and is equipped with a metal adapter at the tip that connects to dialyzer tubing.

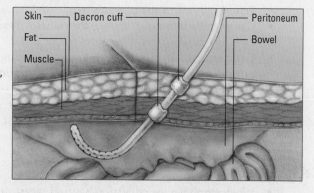

Swan neck catheter

To insert a Swan neck (or flanged collar) catheter, the doctor positions the collar just below the dermis so that the device extends through the abdominal wall. He keeps the distal end of the cuff from extending into the peritoneum, where it could cause adhesions.

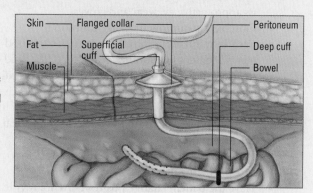

TWH catheter

To insert a TWH catheter, the doctor rolls up the flexible disk section of the implant, inserts it into the peritoneal cavity, and retracts it against the abdominal wall. The implant's first cuff rests just outside the peritoneal membrane and its second cuff rests just under the skin. Because the TWH catheter doesn't float freely in the peritoneal cavity, it prevents inflowing dialyzing solution from being directed at the sensitive organs, which increases patient comfort during dialysis.

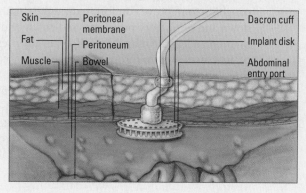

urinate, perform straight catheterization, as ordered, to drain the bladder.
- During dialysis, monitor the patient's vital signs every 10 minutes until they stabilize, then every 2 to 4 hours or as ordered. Report any abrupt or significant changes.
- Periodically check the patient's weight and report any gain.
- Using sterile technique, change the catheter dressing every 24 hours or whenever it becomes wet or soiled.
- To determine whether a wet abdominal dressing around the catheter site is from leakage of dialysate or wound drainage, use a dextrose test strip. Because of its high dextrose content, dialysate reacts positively while wound drainage doesn't.
- Monitor the patient for signs of infection. (See *Check for signs of peritonitis*.)

Collecting the empties
- When emptying the collection bag and measuring the solution, wear protective eyewear and gloves.
- Observe the outflow drainage for blood.
- Keep in mind that drainage is commonly blood-tinged after catheter placement but should clear after a few fluid exchanges. Notify the practitioner of bright red or persistent bleeding.
- Watch the patient for respiratory distress, which may indicate fluid overload or leakage of dialyzing solution into the pleural space. If it's severe, drain the patient's peritoneal cavity and call the practitioner.
- Periodically check the outflow tubing for clots or kinks that may be obstructing drainage.
- Have the patient change position often. Provide passive range-of-motion (ROM) exercises and encourage deep breathing and coughing to improve comfort, reduce the chance of skin breakdown and respiratory problems, and enhance dialysate drainage.
- Maintain adequate nutrition, following any prescribed diet. The patient loses protein through the dialysis procedure and, therefore, requires protein replacement.
- To prevent fluid imbalance, calculate the patient's fluid balance at the end of each dialysis session or after every 8-hour period in a longer session. Include oral and I.V. fluid intake as well as urine output, wound drainage, and perspiration. Record and report any significant imbalance, whether positive or negative.

Take charge!

Check for signs of peritonitis

If you detect signs or symptoms of peritonitis, notify the practitioner and send a dialysate specimen to the laboratory for smear and culture.

Watch closely for these signs and symptoms:
- fever
- persistent abdominal pain and cramping
- slow or cloudy dialysis drainage
- swelling and tenderness around the catheter
- increased WBC count.

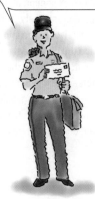

Return to sender! The patient loses protein through dialysis and requires protein replacement.

Renal system disorders

The most common renal disorders seen in critical care units include acute kidney injury (AKI) and acute tubular necrosis.

Acute kidney injury

AKI is the sudden interruption of renal function resulting from:
- obstruction
- reduced circulation
- renal parenchymal disease.

AKI is sometimes reversible, but if it's left untreated, permanent damage can lead to chronic renal failure. As a critical care nurse, you play a vital role in assessing and treating patients with AKI.

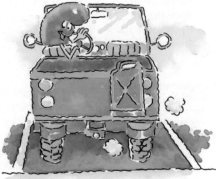

AKI is sometimes reversible.

What causes it

Acute AKI may be classified as prerenal, intrarenal, or postrenal. Each type has different causes. (See *Causes of AKI*, page 538.)

How it happens

Each classification of AKI—prerenal, intrarenal, and postrenal—has its own pathophysiology:
- *Prerenal failure* results from conditions that diminish blood flow to the kidneys (hypoperfusion). Examples include hypovolemia, hypotension, vasoconstriction, or inadequate cardiac output. One condition, prerenal azotemia (excess nitrogenous waste products in the blood), accounts for 40% to 80% of all cases of AKI. Azotemia occurs as a response to renal hypoperfusion. Typically, it can be rapidly reversed by restoring renal blood flow and glomerular filtration.
- *Intrarenal failure*, also called *intrinsic* or *parenchymal* kidney injury, results from damage to the filtering structures of the kidneys, usually from acute tubular necrosis, a disorder that causes cell death, or from nephrotoxic substances, such as certain antibiotics or radiologic dyes.
- *Postrenal failure* results from bilateral obstruction of urine outflow, as in prostatic hyperplasia or bladder outlet obstruction.

Causes of AKI

AKI is classified as prerenal, intrarenal, or postrenal. All conditions that lead to prerenal failure impair blood flow to the kidneys (renal perfusion), resulting in a decreased GFR and increased tubular resorption of sodium and water. Intrarenal failure results from damage to the kidneys. Postrenal failure results from obstructed urine flow. The causes of each type of AKI are listed here.

Prerenal failure	Intrarenal failure	Postrenal failure
Cardiovascular disorders	**Acute tubular necrosis**	**Bladder obstruction**
• Arrhythmias • Cardiac tamponade • Cardiogenic shock • Heart failure • Myocardial infarction	• Ischemic damage to renal parenchyma from unrecognized or poorly treated prerenal failure • Nephrotoxins, including analgesics; anesthetics such as methoxyflurane; antibiotics such as gentamicin (Garamycin); heavy metals such as lead; radiographic contrast media; and organic solvents	• Anticholinergic drugs • Autonomic nerve dysfunction • Infection • Tumor
Hypovolemia		**Ureteral obstruction**
• Burns • Dehydration • Diuretic overuse • Hemorrhage • Hypovolemic shock • Trauma	• Obstetric complications, such as eclampsia, postpartum renal failure, septic abortion, and uterine hemorrhage • Myoglobin release, such as crush injury, myopathy, sepsis, and transfusion reaction	• Blood clots • Calculi • Edema vor inflammation • Necrotic renal papillae • Retroperitoneal fibrosis or hemorrhage • Surgery (accidental ligation) • Tumor • Uric acid crystals
Peripheral vasodilation	**Other parenchymal disorders**	
• Antihypertensive drugs • Sepsis	• Acute glomerulonephritis • Acute interstitial nephritis • Acute pyelonephritis	**Urethral obstruction**
Renovascular obstruction	• Bilateral renal vein thrombosis • Malignant nephrosclerosis	• Prostatic hyperplasia or tumor • Strictures
• Arterial embolism • Arterial or venous thrombosis • Tumor	• Papillary necrosis • Periarteritis nodosa (inflammatory disease of the arteries) • Renal myeloma	
Severe vasoconstriction	• Sickle cell disease • Systemic lupus erythematosus • Vasculitis	
• Disseminated intravascular coagulation • Eclampsia • Malignant hypertension • Vasculitis		

Going through phases

With treatment, the patient passes through three distinct phases:
1. oliguric (decreased urine output)
2. diuretic (increased urine output)
3. recovery.

Output down

Oliguria is a decreased urine output (less than 400 ml/24 hours).
Prerenal oliguria results from decreased blood flow to the kidney.

Before damage occurs, the kidney responds to decreased blood flow by conserving sodium and water. Once damage occurs, the kidney's ability to conserve sodium is impaired. Untreated prerenal oliguria may lead to acute tubular necrosis.

During this phase, BUN and creatinine rise, and the ratio of BUN to creatinine falls from 20:1 (normal) to 10:1. Hypervolemia also occurs, causing edema, weight gain, and elevated blood pressure.

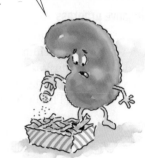

Output up

The diuretic phase is marked by urine output that can range from normal (1 to 2 L per day) to as great as 4 to 5 L per day. High urine volume has two causes, including:
- the kidney's inability to conserve sodium and water
- osmotic diuresis produced by high BUN levels.

During the diuretic phase, which lasts several days to 1 week, BUN and creatinine levels slowly increase and hypovolemia and weight loss result. These conditions can lead to deficits of potassium, sodium, and water that can be deadly if left untreated. If the cause of the diuresis is corrected, azotemia gradually disappears and the patient improves greatly—leading to the recovery stage.

On the road to recovery . . .

The recovery phase is reached when BUN and creatinine levels return to normal and urine output is between 1 and 2 L per day.

It gets complicated . . .

Primary damage to the renal tubules or blood vessels results in kidney failure (intrarenal failure). The causes of intrarenal failure are classified as nephrotoxic, inflammatory, or ischemic.

Irreparable damage

When nephrotoxicity or inflammation causes the damage, the delicate layer under the epithelium (basement membrane) becomes irreparably damaged, commonly proceeding to chronic renal failure.

Severe or prolonged lack of blood flow (ischemia) may lead to renal damage (ischemic parenchymal injury) and excess nitrogen in the blood (intrinsic renal azotemia).

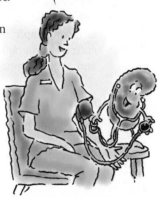

What to look for

The signs and symptoms of prerenal failure depend on the cause. If the underlying problem is a decrease in blood pressure and volume, the patient may have:
- oliguria
- tachycardia
- hypotension

- dry mucous membranes
- flat jugular veins
- lethargy progressing to coma
- decreased cardiac output and cool, clammy skin in a patient with heart failure.

Negative progress

As AKI progresses, the patient may show signs and symptoms of uremia, including:
- confusion
- GI complaints
- fluid in the lungs
- infection.

About 5% of all hospitalized patients develop AKI. The condition is usually reversible with treatment; however, if it isn't treated, it may progress to end-stage renal disease, excess urea in the blood (prerenal azotemia or uremia), and death.

What tests tell you

These tests are used to diagnose AKI:
- Blood studies reveal elevated BUN, serum creatinine, and potassium levels and decreased blood pH, bicarbonate, HCT, and Hb levels.
- Urine studies show casts, cellular debris, decreased specific gravity, and, in glomerular diseases, proteinuria and urine osmolality close to serum osmolality. Urine sodium level is less than 20 mEq/L if oliguria results from decreased perfusion and more than 40 mEq/L if it results from an intrarenal problem.
- Arterial blood gas analysis reveals decreased pH and bicarbonate levels, indicating metabolic acidosis.
- Creatinine clearance testing is used to measure the GFR and estimate the number of remaining functioning nephrons.
- ECG shows tall, peaked T waves, a widening QRS complex, and disappearing P waves if increased blood potassium (hyperkalemia) is present.
- Other studies used to determine the cause of AKI include kidney ultrasonography, plain films of the abdomen, KUB radiography, excretory urography, renal scan, retrograde pyelography, CT scan, and nephrotomography.

How it's treated

Supportive measures include a diet high in calories and low in protein, sodium, and potassium, with supplemental vitamins and restricted fluids. Meticulous electrolyte monitoring is essential to detect hyperkalemia.

Send in the drugs

Drug therapy for AKI may include:

- sodium bicarbonate and hypertonic glucose and insulin infusions administered I.V., sodium polystyrene sulfonate (Kayexalate) by mouth or by enema, and calcium gluconate (in an emergency) to reduce potassium levels
- diuretics to manage hypervolemia
- fluid replacement to correct hypovolemia.

Overload overview

Even with treatment, an elderly patient is susceptible to volume overload, possibly precipitating acute pulmonary edema, hypertensive crisis, hyperkalemia, and infection.

If hyperkalemia can't be reduced with drugs, acute therapy may include dialysis. To control uremic symptoms, hemodialysis or peritoneal dialysis may be necessary. CVVH is an alternative hemodialysis technique for treatment of AKI.

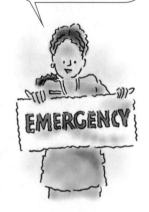

Calcium gluconate may be given in an emergency to reduce your patient's potassium levels.

What to do

- If the patient is to receive a diuretic, be sure to obtain a urine sample for urine studies before giving the diuretic because these drugs can alter urine results.
- Measure and record the patient's intake and output hourly, including wound drainage, NG tube output, and diarrhea. Insert an indwelling urinary catheter if indicated. Assess skin turgor; evidence of peripheral, sacral, or periorbital edema; and degree of pitting, if any. Monitor the patient's daily weight for trends.
- Check urine specific gravity and osmolality, as ordered. With prerenal failure, urine specific gravity is typically greater than 1.020 and urine osmolality is increased up to 500 mOsm; with intrarenal failure, specific gravity is typically less than 1.010 and osmolality is approximately 350 mOsm.
- If the patient is hemodynamically unstable, the insertion of a PA catheter may be used to assess the patient's hemodynamic status. Monitor parameters, as ordered.
- Assess Hb levels and HCT and replace blood components, as ordered.

Whole lotta blood

- Don't use whole blood to transfuse the patient if he's prone to heart failure and can't tolerate extra fluid volume. Packed RBCs deliver the necessary blood components without added volume.

- Assess the patient's cardiopulmonary status often, including heart and breath sounds. Monitor his cardiac rhythm. Report any short-ness of breath, crackles, gallops, pericardial friction rub, tachycar-dia, or the presence of S_3 heart sounds because these may be signs of fluid overload.
- Monitor the patient's level of consciousness at least every 2 to 4 hours, or more often if indicated.
- Maintain proper electrolyte balance. Strictly monitor the patient's potassium levels, especially during emergency treatment to reduce potassium levels. Avoid administering drugs containing potassium.
- Watch the patient for symptoms of hyperkalemia (malaise, anorexia, paresthesia, or muscle weakness) and ECG changes (tall, peaked T waves; widening QRS complex; and disappearing P waves) and report them immediately.
- Provide a high-calorie, low-protein, low-potassium, low-sodium diet, with vitamin supplements. Give anorectic patients small, frequent meals.
- Use sterile technique when performing procedures because a criti-cally ill patient with renal failure is highly susceptible to infection.
- Encourage coughing and deep breathing and perform passive ROM exercises to reduce complications of bed rest.
- Consult the pharmacy regarding modifying the dose to account for the patient's impaired renal function.

Dry no more

- Use a lubricating lotion to combat dry skin. Provide mouth care frequently because mucous membranes become dry.
- Assess the patient for signs and symptoms of GI bleeding. Administer drugs carefully, especially antacids and stool softeners. Use aluminum hydroxide–based antacids; magnesium-based ant-acids can cause serum magnesium levels to increase critically.
- Use appropriate safety measures, such as side rails or assistance with ambulation, because the patient with central nervous system involvement may be dizzy or confused. Institute bleeding precau-tions to minimize the patient's risk for bleeding.
- Provide appropriate care to a patient receiving hemodialysis, peri-toneal dialysis, or CRRT. Provide emotional support to the patient and his family and explain diagnostic tests, treatments, and proce-dures. Caring for the patient with AKI requires the involvement of a multidisciplinary team. (See *Meet the team*.)

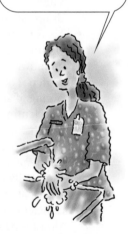

Use sterile technique when performing procedures on a critically ill patient with renal failure. He's at high risk for infection.

Acute tubular necrosis

Acute tubular necrosis (also called *acute tubulointerstitial nephritis*) causes 75% of all cases of AKI. This disorder destroys the tubular

Meet the team

Because AKI affects multiple body systems, a multidisciplinary approach to care is needed, with the critical care nurse coordinating care.

Here's how other members of the multidisciplinary team contribute to your patient's care:

- A nephrologist can evaluate and manage the patient's kidney function.
- A respiratory or cardiology specialist may be involved to deal with complications.
- A nutritional therapist may recommend restrictions or supplements.
- A physical or occupational therapist may help the patient with energy conservation and rehabilitation.
- A pharmacist can assist with medication dosing.
- If a prolonged hospital stay is expected and the patient requires long-term care or home care, social services should be consulted early in the patient's care.
- The patient and his family may benefit from spiritual counseling.

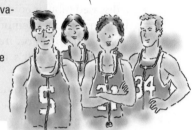

Go team! You need to coordinate care for a patient with AKI.

segment of the nephron, causing renal failure and uremia (excess by-products of protein metabolism in the blood). Because acute tubular necrosis can be fatal in up to 40% to 70% of cases, prevention, prompt recognition, and intervention by the critical care nurse are vital.

What causes it

Acute tubular necrosis may follow two types of kidney injury:

1. *Ischemic* injury, the most common cause, interrupts blood flow to the kidneys. The longer the blood flow is interrupted, the worse the kidney damage.
2. *Nephrotoxic* injury usually affects debilitated patients, such as the critically ill and those who have undergone extensive surgery.

Blood disruption

In ischemic injury, blood flow to the kidneys may be disrupted by:

- circulatory collapse
- severe hypotension
- trauma
- hemorrhage
- dehydration
- cardiogenic or septic shock
- surgery
- anesthetics
- transfusion reactions.

Toxic talk

Nephrotoxic injury can result from:
- ingesting or inhaling toxic chemicals, such as carbon tetrachloride, heavy metals, and methoxyflurane anesthetics
- a hypersensitivity reaction of the kidneys to such substances as antibiotics and radiographic contrast agents.

Cause and effect

Some specific causes of acute tubular necrosis and their effects include:
- a diseased tubular epithelium that allows glomerular filtrate to leak through the membranes and be resorbed into the blood
- obstructed urine flow from the collection of damaged cells, casts, RBCs, and other cellular debris in the tubules
- ischemic injury to glomerular epithelial cells, causing cellular collapse and poor glomerular capillary permeability
- ischemic injury to the vascular endothelium, eventually causing cellular swelling and tubular obstruction.

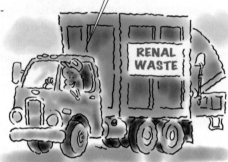

Nephrotoxic injury can result from ingesting or inhaling toxic chemicals.

How it happens

Deep or shallow lesions may occur in acute tubular necrosis.

Lesion lesson

With ischemic injury, necrosis creates deep lesions, destroying the tubular epithelium and basement membrane (the delicate layer underlying the epithelium). Ischemic injury causes patches of necrosis in the tubules. Ischemia can also cause lesions in the connective tissue of the kidney.

With nephrotoxic injury, necrosis occurs only in the epithelium of the tubules, leaving the basement membrane of the nephrons intact. This type of damage may be reversible. (See *A close look at acute tubular necrosis.*)

Toll-taking

Toxicity takes a toll on renal structures. Nephrotoxic agents can injure tubular cells by:
- direct cellular toxic effects
- coagulation and destruction (lysis) of RBCs
- oxygen deprivation (hypoxia)
- crystal formation of solutes.

A close look at acute tubular necrosis

In acute tubular necrosis caused by ischemia, patches of necrosis occur, usually in the straight portions of the proximal tubules.

In areas without lesions, tubules are usually dilated. In acute tubular necrosis caused by nephrotoxicity, the tubules have a more uniform appearance.

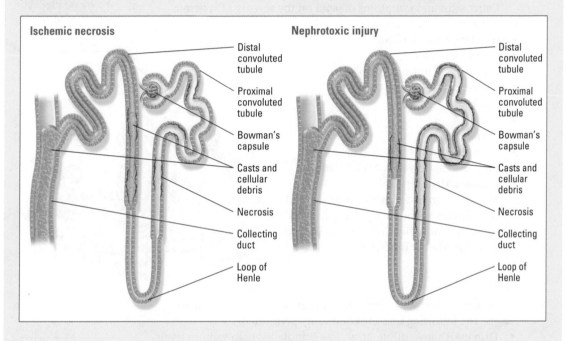

Ischemic necrosis

- Distal convoluted tubule
- Proximal convoluted tubule
- Bowman's capsule
- Casts and cellular debris
- Necrosis
- Collecting duct
- Loop of Henle

Nephrotoxic injury

- Distal convoluted tubule
- Proximal convoluted tubule
- Bowman's capsule
- Casts and cellular debris
- Necrosis
- Collecting duct
- Loop of Henle

Getting complicated

There are several common complications of acute tubular necrosis:
- Infections (frequently septicemia) complicate up to 70% of all cases and are the leading cause of death.
- GI hemorrhage, fluid and electrolyte imbalance, and cardiovascular dysfunction may occur during the acute or recovery phase.
- Neurologic complications are common in elderly patients and occur occasionally in younger patients.
- Excess blood calcium (hypercalcemia) may occur during the recovery phase.

What to look for

Early-stage acute tubular necrosis may be hard to spot because the patient's primary disease may obscure the signs and symptoms. The first recognizable sign may be decreased urine output, usually less than 400 ml/24 hours.

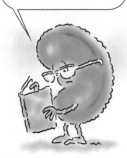

Common complications of acute tubular necrosis include infections, GI hemorrhage, and hypercalcemia.

Difficult to detect

Acute tubular necrosis is difficult to detect in its early stages, so look closely at members of high-risk populations, such as elderly patients or those with diabetes, and be alert for subtle signs and symptoms during your nursing assessments.

Other signs and symptoms depend on the severity of systemic involvement and may include:
- bleeding abnormalities
- vomiting of blood
- dry skin and mucous membranes
- lethargy
- confusion
- agitation
- edema
- fluid and electrolyte imbalances
- muscle weakness with hyperkalemia
- cardiac arrhythmias.

Mortality can be as high as 70%, depending on complications from underlying diseases. The patient with a nonoliguric form of acute tubular necrosis has a better prognosis.

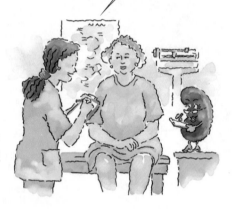

Acute tubular necrosis is difficult to detect in its early stages, so look closely at patients who are members of high-risk groups, such as elderly people.

What tests tell you

Acute tubular necrosis is difficult to diagnose except in advanced stages. The following tests are commonly performed:
- Urinalysis shows dilute urine, low osmolality, high sodium levels, and urine sediment containing RBCs and casts.
- Blood studies reveal high BUN and serum creatinine levels, low serum protein levels, anemia, platelet adherence defects, metabolic acidosis, and hyperkalemia.
- ECG may show arrhythmias from electrolyte imbalances and, with hyperkalemia, a widening QRS complex; disappearing P waves; and tall, peaked T waves.

How it's treated

The patient with acute tubular necrosis requires vigorous supportive measures during the acute phase until normal kidney function is restored. Therapy may include:
- diuretics and fluids to flush tubules of cellular casts and debris and to replace lost fluids (initially)
- emergency I.V. infusion of 50% glucose, regular insulin, and sodium bicarbonate in case of hyperkalemia

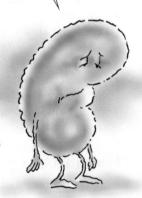

All this talk about vigorous treatment has tired me out!

- sodium polystyrene sulfonates given by mouth or by enema to reduce potassium levels
- calcium channel blockers and prostaglandins, which may aid in treating nephrotoxic acute tubular necrosis.

Furthermore

Treatment for the patient with acute tubular necrosis may also include:
- daily replacement of projected and calculated fluid losses
- transfusion of packed RBCs for anemia
- non-nephrotoxic antibiotics for infection
- hemodialysis or peritoneal dialysis to prevent severe fluid and electrolyte imbalance and uremia.

What to do

- Take steps to maintain the patient's fluid balance. Accurately record intake and output, including wound drainage, NG tube output, and hemodialysis or peritoneal dialysis balances. Weigh the patient daily.
- Assist with insertion of a central venous or PA catheter to monitor fluid status. Monitor hemodynamic parameters as indicated.
- Watch the patient for fluid overload, a common complication when infusing large fluid volumes.
- Monitor Hb levels and HCT and administer blood products, as needed. Use fresh packed RBCs instead of whole blood to prevent fluid overload and heart failure.
- Maintain electrolyte balance. Monitor laboratory results and report imbalances.
- Monitor the patient's vital signs, oxygen saturation, cardiac rhythm, and cardiopulmonary status. Treat hypotension immediately to avoid renal ischemia. Monitor vital signs closely. Fever and chills may signal the onset of an infection, which is the leading cause of death in acute tubular necrosis. (See *Temperature regulation in elderly patients*, page 548.)
- Check for potassium content in prescribed drugs (e.g., potassium penicillin). Provide dietary restriction of foods containing sodium and potassium, such as bananas, orange juice, and baked potatoes.
- Provide adequate calories and essential amino acids while restricting protein intake to maintain an anabolic state. Total parenteral nutrition may be indicated for a critically ill and debilitated or catabolic patient.
- Use sterile technique, especially when handling catheters, because the critically ill or debilitated patient is vulnerable to infection.
- Administer sodium bicarbonate, as ordered, for acidosis or assist with dialysis in severe cases.

- Provide the patient with reassurance and emotional support. Encourage him and his family to verbalize their concerns. Fully explain each procedure.
- To prevent acute tubular necrosis, make sure the patient is well hydrated before surgery or after X-rays requiring use of a contrast medium. Administer mannitol, as ordered, to the high-risk criti- cally ill patient before and during these procedures. Administer nephrotoxic drugs cautiously and avoid using contrast dyes in the high-risk patient.

Quick quiz

1. The kidneys secrete erythropoietin when:
    A. oxygen supply in tissue decreases.
    B. calcium levels are insufficient.
    C. vitamin D becomes inactive.
    D. pH level drops below 7.35.

Answer: A. The kidneys secrete erythropoietin when the oxygen supply in tissue decreases.

2. In peritoneal dialysis, particles move through a semipermeable membrane from an area of high solute concentration to an area of low solute concentration in a process called:
    A. diffusion.
    B. active transport.
    C. permission.
    D. osmosis.

Answer: A. Diffusion is the movement of particles through a semi- permeable membrane from an area of high solute concentration to an area of low solute concentration. In peritoneal dialysis, waste products and excess electrolytes in the blood cross through the semi- permeable peritoneal membrane into the dialysate through diffusion.

3. Prerenal failure results from:
    A. bilateral obstruction of urine outflow.
    B. conditions that diminish blood flow to the kidneys.
    C. damage to the kidneys.
    D. ischemic damage to renal parenchyma.

Answer: B. Prerenal failure is caused by any condition that reduces blood flow to the kidneys, such as hypotension, hypovolemia, vaso- constriction, and inadequate cardiac output.

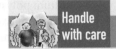
Handle with care

Temperature regulation in elderly patients

The aging process changes a person's temperature regulation system, making tempera- ture an unreliable sign of infection. Even with a clinical infection, an older person may regis- ter no fever. Furthermore, an older adult is at higher risk for infection because of age-related changes in immunity and increased incidence of hospitalization, which can lead to nosocomial infections.

4. Acute tubular necrosis following ischemic renal injury may be due to:
    A. fluid volume overload.
    B. inhaling toxic chemicals.
    C. a hypersensitivity reaction to radiographic contrast agents.
    D. severe hypotension.

Answer: D. Acute tubular necrosis may follow ischemic or nephro-toxic injury to the kidney. Ischemic injury may be caused by severe hypotension as well as circulatory collapse, trauma, hemorrhage, de-hydration, surgery, anesthetics, transfusion reactions, and cardiogenic or septic shock.

Scoring

☆☆☆   If you answered all four questions correctly, take a dip in a kidney-shaped pool. Your information-filtering system is intact.

☆☆   If you answered three questions correctly, try to resorb what you've read. With a little concentration, you can detoxify your thinking and restore balance through work and play regulation.

☆   If you answered fewer than three questions correctly, don't expel yourself. Reread the chapter to flush out the facts and then take the test again.

Suggested References

Bellomo, R., Kellum, J. A., & Ronco, C. (2012). Acute kidney injury. *The Lancet, 380*(9843), 756–766.

Burns, S. M., & Chulay, M. (2010). *AACN essentials of critical care nursing* (2nd ed.). New York, NY: McGraw-Hill.

Jarvis, C. (2011). *Physical examination and health assessment* (6th ed.). St. Louis, MO: Mosby.

McCance, K. L., & Huether, S. E. (Eds.). (2013). *Pathophysiology: The biologic basis for disease in adults and children* (7th ed.). St. Louis, MO: Mosby.

Schneider, A. G., Bellomo, R., Bagshaw, S. M., Glassford, N. J., Lo, S., Jun, M., . . . Gallagher, M. (2013). Choice of renal replacement therapy modality and dialysis dependence after acute kidney injury: A systematic review and meta-analysis. *Intensive Care Medicine, 39*(6), 987–997.

Chapter 8

Endocrine system

Just the facts

In this chapter, you'll learn:

♦ structure and function of the endocrine system

♦ assessment of the endocrine system

♦ diagnostic tests and treatments for critically ill patients

♦ endocrine system disorders and related nursing care.

Understanding the endocrine system

The endocrine system regulates and integrates the body's metabolic activities and maintains internal homeostasis. It has three major components:

1. glands, which are specialized organs that produce, store, and secrete hormones and chemical transmitters into the bloodstream to regulate body functions
2. hormones, which are chemical substances secreted by glands in response to stimulation from the nervous system, other hormones, and other sites
3. receptors, which are protein molecules that trigger specific physiologic changes in target cells in response to hormonal stimulation.

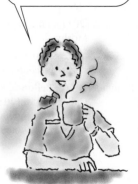

Simply put, the endocrine system regulates metabolism and maintains homeostasis.

Glands

The major glands of the endocrine system are the: (See *Endocrine gland sites*.)

• pituitary gland
• thyroid gland
• parathyroid glands
• adrenal glands
• pancreas

Endocrine gland sites

The illustration below shows the location of the major endocrine glands (except the gonads).

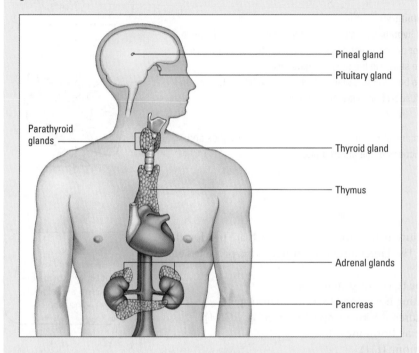

- Pineal gland
- Pituitary gland

Parathyroid glands

- Thyroid gland

- Thymus

- Adrenal glands

- Pancreas

- thymus
- pineal gland
- gonads.

Pituitary gland

The pituitary gland rests in the sella turcica, a depression in the sphenoid bone at the base of the brain. It's connected by the infundibulum to the hypothalamus, from which it receives chemical and nervous stimulation. (See *Understanding the hypothalamus*, page 552.)

Powerful pea

The pea-sized pituitary gland has two regions, or lobes: posterior and anterior. The posterior pituitary lobe stores and releases

Understanding the hypothalamus

The hypothalamus integrates the endocrine and autonomic nervous systems. It controls some endocrine gland functions through neural and hormonal stimulation.

Pathways to the posterior pituitary

Neural pathways connect the hypothalamus to the posterior pituitary gland. These neurons stimulate the posterior pituitary gland to secrete two effector hormones—ADH and oxytocin—which are stored in the posterior pituitary.

When ADH is secreted, the body retains water. Oxytocin stimulates uterine contractions during labor and milk secretion in lactating women.

Inhibition and stimulation

The hypothalamus produces many other inhibiting and stimulating hormones and other factors that regulate functions of the anterior pituitary.

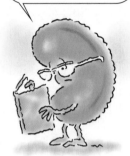

The hypothalamus integrates the endocrine and autonomic nervous systems.

oxytocin and antidiuretic hormone (ADH), which are produced by the hypothalamus. The larger anterior pituitary lobe produces at least six hormones:

1. growth hormone (GH), or somatotropin
2. thyroid-stimulating hormone (TSH), or thyrotropin
3. corticotropin (adrenal corticotropic hormone or ACTH)
4. follicle-stimulating hormone (FSH)
5. luteinizing hormone (LH)
6. prolactin.

Thyroid gland

The thyroid gland is directly beneath the larynx and partly in front of the trachea. It has two lobes—one on either side of the trachea—connected by a strip of tissue called the *isthmus*, which gives the gland a butterfly shape. (See *A close look at the thyroid gland*.)

Metabolism master

The thyroid gland regulates the body's metabolism and produces three hormones:

1. triiodothyronine (T_3)
2. thyroxine (T_4)
3. calcitonin.

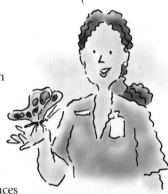

The thyroid gland is shaped like a butterfly . . . I'm sure it isn't as colorful though.

A close look at the thyroid gland

This illustration shows the structure and location of the thyroid gland.

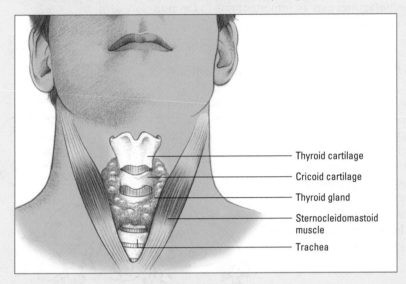

Thyroid cartilage

Cricoid cartilage

Thyroid gland

Sternocleidomastoid muscle

Trachea

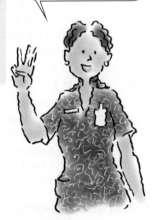

Three thyroid hormones regulate metabolism and blood calcium levels: T_3, T_4, and calcitonin.

T_3 and T_4 work together to regulate cellular metabolism. Calcitonin maintains blood calcium levels by inhibiting calcium release from bone.

Parathyroid glands

There are four parathyroid glands, one in each corner of the thyroid gland. Together, they produce parathyroid hormone (PTH) or parathormone, which maintains the body's calcium levels by traveling to three target tissue types:
1. bone to regulate the deposit and resorption of calcium from bone
2. GI tissue to influence the absorption of calcium from the small intestine
3. renal tissue to regulate the excretion of calcium.

Adrenal glands

There are two adrenal glands, one above each kidney. Each adrenal gland has an inner layer (the medulla) and an outer layer (the cortex).

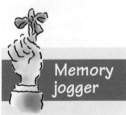

Memory jogger

To remember the location of the adrenal glands, think "add-renal" because they're "added" to the renal organs, the kidneys.

Innie

The adrenal medulla produces catecholamines (primarily epinephrine and norepinephrine) and is considered a neuroendocrine structure because catecholamines play an important role in the autonomic (involuntary) nervous system.

Outie

The adrenal cortex is the larger, outer layer and has three zones, or cell layers:

1. zona glomerulosa, the outermost zone, which produces mineralocorticoids, primarily aldosterone
2. zona fasciculata, the middle and largest zone, which produces the glucocorticoids cortisol (hydrocortisone), cortisone, and corticosterone and small amounts of the sex hormones androgen and estrogen
3. zona reticularis, the innermost zone, which produces mainly glucocorticoids and some sex hormones.

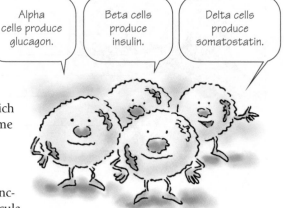

Alpha cells produce glucagon.

Beta cells produce insulin.

Delta cells produce somatostatin.

Pancreas

The pancreas has endocrine and exocrine functions. Endocrine means released into the circulatory system and therefore the hormone can act on tissue all over the body. Exocrine means released via a duct and therefore it acts locally. It's located behind the stomach, extending to the spleen and within the duodenal curve.

Visit the islets of Langerhans

The islets of Langerhans distributed in the distal pancreas perform the endocrine function and contain alpha, beta, and delta cells. Alpha cells produce glucagon; beta cells, insulin; and delta cells, somatostatin.

Thymus

The thymus is located behind the sternum and contains lymphatic tissue. This gland produces hormones (thymosin and thymopoietin), but its major role is related to the immune system: It produces T cells, which are involved in cell-mediated immunity.

Pineal gland

The tiny pineal gland lies at the back of the third ventricle of the brain. It produces the hormone melatonin, which regulates a person's sleep–wake cycles and plays a role in mood regulation and the female reproductive cycle.

Gonads

The gonads include the:
- ovaries (in females)
- testes (in males).

Feminine function

The ovaries promote the development and maintenance of female sex-related traits, regulate the menstrual cycle, and maintain the uterus for pregnancy. With the help of other hormones, they also prepare the mammary glands for lactation.

Masculine mode

The testes produce spermatozoa and the male sex hormone testosterone. Testosterone stimulates and maintains male sex-related traits.

Hormones

Hormones can be structurally classified into three types:
1. amines
2. polypeptides
3. steroids.

Amenable amines

Amines are derived from tyrosine, an essential amino acid found in most proteins. They include the thyroid hormones (T_3 and T_4) and the catecholamines (epinephrine, norepinephrine, and dopamine). Amines bind to receptor sites on cell walls, which enables them to produce rapid changes within the cell. Think amine means quick response.

Poly want a peptide?

Polypeptides are protein compounds made of many amino acids connected by peptide bonds. More complex molecules than amines, the polypeptides have a slower response. They include:
- anterior pituitary hormones (somatotropin [GH], TSH, corticotropin, FSH, LH, melanocyte-stimulating hormone, and prolactin)
- posterior pituitary hormones (ADH and oxytocin)
- PTH
- pancreatic hormones (insulin and glucagon).

Steroidal secretions

Steroids, derived from cholesterol, include:
- adrenocortical hormones (aldosterone and cortisol) secreted by the adrenal cortex
- sex hormones (estrogen and progesterone in females and testosterone in males) secreted by the gonads.

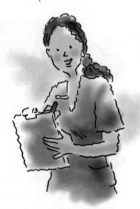

Amines are derived from tyrosine, an essential amino acid found in most proteins.

Hormone release and transport

All hormone release results from endocrine gland stimulation, but release patterns vary greatly:
- Corticotropin (secreted by the anterior pituitary lobe) and cortisol (secreted by the adrenal cortex) are released in irregular spurts in response to body rhythm cycles, with levels peaking in the early morning.
- Secretion of PTH (by the parathyroid gland) and prolactin (by the anterior pituitary) occurs fairly evenly throughout the day.
- Secretion of insulin by the pancreas has both steady and sporadic release patterns in response to glucose levels. (See *Endocrine changes with aging*.)

Hormone function

When a hormone reaches its target site, it binds to a specific receptor on the cell membrane or in the cell:
- Polypeptides and some amines bind to membrane receptor sites.
- Smaller, more lipid-soluble steroids and thyroid hormones diffuse through cell membranes and bind to intracellular receptors.

Handle with care

Endocrine changes with aging

A common endocrine change in older adults is a decreased ability to tolerate stress.

Age matters

When stress stimulates an older person's pancreas, the blood glucose concentration increases more and remains elevated longer than in a younger adult. Such diminished glucose tolerance is a normal part of aging. Keep this in mind when evaluating an older person for diabetes.

If coma develops

Older adults rarely become ketoacidotic, even with extremely elevated blood glucose levels. When coma develops, it's usually from hyperosmolar hyperglycemic nonketotic syndrome (HHNS), which can be triggered by acute illness (such as a urinary tract infection or pneumonia) or surgery in older adults.

Other changes

Other normal variations in endocrine function include a decreased cortisol secretion rate and decline in serum aldosterone levels. Changes in endocrine function during menopause vary from woman to woman, but normally, estrogen levels diminish and FSH production increases. In men, testosterone levels decrease at a later age and often at a slower rate.

Right on target!

After binding to the receptor, each hormone produces a unique physiologic change, depending on the target site and the hormone's action at that site. A particular hormone may produce different effects at different target sites.

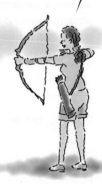

When a hormone reaches its target site, it binds to a receptor on the cell membrane or in the cell.

Hormonal regulation

Hormonal regulation is a complex feedback mechanism involving hormones, the central nervous system, and blood chemicals and metabolites that maintain the body's delicate equilibrium by regulating hormone synthesis and secretion. (Feedback is information sent to endocrine glands that signals the need for changes in hormone levels, either increasing or decreasing hormone production and release.) (See *The feedback loop*, page 558.)

Heart and hormones

The heart has a role in endocrine function. In the walls of the atria, there are cells that produce atrial natriuretic hormone (ANH), also referred to as *atrial natriuretic peptide*. The atria secrete ANH in response to increased atrial wall stretching due to increased blood pressure or blood volume. ANH causes increased renal excretion of sodium and water, thus reducing blood volume and blood pressure.

ANH reduces blood volume and pressure by increasing sodium and water excretion by the kidneys.

Endocrine system assessment

To assess the patient's endocrine system, take an accurate health history and conduct a thorough physical examination. When an acutely ill patient with an endocrine disorder arrives in the critical care unit, the information you obtain from the health history, physical examination, and diagnostic tests are used to treat and stabilize the patient. After the patient is stable, you may obtain additional data.

Health history

Because the endocrine system interacts with all other body systems, conduct a complete body systems review. Ask the patient about overall patterns of health and illness.

The feedback loop

This diagram depicts the negative feedback mechanism that regulates the endocrine system.

From simple ...

Simple feedback occurs when the level of one substance regulates the secretion of hormones (simple loop). For example, a low serum calcium level stimulates the parathyroid gland to release PTH. PTH, in turn, promotes resorption of calcium. A high serum calcium level inhibits PTH secretion.

... to complex

When the hypothalamus receives negative feedback from target glands, the mechanism is more complicated (complex loop). *Complex feedback* occurs through an axis established between the hypothalamus, pituitary gland, and target organ. For example, secretion of corticotropin-releasing hormone from the hypothalamus stimulates release of corticotropin by the pituitary, which, in turn, stimulates cortisol secretion by the adrenal gland (the target organ). A rise in serum cortisol levels inhibits corticotropin secretion by decreasing corticotropin-releasing hormone.

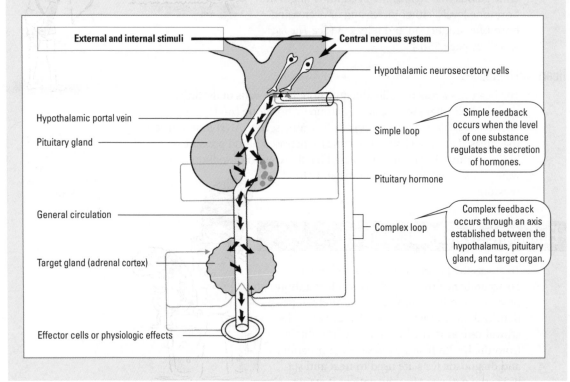

Current health status

Ask the patient to describe his chief complaint. Common complaints associated with endocrine disorders include fatigue, weakness, weight changes, mental status changes, polyuria, polydipsia, and abnormalities of sexual maturity and function.

Ask questions

Be sure to ask the patient these questions:
- Have you noticed any changes in your skin?
- Do you bruise more easily than you used to?
- Have you noticed any change in the amount or distribution of your body hair?
- Do your eyes burn or feel gritty when you close them?
- How good is your sense of smell?

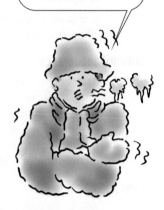

Intolerance of cold may indicate hypothyroidism . . .

Previous health status

Ask about the patient's medical history. You may identify insidious and vague symptoms of endocrine dysfunction if the patient has had a skull fracture, surgery, complications of surgery, or brain infection, such as meningitis or encephalitis.

Family history

Ask about the patient's family history because some endocrine disorders, such as diabetes mellitus and thyroid disease, are inherited or have strong familial tendencies.

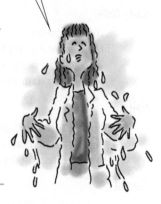

. . . and intolerance of heat may indicate hyperthyroidism.

Lifestyle patterns

Ask the patient about temperature intolerance, which may indicate certain thyroid disorders. For example, intolerance of cold may indicate hypothyroidism and intolerance of heat, hyperthyroidism.

Physical assessment

Include a total body evaluation and complete neurologic assessment in the physical examination because the hypothalamus plays an important role in regulating endocrine function.

Permissive condition

If the patient's condition permits, begin by measuring height, weight, and vital signs. Measure blood pressure with the patient lying, sitting, and standing. Compare the findings with normal expected values and the patient's baseline measurements, if available. Then use inspection, palpation, and auscultation to obtain the most objective findings.

Inspection

Systematically inspect the patient's overall appearance and examine all areas of the body.

Outward appearance

Assess the patient's physical appearance and mental and emotional status. Note such factors as affect, speech, level of consciousness (LOC), orientation, appropriateness and neatness of dress and grooming, and activity level. Evaluate general body development, including posture, body build, proportionality of body parts, and distribution of body fat.

Skin deep

Assess the patient's overall skin color and inspect the skin and mucous membranes for lesions or areas of increased, decreased, or absent pigmentation. As you do so, be sure to consider racial and ethnic variations. In a dark-skinned patient, color variations are best assessed in the sclera, conjunctiva, mouth, nail beds, and palms. Next, assess the patient's skin texture and hydration.

Hairy topic

Inspect the hair for amount, distribution, condition, and texture. Observe scalp and body hair for abnormal patterns of growth or hair loss. Remember to consider normal racial, ethnic, and sex-related differences in hair growth and texture.

Nail it

Next, check the patient's fingernails for cracking, peeling, separation from the nail bed (onycholysis), and clubbing; observe the toenails for fungal infection, ingrown nails, discoloration, length, and thickness.

Face it

Assess the patient's face for overall color and the presence of erythematous areas, especially in the cheeks. Note facial expression. Is it pained and anxious, dull and flat, or alert and interested? Note the shape and symmetry of the eyes and look for eyeball protrusion (exophthalmos), incomplete eyelid closure, and periorbital edema. Have the patient extend his tongue and inspect it for color, size, lesions, positioning, and tremors or unusual movements.

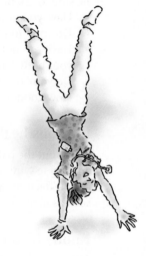

Inspect the patient's outward appearance from head to toe.

Neck check

While standing in front of the patient, examine the neck—first with it held straight, then slightly extended. Check for neck symmetry and midline positioning and for symmetry of the trachea.

Use tangential lighting directed downward from the patient's chin to see the thyroid gland. An enlarged thyroid may be diffuse and asymmetrical.

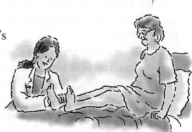

Examine the patient's feet for size and other characteristics.

Chest check

Evaluate the overall size, shape, and symmetry of the patient's chest, noting any deformities. In females, assess the breasts for size, shape, symmetry, pigmentation (especially on the nipples and in skin creases), and nipple discharge (galactorrhea). In males, observe for bilateral or unilateral breast enlargement (gynecomastia) and nipple discharge.

Go to extremes

Inspect the patient's extremities. Check the arms and hands for tremors. To do so, have the patient hold both arms outstretched in front with the palms down and fingers separated. Place a sheet of paper on the outstretched fingers and watch for trembling.

Note any muscle wasting, especially in the upper arms. Have the patient grasp your hands to assess the strength and symmetry of his grip.

Next, inspect the legs for muscle development, symmetry, color, and hair distribution. Examine the feet for size and note lesions, corns, calluses, and marks from socks or shoes. Inspect the toes and the spaces between them for maceration and fissures.

Palpation

Palpate the thyroid gland if possible. When you can palpate it, the gland should be smooth, finely lobulated, nontender, and either soft or firm. You should be able to feel the gland's sections. (See *Palpating the thyroid*, page 562.)

A thyroid nodule feels like a knot, protuberance, or swelling; a firm, fixed nodule may be a tumor. Be careful not to confuse thick neck musculature with an enlarged thyroid or a goiter.

Search for signs

Attempt to elicit Chvostek's sign and Trousseau's sign if you suspect a patient has hypocalcemia (low serum calcium levels) related to deficient or ineffective PTH secretion from hypoparathyroidism or surgical removal of the parathyroid glands.

To elicit Chvostek's sign, tap the facial nerve in front of the ear with a finger; if the facial muscles contract toward the ear, the test is positive for hypocalcemia.

Palpating the thyroid

To palpate the thyroid, follow these steps:
• Stand in front of the patient and place your index and middle fingers below the cricoid cartilage on both sides of the trachea.
• Palpate for the thyroid isthmus as he swallows.
• Then ask the patient to flex his neck toward the side being examined as you gently palpate each lobe.

In most cases, only the isthmus connecting the two lobes is palpable. However, if the patient has a thin neck, you may feel the whole gland. If he has a short, stocky neck, you may have trouble palpating even an enlarged thyroid.

Right and left

To locate the right lobe, follow these steps:
• Use your right hand to displace the thyroid cartilage slightly to your left.
• Hook your left index and middle fingers around the sternocleidomastoid muscle, as shown at right, to palpate for thyroid enlargement.

Then examine the left lobe by using your left hand to displace the thyroid cartilage and your right hand to palpate the lobe.

Palpating the right lobe

Sternocleidomastoid muscles

Thyroid cartilage

Thyroid gland

Isthmus

Trachea

To elicit Trousseau's sign, place a blood pressure cuff on the arm and inflate it above the patient's systolic pressure. In a positive test, the patient exhibits carpal spasm (ventral contraction of the thumb and digits) within 3 minutes.

Auscultation

If you palpate an enlarged thyroid, auscultate the gland for systolic bruits, a sign of hyperthyroidism. Bruits are heard when accelerated blood flow through the thyroid arteries produces vibrations.

Two techniques

To auscultate for bruits, place the bell of the stethoscope over one of the lateral lobes of the thyroid and then listen carefully for a low, soft, rushing sound. To ensure that tracheal sounds don't obscure bruits, have the patient hold his breath while you auscultate.

To distinguish a bruit from a venous hum, first listen for the rushing sound, then gently occlude the jugular vein with your fingers

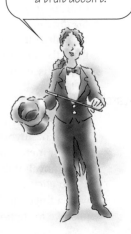

Abracadabra! A venous hum disappears during venous compression, a bruit doesn't.

on the side you are auscultating, and listen again. A venous hum (produced by jugular blood flow) disappears during venous compression, a bruit doesn't.

Diagnostic tests

Various tests are used to suggest, confirm, or rule out an endocrine disorder. Some test results also identify a dysfunction as hyperfunction or hypofunction or indicate whether a problem is primary, secondary, or functional. (See *Common endocrine laboratory studies*, pages 564 to 566.) Endocrine function is tested through direct and indirect testing and imaging studies.

Direct and indirect testing

Direct and indirect testing measure hormone levels or substances controlled by hormones. When test results are borderline, provocative testing may be done. (See *Provocative testing*.)

Direct testing

The most common method, direct testing, is used to measure hormone levels in the blood or urine. Accurate measurement requires special techniques because the body contains only minute amounts of hormones.

Methods of direct testing used to measure hormone levels in the blood and urine are:
- immunoradiometric assays (IRMAs)
- radioimmunoassay (RIA)
- 24-hour urine testing (needed to evaluate when the levels increase and decrease throughout the day).

IRMA and ICMA

IRMAs measure peptide and protein hormone levels using a receptor antiserum labeled with radioiodine.

Immunochemiluminometric assays (ICMAs) use a chemical reagent that emits a specific light wavelength when activated by a particular substance. IRMA and ICMA tests are more specific, stable, precise, and easier to use than RIAs.

Turn up the radioimmunoassay

RIA determines many hormone levels by incubating blood or urine (or a urine extract) with the hormone's antibody and a radiolabeled hormone tracer (antigen). Antibody-tracer complexes are then measured.

For example, charcoal absorbs and removes a hormone not bound to its antibody-antigen complex. Measuring the remaining

Provocative testing

Provocative testing is used to determine an endocrine gland's reserve function when other tests show borderline hormone levels or don't quite pinpoint the site of the abnormality. For instance, an abnormally low cortisol level may indicate adrenal hypofunction or indirectly reflect pituitary hypofunction.

Provocative principle
Provocative testing works on this principle: Stimulate an underactive gland and suppress an overactive gland, depending on the patient's suspected disorder. A hormone level that doesn't increase with stimulation confirms primary hypofunction. Hormone secretion that continues after suppression confirms hyperfunction.

Common endocrine laboratory studies

When a patient exhibits signs and symptoms of an endocrine disorder, laboratory studies provide valuable clues to the possible cause, as shown in the table below. (*Note:* Keep in mind that abnormal findings may stem from a problem unrelated to the endocrine system.) Remember that values differ among laboratories; check the normal range for the specific laboratory.

Test and purpose	Normal findings	Abnormal findings	Possible causes of abnormal findings
Blood tests			
Calcium Used to detect bone and para-thyroid disorders	8.2 to 10.2 mg per dl	Above normal level	Parathyroid tumors, hyperparathyroidism
		Below normal level	Hypoparathyroidism
Catecholamine Used to assess adrenal medulla function Epinephrine, supine	0 to 110 pg per ml	Above normal level	Pheochromocytoma
Epinephrine, standing	0 to 140 pg per ml		
Norepinephrine, supine	70 to 750 pg per ml		
Norepinephrine, standing	200 to 1,700 pg per ml		
Cortisol Used to evaluate adrenocortical function	8 a.m.: 9 to 35 mcg per dl 4 p.m.: 3 to 12 mcg per dl (Usually, the 4 p.m. level is half the 8 a.m. level.)	Above normal level	Cushing's disease, Cushing's syndrome
		Below normal level	Addison's disease
Glucose tolerance test, oral Used to detect diabetes mellitus and hypoglycemia	160 to 180 mg per dl within 1 hour of oral glucose test dose; returns to fasting levels or lower within 3 hours	Above normal level	Cushing's disease, pheochro-mocytoma, diabetes mellitus
		Below normal level	Addison's disease, hypo-thyroidism, hypopituitarism, hypoglycemia
Glycosylated hemoglobin Used to monitor the degree of glucose control in diabetes mel-litus over 3 months	<6% of total hemo-globin—good control	Above normal level	Uncontrolled diabetes mellitus

Common endocrine laboratory studies *(continued)*

Test and purpose	Normal findings	Abnormal findings	Possible causes of abnormal findings
Blood tests (continued)			
Gonadotropin (FSH, LH) Used to distinguish a primary gonadal problem from pituitary insufficiency	*Males* FSH: 5 to 20 mIU per ml LH: 5 to 20 mIU per ml	Above normal level	Primary gonadal failure
	Females FSH: Follicular phase, 5 to 20 mIU per ml Midcycle peak, 15 to 30 mIU per ml Luteal phase, 5 to 15 mIU per ml Postmenopausal, >50 mIU/ml LH: Follicular phase, 5 to 15 mIU per ml Midcycle peak, 30 to 60 mIU per ml Luteal phase, 5 to 15 mIU per ml Postmenopausal, 50 to 100 mIU per ml	Below normal level	Pituitary insufficiency
GH radioimmunoassay Used to evaluate GH oversecretion	*Males:* <5 ng/ml	Above normal level	Pituitary or hypothalamic tumor; diabetes mellitus
	Females: <10 ng/ml	Below normal level	Pituitary infarction
Insulin-induced hypoglycemia Used to detect hypopituitarism	GH increase two to three times greater than baseline.	Below normal level of GH	Hypopituitarism
Parathyroid hormone Used to evaluate parathyroid function	10 to 50 pg per ml	Above normal level	Hyperparathyroidism
		Below normal level	Hypoparathyroidism

(continued)

Common endocrine laboratory studies *(continued)*

Test and purpose	Normal findings	Abnormal findings	Possible causes of abnormal findings
Blood tests (continued)			
Phosphorus Used to detect parathyroid disorders and renal failure	2.7 to 4.5 mg per dl	Above normal level	Hypoparathyroidism, renal failure, diabetic ketoacidosis (DKA)
		Below normal level	Hyperparathyroidism
Thyroid-stimulating hormone Used to detect primary hypothyroidism	<15 IU/ml	Above normal level	Hypothyroidism, thyroid cancer
		Below normal level	Hyperthyroidism
T_4 radioimmunoassay Used to evaluate thyroid function and monitor iodine or antithyroid therapy	5 to 15 mcg per dl	Above normal level	Hyperthyroidism
		Below normal level	Hypothyroidism
T_3 radioimmunoassay Used to detect hyperthyroidism if T_4 levels are normal	80 to 200 ng per dl	Above normal level	Hyperthyroidism
		Below normal level	Hypothyroidism
Urine studies			
Cortisol Used to measure free cortisol to evaluate adrenocortical function	<50 mg/24 hour	Above normal level	Cushing's disease
17-hydroxycorticosteroid Used to evaluate adrenal function	*Males:* 4.5 to 12 mg per 24 hour	Above normal level	Cushing's syndrome, pituitary tumor
	Females: 2.5 to 10 mg per 24 hour	Below normal level	Hypopituitarism, Addison's disease
17-ketosteroid Used to evaluate adrenocortical and gonadal function	*Males:* 10 to 25 mg per 24 hour	Above normal level	Congenital adrenal hyperplasia
	Females: 4 to 6 mg per 24 hour	Below normal level	Adrenal insufficiency

radiolabeled complex indicates the extent to which the sample hormone blocks binding, compared with a standard curve showing reactions with known hormone quantities. Although the RIA method provides reliable results, it doesn't measure every hormone.

All-day affair

A 24-hour urine test may be ordered to confirm adrenal, renal, and gonadal disorders. Because these hormones are secreted at varying rates during the day, a 24-hour total is more reflective of function. Metabolite measurement is used to evaluate hormones excreted in virtually undetectable amounts.

Nursing considerations

For direct testing, hormone measurement may include serum or urine collection. Provide appropriate teaching:

- Venipuncture will be done to collect blood. Tell the patient when this will be done and who will do it.
- Accurate testing may require several blood samples taken at different times of the day because physiologic factors—such as stress, diet, episodic secretions, and body rhythms—can change circulating hormone levels.
- Urine is collected for 24 hours using the appropriate collection device. If a specimen is accidentally discarded, the collection must be restarted.

Indirect testing

Indirect testing is used to measure the substance controlled by a hormone—not the hormone itself. For example, glucose measurements are used to evaluate insulin levels and calcium measurements are used to assess PTH activity. Although RIAs measure these substances directly, indirect testing is easier and less costly.

Not so fast

Glucose levels obtained indirectly accurately reflect insulin's effectiveness. Even so, various factors that affect calcium may alter PTH levels and, thus, results of indirect testing.

For example, abnormal protein levels can lead to seemingly abnormal calcium levels because nearly half of calcium binds to plasma proteins. Therefore, other possibilities must be ruled out before assuming that an abnormal calcium level reflects a PTH imbalance.

Nursing considerations

For indirect testing, hormone measurement may include serum or urine collection. Provide appropriate teaching:

- Venipuncture will be done to collect blood. Tell the patient when this will be done and who will do it.

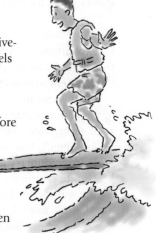

Thinking imbalance? Rule out other possible causes of abnormal calcium levels before you assume it's PTH imbalance.

- Accurate testing may require several blood samples taken at different times of the day because physiologic factors—such as stress, diet, episodic secretions, and body rhythms—can change circulating hormone levels.
- Urine is collected for 24 hours using the appropriate collection device. If a specimen is accidentally discarded, the collection must be restarted.

Imaging studies

Imaging studies are done with or after other tests. Some X-ray studies are performed at the bedside in the critical care unit. Computed tomography (CT) scans, magnetic resonance imaging (MRI), and nuclear medicine scans are done in the department, and the nurse accompanies and monitors an unstable patient.

X-rays

Routine X-rays are used to evaluate how an endocrine dysfunction affects body tissues, although they don't reveal endocrine glands. For example, a bone X-ray, routinely ordered for a suspected parathyroid disorder, can show the effects of a calcium imbalance.

Nursing considerations
- Explain the procedure to the patient.
- Radiographic studies require no special pretest or posttest care.

CT scan and MRI

CT scan and MRI are used to assess an endocrine gland by providing high-resolution, tomographic, three-dimensional (3-D) images of the gland's structure and may be used to identify tumors.

Nursing considerations
- Explain the procedure to the patient.
- Confirm that the patient isn't allergic to iodine or shellfish. A patient with such allergies may have an adverse reaction to the contrast medium. If the patient has an allergy, a pretest allergy preparation may be given.
- If contrast medium is ordered, explain that it's injected into an existing I.V. line or that a new line may be inserted.
- Preprocedure testing should include evaluation of renal function (serum creatinine and blood urea nitrogen [BUN] levels) because the contrast medium can cause acute renal failure.
- After the procedure, encourage oral fluid intake to flush the contrast medium out of the patient's body, unless contraindicated or

if the patient is on nothing-by-mouth status. The practitioner may write an order to increase I.V. fluids.
* Check serum creatinine and BUN levels after the procedure.

Nuclear medicine studies

Nuclear medicine studies include radionuclide thyroid imaging.

Evaluate and assess

Radionuclide thyroid imaging is done to:
* evaluate thyroid function
* assess size, structure, and position of the thyroid gland.
   Such testing typically follows discovery of a palpable mass, enlarged gland, or asymmetrical goiter. After oral administration or I.V. injection of a radioisotope (such as iodine 131 [^{131}I], iodine 123, or technetium-99m pertechnetate), images are taken of the thyroid gland.

Hot spots and cold spots

With radionuclide thyroid imaging, hyperfunctioning nodules (areas of excessive iodine uptake) appear as black regions called *hot spots*. Hypofunctioning nodules (areas of little or no iodine uptake) appear as white or light gray regions called *cold spots*. Biopsy may be performed on the lesion to rule out malignancy.

Nursing considerations
* Explain the procedure to the patient.
* Confirm that the patient isn't allergic to iodine or shellfish. A patient with such allergies may have an adverse reaction to the contrast medium or radioactive isotope. If the patient has an allergy, a pretest allergy preparation may be given.
* If I.V. radioisotope is ordered, explain that it's injected into an existing I.V. line or that a new line may be inserted.
* After the procedure, encourage oral fluid intake to flush the radioisotope out of the patient's body, unless contraindicated or if the patient is on nothing-by-mouth status. The practitioner may write an order to increase I.V. fluids.

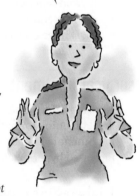

Radionuclide thyroid imaging is ordered after a palpable mass, enlarged gland, or asymmetrical goiter is found.

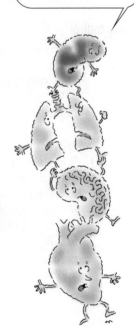

Endocrine dysfunction can affect all body systems. Whoa!

Treatments

Endocrine dysfunction can affect all body systems and, if not corrected, can be life-threatening. Treatment of an acutely ill patient with an endocrine disorder is a complex process that may include drug therapy, nonsurgical treatments, and surgical procedures such as pancreas transplantation.

Drug therapy

Drugs are commonly used to treat endocrine disorders, such as adrenal crisis, DKA, myxedema coma, and thyrotoxic crisis. Some drug therapies commonly used to treat critical care patients with acute endocrine disorders include:

- insulin therapy
- antithyroid medications
- thyroid replacement medications
- corticosteroids
- ADH. (See *Common endocrine medications.*)

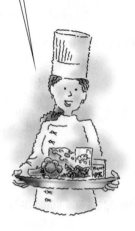

Meal planning aids control of the body's major glucose source.

Nonsurgical treatments

Nonsurgical treatments for patients with endocrine disorders include meal planning for patients with diabetes and using a hyperthermia-hypothermia blanket to treat patients with hyperthermia due to an increased hypermetabolic state in thyrotoxic crisis.

Diabetes meal planning

Meal planning is the cornerstone of diabetes care because it directly controls the body's major glucose source. The American Dietetic Association and the American Diabetes Association recommend an individual nutritional assessment to determine appropriate medical nutrition therapy.

Taking control

When the patient's condition is stable, schedule a consultation with the dietitian or diabetes educator. The patient's food intake can be carefully controlled to prevent widely fluctuating blood glucose levels. Adherence to a meal plan to avoid hypoglycemia is even more important if the patient is taking insulin or sulfonylureas.

Nursing considerations
- When the patient is stable, explain the need for a special meal plan to control blood glucose levels. Arrange for a dietitian to teach the patient how to plan meals. The dietitian may recommend the food exchange system. This method, based on the carbohydrate, fat, and protein content of six basic food groups, allows greater flexibility in meal planning. Exchange groups include dairy products, vegetables, fruits, breads, meats, and fats.

Common endocrine medications

Drugs	Indications	Adverse reactions	Practice pointers
Oral antidiabetics			
Sulfonylureas Glipizide (Glucotrol) Glyburide (DiaBeta)	• Type 2 diabetes	• Hypoglycemia • Dizziness • Agranulocytosis • Nausea • Thrombocytopenia • Rash	• Check for signs and symptoms of hypoglycemia and hyperglycemia. • Monitor blood glucose levels. An increased risk of hypoglycemia exists when given in combination with insulin.
Biguanides Metformin (Glucophage)	• Type 2 diabetes	• Diarrhea • Flatulence • Headache • Lactic acidosis • Nausea and vomiting	• Give drug with meals. • Assess renal function. • Monitor for lactic acidosis, especially in patients with renal insufficiency. • Be aware that contrast dye may increase risk of lactic acidosis. Stop metformin 48 hours before procedure using contrast dye. Assess renal function prior to resuming treatment.
Thiazolidinediones Pioglitazone (Actos) Rosiglitazone (Avandia)	• Type 2 diabetes	• Edema • Headache • Hypoglycemia (rare if used as a single agent) • Myalgia • Pharyngitis • Upper respiratory infection • Weight gain	• Monitor liver function studies. • Don't use in patients with active liver disease. • Use cautiously in patients with edema or heart failure. • Avandia has been associated with increased risk for stroke or heart attack. It isn't recommended for use with insulin. • Actos has been associated with a substantial increase in risk for bladder cancer.
Alpha glucosidase inhibitors Acarbose (Precose)	• Type 2 diabetes	• Abdominal pain • Diarrhea • Flatulence	• Acarbose alone doesn't cause hypoglycemia; however, when given with a sulfonylurea or insulin, it may increase the hypoglycemic potential of the sulfonylurea. If hypoglycemia occurs, treat with glucose (dextrose) rather than sucrose because acarbose blocks sucrose uptake.

(continued)

Common endocrine medications *(continued)*

Drugs	Indications	Adverse reactions	Practice pointers
Insulins			
Rapid-acting: Lispro Short-acting: Regular Intermediate-acting: NPH Long-acting: Ultralente	• All types of diabetes	• Hypoglycemia • Weight gain	• Monitor for hypoglycemia. • Monitor blood glucose levels. • Educate the patient about the symptoms and treatment of hypoglycemia and hyperglycemia. • Use regular humulin insulin only with continuous insulin infusion and administer on I.V. infusion pump.
Antithyroid medications			
Thyroid hormone antagonist Propylthiouracil	• Hyper-thyroidism	• Arthralgia • Diarrhea • Drowsiness • Nausea and vomiting • Headache • Loss of taste perception • Myxedema coma • Systemic lupus erythematosus–like syndrome • Vertigo • Agranulocytosis • Leukopenia • Hepatotoxicity	• Use cautiously with anticoagulants because bleeding risk is increased. • Instruct the patient to report any signs of bleeding. • Monitor the effects of cardiac medications after hyperthyroidism is corrected; cardiac medication dosages may need to be decreased. • Be aware that frequent thyroid tests may be necessary initially to adjust dosing. • Educate the patient about symptoms of hypothyroidism (myxedema coma).
Thyroid replacement medications			
Thyroid hormone Levothyroxine (Synthroid)	• Hypo-thyroidism	• Hypertension • Insomnia • Intolerance to heat • Menstrual irregularities • Nervousness • Tachycardia • Thyrotoxicosis • Weight loss • Tremor	• Instruct the patient to avoid aluminum- and magnesium-containing antacids, which decrease T_4 absorption. • Be aware that requirements for antidiabetic medications may change with treatment. • Instruct patient to take medications in the early morning on an empty stomach. • Keep in mind that frequent thyroid tests may be necessary initially to adjust dosing. • Monitor for toxicity. • Teach the patient about symptoms of toxicity (thyrotoxicosis symptoms). • Use cautiously in elderly patients and in those with renal impairment or cardiovascular disorders. • Monitor for cardiac arrhythmias such as tachycardia.

Common endocrine medications *(continued)*

Drugs	Indications	Adverse reactions	Practice pointers
Corticosteroids			
Glucocorticoid Hydrocortisone	• Acute adrenal crisis	• Cataracts • Delirium and hallucinations • Diabetes mellitus • Hirsutism • Hypertension • Increased appetite • Insomnia • Muscle wasting • Peptic ulcer • Seizures • Delayed wound healing	• Avoid abrupt cessation because the adrenal gland is suppressed during steroid use. • Be aware that drug-induced diabetes can result. • Use cautiously if the patient is on concomitant anticoagulant therapy. Prothrombin time results may differ after steroids are initiated. • Use cautiously if potassium-depleting diuretics are used. Steroids can worsen hypokalemia. • Keep in mind that initial signs of infection may be masked due to the drug's anti-inflammatory effects. • Administer with food or milk to avoid GI distress. • Monitor blood pressure, weight, serum glucose level, and serum electrolyte level.

Hyperthermia-hypothermia blanket

A hyperthermia-hypothermia blanket is used to increase, decrease, or maintain body temperature through conductive heat or cold transfer between the blanket and patient. It can be operated manually or automatically.

Common for cooling

The therapeutic blanket is most commonly used to reduce high fever resulting from infectious and inflammatory processes and hypermetabolic states such as thyrotoxic crisis. The treatment may be initiated when more conservative measures, such as baths, ice packs, and antipyretics, are unsuccessful.

It's also used to:
- maintain normal temperature during surgery or shock
- induce hypothermia during surgery or following cardiac arrest by decreasing metabolic activity, thereby reducing oxygen requirements
- provide warmth in cases of severe hypothermia.

Nursing considerations
- Explain the procedure to the patient. Follow your facility's policy and procedure and the manufacturer's instructions for proper use of the blanket.

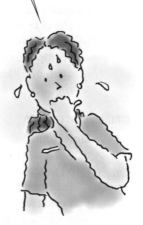

Whew! A hyperthermia-hypothermia blanket is most commonly used to reduce high fever.

- Record baseline vital signs and monitor temperature, pulse, respirations, blood pressure, and cardiac rhythm during the treatment.
- For automatic operation, insert the thermistor probe in the patient's rectum and tape it in place to prevent accidental dislodgment.
- Assess for skin breakdown and reposition the patient every 1 to 2 hours, unless contraindicated. Keep the patient's skin, bedclothes, and blanket free from perspiration and condensation.
- Shivering increases metabolic demand and oxygen consumption and elevates body temperature. Collaborate with the physician to plan for medication or modification of the temperature to deal with shivering before it occurs.
- To prevent complications, such as premature ventricular contractions, avoid lowering the patient's temperature more than 1° every 15 minutes.
- Document the procedure, the patient's tolerance of the treatment, any complications, and interventions.

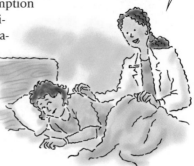

If the patient shivers excessively during hypothermia treatment, stop the procedure and tell the practitioner immediately.

Surgery

In the critical care unit, you may care for patients with end-stage pancreatic disease requiring transplantation surgery.

Pancreas transplantation

Pancreas transplantation involves the replacement of a person's pancreas with a donor pancreas.

Indications for transplantation

Pancreas transplantation is indicated for patients with end-stage pancreatic disease, primarily type 1 diabetes mellitus. Such patients generally have serious complications of the disease, including neuropathies and macrovascular and microvascular disease.

The risks associated with transplantation surgery and immunosuppressive therapy are less than those associated with the disease complications. The goal of pancreas transplantation is to restore blood glucose levels to normal and limit the progression of complications.

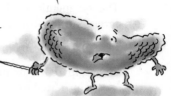

The goals of pancreas transplantation are to restore blood glucose levels and limit complications.

Common concurrence

Most commonly, pancreas transplantation is done along with renal transplantation. This procedure is called *simultaneous pancreas-kidney (SPK) transplantation*. (See *SPK transplantation*.)

Pancreas transplantation can also be done after renal transplantation using a procedure called *pancreas-after-kidney transplantation*. In other cases, a single transplant procedure, called *pancreas transplant alone*, is done.

SPK transplantation

This illustration depicts SPK transplantation, in which a donor pancreas is anasto-mosed using the systemic bladder technique.

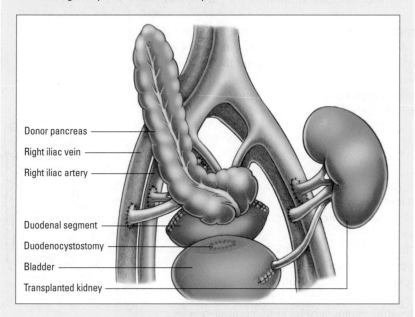

Donor pancreas
Right iliac vein
Right iliac artery

Duodenal segment
Duodenocystostomy
Bladder
Transplanted kidney

It's complicated

Possible surgical complications include:
- graft thrombosis
- infection
- pancreatitis
- intrapancreatic abscess
- leakage at the anastomosis site
- organ rejection.

When to say no

Contraindications for pancreas transplantation include:
- heart disease that can't be controlled
- active infection
- malignancy within the last 3 years
- current and active substance abuse
- history of noncompliance or significant psychiatric illness
- irreversible liver or lung dysfunction
- other systemic illnesses that would delay or prevent recovery.

Nursing considerations

Before surgery
- Prepare the patient thoroughly for the procedure and prolonged recovery period. Provide emotional support for the patient and his family.
- Review the transplant procedure. If the patient is undergoing SPK transplantation, describe the dialysis procedure that may be required for a short time after transplantation until the new kidney begins to function.
- Discuss the immunosuppressant drugs that are to be taken and describe potential adverse effects.

The pancreas is in

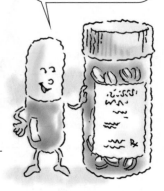

Discuss immunosuppressant drugs and their possible adverse effects with the patient.

After surgery
- Assess vital signs, cardiac rhythm, and cardiopulmonary and hemodynamic status closely at least every 15 minutes in the initial postoperative period and then hourly or as indicated by the patient's condition.
- If the patient is intubated and on a ventilator, assist with extubation as soon as possible, administer supplemental oxygen, and assess respiratory status, including breath sounds and oxygen saturation.
- Monitor hemodynamic parameters, including central venous pressure, pulmonary artery pressure, and pulmonary artery wedge pressure for changes indicating shifts in fluid volume because the patient is at high risk for fluid and electrolyte imbalance.
- Administer fluid replacement as ordered and carefully monitor intake and output, including urine and nasogastric (NG) tube or wound drainage. Weigh the patient daily and report any rapid gain, which indicates fluid retention.
- In the immediate postoperative period, assess renal and endocrine function and the need for insulin. Monitor laboratory test results, especially BUN, creatinine, serum amylase, and blood glucose levels.
- Because your transplant patient's immune system is suppressed by medications, he's at high risk for infection. Maintain strict infection control precautions such as meticulous hand washing. Monitor for signs of infection and rejection, including low-grade fever; elevated white blood cell count; swelling of the graft area; and increased serum amylase, lipase, and glucose levels. Administer antibiotics and immunosuppressant medications as ordered.

Endocrine system disorders

Some common endocrine disorders you may encounter in the critical care environment are acute adrenal crisis, diabetes insipidus, diabetes mellitus, DKA, HHNS, myxedema coma, syndrome of inappropriate antidiuretic hormone (SIADH), and thyroid storm.

Addison's disease

Addison's disease, also called *adrenal hypofunction* or *adrenal insufficiency*, occurs in two forms: primary and secondary. This relatively uncommon disorder occurs in people of all ages and both sexes. Either primary or secondary Addison's disease can progress to adrenal crisis.

Acute adrenal crisis, also called *addisonian crisis*, is a deficiency of mineralocorticoids and glucocorticoids that requires immediate treatment. (See *Understanding adrenal crisis*, page 578.)

What causes it

Causes of Addison's disease are classified according to whether they result in primary or secondary hypofunction.

Who's on first?

In primary hypofunction, the cause lies with the adrenal glands when approximately 90% of the gland is destroyed, apparently through an autoimmune process.

Other causes of primary hypofunction include:
- tuberculosis
- bilateral adrenalectomy
- hemorrhage into the adrenal glands
- neoplasms
- infections.

What's on second?

In secondary hypofunction, the cause lies outside the adrenal gland and includes:
- pituitary gland malfunction (decreased secretion of ACTH)
- abrupt steroid withdrawal (Long-term treatment with steroid medication suppresses the secretion of corticotropin by the pituitary and leaves it unable to quickly resume production.)
- removal of a corticotropin-secreting tumor.

Understanding adrenal crisis

Adrenal crisis (acute adrenal insufficiency) is the most serious complication of Addison's disease. It may occur gradually or suddenly.

Who's at risk
This potentially lethal condition usually develops in patients who:
• don't respond to hormone replacement therapy
• undergo extreme stress without adequate glucocorticoid replacement
• abruptly stop hormone therapy

• undergo trauma
• undergo bilateral adrenalectomy
• develop adrenal gland thrombosis after a severe infection (Waterhouse-Friderichsen syndrome).

What happens
In adrenal crisis, destruction of the adrenal cortex leads to a rapid decline in the steroid hormones cortisol and aldosterone. This directly affects the liver, stomach, and kidneys. The flowchart below depicts what happens in adrenal crisis.

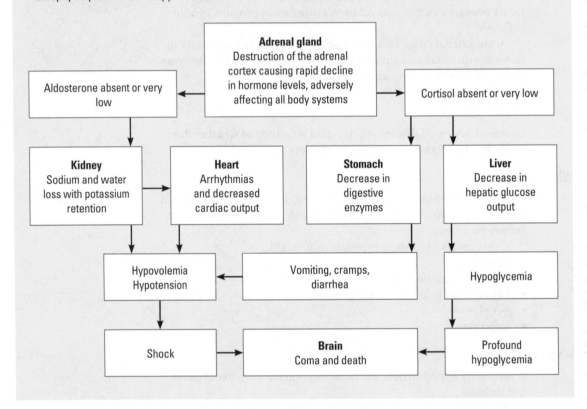

How it happens

Addison's disease is characterized by decreased secretion of the adrenal hormones glucocorticoids (cortisol and aldosterone), mineralocorticoids, and androgens. Addisonian crisis can occur with severe stress, such as illness, surgery, sepsis, trauma, and abrupt discontinuation of steroid therapy.

Release the aldosterone!

Aldosterone release occurs in response to hypovolemia as the body attempts to maintain vascular volume. Aldosterone causes the renal tubules to resorb sodium. As sodium is resorbed, water naturally follows and is resorbed. Vascular volume and blood pressure increase. Cortisol release causes an increase in glucose production as the body attempts to supply the body with this fuel.

Emergency!

In acute addisonian crisis, both hormones are suddenly depleted. Here's what happens:
1. First, blood pressure drops due to hypovolemia and hyponatremia. Standard pressor therapy is difficult to regulate because the response to catecholamines is unpredictable.
2. Second, blood glucose plummets, and coma and death ensue if immediate treatment isn't available.

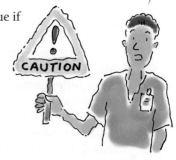

With acute addisonian crisis, coma and death ensue without immediate treatment.

What to look for

Typical clinical features of Addison's disease include:
- profound hypotension
- dehydration
- profound weakness and fatigue
- nausea and vomiting
- hypoglycemia
- neurologic changes
- hyperkalemia
- hyponatremia
- hypercalcemia
- tachycardia.

What tests tell you

In a patient with typical addisonian symptoms, these findings strongly suggest acute adrenal insufficiency:
- Plasma cortisol is decreased.
- Serum sodium and fasting blood glucose levels are decreased.
- Corticotropin is increased.
- Serum potassium level is increased.
- Serum BUN level is increased.
- Various radiologic tests identify adrenal gland size such as X-rays that show adrenal calcification.

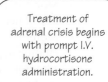

Treatment of adrenal crisis begins with prompt I.V. hydrocortisone administration.

How it's treated

Treatment for the patient with adrenal crisis is prompt I.V. bolus administration of 100 mg of hydrocortisone, followed by

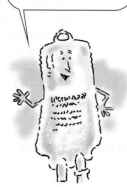

hydrocortisone diluted with normal saline with added electrolytes given as an I.V. infusion until the patient's condition stabilizes.

Furthermore . . .

Further treatment includes:
- aggressive fluid replacement with up to 5 L of I.V. saline with electrolyte replacement, such as sodium and potassium
- vasopressors (if the patient doesn't respond to the initial treatment), such as epinephrine or norepinephrine, titrated to the patient's blood pressure
- hormone replacement, such as hydrocortisone or fludrocortisone
- blood glucose management with I.V. dextrose solution
- maintenance corticosteroid (hydrocortisone) replacement when the patient's condition is stable.

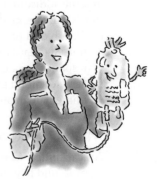

Monitor the patient's blood glucose levels and administer I.V. glucose if necessary.

What to do

- Explain all procedures and tests to the patient and his family.
- Monitor the patient's vital signs and oxygen saturation closely. Assist with insertion of a pulmonary artery catheter as indicated for fluid status evaluation. Assess hemodynamic parameters and monitor for shock.
- Assess the patient's respiratory status and auscultate breath sounds for crackles, which may indicate fluid overload.
- Monitor cardiac rhythm and assess for possible arrhythmias secondary to electrolyte imbalance (evidenced by tall, tented T waves and widening QRS complex associated with hyperkalemia).
- Monitor the patient's intake and output, fluid replacement therapy, and daily weight.
- Monitor the patient's blood glucose levels and administer I.V. glucose if necessary.
- Monitor electrolytes for sodium and potassium imbalances, including hyponatremia and hyperkalemia during crisis.
- Monitor renal function studies and laboratory test results, including hemoglobin (Hb) and hematocrit, serum electrolytes, and blood glucose levels.
- Monitor the patient's NG tube in case of vomiting.
- Institute emergency measures if needed, such as mechanical ventilation in case of cardiopulmonary arrest.
- Maintain a quiet environment.
- Maintain standard infection control measures.

Diabetes insipidus

Diabetes insipidus is a water metabolism disorder caused by deficiency of ADH. ADH is also called *vasopressin*. The absence of ADH allows filtered water to be excreted in the urine instead of being reabsorbed. Diabetes insipidus causes excessive urination (polyuria) and excessive thirst (polydipsia) and large fluid intake.

What causes it

Possible causes of diabetes insipidus include:
- pituitary tumor
- hypothalamic tumor
- cranial trauma (basilar skull fracture)
- cranial surgery
- stroke
- certain medications (lithium [Eskalith], phenytoin [Dilantin], and alcohol)
- rare genetic form of an X-linked recessive trait
- other idiopathic, nephrogenic, or neurogenic causes.

How it happens

Diabetes insipidus is a syndrome resulting from a lack of ADH secretion. ADH is a hormone released by the posterior pituitary in response to increased serum osmolality. It controls the body's ability to retain water.

Three forms

There are three forms of diabetes insipidus:
1. neurogenic
2. nephrogenic
3. psychogenic.

Some nerve!

Neurogenic or central diabetes insipidus is caused by inadequate synthesis or release of ADH. It occurs when trauma or an organic lesion of the hypothalamus, infundibular stem, or posterior pituitary partially or completely blocks ADH synthesis, transport, or release. Causes of organic lesions include brain tumors, hypophysectomy, aneurysms, thrombosis, and infection.

The onset of neurogenic diabetes insipidus is acute and involves:
- progressive loss of nerve tissue and increased diuresis
- normal diuresis
- polyuria and polydipsia due to permanent loss of the ability to secrete adequate ADH.

Kidney cause

Nephrogenic diabetes insipidus is caused by resistance of the kidney to the effects of ADH. It's caused by certain medications (lithium) and conditions as pyelonephritis, polycystic disease, and intrinsic renal disease.

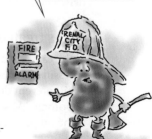

Oh no! Nephrogenic diabetes insipidus is caused by inadequate renal response to ADH.

Fluid overflow

Psychogenic diabetes insipidus is caused by extremely large fluid intake, which may be idiopathic or related to psychosis or sarcoidosis. The polydipsia and resultant polyuria wash out ADH more quickly than it can be replaced.

Chronic polyuria can overwhelm the renal medullary concentration gradient, rendering patients partially or totally unable to concentrate urine. Regardless of the cause, insufficient ADH causes the immediate excretion of large volumes of dilute urine and consequent plasma hyperosmolality.

What to look for

Your assessment findings in a patient with diabetes insipidus may include:

- abrupt onset of increased urine output (polyuria), sometimes producing nearly colorless urine up to 4 to 16 L urine per day
- extreme thirst (polydipsia) leading to fluid intake of 5 to 20 L per day
- weight loss
- dizziness, weakness
- nocturia leading to sleep disturbance and fatigue
- signs of dehydration, such as fever and dry skin and mucous membranes
- hypotension and tachycardia
- change in LOC
- fatigue.

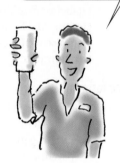

Most signs and symptoms of diabetes insipidus are related to fluid intake and output.

What tests tell you

Diagnostic testing may reveal these findings:

- Urinalysis shows almost colorless urine with low urine osmolality (50 to 200 mOsm per kg).
- Serum osmolality is increased (greater than 300 mOsm/kg).
- Urine specific gravity is decreased (less than 1.005).
- Serum sodium is greater than 147 mEq/L.
- A dehydration test or water deprivation test identifies vasopressin deficiency, which differentiates nephrogenic from pituitary effects.

How it's treated

Until the cause of diabetes insipidus is identified and eliminated, vasopressin or a vasopressin stimulant is given to control fluid balance and prevent dehydration. Treatment measures include:

- hypotonic I.V. solution administration (1 ml for every 1 ml of urine output) to replace free water lost in urine

- medications (subcutaneous [subQ] or I.M. vasopressin aqueous preparations; subQ, I.V., or nasal spray desmopressin acetate [DDAVP] to maintain volume)
- thiazide diuretics for patients with nephrogenic diabetes insipidus
- transsphenoidal hypophysectomy for patients with pituitary tumors.

What to do

- Vasopressin administration can cause hypertension, angina, and myocardial infarction (MI) due to the vasoconstrictive effects of the drug. Monitor the patient's cardiac status closely, including vital signs, cardiac rhythm, and hemodynamic parameters.
- Monitor urine output and urine specific gravity.
- Monitor other output sources such as drainage tubes.
- Monitor daily weights, serum laboratory test results, and skin turgor.
- Assess the patient's LOC.
- Assess the patient receiving vasopressin for signs of water intoxication, including drowsiness, headache, light-headedness, seizure, or coma. Notify the practitioner immediately if any occur.

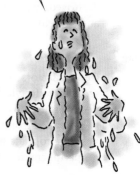

Treatment measures for the patient with diabetes insipidus include controlling fluid balance and preventing dehydration.

Diabetes mellitus

Diabetes mellitus is a chronic disease of absolute or relative insulin deficiency or resistance. It's characterized by disturbances in carbohydrate, protein, or fat metabolism.

Diabetes is the leading cause of blindness in adults. It's also a major risk factor for MI, stroke, renal failure, and peripheral vascular disease.

What causes it

Diabetes is classified as type 1 or type 2.

Virus or environment

The cause of type 1 diabetes is thought to be an autoimmune process that's triggered by a virus or environmental factor. However, the cause of the idiopathic form isn't known; patients with this form exhibit no evidence of an autoimmune process.

Lifestyle and heredity

The cause of type 2 diabetes is thought to be beta cell exhaustion due to lifestyle habits and hereditary factors. Risk factors thought to contribute to the development of type 2 diabetes include:

- obesity
- family history

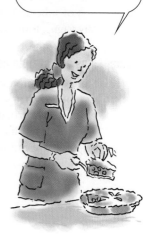

Lifestyle habits and hereditary factors can cause type 2 diabetes.

- Black, Hispanic, or Native American ethnicity
- history of gestational diabetes during pregnancy.

How it happens

When a person is genetically susceptible to type 1 diabetes, a triggering event, possibly a viral infection, causes production of autoantibodies against the beta cells of the pancreas. The resultant destruction of the beta cells leads to a decline and ultimate absence of insulin secretion. After more than 90% of the beta cells are destroyed, hyperglycemia, enhanced lipolysis (decomposition of fat), and protein catabolism result.

Take 2

Genetic factors are significant in type 2 diabetes, and obesity and a sedentary lifestyle accelerate its onset. Type 2 diabetes is a chronic disease caused by one or more dysfunctions, including:

- impaired insulin secretion
- inappropriate hepatic glucose production
- peripheral insulin receptor insensitivity.

Compliance or resistance

Patients with type 1 diabetes require insulin to prevent death. Type 2 diabetes is sometimes called an *insulin-resistant disease*. In this type of diabetes, beta cells secrete higher and higher levels of insulin to move glucose into the cell and, over time, the cells become exhausted.

What to look for

Patients with type 1 diabetes usually report rapid muscle wasting and loss of subcutaneous fat. With type 2 diabetes, symptoms are generally vague, long-standing, and develop gradually.

Similar signs and symptoms

Signs and symptoms of hyperglycemia reported by patients with type 1 or type 2 diabetes include:

- excessive urination (polyuria)
- excessive thirst (polydipsia)
- excessive eating (polyphagia)
- weight loss

- fatigue
- weakness
- vision changes
- frequent skin infections
- dry, itchy skin
- vaginal infections or discomfort.

What tests tell you

Test results indicate diabetes when they occur on two separate occasions:
- Fasting serum glucose level is greater than 126 mg/dl.
- A 2-hour oral glucose tolerance test is greater than 200 mg/dl with a 75-g carbohydrate load.
- A nonfasting draw of serum glucose is greater than 200 mg/dl at any time of the day.

Other results

Other diagnostic tests used to assess and manage diabetes include urinalysis (showing the presence of acetone) and an A_{1c} or glycosylated Hb test, which reflects serum glucose levels over a 3-month period (the lifespan of a red blood cell).

When glucose enters the blood, it binds with Hb. The A_{1c} test is used to measure the percentage of glucose bound to Hb. People without diabetes average 4% to 6% glucose. For people with diabetes, the goal is to achieve 7% glucose or less. The closer the result is to the normal range, the lower the likelihood of developing complications in the long run.

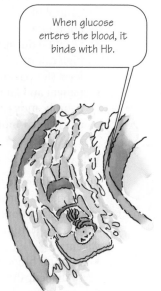

When glucose enters the blood, it binds with Hb.

How it's treated

The goal of effective treatment for patients with all types of diabetes is to optimize blood glucose control and decrease the vascular complications, such as blindness, renal failure, cardiovascular disease, and peripheral vascular disease, and neuropathy.

Type 1 treatment

Treatment for patients with type 1 diabetes includes:
- insulin replacement
- meal planning
- exercise
- pancreas transplantation.

Type 2 treatment

Treatment for patients with type 2 diabetes includes:

- lifestyle modification to include reduced calorie diet, weight reduction, and exercise to reduce insulin resistance and increase glucose utilization.
- oral antidiabetic drugs to stimulate endogenous insulin production, increase insulin sensitivity in cells, suppress hepatic gluconeogenesis, and delay GI carbohydrate absorption
- insulin therapy if control isn't achieved with oral agents.

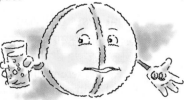

If type 2 diabetes isn't controllable with oral antidiabetic drugs, insulin therapy is used.

Types 1 and 2 treatment

Treatment for patients with either type 1 or type 2 diabetes includes:

- careful monitoring of blood glucose levels
- individualized meal planning designed to meet nutritional needs, control blood glucose and lipid levels, and reach and maintain appropriate body weight
- weight reduction (for an obese patient with type 2 diabetes) or high caloric allotment depending on the growth stage and activity level (for patients with type 1 diabetes)
- patient and family education about the disease process, possible complications, nutritional management, exercise regimen, blood glucose self-monitoring, and insulin or oral medications.

What to do

In the critical care unit, you may care for patients who have a history of diabetes but are admitted to the unit because of surgery or another medical condition. Some medical conditions, such as stroke or renal failure, result from diabetic effects on the cardiovascular or renal systems.

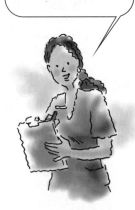

Patients in critical care units may have diabetes but are usually there because of surgery or another medical condition.

- Monitor blood glucose levels and assess for acute complications of diabetic therapy, especially DKA and hypoglycemia (blood glucose less than 50 mg/dl); signs and symptoms include tachycardia, pallor, diaphoresis, weakness, vagueness, slow cerebration, dizziness, irritability, seizure, and coma. Some medications, such as beta-adrenergic blockers, can mask the symptoms of a hypoglycemic reaction, so more frequent blood glucose monitoring may be necessary.
- Treatment for a hypoglycemic reaction is glucose. If the patient can swallow, provide oral glucose or a sucrose-containing drink followed by a snack of a complex carbohydrate and a protein. If the patient can't drink, give a bolus of 25 g of 50% dextrose. Obtain blood glucose measurements before administering glucose, if possible, to confirm the diagnosis. Document blood glucose levels after treatment as well as the patient's response to treatment.

- Assess for diabetic effects on the cardiovascular system, such as stroke, acute coronary syndromes, peripheral vascular impairment, and peripheral neuropathy. Assess cardiovascular and neurovascular status and fluid balance and monitor for cardiac arrhythmias.
- Be aware that more frequent blood glucose monitoring and insulin dose adjustments may be necessary during periods of physiologic stress, such as acute illness and surgery, because blood glucose levels increase as a result of elevated stress hormones (such as epinephrine and cortisol).
- Studies have demonstrated improved outcomes, fewer infections, and decreased risk for cardiac events in critical care patients whose glucose is maintained at less than 150 mg/dl.

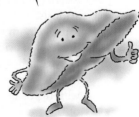

Monitor blood glucose more often and adjust the insulin dose if necessary when the patient is under stress. I try to find ways to relieve my stress.

Diabetic ketoacidosis

DKA is an acute complication of hyperglycemic crisis in patients with diabetes. It's a life-threatening complication that's most common in patients with type 1 diabetes and is sometimes the first evidence of the disease.

What causes it

DKA may result from:
- infection
- illness
- surgery
- stress
- insufficient or absent insulin.

How it happens

In DKA, production by the liver and release of glucose into the blood (gluconeogenesis) is increased, and uptake of glucose by the cells is decreased by the lack of insulin.

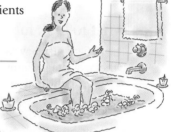

When glucose is lacking, I convert glycogen to glucose for release into the bloodstream.

What happens?

When the cells don't receive fuel (glucose), the liver responds by converting glycogen to glucose for release into the bloodstream. When all excess glucose molecules remain in the serum, osmosis causes fluid shifts. The cycle continues until fluid shifts in the brain cause coma and death. In the absence of endogenous insulin, the body breaks down fats for energy. In the process, fatty acids develop too rapidly and are converted to ketones, resulting in severe metabolic acidosis.

Acidosis also affects potassium levels. For every 0.1 change in pH, there's a reciprocal 0.6 change in potassium. As acidosis worsens, blood glucose levels increase and hyperkalemia worsens. The cycle continues until coma and death occur.

As with diabetes, the liver responds to the lack of fuel (glucose) in cells by converting glycogen to glucose for release into the bloodstream. Excess glucose molecules in the serum trigger osmosis and fluid shifts from the cells and extracellular spaces into the vascular circulation.

What to look for

The patient may have a rapid onset of drowsiness, stupor, and coma. Other assessment findings include:
- severe dehydration
- rapid and deep breathing (Kussmaul's respirations) as compensation for acidosis
- fruity breath odor due to acetone
- polyuria, polydipsia, and polyphagia
- weight loss
- muscle wasting
- vision changes
- recurrent infections
- abdominal cramps
- nausea and vomiting
- leg cramps.

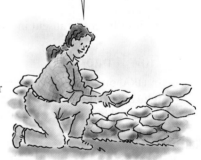

There's a stack of findings used to diagnose DKA.

What tests tell you

A wide range of findings are used to diagnosis DKA:
- Serum glucose is elevated (200 to 800 mg per dl). Patients in coma may have serum glucose levels greater than 1,000 mg/dl.
- Serum ketone level is increased.
- Urine acetone test is positive.
- Arterial blood gas (ABG) analysis reveals metabolic acidosis.
- Initially, normal potassium level or hyperkalemia, depending on the level of acidosis; hypokalemia follows.
- Electrocardiogram (ECG) findings show changes related to hyperkalemia (tall, tented T waves and widened QRS complex); later, with hypokalemia, ECG shows flattened T wave and the presence of U wave.
- Serum osmolality is elevated.

How it's treated

Treatment goals for the patient with DKA include stop gluconeogenesis, rehydration, control of glucose levels, and restoration of electrolyte and acid–base balance. If the patient is comatose, airway support and mechanical ventilation may be indicated.

What to do

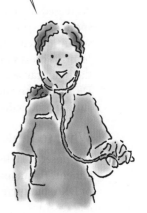

Monitor the patient's vital signs because changes reflect hydration status.

- Simultaneously, correct dehydration, using non-dextrose-based I.V. fluids and stop production of glucose by administering I.V. insulin therapy.
- Replace electrolytes based on laboratory test results.
- Monitor blood glucose levels. As blood glucose level nears 250 mg/dl, give dextrose-based I.V. fluid to prevent hypoglycemia.
- Monitor potassium levels. As blood glucose level normalizes, potassium moves back into the intracellular space. Add potassium as ordered to I.V. fluid to prevent hypokalemia.
- Monitor ABG levels. As blood glucose level normalizes, acidosis is corrected.
- Assess the patient's LOC and ability to maintain a patent airway. Monitor respiratory status, including breath sounds and oxygen saturation. Monitor cardiac rhythm for arrhythmias that may result from electrolyte imbalance.
- Monitor the patient's vital signs because changes reflect hydration status.
- Monitor blood glucose and serum electrolyte levels, especially potassium levels and ABG results.

Stop gluconeogenesis by administering regular insulin I.V. as ordered, usually as a bolus dose and then by continuous I.V. infusion, using an I.V. infusion pump. Blood glucose levels must be reduced gradually to prevent cerebral fluid shifting and subsequent cerebral edema. Anticipate potassium replacement after insulin therapy is initiated.

- Administer I.V. fluid replacement initially with 1 to 2 L normal saline and then half-normal saline. When the patient's blood glucose levels reach 250 mg/dl, anticipate the addition of glucose to the fluid replacement to prevent hypoglycemia.
- When the patient is stable, consult the diabetes educator to assist with patient teaching.

Hyperosmolar hyperglycemic nonketotic syndrome

HHNS is an acute hyperglycemic crisis accompanied by hyperosmolality and severe dehydration without ketoacidosis. If not treated properly, it can cause coma or death.

HHNS is most common in patients with type 2 diabetes (usually middle-aged or older) but can occur in anyone whose insulin tolerance is stressed and in patients who have undergone certain therapeutic procedures, such as peritoneal dialysis, hemodialysis, or total parenteral nutrition.

What causes it

Causes of HHNS include illness, infection, and stress.

How it happens

With HHNS in patients with type 2 diabetes, glucose production and release into the blood is increased or glucose uptake by the cells is decreased. When the cells don't receive fuel (glucose), the liver responds by converting glycogen to glucose for release into the bloodstream. When all excess glucose molecules remain in the serum, osmosis causes fluid shifts. The cycle continues until fluid shifts in the brain cause coma and death. The difference between HHNS and DKA is that the body does not convert to fat metabolism and the resulting production of ketones, so acidosis does not occur.

What to look for

The onset of HHNS is usually gradual and may not be noticed by the patient. The manifestations of HHNS are similar to those of DKA, but there are differences. (See *Comparing HHNS and DKA.*)

> As HHNS progresses, your assessment may turn up these findings.

Making progress

As HHNS progresses, assessment findings may include:
- severe dehydration
- hypotension and tachycardia
- diaphoresis
- tachypnea
- polyuria, polydipsia, and polyphagia
- lethargy and fatigue
- vision changes
- rapid onset of lethargy
- stupor and coma
- neurologic changes.

What tests tell you

Diagnosing HHNS begins with serum glucose testing but also involves several other evaluations.
- Serum glucose level is elevated, sometimes 800 to 2,000 mg per dl.
- Ketones are absent, so there's no acidosis and urine and serum ketone results are negative.

Comparing HHNS and DKA

HHNS and DKA are both acute complications of diabetes. They share some similarities but are two distinct conditions. Use this flowchart to determine which condition your patient has.

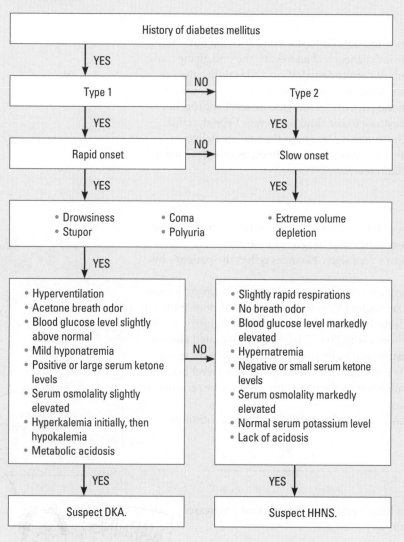

- Urine glucose levels are positive.
- Serum osmolality is increased.
- Serum sodium levels are elevated and the serum potassium level is usually normal.
- ABG results are usually normal, without evidence of acidosis.

How it's treated

Treatment for patients with HHNS is focused on correcting fluid volume deficits and electrolyte imbalances and addressing the underlying cause:
- I.V. fluids are given to correct dehydration and stabilize the cardiovascular system. Administer isotonic or half-normal saline as ordered. When the patient's blood glucose level approaches 250 mg/dl, add dextrose to the fluid to prevent hypoglycemia.
- I.V. insulin and electrolyte replacement therapy are delivered.
- Blood glucose levels are monitored. As blood glucose levels normalize, so do sodium levels.

What to do

- Assess the patient's LOC and ability to maintain a patent airway. Monitor respiratory status and oxygen saturation.
- Monitor the patient's vital signs. Changes reflect the patient's hydration status.
- Monitor the patient's blood glucose and serum electrolyte levels.
- Administer regular insulin I.V. as ordered, by continuous infusion, and titrate the dosage based on the patient's blood glucose levels.
- Remember, the patient with HHNS has severely elevated glucose levels, but less insulin is usually needed (compared with that required by patients with DKA) to reduce the glucose level because the patient typically secretes some insulin and may be sensitive to additional doses.
- Provide patient and family education to foster prevention of future episodes.

Myxedema coma

Myxedema coma is a life-threatening disorder that progresses from hypothyroidism.

What causes it

Causes of hypothyroidism include:
- pituitary failure to produce TSH
- hypothalamic failure
- chronic autoimmune thyroiditis (Hashimoto's disease)
- amyloidosis and sarcoidosis

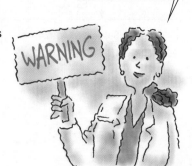

Myxedema coma is a life-threatening form of hypothyroidism.

- inability to synthesize hormones
- use of antithyroid hormones
- post thyroidectomy effects
- post radiation therapy effects.

How it happens

There are two classifications of hypothyroidism: primary and secondary. Primary hypothyroidism originates as a disorder of the thyroid gland. Secondary hypothyroidism is caused by a failure to stimulate normal thyroid function or an inability to synthesize thyroid hormones due to an iodine deficiency (usually dietary) or use of antithyroid medications.

A myx of causes

Myxedema coma can result from either primary or secondary hypothyroidism and progresses slowly and gradually. It's usually precipitated by infection, exposure to cold, or sedative use. Cellular metabolism decreases to a fatal level if the patient with myxedema coma is left untreated.

What to look for

The progression to myxedema coma is usually gradual but may develop abruptly if stress aggravates severe or prolonged hypothyroidism.

Inspect and assess

Periorbital edema; dry, flaky skin; thick, brittle nails; and sacral or peripheral edema may be present in the patient with myxedema coma. Cardiac assessment may reveal muffled or S_3 heart sounds. In addition, look for changes in the patient's overall appearance and behavior, including:
- decreased mental ability (slight mental slowing to severe obtundation)
- thick and dry tongue
- hoarseness
- slow and slurred speech.

What else?

Assessment findings also include:
- progressive stupor
- significantly depressed respirations and adventitious breath sounds
- hypoglycemia
- hyponatremia
- hypotension and bradycardia
- severe hypothermia without shivering
- decreased deep tendon reflexes
- alopecia
- rough, dry skin.

What tests tell you

Several test findings are useful in diagnosing myxedema coma:

- Serum levels of T_3 and T_4 are decreased.
- Serum levels of TSH are increased.
- Radioactive iodine (^{131}I) testing reveals low serum levels of thyroid hormones.
- Radioisotope scanning of thyroid tissue is used to identify ectopic thyroid tissue.
- A CT scan, MRI, or skull X-ray may disclose an underlying cause, such as pituitary or hypothalamic lesions.
- Chest X-ray may show pleural effusion.

How it's treated

Rapid treatment may be necessary for patients in myxedema coma, including:

- administration of I.V. hydrocortisone and I.V. levothyroxine (a thyroid agent)
- possible ventilatory support if the patient is comatose
- I.V. fluid replacement
- warming devices
- maintenance thyroid replacement.

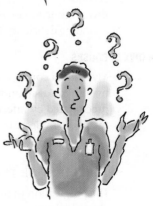

In myxedema coma, a CT scan, MRI, or skull X-ray may disclose an underlying cause, such as pituitary or hypothalamic lesions.

What to do

- Assess the patient's LOC and ability to maintain a patent airway.
- Monitor the patient's respiratory status, adequacy of ventilation and oxygen saturation, and ABG levels. Administer supplemental oxygen as ordered and anticipate the need for intubation and mechanical ventilation.
- Monitor vital signs and cardiac arrhythmias. Auscultate for muffled heart sounds or changes such as S_3.
- Monitor temperature closely until the patient is stable and institute warming measures such as applying a warming blanket.
- Administer medications as ordered. Use CNS depressants cautiously as patient with hypothyroidism are sensitive to the depressant effects.
- Administer I.V. fluids as ordered and monitor fluid balance status, serum electrolytes, and blood glucose levels.
- Assess for possible sources of infection—such as blood, sputum, and urine—and provide meticulous skin care.

Syndrome of inappropriate antidiuretic hormone

SIADH is a relatively common complication of surgery or critical illness.

What causes it

The most common cause of SIADH is oat-cell lung cancer, which secretes ADH or a vasopressor-like substance that the body responds to as if ADH were secreted.

Many other possibilities

Other causes include:
- neoplastic diseases (pancreatic, brain, and prostatic tumors; Hodgkin's disease; and thymoma)
- brain abscess
- stroke
- Guillain-Barré syndrome
- pulmonary disorders
- adverse effects of medications (chlorpropamide, tolbutamide, vincristine, cyclophosphamide, haloperidol, carbamazepine, clofibrate, morphine, and thiazides)
- adrenal insufficiency
- anterior pituitary insufficiency.

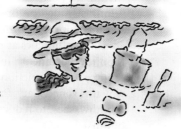

In SIADH, excessive ADH is secreted and the body responds by retaining water. It isn't what you want for bathing suit season.

How it happens

In SIADH, ADH is secreted excessively and the body responds by retaining water. Fluid shifts within compartments cause decreased serum osmolality.

What to look for

Most commonly, a patient with SIADH complains of anorexia, nausea, and vomiting. Despite these symptoms, the patient may report weight gain. Assessment findings may also include:
- thirst
- neurologic changes—such as lethargy, headache, and emotional and behavioral changes—and sluggish deep tendon reflexes
- tachycardia associated with increased fluid volume
- hyponatremia.

What tests tell you

Diagnosis of SIADH involves both blood and urine testing:
- Serum osmolality is decreased (less than 280 mOsm/kg).
- Urine sodium is increased (greater than 20 mEq/day).
- Serum sodium level is decreased.
- ADH level is elevated.

How it's treated

Treatment is based on the underlying cause and the patient's symptoms.

First thing first

Treatment begins with restricting fluid intake to 500 to 1,000 ml per day. Other measures may include administration of 200 to 300 ml of 3% to 5% sodium chloride solution for patients with severe hyponatremia. A loop diuretic may also be ordered to reduce the risk for heart failure after administration of hypertonic sodium chloride solution.

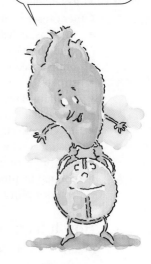

Help me, please! The patient may need a loop diuretic to reduce the risk for heart failure.

What to do

- Assess the patient's neurologic, cardiac, and respiratory status.
- Implement seizure and safety precautions if the patient's serum sodium levels are dangerously low. Monitor serum electrolyte levels.
- Monitor the patient's vital signs, oxygen saturation, and cardiac rhythm for potential arrhythmias.
- Administer medications and I.V. fluids as ordered. If hypertonic sodium chloride is ordered, monitor for fluid overload and administer diuretics as ordered.
- Monitor the patient's intake and output and daily weight.
- Enforce fluid restrictions and explain to the patient and his family why this is necessary. Provide frequent oral care avoiding drying mouthwashes, to reduce the discomfort of dry mouth and sense of thirst.

Thyroid storm

Thyroid storm, also called *thyrotoxic crisis*, is a life-threatening emergency in a patient with hyperthyroidism. Thyroid storm may be the initial symptom in a patient with hyperthyroidism that hasn't been diagnosed.

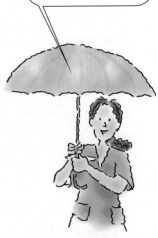

Thyroid storm is a life-threatening emergency in a patient with hyperthyroidism.

What causes it

The onset of thyroid storm is almost always abrupt and evoked by a stressful event, such as trauma, surgery, or infection.

Not-so-common causes

Other, less common causes include:
- metastatic carcinoma of the thyroid
- pituitary tumor secreting TSH
- DKA
- poor compliance with antithyroid therapy.

How it happens

Thyroid storm develops when there's a surge of thyroid hormones. Hyperthyroidism can result from genetic and immunologic factors.

Graves' is grave

Graves' disease—the most common form of hyperthyroidism—is an autoimmune process in which the body makes an antibody similar to TSH and the thyroid responds to it. Overproduction of T_3 and T_4 increases adrenergic activity and severe hypermetabolism results. This can rapidly lead to cardiac, sympathetic nervous system, and GI collapse.

What to look for

A patient in thyroid storm initially shows marked tachycardia, vomiting, and stupor. Other findings may include:

- irritability and restlessness
- vision disturbances such as diplopia
- tremor
- tachycardia and cardiac arrhythmia
- weakness
- heat intolerance
- angina
- shortness of breath
- cough
- swollen extremities
- exophthalmos.

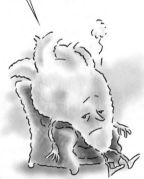

Without treatment, thyroid storm can lead to vascular collapse, hypotension, coma, and death.

Raise the flag

On palpation, an enlarged thyroid may be felt. Any change in LOC and increasing temperature in a patient with hyperthyroidism should raise red flags. Fever, typically above 100.4°F (38°C), begins insidiously and rises rapidly to a lethal level. Without treatment, the patient may experience vascular collapse, hypotension, coma, and death.

What tests tell you

These diagnostic test findings may indicate impending thyroid storm:

- Serum T_3 and T_4 levels are elevated.
- TSH level is decreased.
- Radioisotope scanning shows increased uptake.
- CT scan or MRI may disclose an underlying cause such as pituitary lesion.
- A 12-lead ECG may show supraventricular tachycardia and premature atrial and ventricular contractions.

How it's treated

Immediate treatment for a patient with thyroid storm is necessary to prevent death and includes:

- beta-adrenergic blockers to block adrenergic effects
- propylthiouracil and methimazole to block thyroid hormone synthesis
- possible corticosteroid administration to block conversion of T_3 and T_4
- avoidance of aspirin because salicylates block binding of T_3 and T_4
- cooling measures such as use of a hyperthermia-hypothermia blanket.

What to do

- Assess the patient's LOC and cardiopulmonary status.
- Monitor the patient's vital signs and core body temperature and institute cooling measures such as use of a hyperthermia-hypothermia blanket.
- Monitor ECG readings. Increased adrenergic activity may produce arrhythmias.
- Monitor the patient for signs of heart failure.
- Monitor I.V. fluids and fluid and electrolyte balance.
- Monitor the patient for high blood glucose levels. Excessive thyroid activity can lead to glyconeogenesis.
- Provide a quiet environment.

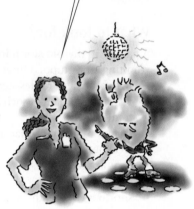

Monitor ECG readings because increased adrenergic activity can produce arrhythmias.

Quick quiz

1. Pituitary hormones are controlled by the:
    A. hypothalamus.
    B. midbrain.
    C. adrenal glands.
    D. target organs.

Answer: A. The hypothalamus receives, integrates, and directs hormone secretion.

2. Which dysfunction should you address first in a patient with DKA?
    A. Acidosis
    B. Hyperkalemia
    C. Hyperglycemia
    D. Hypovolemia

Answer: D. Hypovolemia may be severe and should be addressed first, followed by hyperglycemia, and then hyperkalemia. Acidosis is corrected by correcting the other imbalances.

3.   What's an appropriate treatment measure for a patient with addisonian crisis?
   A.   I.V. fluid replacement
   B.   I.V. corticosteroids
   C.   Blood glucose management
   D.   All of the above

Answer: D. All of the therapies indicated are first-line treatment measures during addisonian crisis.

4.   A patient is experiencing thyroid storm. Which drug is contraindicated?
   A.   I.V. beta-adrenergic blockers
   B.   Aspirin
   C.   Propylthiouracil
   D.   Corticosteroids

Answer: B. Aspirin is contraindicated in patients with thyroid storm because it blocks the binding of T_3 and T_4.

5.   Which sign is manifested in patients with diabetes insipidus?
   A.   Decreased urine output
   B.   Increased serum osmolality
   C.   Increased urine osmolality
   D.   Increased urine specific gravity

Answer: B. Urine output increases with diabetes insipidus; therefore, serum osmolality is increased.

Scoring

☆☆☆   If you answered all five questions correctly, give yourself a gland! Your endocrine energy is practically radioactive.

☆☆   If you answered four questions correctly, don't worry about your target cells. Your knowledge receptors are still uptaking information.

☆   If you answered fewer than four questions correctly, quit the hemming and hormoning and review the chapter.

Suggested References

Fischbach, F. T. (2009). *A manual of laboratory and diagnostic tests* (8th ed.). Philadelphia, PA: Lippincott Williams & Wilkins.

Goldman, L., & Schafer, A. I. (Eds.). (2012). *Goldman's Cecil medicine.* Philadelphia, PA: Elsevier Saunders.

Kitabchi, A. E., Hirsch, I. B., & Emmett, M. (2014). *Diabetic ketoacidosis and hyperosmolar hyperglycemic state in adults: Clinical features, evaluation and diagnosis.* Retrieved from http://www.uptodate.com/contents/diabetic-ketoacidosis-and-hyperosmolar-hyperglycemic-state-in-adults-clinical-features-evaluation-and-diagnosis

McCulloch, D. K. (2014). *Initial management of blood glucose in adults with type 2 diabetes mellitus.* Retrieved from http://www.uptodate.com/contents/initial-management-of-blood-glucose-in-adults-with-type-2-diabetes-mellitus

Urden, L. D., Stacy, K. M., & Lough, M. E. (2006). *Critical care nursing. Diagnosis and management.* St. Louis, MO: Mosby.

Chapter 9

Hematologic and immune systems

Just the facts

In this chapter, you'll learn:

♦ structure and function of the hematologic and immune systems

♦ assessment of the hematologic and immune systems

♦ diagnostic tests and treatments for critically ill patients

♦ hematologic and immune systems disorders and related nursing care.

Understanding the hematologic and immune systems

The hematologic system consists of the blood and bone marrow. The immune system consists of specialized cells, tissues, and organs found throughout the body.

Transport and delivery

Functions of the hematologic system include:
- transporting blood cells and immunity-related cells, hormones, and gases throughout the body
- delivering oxygen and nutrients to all body tissues
- removing wastes collected from cells and tissues.

Defense! Defense!

The immune system defends the body against invasion by harmful organisms and chemical toxins. The blood plays an important part in this protective system.

Kin systems

The hematologic and immune systems are distinct, yet closely related. Their cells share a common origin in the bone

Cells of the hematologic and immune systems originate in the same place and travel together.

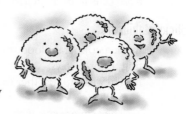

marrow, and the immune system uses the bloodstream to transport defensive components to the site of an invasion.

Hematologic system

The hematologic system consists of various formed elements, or blood cells, suspended in a fluid called *plasma*.

Formed elements in the blood include:
- red blood cells (RBCs), or erythrocytes
- platelets
- white blood cells (WBCs), or leukocytes.

RBCs and platelets function entirely within blood vessels. WBCs act mainly in the tissues outside the blood vessels.

Red blood cells

RBCs transport oxygen and carbon dioxide to and from body tissues. They contain hemoglobin (Hb), the oxygen-carrying molecule that gives blood its red color. The RBC surface carries antigens (substances that trigger immune responses), which determine a person's blood group or blood type.

Days of their lives

RBCs have an average life span of 120 days. Bone marrow releases RBCs into circulation in an immature form as reticulocytes. The reticulocytes mature into RBCs in about 1 day. The spleen sequesters, or isolates, old, worn-out RBCs, removing them from circulation.

The rate of reticulocyte release usually equals the rate of old RBC removal. When RBC depletion occurs (e.g., with hemorrhage), the bone marrow is stimulated by erythropoietin to increase reticulocyte production and maintain the normal RBC count.

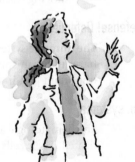

The rate of reticulocyte release equals the rate of RBC removal. That makes sense!

Platelets

Platelets are small, colorless, disk-shaped cytoplasmic fragments split from cells in bone marrow called *megakaryocytes*.

Sticky stabilizers

In the peripheral blood, the sticky platelets contribute to blood clotting in three ways:
1. They clump together to plug small defects in small blood vessel walls.
2. They congregate at an injury site in a larger vessel and close the wound so a clot can form.

3. They release substances that stabilize the clot. For example, they release serotonin, which reduces blood flow by vasoconstriction, and thromboplastin, an enzyme essential to clotting.

White blood cells

Five types of WBCs participate in the body's defense and immune systems. They are:

1. neutrophils
2. eosinophils
3. basophils
4. monocytes
5. lymphocytes.

    The WBCs are classified as either granulocytes or agranulocytes.

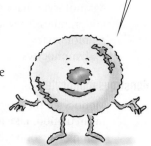

A granulocyte contains a single multilobed nucleus and granules.

Granulocytes

Granulocytes are polymorphonuclear leukocytes. Each contains a single multilobular nucleus and granules in the cytoplasm. Each type of granulocyte exhibits different properties, and each is activated by different stimuli. The granulocytes include:

*   neutrophils
*   eosinophils
*   basophils.

Neutrophils engulf, ingest, and digest

The most abundant granulocytes—the neutrophils—account for 47.6% to 76.8% of circulating WBCs. Neutrophils are phagocytic, meaning they engulf, ingest, and digest foreign materials. They leave the bloodstream by passing through the capillary walls into the tissues (a process called *diapedesis*), then migrate to accumulate at infection sites.

Replacement bands

Worn-out neutrophils form the main component of pus. Bone marrow produces their replacements, which are immature neutrophils called *bands*. In response to infection, bone marrow produces many immature cells and releases them into circulation, elevating the band count.

Ingestion by eosinophils

Eosinophils account for 0.3% to 7% of circulating WBCs. Eosinophils migrate from the bloodstream by diapedesis in response to an allergic reaction. Eosinophils accumulate in loose connective tissue, where they're involved in ingesting antigen-antibody complexes.

Basophils secrete histamine

The least common granulocyte—basophils—usually make up fewer than 2% of circulating WBCs. They possess little or no phagocytic ability. The basophils cytoplasmic granules secrete histamine, bradykinin, and heparin in response to certain inflammatory and immune stimuli. This increases vascular permeability and eases fluid passage from capillaries into body tissues.

Agranulocytes

Agranulocytes have nuclei without lobes and lack specific cytoplasmic granules. They include:
- monocytes
- lymphocytes.

Monstrous monocytes

Monocytes, the largest WBCs, constitute only 0.6% to 9.6% of WBCs in circulation. Like neutrophils, monocytes enlarge and mature, becoming macrophages, or histiocytes. As macrophages, monocytes may roam freely through the body when stimulated by inflammation. Usually, they remain immobile, populating most organs and tissues.

Defense against infection

Monocytes are part of the reticuloendothelial system, which defends the body against infection and disposes of cell breakdown products. Macrophages concentrate in structures that filter large amounts of body fluid, such as the liver, spleen, and lymph nodes, where they defend against invading organisms.

Macrophages are efficient phagocytes (cells that ingest microorganisms, cellular debris such as worn-out neutrophils, and necrotic tissue). When mobilized at an infection site, they phagocytize cellular remnants and promote wound healing.

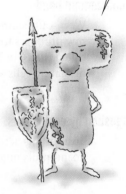

T lymphocytes attack infected cells directly.

Lymphocytes: Least but not last

Lymphocytes, the smallest and the second most numerous (16.2% to 43%) of the WBCs, originate from stem cells in the bone marrow. There are two types of lymphocytes:
1. T lymphocytes, which attack infected cells directly
2. B lymphocytes, which produce molecules called *antibodies* that attack specific antigens.

Blood clots

Hemostasis (blood clotting) is the complex process by which platelets, plasma, and coagulation factors interact to control bleeding.

Extrinsic coagulation cascade

When a blood vessel ruptures, local vasoconstriction (decrease in the caliber of blood vessels) and platelet clumping (aggregation) at the injury site initially prevent hemorrhage. This initial activation of the coagulation system, called the *extrinsic cascade*, requires the release of tissue thromboplastin from the damaged cells.

Intrinsic clotting cascade

Formation of a more stable clot requires initiation of the complex clotting mechanisms known as the *intrinsic cascade system*. This clotting system is activated by a protein called *factor XII*, which is one of 13 substances necessary for coagulation and derived from plasma and tissue.

The final result of the intrinsic and extrinsic cascade is a fibrin clot, an accumulation of a fibrous, insoluble protein at the injury site. (See *Understanding clotting*, page 606.)

Blood groups

A person's blood is one of four blood types: A, B, AB, and O.

A is for antigen . . .

In type A blood, A antigens appear on RBCs. Type B blood contains B antigens. Type AB blood contains both antigens. Type O blood has neither antigen.

Testing, testing: A, B, AB, O

Testing for the presence of A and B antigens on RBCs is the most important system for classifying blood. Plasma may contain antibodies that interact with these antigens, causing the cells to agglutinate, or combine into a mass. Plasma can't contain antibodies to its own cell antigen or it would destroy itself. For example, type A blood has A antigens but no A antibodies; however, it does have B antibodies.

Crossmatching for compatibility

Precise blood typing and crossmatching (mixing and observing for agglutination of donor cells) are essential, especially before blood

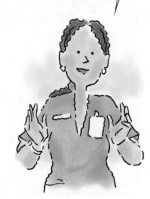

Plasma can't contain antibodies to its own cell antigen or it would destroy itself.

Understanding clotting

When a blood vessel is severed or injured, clotting begins within minutes to stop blood loss. Coagulation factors are essential to normal blood clotting. Absent, decreased, or excess coagulation factors can cause a clotting abnormality. Coagulation factors are commonly designated by Roman numerals.

Two pathways to clotting

Clotting is initiated through two different pathways, the intrinsic pathway or the extrinsic pathway. The intrinsic pathway is activated when plasma comes in contact with damaged vessel surfaces. The extrinsic pathway is activated when tissue thromboplastin, a substance released by damaged endothelial cells, comes in contact with one of the clotting factors.

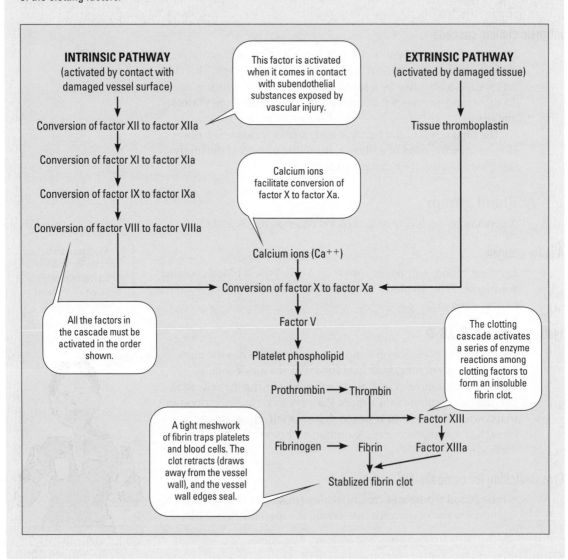

Compatible blood types

Precise blood typing and crossmatching can prevent the transfusion of incompatible blood, which can be fatal. Usually, typing the recipient's blood and crossmatching it with available donor blood takes less than 1 hour.

Matchmaking

Agglutinogen (an antigen in RBCs) and agglutinin (an antibody in plasma) distinguish the four ABO blood groups. This table depicts ABO compatibility from the perspectives of recipients and donors.

Blood group	Antibodies in plasma	Compatible RBC group	Compatible plasma
Recipient			
O	Anti-A and anti-B	O	O, A, B, AB
A	Anti-B	A, O	A, AB
B	Anti-A	B, O	B, AB
AB	Neither anti-A nor anti-B	AB, A, B, O	AB
Donor			
O	Anti-A and anti-B	O, A, B, AB	O
A	Anti-B	A, AB	A, O
B	Anti-A	B, AB	B, O
AB	Neither anti-A nor anti-B	AB	AB, A, B, O

transfusions. A donor's blood must be compatible with a recipient's or the result can be fatal. The following blood groups are compatible:

- type A with type A or O
- type B with type B or O
- type AB with type A, B, AB, or O
- type O with type O only. (See *Compatible blood types*.)

Factor in Rh

Rh typing is used to determine whether a substance, called an *Rh factor*, is present or absent in a person's blood. Of the eight types of Rh antigens, only C, D, and E are common. The presence or absence of the D antigen determines whether a person has Rh-positive or Rh-negative blood.

Blood typically is Rh-positive, meaning it contains Rh D antigen. Blood without the Rh D antigen is Rh-negative. Anti-Rh antibodies occur only in a person who has become sensitized to the Rh factor.

Anti-Rh antibodies can only appear in the blood of an Rh-negative person after introduction of Rh-positive RBCs into the bloodstream such as from transfusion of Rh-positive blood. An Rh-negative female who carries an Rh-positive fetus may also acquire anti-Rh antibodies.

A person with Rh-negative blood should only receive a transfusion with Rh-negative blood. Repeated transfusions of Rh-positive blood to an Rh-negative patient puts the patient at risk for hemolysis and agglutination.

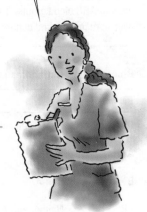

Anti-Rh antibodies occur in an Rh-negative person after Rh-positive RBCs are introduced into the bloodstream.

Immune system

The organs and tissues of the immune system are involved with the growth, development, and dissemination of lymphocytes. (See *Organs and tissues of the immune system.*)

Immunity divided by 3

The immune system has three major divisions:
1. central lymphoid organs and tissues
2. peripheral lymphoid organs and tissues
3. accessory lymphoid organs and tissues.

Central lymphoid organs and tissues

The bone marrow and thymus play roles in developing B cells and T cells, which are the two major types of lymphocytes.

Bone marrow

The bone marrow contains stem cells, which are multipotential, meaning they may develop into several different cell types. The immune system and blood cells develop from stem cells in a process called *hematopoiesis*.

Stemming from stem cells

Soon after differentiation from the stem cells, some of the cells become part of the immune system and sources of lymphocytes; others develop into phagocytes, which ingest microorganisms and cellular debris.

Organs and tissues of the immune system

The immune system includes cells that circulate in the bloodstream as well as organs and tissues in which lymphocytes predominate. This illustration depicts the central, peripheral, and accessory lymphoid organs and tissues.

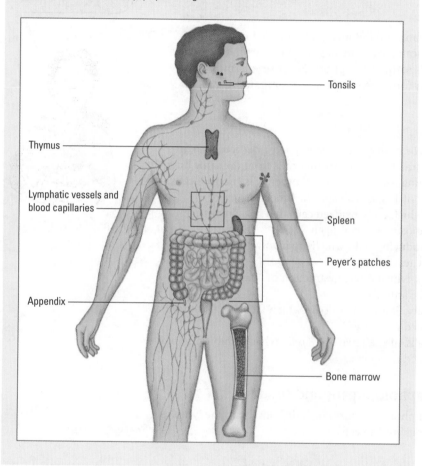

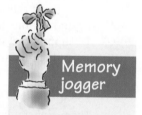

Memory jogger

To help you remember where lymphocytes mature, remember:

B cells mature in the

Bone marrow

T cells mature in the

Thymus.

To B or to be T

The lymphocytes further differentiate into either B cells (which mature in the bone marrow) or T cells (which travel to the thymus and mature). B cells and T cells are distributed throughout the lymphoid organs, especially the lymph nodes and spleen.

B cells don't attack pathogens themselves but instead produce antibodies, which attack pathogens or direct other cells, such as phagocytes, to attack them. This response is regulated by T cells and their products, lymphokines, which determine the immunoglobulin class a B cell will manufacture.

Thymus

In a fetus or an infant, the thymus is a two-lobed mass of lymphoid tissue located over the base of the heart in the mediastinum. The thymus forms T lymphocytes for several months after birth and gradually atrophies until only a remnant persists in adults.

Teaching T cells

In the thymus, T cells undergo a process called *T-cell education,* in which the cells "learn" to recognize other cells from the same body (self cells) and distinguish them from all other cells (nonself cells). There are five types of T cells with specific functions:

1. memory cells, which are sensitized cells that remain dormant until second exposure to an antigen
2. lymphokine-producing cells, which are involved in delayed hypersensitivity reactions
3. cytotoxic T cells, which direct destruction of an antigen or the cells carrying the antigen
4. helper T cells, also known as *T4 cells,* which facilitate the humoral and cell-mediated responses
5. suppressor T cells, also known as *T8 cells,* which inhibit humoral and cell-mediated responses.

Peripheral lymphoid organs and tissues

The peripheral lymphoid structures include lymph and the lymphatic vessels, lymph nodes, and spleen.

Lymph

Lymph is a clear fluid that bathes body tissues. It contains a liquid portion that resembles blood plasma.

Lymphatic vessels

The lymphatic vessels form a network of thin-walled channels that drain lymph from body tissues. Lymph seeps into the lymphatic vessels through their thin walls. (See *Lymphatic vessels and lymph nodes.*)

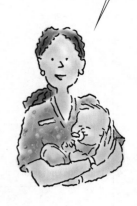

The thymus forms T lymphocytes until several months after birth and then gradually atrophies.

Lymphatic vessels and lymph nodes

The primary lymphatic vessels and structures of a lymph node are depicted below.

Into the nodes

Afferent lymphatic vessels carry lymph into the subcapsular sinus (or cavity) of the lymph node. From there, lymph flows through cortical sinuses and smaller radial medullary sinuses.

Phagocytic cells in the deep cortex and medullary sinuses attack antigens in lymph. Antigens may also be trapped in the follicles of the superficial cortex.

Back into the vessels

Cleansed lymph leaves the node through efferent lymphatic vessels at the hilum (a depression at the exit or entrance of the node). The efferent vessels drain into lymph node chains that, in turn, empty into large lymph vessels, or trunks, that drain into the subclavian vein of the vascular system.

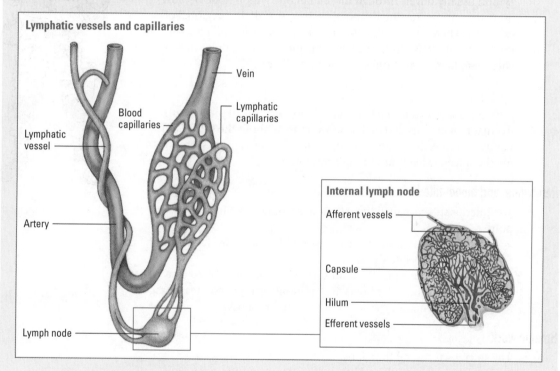

Lymphatic vessels and capillaries

Vein

Blood capillaries

Lymphatic capillaries

Lymphatic vessel

Artery

Lymph node

Internal lymph node

Afferent vessels

Capsule

Hilum

Efferent vessels

Fluid enters but can't exit

Lymphatic capillaries are located throughout most of the body. They're wider than blood capillaries and permit interstitial fluid to flow into them but not out.

Lymph nodes

Lymph nodes are small, oval-shaped structures along the lymphatic vessels. They're most abundant in the head, neck, axillae, abdomen, pelvis, and groin. Lymph nodes remove and destroy antigens circulating in the blood and lymph.

From vessels to nodes

Afferent lymphatic vessels, which resemble veins, carry lymph into the lymph nodes; the lymph slowly filters through the node and is collected into efferent lymphatic vessels.

Node to node

Lymph usually travels through more than one lymph node because numerous nodes line the lymphatic vessels that drain a region. For example, axillary nodes filter drainage from the arms and femoral nodes filter drainage from the legs. This prevents organisms that enter peripheral areas from entering central areas.

Spleen

A person's spleen is in the left upper abdominal quadrant beneath the diaphragm. This dark red, oval structure is about the size of a fist. Bands of connective tissue from the dense fibrous capsule surrounding the spleen extend into the spleen's interior.

Red, white, and blood-filled

The interior spleen, called the *splenic pulp*, contains white and red pulp:

- White pulp contains compact masses of lymphocytes surrounding branches of the splenic artery.
- Red pulp is a network of blood-filled sinusoids supported by a framework of reticular fibers and mononuclear phagocytes, along with some lymphocytes, plasma cells, and monocytes.

Splenic work

The spleen has several functions:

- Its phagocytes engulf and break down worn-out RBCs, causing the release of Hb, which then breaks down into its components. These phagocytes also selectively retain and destroy damaged or abnormal RBCs and cells with large amounts of abnormal Hb.
- It filters and removes bacteria and other foreign substances that enter the bloodstream; these substances are promptly removed by splenic phagocytes.
- Splenic phagocytes interact with lymphocytes to initiate an immune response.
- It stores blood and 20% to 30% of platelets.

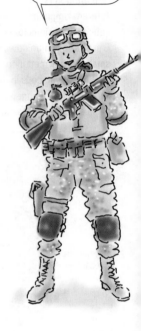

Lymph nodes filter out and destroy circulating antigens.

Accessory lymphoid organs and tissues

The tonsils, adenoids, appendix, and Peyer's patches are the accessory lymphoid organs and tissues. They remove foreign debris in much the same way lymph nodes do. They're located in areas where microbial access is more likely to occur.

Immunity

Immunity is the body's capacity to resist invading organisms and toxins, thereby preventing tissue and organ damage.

Elimination and preservation

The cells and organs of the immune system recognize, respond to, and eliminate foreign substances (antigens), such as bacteria, fungi, viruses, and parasites. They also preserve the body's internal environment by scavenging dead or damaged cells.

The immune system has three basic defensive functions:
- protective surface phenomena
- general host defenses
- specific immune responses.

Protective surface phenomena

Protective surface phenomena are physical, chemical, and mechanical barriers that prevent organisms from entering the body. Such phenomena include organs, structures, and processes of many body systems:
- integumentary
- respiratory
- GI
- genitourinary.

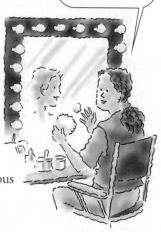

The skin and mucous membranes prevent microbial invasions.

Skin-deep defenses

Intact and healing skin and mucous membranes physically defend against microbial invasion by preventing attachment of microorganisms. Skin desquamation (normal cell turnover) and low pH further impede bacterial colonization.

Antibacterial substances, such as the enzyme lysozyme (in tears, saliva, and nasal secretions) chemically protect seromucous surfaces, such as the conjunctiva of the eye and oral mucous membranes.

Defensive breathing

In the respiratory system, turbulent airflow through the nostrils and nasal hairs filters foreign materials. Nasal secretions contain an immunoglobulin that discourages microbe adherence, and the mucous layer lining the respiratory tract is continually sloughed off and replaced.

GI system GIs

Bacteria that enter the GI system are mechanically removed through salivation, swallowing, peristalsis, and defecation. In addition, the low pH of gastric secretions is bactericidal, making the stomach virtually free from live bacteria. In addition, resident bacteria in the intestines prevent colonization by other microorganisms, protecting the rest of the GI system through a process called *colonization resistance*. In patients who have been on long-term broad-spectrum antibiotics, some of this natural defense is lost. Attempts at replacing this defense (probiotics) have had mixed results.

Urinary sterility

The urinary system is sterile except for the distal end of the urethra and the urinary meatus. Urine flow, low urine pH, immunoglobulin, and the bactericidal effects of prostatic fluid impede bacterial colonization. A series of sphincters also inhibits upward bacterial migration into the urinary tract.

> Resident bacteria in the intestines protect the GI system through a process called colonization resistance.

General host defenses

When an antigen does penetrate the skin or mucous membrane, the immune system launches a nonspecific cellular response to identify and remove the invader.

First response

The first nonspecific response against an antigen, the inflammatory response, involves vascular and cellular changes that eliminate dead tissue, microorganisms, toxins, and inert foreign matter. (See *Understanding inflammation*.)

Next effect

Phagocytosis occurs after inflammation or during chronic infection. In this nonspecific response, neutrophils and macrophages engulf, digest, and dispose of the antigen.

Specific immune responses

All foreign substances elicit the same general host defenses. In addition, particular microorganisms or molecules activate specific immune responses produced by lymphocytes (B cells and T cells) and can initially involve specialized sets of immune cells. Such specific responses are classified as either:
- humoral immunity
- cell-mediated immunity.

Understanding inflammation

The inflammatory response to an antigen involves vascular and cellular changes that eliminate dead tissue, microorganisms, toxins, and inert foreign matter. This nonspecific immune response aids tissue repair in a stepwise fashion.

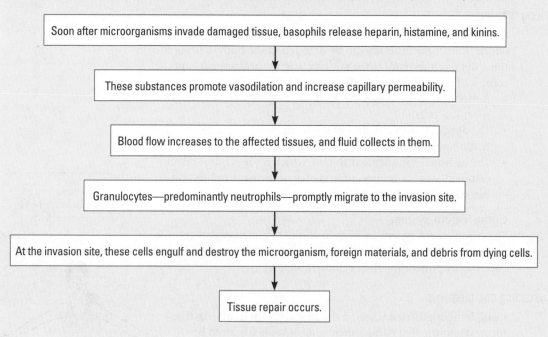

Soon after microorganisms invade damaged tissue, basophils release heparin, histamine, and kinins.

⬇

These substances promote vasodilation and increase capillary permeability.

⬇

Blood flow increases to the affected tissues, and fluid collects in them.

⬇

Granulocytes—predominantly neutrophils—promptly migrate to the invasion site.

⬇

At the invasion site, these cells engulf and destroy the microorganism, foreign materials, and debris from dying cells.

⬇

Tissue repair occurs.

Humoral immunity

In humoral immunity, an invading antigen causes B cells to divide and differentiate into plasma cells. Each plasma cell then produces and secretes a large amount of antigen-specific immunoglobulin into the bloodstream.

Each of the five types of immunoglobulins (IgA, IgD, IgE, IgG, and IgM) has a specific function:
- IgA, IgG, and IgM guard against viral and bacterial invasion.
- IgD is an antigen receptor of B cells.
- IgE causes an allergic response.

Defense depends on the antigen

Depending on the antigen, immunoglobulins work in one of several ways:
- They can disable certain bacteria by linking with toxins that the bacteria produce; these immunoglobulins are called *antitoxins*.

- They can opsonize (coat) bacteria, making them targets for scavenging by phagocytosis.
- Most commonly, they link to antigens, causing the immune system to produce and circulate enzymes called *complements*.

Telling time lag

After an initial exposure to an antigen, a time lag occurs during which little or no antibody can be detected in the body. During this time, the B cell recognizes the antigen, and the antigen-antibody complex forms. The complex has several functions:
- A macrophage processes the antigen and presents it to antigen-specific B cells.
- The antibody activates the complement system, causing an enzymatic cascade that destroys the antigen.
- The activated complement system, which bridges humoral and cell-mediated immunity, attracts phagocytic neutrophils and macrophages to the antigen site.

Complement system

The complement system consists of about 25 enzymes that complement the work of antibodies by aiding phagocytosis or destroying bacteria (by puncturing their cell membranes).

Cascading complements

Complement proteins travel in the bloodstream in an inactive form. When the first complement substance is triggered by an antibody interlocked with an antigen, it sets in motion a ripple effect. As each component is activated in turn, it acts on the next component in a controlled sequence called the *complement cascade*.

Attack complex

The complement cascade leads to formation of the membrane attack complex, which enters the membrane of a target cell and creates a channel through which fluids and molecules flow in and out. The target cell then swells and eventually bursts.

Complementary effects

Effects of the complement cascade also include:
- the inflammatory response (resulting from release of the contents of mast cells and basophils)
- stimulation and attraction of neutrophils (which participate in phagocytosis)
- coating of target cells by C3b (an inactivated fragment of the complement protein C3), making them attractive to phagocytes.

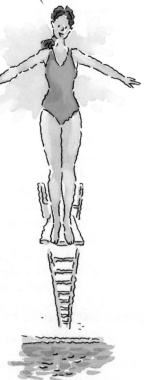

The complement cascade causes a ripple effect.

Cell-mediated immunity

Cell-mediated immunity protects the body against bacterial, viral, and fungal infections and provides resistance against transplanted cells and tumor cells.

T cells destroy and survey

In cell-mediated immunity, a macrophage processes the antigen, which is then presented to T cells. Some T cells become sensitized and destroy the antigen; others release lymphokines, which activate macrophages that destroy the antigen. Sensitized T cells then travel through the blood and lymphatic systems, providing ongoing surveillance for specific antigens.

Hematologic and immune systems assessment

Many signs and symptoms of hematologic disorders are nonspecific and difficult to assess. Others are more specific; use these to focus on possible disorders. Assess the hematologic system if the patient reports any of these specific signs or symptoms, including:

- abnormal bleeding
- bone and joint pain
- exertional dyspnea
- unexplained ecchymoses
- fatigue and weakness
- fever
- lymphadenopathy
- petechiae
- shortness of breath
- chills
- night sweats.

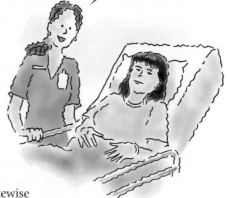

If the patient reports the specific signs or symptoms discussed here, assess for hematologic disorders.

Immune challenges

Accurately assessing a patient's immune system can likewise challenge your skills. Immune disorders sometimes produce characteristic signs—such as butterfly rash in systemic lupus erythematosus (SLE)—but they usually cause vague symptoms, such as fatigue or dyspnea, which initially seem related to other body systems. For this reason, assess the immune system whenever a patient reports such symptoms as:

- malaise
- fatigue
- frequent or recurrent infections
- slow wound healing.

Health history

Start your assessment by taking a thorough patient history. Gather information about the patient's current and previous illnesses. Also ask about the patient's family and social histories.

Current health status

Ask the patient how long he has had the problem, when it began, and how suddenly or gradually. Ask if it occurs continuously or intermittently. If intermittently, how frequent and how long is each episode?

Next, determine the location and character of the problem and precipitating conditions. Ask if anything makes the problem better or worse. Also ask about other signs and symptoms that occur at the same time as the primary ones.

Previous health status

Examine the patient's medical history for additional clues to his present condition. Look for information about allergies, immunizations, previously diagnosed illnesses (childhood and adulthood), past hospitalizations and surgeries, and current medications he uses, both prescription and over-the-counter.

Look back

Look at the patient's history for information about past disorders (such as acute leukemia, Hodgkin's disease, sarcoma, and rheumatoid arthritis) that required aggressive immunosuppressant or radiation therapies. Such treatment can diminish blood cell production. Has the patient received any blood products? If so, note when and how often blood product transfusions were used to assess the patient's risk of harboring a blood-borne infection or risk for antibody development, or cytomegalovirus (CMV).

Family history

Some hematologic disorders are inherited. Ask about deceased family members; note their ages at death and causes. Note any inheritable hematologic disorders; a genetics counselor may plot them on a family genogram to determine the patient's inheritance risk.

Lifestyle patterns

The patient may be reluctant to discuss certain habits or lifestyles. Take steps to develop trust between you and the patient to increase cooperation. Inquire about alcohol intake, diet, sexual habits, and

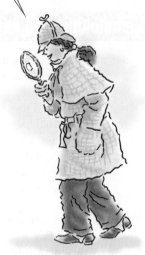

Examine the patient's medical history to find clues about his present condition.

possible drug abuse, all of which can impair hematologic or immune function.

Work and service

Make sure you gather a comprehensive occupational and military service history. Exposure to certain hazardous substances can cause bone marrow dysfunction, especially leukemia.

Physical assessment

Because hematologic and immune disorders can involve almost every body system, perform a complete physical examination.

Assessing vital signs

Vital signs can provide important clues about the patient's hematologic and immune system health.

Thermo-measurement

Take the patient's temperature. Frequent fevers can indicate a poorly functioning immune system. Patients with cancer may not be able to respond with a high-grade fever. Subnormal temperatures usually accompany gram-negative infections.

Heart and BP checks

Note the patient's heart rate. The heart may pump harder or faster to compensate for a decreased oxygen supply resulting from anemia or decreased blood volume from bleeding. This problem can cause tachycardia, palpitations, or arrhythmias.

Measure the patient's blood pressure while lying, sitting, and standing. Check for orthostatic hypotension, which may be caused by septicemia or hypovolemia. Always compare previous history of blood pressure for trends.

O₂ inquiry

Check the patient's breathing and oxygen saturation. If he's having difficulty meeting the body's oxygen needs, he may have pronounced tachypnea.

Size up

Next, measure the patient's height and weight. Compare the findings with normal values for the patient's bone structure. Weight loss may result from anorexia or other GI problems related to immune disorders.

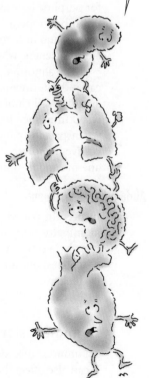

Because hematologic and immune disorders can involve almost every body system, perform a complete physical examination.

Hematologic inspection

Next, concentrate on areas most relevant to a hematologic disorder, including the:

- skin
- mucous membranes
- fingernails
- eyes
- lymph nodes
- liver and spleen.

Skin-deep assessment

The patient's skin color directly reflects body fluid composition. Observe for pallor, cyanosis, or jaundice. Check for erythema and plethora (ruddy color), which appear with local inflammation and polycythemia, respectively. Assess the mucous membranes for jaundice, bleeding, redness, swelling, or ulceration.

Examine skin, nails, and eyes

If you suspect a blood-clotting abnormality, check the patient's skin for purpuric lesions, which may vary in size and usually result from thrombocytopenia. Also, inspect for abnormalities, such as telangiectases, and note their locations. Check the patient's skin for dryness and coarseness, which may indicate iron deficiency anemia.

Note abnormalities in the patient's nails. Longitudinal striations can indicate anemia. Spoon-shaped nails characterize iron deficiency anemia. Nail clubbing indicates chronic tissue hypoxia, which can result from such hematologic disorders as anemia.

Inspect the patient's eyes for jaundice, which may occur from excessive hemolysis. Retinal hemorrhages and exudates suggest severe anemia and thrombocytopenia.

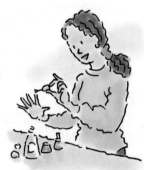

Abnormalities in the patient's nails, such as longitudinal striations, spoon shape, and clubbing, can result from anemia. I'm inspecting for smudges.

Abdominal assessment

Inspect the patient's abdominal area for enlargement, distention, and asymmetry, possibly indicating a tumor. Hepatomegaly and splenomegaly may result from:

- congestion caused by cell overproduction, as in polycythemia or leukemia
- excessive cell destruction, as in hemolytic anemia.

Immune system inspection

An immune disorder can affect the skin and nails as described above. It can also affect the mouth and nose, so assess the nasal cavity for mucous membrane ulceration, which may indicate SLE.

Inspect the oral mucosa. White patches scattered throughout the mouth may indicate candidiasis, and lacy white plaques on the buccal mucosa may be associated with acquired immunodeficiency syndrome (AIDS). Such lesions can also occur in a patient with an immunosuppressive disorder or one who receives chemotherapy.

LOC signs

Evaluate the patient's level of consciousness (LOC) and mental status. Neurologic effects may provide clues to an underlying disease. A patient with SLE may experience altered mentation, depression, or psychosis.

Eyes, fingers, toes, ears, and nose

Observe the patient's eyelids for signs of infection or inflammation. Assess the fundus of the eye; hemorrhage or infiltration may indicate vasculitis.

Assess the patient's peripheral circulation for Raynaud's phenomenon (intermittent arteriolar vasospasm of the fingers or toes and sometimes of the ears and nose). This phenomenon may be caused by SLE or scleroderma.

Urinary system inspection

Because immune dysfunction can affect the urinary system, obtain a urine specimen and evaluate its color, clarity, and odor. Cloudy, malodorous urine may result from a urinary tract infection.

Inspect the urinary meatus. In a patient with WBC deficiency or immunodeficiency, the external genitalia may be focal points for inflammation, which is commonly accompanied by discharge or bleeding related to infection.

Look for lumps

Inspect the lymph node areas where the patient reports swollen glands or lumps for color abnormalities and visible lymph node enlargement. Then inspect all other nodal regions. Proceed from head to toe to avoid missing any region. Normally, lymph nodes can't be seen. Visibly enlarged nodes suggest a current or previous inflammation. Nodes covered with red-streaked skin suggest acute lymphadenitis.

Auscultating the abdomen

With the patient lying down, auscultate the abdomen before palpation and percussion to avoid altering bowel sounds. Listen for a loud, high-pitched, tinkling sound, which heralds the early stages of intestinal obstruction. Lymphoma is a hematologic cause of such obstruction.

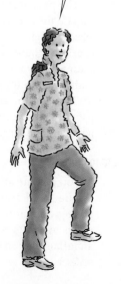

Look from head to toe for lumps or visible lymph node enlargement.

Percussing the liver and spleen

To determine liver and spleen size, and possibly detect tumors, percuss all four quadrants and compare your findings.

Dullness is normal

The normal liver sounds dull. Establish the organ's approximate size by percussing for its upper and lower borders at the midclavicular line. To determine medial extension, percuss to the midsternal landmark.

The normal spleen also sounds dull. Percuss it from the midaxillary line toward the midline. The average-sized spleen lies near the 8th, 9th, or 10th intercostal space. You might mark the liver and spleen borders with a pen for later reference.

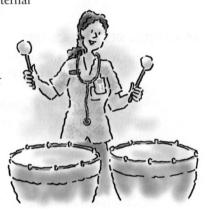

> Percuss all four abdominal quadrants to determine liver and spleen size and to detect tumors.

Palpating lymph nodes, liver, and spleen

Before palpating the lymph nodes, liver, and spleen, make sure the patient is positioned comfortably, draped appropriately, and kept warm. Warm your hands, then palpate using gentle to moderate pressure.

Lymph node palpation

Palpate the patient's neck, axillary, epitrochlear, and inguinal lymph nodes, moving the skin over each area with your finger pads.

Check neck nodes and so on

When palpating nodes in the neck, make sure the patient is sitting.

The patient should remain sitting or should lie down when you palpate the axillary nodes. To check the right axilla, ask the patient to relax the right arm. Use your nondominant hand to support it. Put your other hand as high in the axilla as possible. Palpate against the chest wall for the lateral, anterior, posterior, central, and subclavian nodes. Repeat the procedure for the left axilla.

To assess the epitrochlear nodes, palpate the medial area of the patient's elbow. For the inguinal nodes, palpate below the inguinal ligament and along the upper saphenous vein.

What to look for

As you palpate all nodes, note their location, size, tenderness, texture (hard, soft, or firm), and whether they're movable. For each node group, note current or previous inflammation. Hard or fixed nodes may suggest a tumor. General lymphadenopathy can indicate an inflammation or cancerous condition. (See *Palpating the lymph nodes.*)

Palpating the lymph nodes

When assessing your patient for signs of an immune disorder, palpate the superficial lymph nodes of the head and neck and of the axillary, epitrochlear, inguinal, and popliteal areas, using the pads of your index and middle fingers. Always palpate gently, beginning with light pressure and gradually increasing the pressure.

Head and neck nodes

Head and neck nodes are best palpated with the patient sitting.

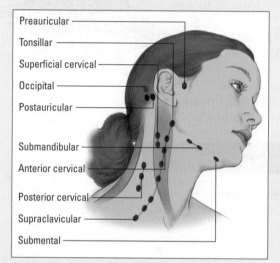

- Preauricular
- Tonsillar
- Superficial cervical
- Occipital
- Postauricular
- Submandibular
- Anterior cervical
- Posterior cervical
- Supraclavicular
- Submental

Axillary and epitrochlear nodes

Palpate the axillary and epitrochlear nodes with the patient sitting. You can also palpate the axillary nodes with the patient lying in a supine position.

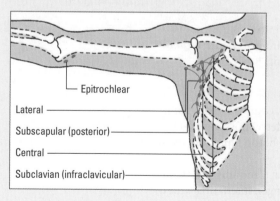

- Epitrochlear
- Lateral
- Subscapular (posterior)
- Central
- Subclavian (infraclavicular)

Inguinal and popliteal nodes

Palpate the inguinal and popliteal nodes with the patient lying in a supine position. You can also palpate the popliteal nodes with the patient sitting or standing.

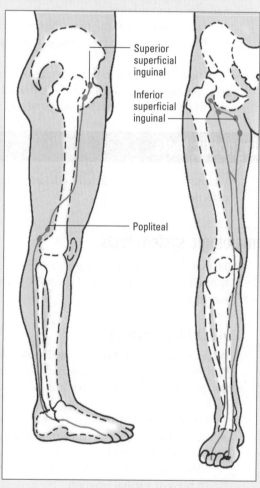

- Superior superficial inguinal
- Inferior superficial inguinal
- Popliteal

Cell-packing problem

As you palpate the patient's nodes, you may discover sternal tenderness. This problem occurs with cell packing in the marrow from anemia, leukemia, and immunoproliferative disorders.

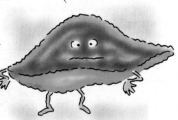

Remember, palpate tender areas last. I'm a sensitive fellow, you know.

Liver and spleen palpation

Accurate liver palpation is difficult and can depend on the patient's size and comfort level and possible fluid accumulation. Lightly palpate all four abdominal quadrants to distinguish tender sites and muscle guarding. Use deeper palpation to delineate abdominal organs and masses.

If necessary, repeat the procedure, checking your hand position and the pressure you exert. Always palpate tender areas last.

Palpate the spleen to detect tenderness and confirm splenomegaly. The spleen must be enlarged about three times normal size to be palpable. (See *Percussing and palpating the spleen.*)

Diagnostic tests

Various tests may be ordered to diagnose hematologic and immune disorders.

Hematologic system tests

Hematologic diagnostic tests allow direct analysis of the blood, its formed elements (cells), and the bone marrow, where blood cells originate.

ABO blood typing

ABO blood typing is used to classify blood into A, B, AB, and O groups according to the presence of major antigens A and B on RBC surfaces and serum antibodies anti-A and anti-B.

Nursing considerations

- Before the patient receives a transfusion, compare current and past ABO typing and crossmatching to detect possible mistaken identification. Both forward and reverse blood typing are required to prevent a lethal reaction.
- If a patient has received blood in the past 3 months, antibodies to this donor blood may develop and linger, interfering with the patient's compatibility testing. This patient will need additional crossmatch testing.

Percussing and palpating the spleen

To assess the spleen, use percussion to estimate its size and palpation to detect tenderness and enlargement. Splenic tenderness may result from infections, which are common in a patient with an immunodeficiency disorder. Splenomegaly may occur with immune disorders that cause congestion by cell overproduction or by excessive demand for cell destruction.

Percussion

To percuss the spleen, follow these steps:

1. Percuss the lowest intercostal space in the left anterior axillary line; percussion notes should be tympanic.

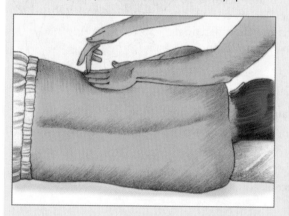

2. Ask the patient to take a deep breath, then percuss this area again. If the spleen is normal in size, the area will remain tympanic. If the tympanic percussion note changes on inspiration to dullness, the spleen is probably enlarged.
3. To estimate spleen size, outline the spleen's edges by percussing in several directions from areas of tympany to areas of dullness.

Palpation

To palpate the spleen, follow these steps:

1. With the patient in a supine position and you at his right side, reach across him to support the posterior lower left rib cage with your left hand. Place your right hand below the left costal margin and press inward.

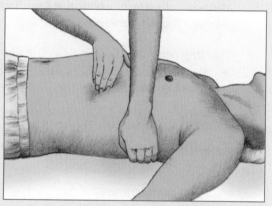

2. Instruct him to take a deep breath. The spleen normally shouldn't descend on deep inspiration below the ninth or tenth intercostal space in the posterior midaxillary line. If the spleen is enlarged, you'll feel its rigid border.

Note: Don't overpalpate the spleen; an enlarged spleen can easily rupture.

Antibody screening test

An antibody screening test—also called an *indirect Coombs test* and *indirect antiglobulin test*—is used to detect unexpected circulating antibodies to RBC antigens in the recipient's or donor's serum before transfusion. Normally, agglutination doesn't occur, indicating that the patient's serum contains no circulating antibodies (other than anti-A and anti-B).

Positive incompatibility

A positive result reveals the presence of unexpected circulating anti-bodies to RBC antigens, indicating donor–recipient incompatibility.

Nursing considerations
- Explain to the patient that the antibody screening test is used to evaluate the possibility of a transfusion reaction.

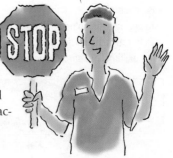

Hold it! Withhold medications that can induce autoimmune hemolytic anemia.

Antiglobulin test

The direct antiglobulin test, also called the *direct Coombs test*, is used to detect immunoglobulins (antibodies) on RBC surfaces. These immunoglobulins coat RBCs when they become sensitized to an antigen such as the Rh factor. The test is used to investigate hemolytic transfusion reactions and aid differential diagnosis of anemias, which may result from an autoimmune reaction or a drug's adverse effect.

Nursing considerations
- As ordered, withhold medications that can induce autoimmune hemolytic anemia.

Coagulation screening tests

Coagulation screening tests are used to detect bleeding disorders and specific coagulation defects.

Nursing considerations
- Explain the test to the patient.
- Allow no more than 4 hours between blood sampling and coagulation testing. Allow only 2 hours between blood centrifugation and coagulation testing because once centrifuged, RBCs lose their buffering effect on the plasma.
- Avoid using hemolyzed plasma, which may decrease clotting times. Place the patient's blood sample on ice immediately after it's collected to preserve its labile factors.

Crossmatching

Crossmatching is used to establish the compatibility or incompatibility of donor and recipient blood and is the final check for such compatibility.

Always necessary, except . . .

Blood is always crossmatched before transfusion, except in extreme emergencies. Because a complete crossmatch may take 45 minutes to

2 hours, an incomplete (10-minute) crossmatch may be acceptable in emergencies. Meanwhile, transfusion can begin with limited amounts of group O negative packed RBCs. When an emergency transfusion is necessary, proceed with special awareness of the complications that may arise because of incomplete typing and crossmatching.

Nursing considerations
- If more than 48 hours have elapsed since a previous transfusion, previously crossmatched donor blood must be crossmatched with a new recipient serum sample to detect newly acquired incompatibilities before transfusion.
- If the recipient hasn't received a transfusion, donor blood need not be crossmatched again for 72 hours.
- If the patient is scheduled for surgery and has received blood during the previous 3 months, his blood must be crossmatched again to detect recently acquired incompatibilities.

D-dimer

D-dimer testing may help diagnose disseminated intravascular coagulation (DIC) by confirming the presence of fibrin split products. Fibrin split products are pieces of clot that enter the circulation after the clot has been broken down. DIC is a process that continually builds and breaks down clots, until all the clotting factors in the body have been depleted. As more clots break down, the D-dimer rises.

Nursing considerations
- Explain the purpose of the test to the patient.
- If the patient is being tested for coagulopathies, apply additional pressure to the venipuncture site to prevent hematoma formation.

Hematocrit

Hematocrit (HCT) test results indicate the percentage of RBCs in whole blood samples. Although normal HCT varies widely, it's roughly three times the person's Hb level and amounts to:
- 42% to 52% in men
- 36% to 48% in women
- 30% to 42% in children.

Below normal HCT suggests anemia or hemodilution; above normal, polycythemia or hemoconcentration due to blood loss.

Nursing considerations
- Explain the purpose of blood studies to the patient.
- Notify the practitioner of significant findings and administer blood products as ordered based on test results.

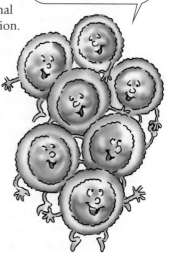

HCT test results indicate the percentage of RBCs in whole blood samples.

Unless the patient has an ischemic cardiac history, HCT less than 21% may not need to be transfused unless the patient is exhibiting signs of decreased tissue perfusion.

Hemoglobin level (total Hb)

Hb—the main component of RBCs—contains *heme*, a complex molecule of iron and porphyrin that gives blood its color, and globin, a simple protein.

O₂ delivery

Hb delivers oxygen from the lungs to the cells and buffers carbon dioxide formed during metabolic activity. A below normal Hb level may result from anemia, recent hemorrhage, or fluid retention causing hemodilution; an above normal Hb level may result from hemoconcentration due to polycythemia or dehydration.

Nursing considerations
- Explain the purpose of blood studies to the patient.
- Notify the practitioner of significant findings and administer blood products as ordered based on test results.
- Unless the patient has an ischemic cardiac history, Hb less than 7 may not need to be transfused unless the patient is exhibiting signs of decreased tissue perfusion.

Partial thromboplastin time

Partial thromboplastin time (PTT) is used to evaluate all intrinsic pathway clotting factors (except factors VII and XIII) by measuring the time needed for a fibrin clot to form after calcium and phospholipid emulsion is added to a plasma sample. PTT is commonly used to monitor heparin therapy.

Normal time

Normally, a fibrin clot forms 25 to 36 seconds after reagent is added. Prolonged times may mean that the plasma sample contains plasma clotting factor deficiencies, heparin, fibrin split products, or circulating anticoagulants that act as antibodies to clotting factors.

Nursing considerations
- Explain to the patient receiving heparin therapy that this test may be repeated at regular intervals to assess his response to treatment.
- Notify the practitioner of test results and adjust the heparin infusion dosage as ordered.
- For a patient on anticoagulant therapy, additional pressure may be needed at the venipuncture site to control bleeding.

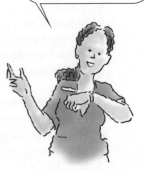

Normally, a fibrin clot forms 25 to 36 seconds after reagent is added. Anything longer can be a problem.

Plasma thrombin time

The plasma thrombin test—also known as the *thrombin clotting time test*—is used to measure how quickly a clot forms after a standard amount of bovine thrombin is added to a platelet-poor plasma sample from the patient and to a normal plasma control sample. It's used to detect a fibrinogen deficiency or defect, diagnose DIC and hepatic disease, and monitor heparin or thrombolytic therapy. Normal test results range from 10 to 15 seconds.

Nursing considerations

- If possible, withhold heparin therapy before the test as ordered. If heparin therapy must be continued, note this on the laboratory request.

Platelet count

Platelet count is used to evaluate platelet (thrombocyte) production, which is necessary for blood clotting. Accurate counts are essential for monitoring chemotherapy and radiation therapy and for assessing the severity of thrombocytosis (abnormally increased platelet count) or thrombocytopenia.

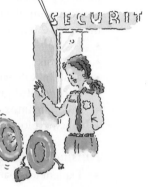

Not so fast . . . nobody gets by unless they're on the list and their I.D. checks out. Many institutions have implemented barcoding and scanners to aid in positive patient identification.

Count down

A normal platelet count varies from 140,000 to 400,000 per µl. A platelet count below 50,000/µl can result in spontaneous bleeding; a count below 5,000/µl usually indicates potential for massive hemorrhage. A decreased platelet count may result from autoimmune processes, some drugs (such as heparin), or infection.

Count up

An increased platelet count may result from hemorrhage, infectious disorders, cancer, iron deficiency anemia, surgery, pregnancy, splenectomy, or an inflammatory disorder.

Nursing considerations

- Explain the purpose of platelet studies to the patient.
- Notify the practitioner of significant findings and administer blood products as ordered based on test results.

Prothrombin time and INR

Prothrombin time (PT) is the time required for a fibrin clot to form in a citrated plasma sample after calcium ion and tissue thromboplastin (factor III) are added. The result is compared to the fibrin clotting time in a control plasma sample.

Indirect test

PT is used to indirectly measure prothrombin and is an excellent screening method for evaluating prothrombin; fibrinogen; and extrinsic coagulation factors V, VII, and X. It's the test of choice for monitoring oral anticoagulant therapy. In a patient receiving an oral anticoagulant, PT usually remains between one and one-half and three times the normal control value.

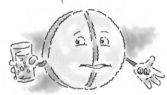

PT is best for monitoring oral anticoagulant therapy.

INR standards

The international normalized ratio (INR) system is the best means of standardizing measurement of PT to monitor oral anticoagulant therapy. Normal INR for those receiving warfarin therapy is 2.0 to 3.0. Increased INR values may indicate:
- DIC
- cirrhosis
- vitamin K deficiency
- uncontrolled oral anticoagulation
- salicylate intoxication
- massive blood transfusion.

Nursing considerations
- Explain to a patient receiving oral anticoagulant therapy that this test may be repeated at regular intervals to assess his response to treatment.
- For a patient on anticoagulant therapy, additional pressure may be needed at the venipuncture site to control bleeding.
- Notify the practitioner of test results; oral anticoagulant therapy dosage adjustments are based on test results.

RBC count

RBC count—also known as *erythrocyte count*—indicates the number of RBCs in whole blood. A depressed RBC count may indicate anemia, fluid overload, recent hemorrhage, or leukemia; an elevated count, dehydration, polycythemia, or acute poisoning.

Nursing considerations
- Explain the purpose of RBC studies to the patient.
- Notify the practitioner of significant findings.

Rh blood typing

The Rh system is used to classify blood according to the presence or absence of antigen D (formerly known as *Rho*) on RBC surfaces. Rh blood typing is used to determine if donors and recipients are compatible before transfusions and to learn whether the patient needs a RhoGAM (Rho[D] immune globulin) injection.

Nursing considerations
- Before the patient receives a transfusion, the Rh factor must be checked along with ABO typing.

Biopsy

Biopsies involve removing small samples of tissue for testing.

Bone marrow aspiration and needle biopsy

In aspiration biopsy, a fluid specimen containing bone marrow cells in suspension is collected. Bone marrow aspiration is an important test for evaluating the blood's formed elements.

Needle biopsy is done to remove a marrow core containing cells but no fluid. The best possible marrow specimens are obtained by using both methods.

Aspire to biopsy

Because most hematopoiesis takes place in bone marrow, histologic and hematologic bone marrow examination yields valuable diagnostic information about blood disorders. Bone marrow aspiration and needle biopsy are used to obtain material for that examination.

Bone marrow biopsy is used to diagnose aplastic, hypoplastic, and vitamin B_{12} deficiency anemias; granulomas; leukemias; lymphomas; myelofibrosis; and thrombocytopenia. It's also used to evaluate chemotherapy effectiveness and to monitor myelosuppression.

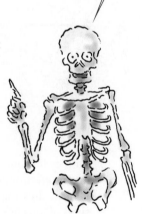

Bone marrow examination yields valuable information about blood disorders.

Nursing considerations
- Describe the procedure and answer the patient's questions. Confirm any medication allergies or past history of hypersensitivity to local anesthetics. Inform the patient that a local anesthetic is used but that he may feel pressure during the biopsy.
- Tell him the test takes 5 to 10 minutes, and test results are usually available in 1 day.
- Tell the patient which bone is to be used for the biopsy. (See *Bone marrow aspiration and biopsy sites*, page 632.)
- Explain to the patient that he may receive I.V. sedation before the procedure.
- Monitor vital signs, oxygen saturation, and cardiac rhythm during and after the procedure. After the procedure, check the biopsy site

Bone marrow aspiration and biopsy sites

The drawings below depict the most common sites for bone marrow aspiration and biopsy. These sites are used because the involved bone structures are relatively accessible and rich in marrow cavities.

Posterior superior iliac crest

The posterior superior iliac crest is the preferred site for aspiration and biopsy because no vital organs or vessels are nearby. The patient lies in a prone or lateral position. The needle is inserted several centimeters lateral to the iliosacral junction and directed downward and toward the anterior inferior spine or entered a few centimeters below the crest at a right angle to the surface of the bone.

Spinous process

The spinous process is preferred if multiple punctures are necessary or if marrow is absent at other sites. The patient sits on the edge of the bed, leaning over the bedside stand. The spinous process of the third or fourth lumbar vertebrae is selected; the needle is inserted at the crest or slightly to one side and advanced in the direction of the bone plane.

Sternum

The sternum involves the greatest risk but provides the best access. The patient is in a supine position with a small pillow beneath his shoulders to elevate his chest and lower his head. The doctor secures the needle guard 3 to 4 mm from the tip of the needle to avoid accidentally puncturing the heart or a major vessel. Then he inserts the needle at the midline of the sternum at the second intercostal space.

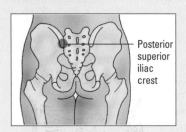

Posterior superior iliac crest

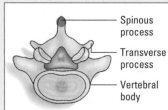

Spinous process

Transverse process

Vertebral body

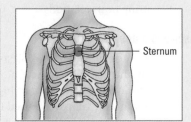

Sternum

for bleeding and inflammation. Monitor for these signs of bleeding or infection: rapid heart rate, low blood pressure, or fever.
- Remove dressing over biopsy site in 24 hours and assess for any signs of infection.

Immune system tests

The practitioner may order various tests to evaluate the patient's immune response. Commonly ordered studies include cellular tests, such as T- and B-lymphocyte assays, to detect immune-mediated disease.

T- and B-lymphocyte surface marker assays

Surface marker assays are used to identify the specific cells involved in the immune response and to examine the balance between the regulatory activities of several interacting cell types, notably T-helper and T-suppressor cells.

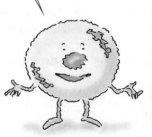

Surface marker assays are used to analyze both normal and malignant cells.

The test involves use of highly specific monoclonal antibodies to define levels of lymphocyte differentiation and to analyze both normal and malignant cells. This information is used to assess immunocompetence in chronic infections; evaluate immunodeficiencies; and classify lymphocytic leukemia, lymphoma, and immunodeficiency disease and AIDS.

Nursing considerations
- Explain the test to the patient.
- Send the sample to the laboratory immediately; don't refrigerate or freeze it.

Treatments

Treatments for patients with hematologic and immune disorders may include drug therapy and transfusion therapy.

Drug therapy

Hematologic drugs include anticoagulants, blood derivatives, hematinics, hemostatics, and heparin antagonists. (See *Common hematologic medications*, pages 634 and 635.)

For patients with some immune disorders, drugs are the primary treatment. For example, epinephrine is the drug of choice for correcting an anaphylactic reaction. For patients with other disorders, drugs are prescribed to treat associated symptoms. (See *Drug therapy in immune disorders*, pages 636 to 638.)

Corticosteroid potentials

Corticosteroids are adrenocortical hormones used to treat patients with immune-mediated disorders because of their potent anti-inflammatory and immunosuppressant effects.

Corticosteroids stabilize the vascular membrane, blocking tissue infiltration by neutrophils and monocytes and thus inhibiting inflammation. They also affect T cells in the bone marrow, causing leukopenia. However, because these drugs aren't cytotoxic, lymphocyte concentration can quickly return to normal within 24 hours after they're withdrawn.

Corticosteroid cautions

Steroids should be used cautiously in patients with GI ulceration, renal disease, hypertension, diabetes mellitus, and psychotic tendencies.

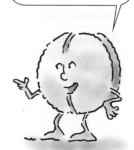

Corticosteroids aren't cytotoxic, so lymphocytes can quickly return to normal afterward. Caution must be used because they can mask infection and delay wound healing if used for prolonged periods of time.

Common hematologic medications

Hematologic drugs include hematinics, which help arrest anemia; anticoagulants and heparin, which impede clotting; hemostatics, which arrest blood flow or reduce capillary bleeding; blood derivatives, which replace blood loss from disease or surgical procedures; and thrombolytic enzymes, which treat thrombotic disorders. This chart outlines common hemolytic drugs, their indications and adverse effects, and practice considerations.

Drugs	Indications	Adverse effects	Practice pointers
Anticoagulants			
Heparin	• Prevention of pulmonary embolism and deep vein thrombosis (DVT) after hip- or knee-replacement surgery • Continuous I.V. or subQ therapy for DVT, myocardial infarction (MI), pulmonary embolism • Disseminated intravascular coagulation, to help stop repeated clotting	• Hemorrhage, thrombocytopenia, chills, fever, pruritus, urticaria, anaphylactoid reactions	• Never administer I.M. • Don't massage the site after subcutaneous (subQ) injection. Rotate injection sites, keeping a record of sites used. • Monitor platelet count and for signs of bleeding. • Check I.V. infusions regularly for underdosing and overdosing. • Measure PTT regularly. Anticoagulation is present when PTT values are one and one-half to two times control values. • Never piggyback other drugs into an infusion line while heparin infusion is running.
Warfarin	• Treatment of pulmonary embolism • Prevention and treatment of DVT, MI, rheumatic heart disease with heart valve damage, atrial arrhythmias	Anorexia, nausea, vomiting, hematuria, hemorrhage, jaundice, urticaria, fever, headache, rash	• PT and INR determinations are essential for proper controls; maintain PT at one and one-half to three times normal and INR at 2.0 to 3.0. • Give drug at the same time daily. • Regularly inspect for bleeding gums, bruises, petechiae, nosebleeds, melena, hematuria, and hematemesis. • Tell the patient to use an electric razor, avoid scratching the skin, and use a soft toothbrush.
Blood derivatives			
Normal serum albumin 5% Normal serum albumin 25%	• Hypovolemic shock • Hypoproteinemia	Vascular overload after rapid infusion, hypotension, nausea, vomiting, dyspnea, pulmonary edema, chills, fever	• Don't give more than 250 g in 48 hours. • Watch for hemorrhage or shock if used after surgery or injury. • Watch for signs of vascular overload (heart failure or pulmonary edema). • Don't use cloudy solutions or those with sediment.

Common hematologic medications *(continued)*

Drugs	Indications	Adverse effects	Practice pointers
Blood derivatives *(continued)*			
Plasma protein fractions	• Hypovolemic shock • Hypoproteinemia	Headache, hypotension or vascular overload after rapid infusion, tachycardia, nausea, vomiting, dyspnea, pulmonary edema, rash, fever, chills, back pain	• Monitor blood pressure; reduce infusion rate if hypotension occurs. • Watch for signs of vascular overload (heart failure or pulmonary edema). • Monitor intake and output; watch for decreased urine output. • Don't give more than 250 g in 48 hours.
Hematinics			
Ferrous sulfate	• Iron deficiency	• Nausea, epigastric pain, vomiting, constipation, black stools, diarrhea, anorexia	• Dilute liquid preparations in orange juice or water, not milk or antacids. Give tablets with orange juice to promote absorption. • Give elixir with a straw to avoid staining teeth. • GI upset is related to dosage; give the drug between meals.
Hemostatics			
Aminocaproic acid	• Excessive bleeding resulting from hyperfibrinolysis	Dizziness, malaise, headache, tinnitus, nausea, cramps, diarrhea, rash	• Monitor coagulation studies, heart rhythm, and blood pressure; notify the practitioner of changes. • Dilute the solution with sterile water for injection, normal saline solution, dextrose 5% in water, or lactated Ringer's solution.
Heparin antagonist			
Protamine	• Heparin overdose	• Bradycardia, circulatory collapse, nausea, vomiting, pulmonary edema, acute pulmonary hypertension, anaphylaxis	• Use cautiously after cardiac surgery. • Give slowly to reduce adverse effects. • Watch for spontaneous bleeding. • Caution in patients with hypersensitivity to fish (increased risk of hypersensitivity)

Transfusion therapy

Transfusion procedures allow administration of a wide range of blood products, such as RBCs, which can revive oxygen-starved tissues; leukocytes, which can combat infections beyond the reach of

(Text continues on page 638.)

Drug therapy in immune disorders

The practitioner may order drug therapy to suppress a patient's immune response. Immune serum studies may be ordered after specific antigens are identified. Immunosuppressants may be used to combat tissue rejection or relieve inflammation. Antiviral agents, which include nucleoside analogs, protease inhibitors, and nonnucleoside reverse transcriptase inhibitors, are used to correct human immunodeficiency virus (HIV) infections. Use this table to find information necessary to administer these drugs.

Drugs	Indications	Adverse effects	Practice pointers
Nucleoside analogs			
Lamivudine	• Treatment of HIV infection in combination with other antivirals	Headache, fatigue, dizziness, insomnia, neutropenia, thrombo-cytopenia, cough, fever, chills, malaise, nausea	• Monitor serum amylase levels. Stop drug if clinical signs and symptoms suggest pancreatitis. • Give with another antiviral. Not indicated for use alone.
Stavudine	• Treatment of HIV-infected patients who have received prolonged zidovudine therapy	Peripheral neuropathy, headache, malaise, insomnia, anxiety, dizziness, chest pain, abdominal pain, diarrhea, nausea, anorexia, weight loss, neutropenia, thrombocytopenia, anemia, rash, hepatotoxicity, chills, fever, pancreatitis	• It may be taken with or without food. • Teach patient signs and symptoms of peripheral neuropathy, which is the major dose-limiting effect. It may not resolve after drug is discontinued. • Monitor liver function tests.
Zidovudine, AZT	• Symptom-producing HIV infection	Headache, seizures, paresthesia, somnolence, anorexia, nausea, vomiting, diarrhea, constipation, severe bone marrow suppression (resulting in anemia), rash, myalgia, fever, increased liver enzymes	• Use cautiously in patients with severe bone marrow depression. • Monitor blood studies every 2 weeks to detect anemia or granulocytopenia. • For I.V. use, dilute before administration. Remove the calculated dose from the vial; add to dextrose 5% in water injection to achieve a concentration not exceeding 4 mg/ml. Infuse over 1 hour at a constant rate. Avoid rapid infusion or bolus injection.
Protease inhibitors			
Saquinavir	• Treatment of advanced HIV infection in combination with other antivirals	Headache, dizziness, chest pain, pancreatitis, pancytopenia, thrombocytopenia, portal hypertension, hyperglycemia, cough, rash	• Watch for adipogenic adverse effects (redistribution of body fat, peripheral wasting, and breast enlargement). • Use cautiously in patients with liver impairment.
Indinavir	• HIV infection	Headache, abdominal pain, nausea, acute renal failure, hemolytic anemia, neutropenia, hepatic failure, hyperglycemia, back pain, insomnia, dizziness, malaise	• Instruct patient to drink at least 6 glasses of water per day. • Give the drug on an empty stomach. • Monitor blood glucose levels.

Drug therapy in immune disorders *(continued)*

Drugs	Indications	Adverse effects	Practice pointers
Protease inhibitors (continued)			
Ritonavir	• HIV infection	Asthenia, generalized tonic-clonic seizure, pancreatitis, thrombocytopenia, leukopenia, hepatitis, diabetes mellitus, hypersensitivity reaction, rash, myalgia, anorexia, abdominal pain, constipation, diarrhea, nausea, vomiting	• Monitor liver function studies and blood glucose levels. • Administer with food.
Nonnucleoside reverse transcriptase inhibitors			
Delavirdine	• HIV infection (especially in patients infected in North America and Europe)	Anxiety, asthenia, fatigue, headache, sinusitis, abdominal pain, nausea, vomiting, rash, cough	• Monitor patient for rash. • Should be used with other antivirals because resistance develops quickly when used as single therapy.
Nevirapine	• Prevention of maternal–fetal transmission of HIV • Adjunct therapy for HIV infection	Headache, fever, nausea, diarrhea, abdominal pain, hepatitis, hepatotoxicity, Stevens-Johnson syndrome, severe hypersensitivity reaction	• Monitor patient for and immediately report blistering rash.
Immune serums			
Hepatitis B immune globulin (HBIG)	• Hepatitis B exposure	Urticaria, pain and tenderness at injection site, anaphylaxis, angioedema	• Obtain a history of allergies and reactions to immunizations. • Inject the drug into the anterolateral aspect of thigh or deltoid area. • Administer with the hepatitis B vaccine for postexposure prophylaxis (needlestick or direct contact).
Immune globulin	• Bone marrow transplant • Hepatitis exposure	Headache, faintness, nausea, vomiting, hip pain, chest pain, chest tightness, dyspnea, urticaria, muscle stiffness (at injection site), anaphylaxis, fever, chills, malaise	• Have epinephrine available in case of anaphylactic reaction to the medication. • Use cautiously in patients with a history of cardiovascular disease of thrombotic episodes.

(continued)

Drug therapy in immune disorders *(continued)*

Drugs	Indications	Adverse effects	Practice pointers
Immunosuppressants			
Cyclosporine	Prophylaxis of organ rejection in kidney, liver, bone marrow, and heart transplants	Tremor, headache, seizures, confusion, hypertension, nephrotoxicity, leukopenia, thrombocytopenia, hepatotoxicity, flushing, acne, infections, increased low-density lipoproteins, anaphylaxis	• Measure oral doses carefully in an oral syringe. To increase palatability, mix with whole milk, chocolate milk, or fruit juice. Use a glass container to minimize adherence to container walls. • Give dose once daily in the morning at the same time each day. • May be taken with meals if drug causes nausea

antibiotics; and clotting factors, plasma, and platelets, which can help patients with clotting disorders live virtually normal lives. Common procedures include factor replacement and exchange transfusions.

Factor replacement

I.V. infusion of deficient clotting elements is a major part of treatment for patients with coagulation disorders. Factor replacement typically corrects clotting factor deficiencies, thereby stopping or preventing hemorrhage.

Products depend on disorders

Various blood products are used, depending on the specific disorder being treated:

- Fresh frozen plasma is used to treat clotting disorders with unknown causes, clotting factor deficiencies resulting from hepatic disease or blood dilution, consumed clotting factors secondary to DIC, and deficiencies of clotting factors for which no specific replacement product exists.
- Cryoprecipitate is used to treat von Willebrand's disease, fibrinogen deficiencies, and factor XIII deficiencies.
- Factor VIII (antihemophiliac factor) concentrate serves as the long-term treatment of choice for patients with hemophilia A.
- Prothrombin complex is given to correct hemophilia B, severe liver disease, and acquired deficiencies for the factors it contains (II, VII, IX, and X).

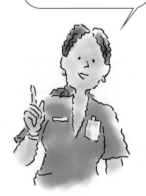

Good news! Transfusion can revive oxygen-starved tissues, combat infections, and aid patients with hemophilia.

Nursing considerations

- Explain the procedure to the patient and assemble equipment.
- Verify the practitioner's order and make sure that the informed consent form was signed.
- Obtain the blood product from the blood bank or pharmacy.
- Identify the patient. It is required that another licensed professional double-check the patient's name, medical record number, and ABO and Rh status (as well as other compatibility factors). This information should be compared with the identification label on the blood product's bag.
- Check the expiration date and inspect the plasma fraction for cloudiness or turbidity.
- Administer fresh frozen plasma within 4 hours because it doesn't contain preservatives.
- Administer platelets using a blood component drip administration set; don't use a microaggregate filter. Infuse 100 ml over 15 minutes.
- Take the patient's vital signs, perform a venipuncture if a line isn't in place, and infuse normal saline solution at a keep-vein-open rate.
- During and after administration, monitor vital signs and watch for signs of anaphylaxis and other allergic reactions and fluid overload.
- Monitor for bleeding, increased pain or swelling at the transfusion site, and fever.
- Monitor the patient's PTT.

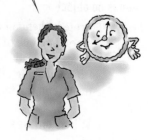

Administer fresh frozen plasma within 4 hours because it doesn't contain preservatives.

Hematologic and immune systems disorders

Hematologic and immune systems disorders commonly seen in the critical care environment include acute leukemia, anaphylaxis, DIC, HIV infection, and idiopathic thrombocytopenic purpura.

Acute leukemia

Leukemia is a group of malignant disorders characterized by abnormal proliferation and maturation of lymphocytes and nonlymphocytic cells leading to suppression of normal cells. It's classified as acute or chronic:

- Acute lymphoblastic leukemia involves abnormal growth of lymphoblasts. It accounts for 80% of all childhood leukemias.
- Acute myelogenous leukemia involves rapid accumulation of myeloblasts. It's one of the most common leukemias in adults.

- Chronic myelogenous leukemia is characterized by myeloproliferation in bone marrow. It's common in middle age but may occur in any age-group.
- Chronic lymphocytic leukemia is characterized by an increase in well-differentiated lymphocytes in the bone marrow and peripheral blood. It's most common in elderly people.

Age is no object

Acute leukemia ranks 20th as the cause of cancer-related deaths among people of all age-groups. Without treatment, acute leukemia invariably leads to death, usually because of complications that result from leukemic cell infiltration of bone marrow or vital organs. With treatment, the prognosis varies.

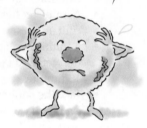

Without treatment, acute leukemia is deadly. With treatment, the prognosis varies.

What causes it

The cause of acute leukemia isn't known. Risk factors seem to include some combination of viruses, genetic and immunologic factors, and exposure to radiation and certain chemicals.

How it happens

Malignant WBC precursors (blasts) proliferate in bone marrow or lymph tissue and accumulate in peripheral blood, bone marrow, and body tissues.

What to look for

Typical clinical features include sudden onset of high fever, night sweats, abnormal bleeding (such as nosebleeds, gingival bleeding, purpura, ecchymoses, and petechiae), easy bruising after minor trauma, and prolonged menses.

Nonspecific signs and symptoms include low-grade fever, night sweats, pallor, and weakness that may persist for days or months before other symptoms appear.

What tests tell you

- Bone marrow aspiration typically shows a proliferation of immature WBCs and is used to confirm the diagnosis.
- Complete blood count (CBC) shows anemia, thrombocytopenia, and neutropenia.
- Differential leukocyte count is used to determine cell type.

How it's treated

Systemic chemotherapy is used to eradicate leukemic cells and induce remission. Chemotherapy varies with the specific disorder. Bone marrow transplants are also an option.

What to do

- Preventing infection is an important part of care for the patient with acute leukemia. Monitor vital signs every 2 to 4 hours. Assess for bleeding and early signs of infection (fever, chills, tachycardia, and tachypnea). Patients with a temperature over 101 °F (38.3 °C) and decreased WBC counts should receive antibiotic therapy promptly.
- Avoid giving aspirin and aspirin-containing drugs.
- Avoid taking rectal temperatures, giving rectal suppositories, and doing digital examinations. Employ measures to prevent constipation.
- Avoid using indwelling catheters and giving I.M. injections.
- Control mouth ulceration by checking the patient's mouth often and by providing frequent mouth care and saline solution rinses.
- Provide psychological support by establishing a trusting relationship to promote communication.

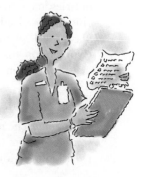

Preventing infection is an important part of care for a patient with acute leukemia.

Anaphylaxis

Anaphylaxis is an exaggerated hypersensitivity reaction to a previously encountered antigen. A severe reaction may precipitate vascular collapse, leading to systemic shock and sometimes death.

What causes it

Causes of anaphylaxis include:
- exposure to sensitizing drugs (such as antibiotics, serums, vaccines, allergen extracts, enzymes, hormones, sulfonamides, local anesthetics, salicylates, polysaccharides, and antineoplastics)
- exposure to diagnostic chemicals (including radiographic contrast media containing iodine)
- foods
- sulfites
- insect venom
- latex.

How it happens

An anaphylactic reaction requires previous sensitization or exposure to the specific antigen. This sensitization causes production of specific IgE antibodies by plasma cells. IgE antibodies then bind to membrane receptors or mast cells and basophils.

Take two

Upon reexposure, the antigens bind to adjacent IgE antibodies or cross-linked IgE receptors, activating a series of reactions that triggers the release of powerful chemical mediators (histamine) from mast cell stores. IgG or IgM enters into the reaction and activates the release of complement fractions.

At the same time, two other chemical mediators, bradykinin and leukotrienes, induce vascular collapse by causing certain smooth muscles to contract and increasing vascular permeability. This collapse leads to decreased peripheral resistance to plasma leakage from the circulation to extravascular tissues. Hypotension ensues, leading to hypovolemic shock and cardiac dysfunction.

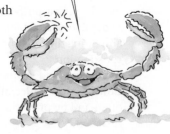

Reexposure to a specific antigen (such as foods like me!) triggers the release of histamine.

What to look for

An anaphylactic reaction usually produces sudden distress within seconds or minutes after exposure to an allergen. (A delayed or persistent reaction may occur up to 24 hours later.)

Signs and symptoms from head to toe

Initial signs and symptoms include a feeling of anxiety and impending doom or fright, weakness, sweating, sneezing, pruritus, urticaria, and angioedema. Cardiovascular signs include hypotension, shock, and arrhythmias. Respiratory signs and symptoms include nasal mucosal edema, profuse watery rhinorrhea, nasal congestion, sudden sneezing attacks, hoarseness, stridor, and dyspnea. GI and genitourinary signs and symptoms include severe stomach cramps, nausea, diarrhea, urinary urgency, and incontinence.

Rapid onset of severe respiratory or cardiovascular reactions are telltale signs of anaphylaxis. It's always an emergency.

What tests tell you

Anaphylaxis can be diagnosed by the rapid onset of severe respiratory or cardiovascular reactions after exposure to an allergen.

How it's treated

Anaphylaxis is always an emergency, requiring an immediate I.M. injection of epinephrine repeated every 5 to 20 minutes as necessary. With cardiac arrest, initiate cardiopulmonary resuscitation.

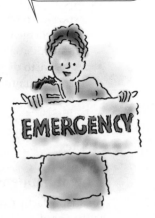

What to do

- Maintain airway patency. Observe for early signs of laryngeal edema (stridor, hoarseness, and dyspnea), which may necessitate endotracheal (ET) intubation, cricothyrotomy, or a tracheostomy.

- Maintain circulatory volume with volume expanders (plasma, saline solution, and albumin) as needed.
- Watch for hypotension and shock. Stabilize the patient's blood pressure with I.V. vasopressors, such as norepinephrine and dopamine. Monitor the patient's cardiac rhythm, vital signs, oxygen saturation, hemodynamic parameters, and urine output as a response index.
- After initial emergency measures, administer other medications as ordered, such as subQ epinephrine solution and I.V. corticosteroids or diphenhydramine.
- Closely monitor a patient undergoing diagnostic tests that use radiographic contrast media, such as cardiac catheterization and angiography.

Disseminated intravascular coagulation

DIC is a grave coagulopathy that accelerates clotting, causing small blood vessel occlusion, organ necrosis, depletion of circulating clotting factors and platelets, and activation of the fibrinolytic system.

These processes in turn can provoke severe hemorrhage. Clotting in the microcirculation usually affects the kidneys and extremities but may occur in the brain, lungs, pituitary and adrenal glands, and GI mucosa.

What causes it

Conditions that can cause DIC include:
- infection
- obstetric complications
- neoplastic disease
- disorders that produce necrosis, such as extensive burns, trauma, brain tissue destruction, transplant rejection, and hepatic necrosis
- heat stroke
- shock
- poisonous snakebite
- cirrhosis
- fat embolism
- incompatible blood transfusion
- cardiac arrest
- surgery necessitating cardiopulmonary bypass
- severe venous thrombosis.

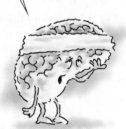

DIC can be caused by brain tissue destruction? I don't like the sound of that!

How it happens

Regardless of how DIC begins, the typical accelerated clotting causes generalized activation of prothrombin and a consequent excess of thrombin.

Clotting and coagulating

Excess thrombin converts fibrinogen to fibrin, producing fibrin clots in the microcirculation. This process consumes large amounts of coagulation factors, causing hypoprothrombinemia, thrombocytopenia, and deficiencies in factors V and VIII.

Circulating thrombin activates the fibrinolytic system, which lyses fibrin clots into fibrin degradation products. Hemorrhage may be the result of the anticoagulant activity of fibrin degradation products as well as depletion of plasma coagulation factors.

What to look for

Abnormal bleeding without a history of serious hemorrhagic disorder can signal DIC.

Blood out of place

Principal signs of such bleeding include cutaneous oozing, petechiae, ecchymoses, hematomas, bleeding from sites of surgical or invasive procedures, and bleeding from the GI tract.

Other signs and symptoms

Also, assess the patient for acrocyanosis. Related or possible signs and symptoms include dyspnea; oliguria; seizures; coma; shock; failure of major organ systems; and severe muscle, back, and abdominal pain.

What tests tell you

Laboratory findings supporting a tentative diagnosis include:
- decreased platelets (less than 100,000/μl)
- decreased fibrinogen level (less than 150 mg/dl)
- increased fibrin degradation products (often greater than 100 mcg/ml)
- prolonged PT (greater than 15 seconds)
- prolonged PTT (greater than 60 seconds)
- decreased urine output (less than 30 ml/hour), elevated blood urea nitrogen level (greater than 25 mg/dl), and elevated serum creatinine level (greater than 1.3 mg/dl).

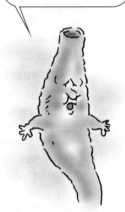

Look for evidence of unusual bleeding, such as cutaneous oozing; petechiae; ecchymoses; hematomas; and bleeding from surgical sites, invasive procedures, or even the GI tract.

How it's treated

Effective treatment for patients with DIC requires prompt recognition and adequate attention to the underlying disorder. Treatment may be generally supportive or highly specific.

If the patient isn't actively bleeding, supportive care alone may reverse DIC. However, active bleeding may require I.V. heparin and administration of blood, fresh frozen plasma, platelets, or packed RBCs to support hemostasis. (See *Understanding DIC and its treatment*, page 646.)

What to do

- Monitor the patient's cardiac, respiratory, and neurologic status closely, at least every 30 minutes initially. Assess breath sounds and monitor vital signs and cardiac rhythm.
- Assess the patient for signs of hemorrhage and hypovolemic shock. Observe the patient's skin color and check peripheral circulation and capillary refill. Inspect skin and mucous membranes for signs of bleeding.
- Check all I.V. and venipuncture sites often. Apply pressure to injection sites for at least 15 minutes.
- Administer supplemental oxygen as ordered. Monitor oxygen saturation and blood gas results, assess for hypoxemia, and anticipate the need for ET intubation and mechanical ventilation.
- Keep the patient as quiet and comfortable as possible to minimize oxygen demands. Place the patient in semi-Fowler's position, as tolerated, to maximize chest expansion.
- Monitor the patient's diagnostic laboratory values and administer blood, fresh frozen plasma, or platelets as ordered.
- Monitor the patient's intake and output hourly, especially when administering blood products. Watch for transfusion reactions and signs of fluid overload.
- Assess the patient for potential complications of DIC, including pulmonary emboli due to accelerated clotting, acute tubular necrosis, or multiple organ failure.
- Provide emotional support to the patient and his family.

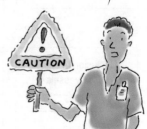

Assess the patient with DIC for signs of hemorrhage and hypovolemic shock.

HIV infection

HIV infection is characterized by progressive decline of immune function that, if left untreated, results in susceptibility to opportunistic infections and malignancies. The most profound state of immunodeficiency caused by HIV is AIDS.

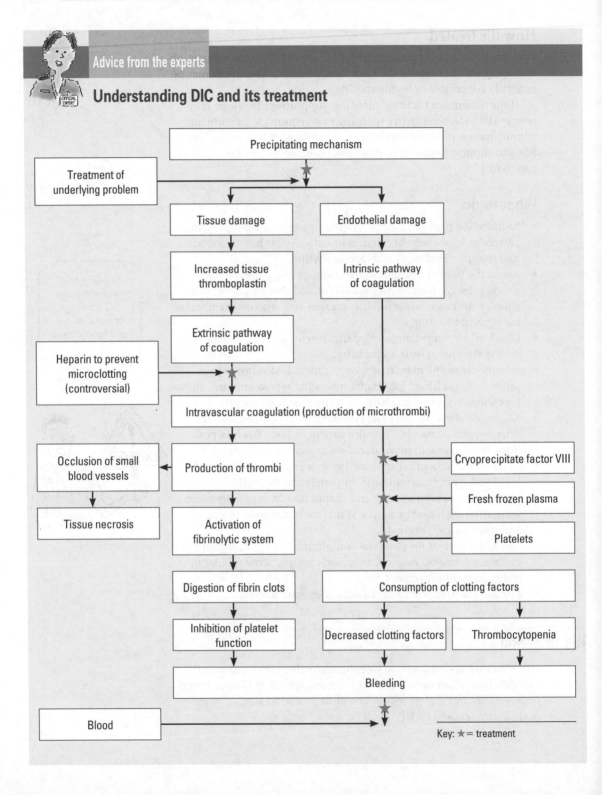

Advice from the experts

Understanding DIC and its treatment

Precipitating mechanism

Treatment of underlying problem

Tissue damage

Endothelial damage

Increased tissue thromboplastin

Intrinsic pathway of coagulation

Extrinsic pathway of coagulation

Heparin to prevent microclotting (controversial)

Intravascular coagulation (production of microthrombi)

Occlusion of small blood vessels

Production of thrombi

Cryoprecipitate factor VIII

Fresh frozen plasma

Platelets

Tissue necrosis

Activation of fibrinolytic system

Digestion of fibrin clots

Consumption of clotting factors

Inhibition of platelet function

Decreased clotting factors

Thrombocytopenia

Bleeding

Blood

Key: ★ = treatment

The Centers for Disease Control and Prevention (CDC) defines AIDS as a confirmed presence of HIV infection and a CD4$^+$ T cell (helper T) count less than 200/μl or presence of HIV with an opportunistic infection. (See *Conditions associated with AIDS*.)

What causes it

The retrovirus HIV causes AIDS. This virus appears in body fluids, such as blood and semen. Modes of transmission include:

* sexual contact, especially with trauma to the rectal or vaginal mucosa, in patients from any age-group (See *HIV in elderly patients*, page 648.)
* transfusion of contaminated blood or blood products
* use of contaminated needles
* perinatal transmission from mother to fetus.

Conditions associated with AIDS

The CDC lists diseases associated with AIDS under three categories. From time to time, the CDC adds to these lists.

Category A
* Persistent generalized lymph node enlargement
* Acute primary HIV infection with accompanying illness
* HIV infection without symptoms

Category B
* Bacillary angiomatosis
* Oropharyngeal or persistent vulvo-vaginal candidiasis
* Fever or diarrhea lasting longer than 1 month
* Idiopathic thrombocytopenic purpura
* Pelvic inflammatory disease, especially with a tubo-ovarian abscess
* Peripheral neuropathy
* Cervical dysplasia
* Oral leukoplakia (hairy)

* Herpes zoster, with at least two different episodes or involving more than one dermatome
* Listeriosis

Category C
* Candidiasis of the bronchi, trachea, lungs, or esophagus
* Invasive cervical cancer
* Disseminated or extrapulmonary coccidioidomycosis
* Extrapulmonary cryptococcosis
* Chronic interstitial cryptosporidiosis
* CMV disease affecting organs other than the liver, spleen, or lymph nodes
* CMV retinitis with vision loss
* Encephalopathy related to HIV
* Herpes simplex infection with chronic ulcers or herpetic bronchitis, pneumonitis, or esophagitis

* Disseminated or extrapulmonary histoplasmosis
* Chronic intestinal isosporiasis
* Kaposi's sarcoma
* Burkitt's lymphoma
* Immunoblastic lymphoma
* Primary brain lymphoma
* Disseminated or extrapulmonary *Mycobacterium avium-intracellulare* complex or *Mycobacterium kansasii*
* Pulmonary or extrapulmonary *Mycobacterium tuberculosis*
* Disseminated or extrapulmonary infection with any other species of *Mycobacterium*
* *Pneumocystis carinii* pneumonia
* Recurrent pneumonia
* Progressive multifocal leukoencephalopathy
* Recurrent *Salmonella* septicemia
* Toxoplasmosis of the brain
* Wasting syndrome caused by HIV

How it happens

For patients with AIDS, the number of $CD4^+$ T cells declines, mainly because HIV selectively binds with and destroys them. A substance called *gp 120* binds HIV to $CD4^+$ T-cell receptor sites.

Enter HIV

After binding to a target cell, HIV enters the cell and sheds its envelope. How the virus enters the cell isn't known. After HIV enters the cell, the enzyme reverse transcriptase transcribes the genomic ribonucleic acid into deoxyribonucleic acid (DNA). Afterward, during cell division, a virus-encoded enzyme integrates the DNA into the host genome. At this point, HIV's replication cycle may be suspended until the infected $CD4^+$ T cell is activated.

Critical destruction

Because $CD4^+$ T cells are critically important in the immune response, destruction of even part of their population can cause immunodeficiencies. These immunodeficiencies leave the patient vulnerable to the potentially fatal opportunistic infections and cancers characteristic of AIDS.

What to look for

Signs and symptoms of AIDS vary widely; nonspecific ones include:
- fatigue
- afternoon fevers
- night sweats
- weight loss
- diarrhea
- cough.

That's all 'til later

Patients may be otherwise asymptomatic until the abrupt onset of complications, such as opportunistic infection and HIV encephalopathy (dementia) marked by confusion, apathy, and paranoia. (See *Opportunistic infections in AIDS*.)

What tests tell you

- Enzyme-linked immunosorbent assay (ELISA) is the most widely used test to determine the presence of antibodies for HIV. If the results are positive, the test is repeated. If the results are still positive, the findings are confirmed by another method, usually the Western blot or an immunofluorescence assay.

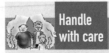

Handle with care

HIV in elderly patients

HIV infection occurs predominantly in young people (in most cases ages 17 to 55). However, incidence is rapidly increasing in people ages 50 and older. This group may not have benefited from HIV-prevention messages, which are commonly targeted at younger people. Make sure you take a sexual history from older patients or inquire about their sexual activity, which may aid in diagnosing the disease.

HIV is picky. It selectively binds with and destroys helper T cells, causing immunodeficiencies.

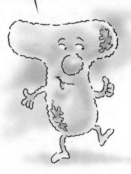

Opportunistic infections in AIDS

The chart below lists microbial forms and specific organisms that cause opportunistic infections in patients with AIDS.

Microbiologic agent	Organism	Infection
Protozoa	*P. carinii*	Pneumocystosis
	Cryptosporidium	Cryptosporidiosis
	Toxoplasma gondii	Toxoplasmosis
	Histoplasma	Histoplasmosis
Fungi	*Candida albicans*	Candidiasis
	Cryptococcus neoformans	Cryptococcosis
Viruses	Herpes	Herpes simplex 1 and 2
	CMV	CMV retinitis
Bacteria	*M. tuberculosis*	Tuberculosis
	M. avium	*M. avium* complex

Note: Other opportunistic conditions include Kaposi's sarcoma, wasting syndrome, and AIDS dementia complex.

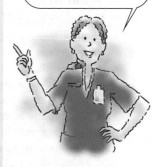

ELISA is the most widely used test to determine the presence of antibodies for HIV, but direct testing is more reliable because it detects HIV itself.

- Direct testing is more reliable because it detects HIV itself. Direct testing includes antigen testing, HIV cultures, nucleic acid probes of peripheral blood lymphocytes, and polymerase chain reaction tests.
- CD4$^+$ T-cell and CD8$^+$ T-cell subset counts are used to evaluate the severity of immunosuppression and response to treatment. Other useful tests may include erythrocyte sedimentation rate, CBC, and p24 antigen and anergy testing.

How it's treated

Although no cure has yet been found, signs and symptoms can be managed with treatment. Primary therapy for HIV infection includes three different types of antiretrovirals used in combination:

- protease inhibitors, such as ritonavir, indinavir, nelfinavir, and saquinavir
- nucleoside reverse transcriptase inhibitors, such as zidovudine, didanosine, zalcitabine, lamivudine, and stavudine
- nonnucleoside reverse transcriptase inhibitors, such as nevirapine and delavirdine.

Other options

Other potential therapies include:
- immunomodulatory drugs designed to boost the weakened immune system
- anti-infective and antineoplastic drugs to combat opportunistic infections and associated cancers.

What to do

- Adhere to standard precautions and anticipate the need for transmission-based precautions if the patient develops another infection.
- Assess the patient's cardiopulmonary status—including breath sounds, vital signs, oxygen saturation, and cardiac rhythm—at least every 2 hours or more often, as needed.
- Report any cough, sore throat, or adventitious sounds that may indicate respiratory infection such as pneumonia. Administer supplemental oxygen as ordered. Anticipate the need for ET intubation and mechanical ventilation if the patient's respiratory status deteriorates.
- Monitor the patient for fever, noting its pattern.
- Assess the patient for tender, swollen lymph nodes and check laboratory values. Watch for signs and symptoms of infection, such as skin breakdown, cough, sore throat, and diarrhea.
- Provide mouth care using normal saline solution or bicarbonate solution. Avoid glycerin swabs that dry mucous membranes.
- Monitor the patient's nutritional status. Although parenteral nutrition may be needed for adequate caloric intake, it provides a potential route for infection.
- For the patient with Kaposi's sarcoma, monitor the progression of lesions and provide meticulous skin care.
- An AIDS diagnosis is profoundly distressing because of the social impact and the discouraging prognosis. Offer support to the patient, his friends, and his family.

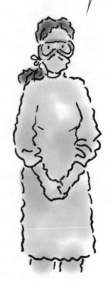

Adhere to standard precautions and anticipate the need for transmission-based precautions if the patient develops another infection.

Idiopathic thrombocytopenic purpura

Idiopathic thrombocytopenic purpura (ITP) results from immunologic platelet destruction. It may be acute (postviral thrombocytopenia) or chronic (Werlhof's disease, purpura hemorrhagica, essential thrombocytopenia, and autoimmune thrombocytopenia).

Acute ITP usually affects children. Chronic ITP mainly affects adults younger than age 50, especially women ages 20 to 40.

What causes it

Acute ITP usually follows a viral infection, such as rubella or chickenpox. Chronic ITP seldom follows infection and is associated with immunologic disorders, such as SLE, or is linked to drug reactions.

How it happens

The platelet membrane is coated with IgG or another antibody and then these sensitized platelets are destroyed. Their destruction is brought about by the reticuloendothelial system of the liver and spleen.

What to look for

Signs and symptoms of ITP include:
- petechiae
- ecchymoses
- mucosal bleeding from the mouth, nose, or GI tract
- purpuric lesions in vital organs (such as the lungs, kidneys, or brain) that may be fatal.

What tests tell you

- A platelet count less than 20,000/µl and prolonged bleeding time suggest ITP.
- Platelets may be abnormal in size and morphologic appearance.
- Anemia may be present.
- Bone marrow studies show an abundance of megakaryocytes and a shortened circulating platelet survival time.

How it's treated

Corticosteroids promote capillary integrity but are only temporarily effective in chronic ITP. Alternative therapy includes:
- immunosuppression
- high-dose I.V. gamma globulin
- splenectomy for which the patient may require blood, blood products, and vitamin K delivery.

What to do

- Monitor the patient's cardiopulmonary status and assess for signs of bleeding. Monitor laboratory results and administer immunoglobulin as ordered.
- Closely monitor patients receiving immunosuppressants for signs of bone marrow depression, infection, mucositis, GI tract ulceration, and severe diarrhea or vomiting.

Quick quiz

1. The spleen must be enlarged about how many times normal size to be palpable?
   A. One
   B. Two
   C. Three
   D. Four

Answer: C. To detect an enlarged spleen on palpation, it must be about three times its normal size.

2. Which is the preferred site for a bone marrow biopsy?
   A. Sternum
   B. Spinous process
   C. Posterior superior iliac crest
   D. Anterior superior iliac crest

Answer: C. The posterior superior iliac crest is the preferred site because no vital organs or vessels are nearby.

3. The drug of choice for a patient experiencing anaphylaxis is:
   A. epinephrine.
   B. aminophylline.
   C. dopamine.
   D. diphenhydramine.

Answer: A. Epinephrine is a bronchodilator that relaxes bronchial smooth muscle by beta$_2$-adrenergic receptor stimulation.

4. Which blood test is used first to identify a response to HIV infection?
   A. Western blot
   B. CD4$^+$ T-cell count
   C. Erythrocyte sedimentation
   D. ELISA

Answer: D. The ELISA is the first screening test for HIV. A Western blot test confirms a positive ELISA test.

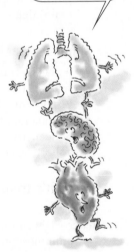

We're next! Read on to learn about multisystem issues.

Scoring

★★★ If you answered all four questions correctly, go have some fun! You're already a bloody genius, Mate!

★★ If you answered three questions correctly, don't despair. No one is immune to an occasional information mismatch.

★ If you answered fewer than three correctly, your oxygen levels may need a boost. Take a break, have a platelet of something nutritious, and get back into circulation as soon as possible.

Suggested References

Feldman, M., Friedman, L. S., & Brandt, L. J. (Eds.). (2010). *Sleisenger and Fordtran's gastrointestinal and liver disease: Pathophysiology, diagnosis, management* (9th ed., Vol. 1). Philadelphia, PA: Elsevier Health Sciences.

Hill, S. R., Carless, P. A., Henry, D. A., Carson, J. L., Hebert, P. C., McClelland, D. B., & Henderson, K. M. (2002). Transfusion thresholds and other strategies for guiding allogeneic red blood cell transfusion. *Cochrane Database of Systematic Reviews*, (2), CD002042.

Hoffman, R., Benz, E. J., & Silberstein, L. E. (2005). *Hematology: Basic principles and practice*. New York, NY: Churchill Livingstone.

Roberts, J. R., & Hedges, J. R. (2009). *Clinical procedures in emergency medicine*. Philadelphia, PA: Elsevier Health Sciences.

Chapter 10

Multisystem issues

Just the facts

In this chapter, you'll learn:

♦ types of multisystem disorders

♦ indications for blood and fluid replacement

♦ treatments specific to multisystem issues

♦ nursing care of the patient with multisystem issues.

A look at multisystem issues

Multisystem issues result from various disorders. For example, a patient may have a head injury that's accompanied by chest and cardiac trauma.

Prompt, efficient, and organized care of multisystem issues requires a multidisciplinary team approach. Typically, assessment, treatment, and care of multisystem issues occur simultaneously.

Shock to the multisystem

Multisystem issues commonly develop in patients experiencing severe sepsis or septic shock. Patients at high risk for septic shock include those with burns; diabetes mellitus; immunosuppression; malnutrition; stress; pancreatitis, chronic cardiac, hepatic, or renal disorders; or a history of excessive antibiotic use. Also at risk are patients who have had invasive diagnostic or therapeutic procedures, surgery, severe burns, or traumatic wounds.

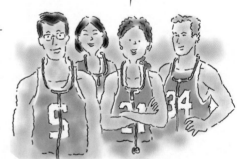

Multisystem issues require a multidisciplinary team!

Assessment

Rapid assessment followed by appropriate interventions influence the outcome of the patient with multisystem issues. General assessment measures should be paired with assessment techniques that are specific to the patient's condition.

History lesson

Begin your assessment by obtaining the patient's history, including:
- chief complaint
- present and previous illnesses
- current medications
- family and social history.

    If the patient is unstable, you may need to wait until he has stabilized to obtain a complete health history.

Is it life-threatening?

Assess the patient for life-threatening problems (such as respiratory distress in the burn victim) and initiate emergency measures such as cardiopulmonary resuscitation (CPR) as appropriate.

The once-over

Your physical examination includes assessment of all body systems, with particular attention to the body systems involved in the multisystem disorder.

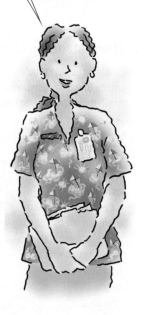

Always assess for life-threatening problems first and initiate emergency measures as needed.

Diagnostic tests

Diagnostics studies are performed to help determine the cause or extent of the patient's multisystem issues. Tests may include laboratory studies (such as hematology, coagulation, chemistry, urine studies, and cultures of blood or body fluids), radiographic studies, electrocardiography, computed tomography (CT) scans, magnetic resonance imaging (MRI), ultrasonography, nuclear medicine scans, and interventional radiologic studies.

Treatment

Treating multisystem issues is a challenge. At times, the causative factors in a patient's deteriorating condition may not be known. As more organ systems are affected, care becomes more complex. Supportive measures are a crucial part of treatment; they include fluid replacement/resuscitation, drug therapy, and blood transfusion.

Fluid replacement

Fluid replacement is a vital part of treating multisystem illnesses. To maintain the patient's health, the fluid and electrolyte balance in the intracellular and extracellular spaces needs to remain relatively constant. Whenever a person experiences an illness or a condition that prevents normal fluid intake or causes excessive fluid loss, I.V. fluid replacement may be necessary.

So predictable

I.V. therapy provides the patient with life-sustaining fluids, electrolytes, and medications and offers the advantage of immediate therapeutic effects. Solutions used for I.V. fluid replacement fall into the broad categories of crystalloids and colloids. (See *Understanding electrolytes*.)

Understanding electrolytes

Electrolytes help regulate water distribution, govern acid–base balance, and transmit nerve impulses. They also contribute to energy generation and blood clotting. The lists here summarize what the body's major electrolytes do. Check the illustration below to see how electrolytes are distributed within the intracellular fluid (ICF) and extracellular fluid (ECF) spaces.

Potassium (K)
- It's the main ICF cation.
- Regulates cell excitability
- Permeates cell membranes, thereby affecting the cells electrical status
- Helps to control ICF osmolality and, consequently, ICF osmotic pressure
- Inverse relationship with sodium; as potassium increases, sodium drops

Magnesium (Mg)
- It's a leading ICF cation.
- Contributes to many enzymatic and metabolic processes, particularly protein synthesis
- Modifies nerve impulse transmission and skeletal muscle response (Unbalanced Mg concentrations dramatically affect neuromuscular processes.)

Phosphorus (P)
- It's a main ICF anion.
- Promotes energy storage and carbohydrate, protein, and fat metabolism
- Acts as a hydrogen buffer

Sodium (Na)
- It's the main ECF cation, comprising 95% of all ECF ions.
- Helps govern normal ECF osmolality (A shift in Na concentrations triggers a fluid volume change to restore normal solute and water ratios.)
- Helps maintain acid–base balance
- Activates nerve and muscle cells
- Influences water distribution (with chloride)

Chloride (Cl)
- It's a main ECF anion.
- Helps maintain normal ECF osmolality
- Affects body pH
- Plays a vital role in maintaining acid–base balance; combines with hydrogen ions to produce hydrochloric acid

Calcium (Ca)
- It's a major cation in teeth and bones; found in fairly equal concentrations in ICF and ECF.

- It's also found in cell membranes, where it helps cells adhere to one another and maintain their shape.
- Acts as an enzyme activator within cells (Muscles must have Ca to contract.)
- Aids coagulation
- Affects cell membrane's permeability and firing level

Bicarbonate (HCO_3^-)
- It's present in ECF.
- Its primary function is regulating acid–base balance.

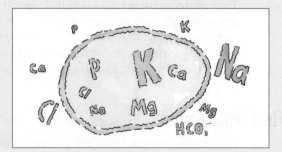

Easy flowing

Crystalloids are solutions with small molecules that flow easily from the bloodstream into cells and tissues. There are three types of crystalloids:

- *Isotonic crystalloids* contain about the same concentration of osmotically active particles as extracellular fluid, so fluid doesn't shift between the extracellular and intracellular areas. Lactated Ringer's solution and 0.9% normal saline are the two most commonly used.
- *Hypotonic crystalloids* are less concentrated than extracellular fluid, so they move from the bloodstream into the cell, causing the cell to swell.
- *Hypertonic crystalloids* are more highly concentrated than extracellular fluid, so fluid is pulled into the bloodstream from the cell, causing the cell to shrink. (See *A look at I.V. solutions*, pages 658 and 659.)

Water movers

Hypertonic solutions called *colloids* may be used to increase blood volume. Colloids draw water from the interstitial space into the vasculature. Examples of colloid solutions are plasma, albumin, hetastarch, and dextran.

The effects of colloids last several days if the lining of the capillaries is normal. The patient needs to be closely monitored during a colloid infusion for increased blood pressure, dyspnea, and bounding pulse, which are signs of hypervolemia.

What to do

- Check the I.V. order for completeness and accuracy. Most I.V. orders expire after 24 hours. A complete order should specify the amount and type of solution, specific additives and their concentrations, and the rate and duration of the infusion.
- Keep in mind the size, age, and history of the patient when giving I.V. fluids to prevent fluid overload.
- Change the site, dressing, and tubing as often as your institution's policy requires. Solutions should be changed at least every 24 hours.
- Monitor the I.V. site for signs of complications, such as infiltration, phlebitis or thrombophlebitis, infection, and extravasation.
- Monitor the patient for signs of complications of I.V. therapy, such as an allergic reaction, air embolism, and fluid overload.
- Monitor intake and output. Notify the practitioner if the patient's urine output falls below 30 ml/hour.

A look at I.V. solutions

This chart shows examples of commonly used I.V. fluids and includes some of the clinical uses and special consideration associated with their use.

Solution	Uses	Special considerations
Isotonic		
Dextrose 5% in water (D₅W)	• Fluid loss and dehydration • Hypernatremia	• Solution is isotonic initially; becomes hypotonic when dextrose is metabolized. • Don't use for resuscitation; can cause hyperglycemia. • Use cautiously in renal or cardiac disease; can cause fluid overload. • Doesn't provide enough daily calories for prolonged use; may cause eventual breakdown of protein.
Normal saline (0.9% NS)	• Shock • Hyponatremia • Blood transfusions • Resuscitation • Fluid challenges • Metabolic alkalosis • Hypercalcemia • Fluid replacement in patients with diabetic ketoacidosis (DKA)	• Because this replaces ECF, use cautiously in patients with heart failure, edema, or hypernatremia; can lead to overload.
Lactated Ringer's solution (LR)	• Dehydration • Burns • Lower GI tract fluid loss • Acute blood loss • Hypovolemia due to third-space shifting	• Electrolyte content is similar to serum but doesn't contain magnesium. • Contains potassium; don't use in patients with renal failure; can cause hyperkalemia. • Don't use in liver disease because the patient can't metabolize lactate; a functional liver converts it to bicarbonate; don't give if patient's pH is greater than 7.5.
Hypotonic		
Half-normal saline (0.45% NS)	• Water replacement • DKA after initial normal saline solution and before dextrose infusion • Hypertonic dehydration • Sodium and chloride depletion • Gastric fluid loss from nasogastric suctioning or vomiting	• Use cautiously; may cause cardiovascular collapse or increased intracranial pressure. • Don't use in patients with liver disease, trauma, or burns.

A look at I.V. solutions

Solution	Uses	Special considerations
Hypertonic		
Dextrose 5% in half-normal saline (D₅½NS)	• DKA after initial treatment with normal saline solution and half-normal saline solution—prevents hypoglycemia and cerebral edema (occurs when serum osmolality is reduced too rapidly)	• In DKA, use only when glucose level falls below 250 mg/dl.
Dextrose 5% in normal saline (D₅NS)	• Hypotonic dehydration • Temporary treatment of circulatory insufficiency and shock if plasma expanders aren't available • Syndrome of inappropriate antidiuretic hormone (or use 3% sodium chloride) • Addisonian crisis	• Use cautiously in cardiac or renal patients because of danger of heart failure and pulmonary edema.
3% sodium chloride (3% NS)	• Severe dilutional hyponatremia • Severe sodium depletion	• Administer cautiously to prevent pulmonary edema. • Observe infusion site closely for signs of infiltration and tissue damage.
Dextrose 10% in water (D₁₀W)	• Used to correct significant hypoglycemia • Administer if the patient's total parenteral nutrition is stopped abruptly (to prevent hypoglycemia).	• Monitor serum glucose levels.

- Monitor the patient for potential fluid and electrolyte disturbances and check serum electrolyte values. (See *Interpreting serum electrolyte test results,* page 660.)
- Documentation for a patient receiving an I.V. infusion should include the date, time, and type of catheter inserted; the site of insertion and its appearance; the type and amount of fluid infused; the patient's tolerance and response to therapy.

Drug therapy

Drug therapy for multisystem issues varies depending on the patient's underlying condition. For example, antibiotics may be used to treat severe sepsis. Fluid resuscitation and vasopressors may be used to treat various types of shock. Corticosteroids and immunosuppressants are used to treat graft-versus-host disease (GVHD). (See *Drug therapy for multisystem disorders,* pages 661 and 662.)

Interpreting serum electrolyte test results

Use the quick-reference chart below to interpret serum electrolyte test results for adult patients.

Electrolyte	Results	Implications	Common causes
Serum sodium	135 to 145 mEq per L	Normal	—
	<135 mEq/L	Hyponatremia	Syndrome of inappropriate antidiuretic hormone
	>145 mEq/L	Hypernatremia	Diabetes insipidus
Serum potassium	3.5 to 5 mEq per L	Normal	—
	<3.5 mEq/L	Hypokalemia	Diarrhea
	>5 mEq/L	Hyperkalemia	Burns and renal failure
Total serum calcium	8.5 to 10.5 mg per dl	Normal	—
	<8.5 mg/dl	Hypocalcemia	Acute pancreatitis
	>10.5 mg/dl	Hypercalcemia	Hyperparathyroidism
Ionized calcium	4.5 to 5.1 mg per dl	Normal	—
	<4.5 mg/dl	Hypocalcemia	Massive transfusion
	>5.1 mg/dl	Hypercalcemia	Acidosis
Serum phosphates	2.5 to 4.5 mg per dl or 1.8 to 2.6 mEq per L	Normal	—
	<2.5 mg/dl or 1.8 mEq/L	Hypophosphatemia	DKA
	>4.5 mg/dl or 2.6 mEq/L	Hyperphosphatemia	Renal insufficiency
Serum magnesium	1.5 to 2.5 mEq per L	Normal	—
	<5 mEq/L	Hypomagnesemia	Malnutrition
	>2.5 mEq/L	Hypermagnesemia	Renal failure
Serum chloride	98 to 108 mEq per L	Normal	—
	<98 mEq/L	Hypochloremia	Prolonged vomiting
	>108 mEq/L	Hyperchloremia	Hypernatremia

Drug therapy for multisystem disorders

Use the chart below as a guide to drug therapy appropriate for multisystem disorders.

Drugs	Indications	Adverse reactions	Practice pointers
Corticosteroids			
Dexamethasone Prednisone	• Inflammatory conditions • Immunosuppression • GVHD	• Euphoria • Insomnia • Seizures • Heart failure or arrhythmias • Thromboembolism • Peptic ulceration • Pancreatitis • Acute adrenal insufficiency	• Use cautiously in patients with myocardial infarction, hypertension, renal disease, or GI ulcer. • Sudden withdrawal after prolonged use may be fatal. • Administer oral drug with milk or food. • Monitor serum electrolytes and blood glucose levels at onset of therapy.
Vasopressors			
Dopamine	• Hypotension • Shock • Decreased cardiac output	• Restlessness • Angina • Headache • Bradycardia, tachycardia, or arrhythmias • Anaphylaxis • Hypotension or hypertension • Extravasation (tissue necrosis and sloughing) if the drug leaks into surrounding tissue at injection site	• Use a central venous catheter. Use a large peripheral vein only in emergency situations and for the shortest time possible. If extravasation occurs in a peripheral vein, stop infusion and treat with phentolamine infiltrate to prevent tissue necrosis. Use a continuous infusion pump to regulate infusion flow rate. • When discontinuing, taper dosage slowly to evaluate stability of blood pressure.
Levophed (Norepinephrine)	• Hypotension • Shock	• Bradycardia, tachycardia, or arrhythmias • Hypotension or hypertension • Headache • Anxiety • Extravasation (tissue necrosis and sloughing) if the drug leaks into surrounding tissue at injection site	• Use a central venous catheter. • Monitor blood pressure closely. • Should not be used as a first-choice agent to increase blood pressure in a severely hypovolemic patient; administer crystalloid fluids first.

(continued)

Drug therapy for multisystem disorders (continued)

Drugs	Indications	Adverse reactions	Practice pointers
Immunosuppressants			
Cyclosporine Tacrolimus	• Prophylaxis of organ rejection	• Headache, tremor, insomnia, paresthesia, delirium, or coma • Peripheral edema • Diarrhea or constipation • Nausea, vomiting, anorexia, abdominal pain, and ascites • Abnormal renal function • Urinary tract infection • Anemia and leukocytosis • Electrolyte imbalance • Pleural effusion, atelectasis, and dyspnea • Photosensitivity • Thrombocytopenia • Nephrotoxicity	• Monitor the patient for signs of neurotoxicity, nephrotoxicity, hyperkalemia, and hypokalemia. • Monitor blood glucose level regularly. • Give drug with adrenal corticosteroids.
Antibiotics			
Ceftizoxime Ceftriaxone	• Serious infections of the lower respiratory and urinary tracts • Intra-abdominal, bone and joint, skin, and gynecologic infections • Bacteremia • Septicemia	• Leukopenia • Serum sickness • Anaphylaxis • Phlebitis or thrombophlebitis • Diarrhea • Thrombocytopenia • Pseudomembranous colitis	• Obtain a specimen for culture and sensitivity tests before giving first dose.
Zosyn (Piperacillin-Tazobactam)	• Appendicitis, peritonitis • Skin infections (cellulitis) • Nosocomial or community-acquired pneumonia	• Diarrhea, constipation • Headache • Nausea, vomiting • Rash, pruritus • Fever	• Assess for previous hypersensitivity reactions to penicillin or cephalosporins. • Monitor renal and blood cell function periodically.

Blood transfusion

Blood transfusions treat decreased hemoglobin (Hb) level and hematocrit (HCT). A whole blood transfusion replenishes the volume and oxygen-carrying capacity of the circulatory system by increasing the mass of circulating red blood cells (RBCs). Because of the risk for circulatory overload, whole blood transfusions are rarely used, except in cases of severe hemorrhage.

Packing it in

Packed RBCs, a blood component from which 80% of the plasma has been removed, are transfused to restore the circulatory system's oxygen-carrying capacity. Hb level below 7 to 10 g per dl of blood is the most common indication for transfusion in the critical care setting. (See *Transfusing blood and blood components*, pages 664 and 665.)

Filtered for patient protection

Packed RBCs contain cellular debris, requiring in-line filtration during administration. Washed packed RBCs, commonly used for patients previously sensitized to transfusions, are rinsed with a special solution that removes white blood cells (WBCs) and platelets, thus decreasing the chance of transfusion reaction.

Self–supplier

In some cases, the patient may receive his own blood during a transfusion, called *autotransfusion* or *autologous transfusion*. In this process, the patient's own blood is collected, filtrated, and reinfused. With the concern over acquired immunodeficiency syndrome and other blood-borne diseases, the use of autologous transfusion is currently on the rise.

Autologous transfusion may be indicated for:
- elective surgery (where the patient donates blood over an extended period of time before surgery)
- nonelective surgery (where the patient's blood is withdrawn immediately before surgery)
- perioperative and emergency blood salvage during and after thoracic or cardiovascular surgery and hip, knee, or liver resection
- perioperative and emergency blood salvage for traumatic injury of the lungs; liver; chest wall; heart; pulmonary vessels; spleen; kidneys; inferior vena cava; and iliac, portal, or subclavian veins.

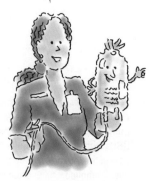

With the concern over blood-borne diseases, the use of autologous transfusion is on the rise.

Refuse to transfuse?

In some cases, a patient may refuse a blood transfusion. For example, a Jehovah's Witness may refuse a transfusion because of his religious beliefs. A competent adult has the right to refuse treatment. You may be able to use other treatment options if the patient refuses the blood transfusion, such as using blood-conservation strategies during surgery or providing erythropoietin, iron, and folic acid supplements preoperatively and postoperatively. Using available alternative treatments supports the patient's right of self-determination and honors the patient's wishes. A court order requiring the patient to undergo the standard treatment can also be obtained in extreme cases.

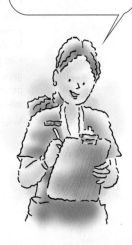

A patient may refuse a transfusion because of religious beliefs. If necessary, a court order that requires the patient to undergo the transfusion may be obtained.

Transfusing blood and blood components

Blood component	Indications	ABO and Rh compatibility	Nursing considerations
Packed RBCs Same RBC volume as whole blood but with most of the plasma removed	• To restore or maintain oxygen-carrying capacity • To correct anemia and surgical blood loss • To increase RBC volume	• ABO compatibility: Type A receives type A or O, type B receives type B or O, type AB receives type AB or O, type O receives type O. • Rh match necessary	• Use a blood administration set to infuse blood within 4 hours. • Administer only with normal saline solution. • Keep in mind that an RBC transfusion isn't appropriate for anemias treatable by nutritional or drug therapies. • Check calcium levels if administering multiple units of RBCs within a 24-hour period. Citrate, used in preserving RBCs, binds to calcium and will cause hypocalcemia.
Leukocyte-poor RBCs Same as packed RBCs with about 70% of the leukocytes removed	• Same as packed RBCs • To prevent febrile reactions from leukocyte antibodies • To treat immunocompromised patients • To restore RBCs to patients who have had two or more nonhemolytic febrile reactions	• Same as packed RBCs • Rh match necessary	• Use blood administration tubing. • It may require a 40-micrometer filter suitable for hard-spun, leukocyte-poor RBCs. • Use only with normal saline solution. • Keep in mind that cells expire 24 hours after washing.
Platelets Platelet sediment from whole blood	• To treat bleeding caused by decreased circulating platelets or functionally abnormal platelets • To improve platelet count preoperatively in a patient whose count is 50,000/μl or less • To prepare for emergency surgery on patients taking platelet inhibitors (such as clopidogrel)	• ABO identical when possible • Rh-negative recipients should receive Rh-negative platelets when possible.	• Use a filtered component drip administration set to infuse. • If ordered, administer prophylactic pretransfusion medications, such as antihistamines or antipyretics, to reduce chills, fever, and allergic reactions. • Complete transfusion within 20 minutes or at the fastest rate the patient can tolerate. • Use single-donor platelets if patient must have repeated transfusions because of the risk of allergic reaction to foreign leukocyte antigens that may be present on leukocytes and platelets. • Keep in mind that platelets shouldn't be used to treat autoimmune thrombocytopenia or thrombocytopenic purpura unless patient has a life-threatening hemorrhage.

Transfusing blood and blood components

Blood component	Indications	ABO and Rh compatibility	Nursing considerations
Fresh frozen plasma (FFP) Noncellular portion of blood, which is separated and frozen after donation	• To correct a coagulation factor deficiency • To replace coagulation factors when a specific factor isn't available • Severe bleeding due to warfarin therapy or urgent reversal of warfarin • To treat thrombotic thrombocytopenic purpura	• ABO compatibility required • Rh match not required	• Use a blood administration set. • Complete transfusion within 20 minutes or at the fastest rate the patient can tolerate. • Monitor patient for signs and symptoms of hypocalcemia. • Remember that FFP must be infused within 6 hours of being thawed.
Cryoprecipitate Plasma that has been centrifuged and the precipitate collected; contains clotting factors only (fibrinogen, factor VIII:c, factor VIII:vWF, factor XIII, and fibronectin)	• To treat factor VIII deficiency and fibrinogen disorders • To treat significant factor XIII deficiency	• ABO compatibility suggested • Rh match not required	• Use a blood administration set to infuse. • Add normal saline solution to each bag of cryoprecipitate, as necessary, to facilitate transfusion. • Keep in mind that cryoprecipitate must be administered within 6 hours of thawing. • Before administering, check lab studies to confirm a deficiency of one of the specific clotting factors present in cryoprecipitate. • Be aware that patients with hemophilia A or von Willebrand's disease should only be treated with cryoprecipitate when appropriate factor VIII concentrates aren't available.
Factor VIII concentrate Recombinant, genetically engineered product; derivative obtained from plasma	• To treat hemophilia A • To treat von Willebrand's disease	• Not required	• Administer by I.V. injection using a filter needle or use the administration set supplied by the manufacturer.
Albumin 5% (buffered saline); albumin 25% (salt poor) A small plasma protein prepared by fractionating pooled plasma	• To replace volume lost because of shock from burns, trauma, surgery, or infections • To treat hypoproteinemia (with or without edema)	• Not required	• Use the administration set supplied by the manufacturer and set rate based on patient condition and response. • Keep in mind that albumin isn't to be used to treat severe anemia. • Administer cautiously in cardiac and pulmonary disease because heart failure may result from volume overload.

Ready to transfuse?

- Make sure that a written order is in the patient's medical record. Confirm that the order and the medical record are labeled with the patient's name and assigned identification number.
- Notify the practitioner if the patient refuses the blood transfusion.
- Obtain baseline vital signs and start an I.V. line if one isn't already started. Use a 20G or larger diameter catheter.

Double-check identity

- Identify the patient and check the blood bag identification number, ABO blood group, Rh compatibility, and expiration date of the blood product. This step should be confirmed by another licensed professional using independent double verification (IDV). Follow your facility's policy for blood administration.
- Obtain the patient's vital signs after the first 15 minutes and then every 30 minutes (or according to the facility's policy) for the remainder of transfusion therapy.
- If administering platelets or FFP, administer each unit immediately after obtaining it.
- Change the filter and tubing after every two units of blood products, unless otherwise indicated by the manufacturer's labeled use or hospital policy.
- Use a blood warmer, as ordered, in special situations, such as when transfusing multiple units of refrigerated blood to a patient with a large volume of blood loss, performing exchange transfusions, or transfusing to a patient with cold agglutinin disease. Always follow the manufacturer's instructions.

Rapid replacement

- For rapid blood replacement, use a pressure bag or rapid transfusion device if necessary. Always follow the manufacturer's instructions for use. Be aware that excessive pressure may develop, leading to broken blood vessels and extravasation with hematoma and hemolysis of the infusing RBCs.
- Many emergency rooms, trauma units, and operating rooms have a massive transfusion protocol that involves administering multiple units of RBCs, platelets, and FFP at once. Follow the physician's orders, the condition of the patient, and your hospital protocol to determine when to give multiple blood products.
- Obtain follow-up laboratory tests as ordered to determine the effectiveness of therapy.

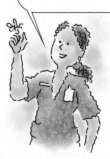

Remember to always replace the filter and tubing if more than 1 hour elapses between transfusions.

- Record the date and time of the transfusion (time started and completed); the type and amount of transfusion product; the type and gauge of the catheter used for infusion; the patient's vital signs before, during, and after transfusion; a verification check of all identification data (including the individuals' names verifying the information); and the patient's response.
- Document the patient's transfusion reaction and the treatment (if any) required. (See *Guide to transfusion reactions*.)

Guide to transfusion reactions

Any patient receiving a transfusion of blood or blood products is at risk for a transfusion reaction. A transfusion reaction may be immediate, occurring during the transfusion or within several hours of the completion of the transfusion, or delayed. This chart describes immediate and delayed reactions.

Reaction	Causes	Signs and symptoms	Prevention	Nursing interventions
Immediate reactions				
Acute hemolytic	Administration of incompatible blood	Chest pain, dyspnea, facial flushing, fever, chills, hypotension, flank pain, bloody oozing at the infusion or surgical incision site, nausea, tachycardia	• Carefully check the patient's identity against the blood or blood product. • Monitor the patient at the start of the transfusion of each unit. • Correctly label all blood samples and blood request forms.	• Monitor the patient carefully for the first 15 minutes of any transfusion. • Administer I.V. fluids, oxygen, epinephrine, and a vasopressor as ordered. • Observe the patient for signs of coagulopathy.
Bacterial contamination	Contamination of blood product	Chills, fever, vomiting, abdominal cramping, diarrhea, shock	• Use sterile technique when collecting or administering blood. • Change the blood tubing and filter after every other unit or when more than 4 hours have elapsed between units. • Transfuse the blood or blood product within 30 minutes of receiving it. • Complete the transfusion of blood within 4 hours.	• Provide broad-spectrum antibiotics, as prescribed. • Monitor the patient for fever for several hours after completion of transfusion. • Obtain blood cultures from a site other than I.V. infusion site. • Keep all blood bags and tubing and send them to the blood bank.

(continued)

Guide to transfusion reactions *(continued)*

Reaction	Causes	Signs and symptoms	Prevention	Nursing interventions
Immediate reactions (continued)				
Febrile nonhemolytic	Bacterial lipopoly-saccharides • Antileukocyte re-cipient antibodies directed against donor WBCs	Fever within 2 hours of transfusion, chills, rigors, headache, palpitation, cough, tachycardia	• Premedicate the pa-tient with antipyretics. • Limit the number of transfusions the patient receives, if possible.	• Relieve the patient's symptoms with an antipyretic. • If the patient requires fur-ther transfusions, consider using a leukocyte removal filter.
Transfusion-related acute lung injury (TRALI)	Granulocyte anti-bodies in the donor or recipient cause complement and histamine release.	Severe respiratory distress within 6 hours of transfusion, fever, chills, cyanosis, hypotension	• There's no known prevention.	• Provide oxygen as needed. • Monitor pulse oximetry. • Prepare for intubation and ventilatory support and hemodynamic monitoring.
Allergic reaction	Allergen in donor blood	Urticaria, fever, nau-sea, vomiting, anaphy-laxis (facial swelling, laryngeal edema, respiratory distress) in extreme cases	• Administer antihis-tamines if the patient has a history of allergic reaction.	Administer antihistamine, corticosteroid, or epineph-rine as ordered. • Prepare for intubation and respiratory support if the patient develops ana-phylaxis.
Hypocalcemia	Rapid infusion of citrate-treated blood; the citrate binds to calcium	Arrhythmias, hypoten-sion, muscle cramps, nausea and vomiting, seizures, prolonged QT interval	• Monitor ionized calcium levels in pa-tients receiving large amounts of transfused blood (i.e., >8 units in a 24-hour period).	• Administer calcium glu-conate I.V., as ordered. • Monitor ECG for arrhythmias or prolonged QT interval. • Monitor patients with an elevated potassium level closely; they're at increased risk for hypocalcemia.
Delayed reactions				
Delayed hemolytic	Production of anti-bodies by RBCs to antigens on trans-fused RBCs	Fever, anemia, jaundice Occurring 5 to 10 days after transfusion	• There's no known prevention.	• Recheck the patient's blood type. • Administer antipyretics for fever.

Guide to transfusion reactions

Reaction	Causes	Signs and symptoms	Prevention	Nursing interventions
Delayed reactions (continued)				
Posttransfusion purpura	Destruction of autologous and allogenic platelets	Thrombocytopenia, bleeding Occurring 7 to 10 days after transfusion	• Limit transfusion in patients with a history of sensitization through pregnancy or previous transfusion.	• Administer high doses of immunoglobulin I.V., as ordered.
GVHD	T-lymphocytes in blood or blood product react against the patient's tissue antigens	Fever, skin rash and desquamation, diarrhea, pancytopenia Occurring 10 to 12 days after transfusion Usually fatal	• Transfuse irradiated blood components to immunocompromised patients.	• Provide supportive care to the patient and his family.

Multisystem disorders

Multisystem disorders include burns, GVHD, hyperthermia, hypothermia, hypovolemic shock, multiple organ dysfunction syndrome (MODS), septic shock, and trauma.

Burns

Burns are tissue injuries caused by contact with thermal, chemical, radiation, or electrical sources or from friction. This leads to varying degrees of cellular skin damage as well as a systemic response that leads to altered body function. A major burn affects every body system and organ, usually requiring painful treatment, skin grafting, and a long period of rehabilitation.

What causes it

Thermal burns, the most common burn type, typically result from:
- residential fires
- automobile accidents
- playing with matches
- improper handling of firecrackers
- scalding accidents and kitchen accidents
- abuse (in children or elderly people)
- clothes that have caught on fire.

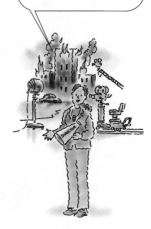

Thermal burns are the most common type of burn. They may result from fires, scalding accidents, and sometimes abuse.

Scorching brews

Chemical burns result from contact, ingestion, inhalation, or injection of acids, alkalis, or vesicants (blistering agents).

It's electric

Electrical burns usually result from contact with faulty electrical wiring and cords or high-voltage power lines.

How it happens

Specific pathophysiologic events depend on the cause and classification of the burn. (See *Visualizing burn depth*.) The injuring agent denatures cellular proteins. Some cells die because of traumatic or ischemic necrosis. Loss of collagen cross-linking also occurs with denaturation, creating abnormal osmotic and hydrostatic pressure gradients that cause intravascular fluid to move into interstitial spaces. Cellular injury triggers the release of mediators of inflammation, contributing to local and, in the case of major burns, systemic increases in capillary permeability.

Visualizing burn depth

It is important to remember that most burns involve tissue damage of multiple degrees and thicknesses. This illustration may help you to visualize burn damage at the various levels.

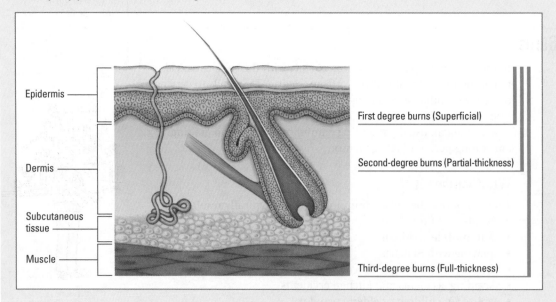

For your epidermis only

A *superficial burn* causes localized injury or destruction to the skin's epidermis by direct contact, such as a chemical spill, or indirect contact, such as sunlight (think "sunburn!"). Although the skin initially remains intact, it is sensitive to further injury. The skin is dry, red, and painful to the touch. This type of burn isn't life-threatening and should heal within 3 to 5 days.

Barrier-breaking blisters

A *superficial partial-thickness burn* involves destruction to the epidermis and the top layer of the dermis. Thin-walled, fluid-filled blisters develop within a few minutes of the injury. As these blisters break, the nerve endings become exposed to the air. Because pain and tactile responses remain intact, subsequent treatments are painful. The barrier function of the skin is lost. It may heal without the need for grafting within 7 to 14 days.

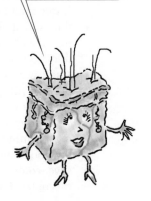

Yowza! Those partial-thickness burns involve blisters and edema!

Deep into the dermis

A *deep partial-thickness burn* involves the epidermis and the full layer of dermis. The patient develops blisters and experiences mild to moderate edema and pain. Compared with a superficial partial-thickness burn, there's less pain sensation with this burn because the sensory neurons have undergone extensive destruction; however, because the barrier function of the skin is lost, sensitivity to pain remains in some areas around the burn. This level of burn may require skin grafts to prevent contractures and scarring.

Third layer, all the way

A *full-thickness burn* extends through the epidermis and dermis and into the subcutaneous tissue layer. It may also involve muscle, bone, and interstitial tissues. The skin is black, dry, and leathery in appearance. Within hours, fluids and protein shift from capillary to interstitial spaces, causing edema. A person's body has an immediate immunologic response to a full-thickness burn, making burn wound sepsis a potential threat. Finally, an increase in calorie demand after a full-thickness burn increases the patient's metabolic rate. This patient will need skin grafts to close the wound beds.

What to look for

Assessment provides a general idea of burn severity. First, determine the depth of tissue damage. A partial-thickness burn damages the epidermis and part of the dermis; a full-thickness burn also affects subcutaneous tissue.

Tracking burn traits

Signs and symptoms depend on the type of burn and may include:

- localized pain and erythema, usually without blisters in the first 24 hours (superficial burn)
- chills, headache, localized edema, and nausea and vomiting (more severe superficial burn)
- thin-walled, fluid-filled blisters appearing within minutes of the injury, with mild to moderate edema and pain (superficial partial-thickness burn)
- white, waxy appearance to damaged area that still blanches to pressure (deep partial-thickness burn)
- white, brown, or black leathery tissue and visible thrombosed vessels due to destruction of skin elasticity (dorsum of hand, most common site of thrombosed veins), without blisters that does not blanch to pressure (full-thickness burn)
- silver-colored, raised or charred area, usually at the site of electrical contact (electrical burn).

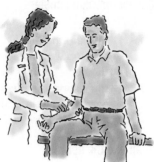

Assessment of the burn will give you an idea of the degree and depth of the tissue damage.

Configure this!

Inspection also reveals the location and extent of the burn. Note the burn's configuration. If the patient has a circumferential burn on an extremity, he run the risk for contracted eschar or interstitial edema constricting the circulation in that extremity. If the patient has burns on his neck, he may suffer airway obstruction; burns on the chest can lead to restricted respiratory excursion.

More to it than just skin

Inspect the patient for other injuries that may complicate recovery such as signs of pulmonary damage from smoke inhalation, including singed nasal hairs, mucosal burns, voice changes, coughing, wheezing, soot in the mouth or nose, and darkened sputum. (See *Understanding the effects of smoke inhalation*.) A burn may occur

---

Understanding the effects of smoke inhalation

Smoke inhalation can cause injury by any combination of these major mechanisms:

1. injury caused by toxic gas exposure
2. injury above the level of the vocal cords due to direct heat or chemicals
3. injury below the level of the vocal cords causing pulmonary edema, pneumonia, and later signs of inflammation.

Thermal injury

Although smoke tends to have a high temperature, it tends to be dry and, therefore, has a low specific heat. This, combined with the excellent heat-exchanging properties of the upper airways, tends to make thermal injuries limited to the supraglottic airways. Thermal injury of the lower respiratory tract may occur in rare situations when there's inhalation of superheated particles or steam.

Understanding the effects of smoke inhalation

Feeling the heat

Heat produces immediate injury to the mucosa, resulting in erythema, ulceration, and edema. This damage may compromise the upper airway lumen if significant edema develops. The presence of external face or neck burns may accentuate anatomic distortion of upper airway structures and further impair gas flow.

Upper airway edema usually appears within 24 hours of injury. Symptoms related to obstruction, such as dyspnea, stridor, and cyanosis, suggest significant anatomic changes, and airway management and intubation is a priority. Upper airway edema usually resolves in 3 to 5 days.

Hypoxic gas inhalation

In a confined space, fire consumes ambient oxygen, and the ambient fraction of inspired oxygen (FIO_2) decreases. The degree to which FIO_2 declines before a fire self-extinguishes is dependent on the type of the fuel. For example, gasoline will self-extinguish at an FIO_2 of 0.15; compounds containing oxygen may burn to an FIO_2 of 0.10 or less.

It's toxic

Hypoxic hypoxemia may be toxic on its own (especially to the nervous system) and may potentiate the toxicities of carbon monoxide (CO) and hydrogen cyanide. Hypoxemia may also trigger an increase in minute ventilation that in turn enhances the amount of smoke inhaled.

Removing the patient from the scene of the exposure and administering supplemental oxygen may help terminate ongoing injury from hypoxic gas inhalation. End-organ damage, particularly to the brain, may persist after removal and may mimic CO or cyanide poisoning.

Direct bronchopulmonary toxin exposure

A large number of the lower molecular weight constituents of smoke, such as acrolein, formaldehyde, chlorine, and nitrous oxide, are toxic to the bronchial mucosa and alveoli. Soot contains elemental carbon and can absorb toxins, thereby increasing their distal delivery. Particles less than 4 micrometers in diameter are more dangerous than the larger particles of black smoke because of their ability to reach the distal airways and alveoli.

Pile of problems

Exposure to these compounds tends to produce acute neutrophilic airway inflammation. Such symptoms as cough, bronchorrhea, dyspnea, and wheezing may not appear until 12 to 36 hours after exposure. Resulting physiologic alterations include disruption of mucociliary transport, increased alveolocapillary permeability, impaired lymphatic flow, worsened ventilation-perfusion ($\dot{V}/\dot{Q}$) matching, and an increased susceptibility to respiratory infections.

Bronchoscopy may reveal erythema, edema, and ulceration of the airways, frequently in association with carbonaceous debris. Acute respiratory distress syndrome (ARDS) may also occur.

Treatment includes administering aerosolized bronchodilators. In addition, intubation and the use of positive end-expiratory pressure may be necessary to manage secretions, maintain small airway patency, minimize the risk for aspiration, and support oxygenation.

Carboxyhemoglobin is not good to have . . .

Smoke inhalation may lead to the absorption of CO and hydrogen cyanide. These molecules impair the delivery and use of oxygen and may result in systemic tissue hypoxia and rapid death. CO poisoning (carboxyhemoglobin in the bloodstream) is the leading cause of smoke-related fatalities, accounting for up to 80% of deaths.

Treating toxins

CO poisoning is treated with maximal oxygen delivery in order to displace CO from Hb and other proteins. Cyanide poisoning, which is rare, is treated by resuscitation, decontamination, and antidotal therapy.

along with other traumas (such as a motor vehicle crash), so don't fixate on the burn and neglect the rest of your assessment.

What tests tell you

An assessment method that can be used to determine the size of a burn is the Rule of Nines chart, which determines the percentage of body surface area (BSA) covered by the burn. (See *Estimating the extent of a burn.*)

Back in the lab

Here are some additional diagnostic test results regarding burns:

- Arterial blood gas (ABG) levels may be normal in the early stages but may reveal hypoxemia and metabolic acidosis later.
- Carboxyhemoglobin level may reveal the extent of smoke inhalation due to the presence of CO.

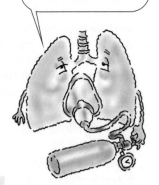

Check a burn victim for pulmonary damage and smoke inhalation. These factors may complicate recovery.

Estimating the extent of a burn

You can estimate the extent of an adult patient's burn by using the Rule of Nines. This method quantifies BSA in multiples of nine, thus the name. To use this method, mentally transfer the burns on your patient to the body charts shown here. Add the corresponding percentages for each body section burned. You can use the total—a rough estimate of burn extent—to calculate fluid replacement needs.

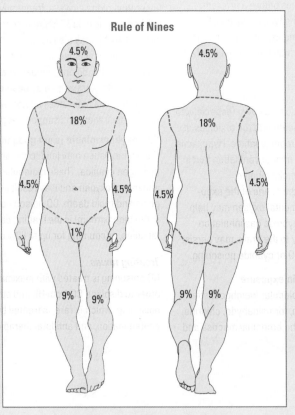

Rule of Nines

4.5%   4.5%

18%   18%

4.5%   4.5%   4.5%   4.5%

1%

9%   9%   9%   9%

- Complete blood count (CBC) may reveal a decreased Hb (due to hemolysis), increased HCT (secondary to hemoconcentration), and leukocytosis (resulting from a systemic inflammatory response or the possible development of sepsis).
- Electrolyte levels may show hyponatremia (from massive fluid shifting) and hyperkalemia (from fluid shifting and cell lysis). Other laboratory tests may reveal elevated blood urea nitrogen (BUN) levels (secondary to fluid loss or increased protein breakdown) and decreased total protein and albumin (resulting from plasma proteins leaking into the interstitial spaces).
- Creatine kinase (CK) and myoglobin levels may be elevated. Keep in mind that CK and myoglobin are helpful indicators of muscle damage. Therefore, the higher the CK or myoglobin level, the more extensive the muscle damage. The presence of myoglobin in urine may lead to acute tubular necrosis.

How it's treated

Initial burn treatments are based on the type of burn and include:
- stopping the burning process; removing any items that retain heat, such as clothing and jewelry (with chemical burns, immediately neutralize by flushing with copious amounts of water)
- maintaining an open airway; assessing airway, breathing, and circulation (ABCs)
- administering supplemental humidified oxygen
- covering partial-thickness burns that are over 30% of BSA or full-thickness burns that are over 5% of BSA with a clean, dry, sterile bed sheet (because of the drastic reduction in body temperature, don't cover large burns with saline-soaked dressings)
- fluid replacement (see *A closer look at fluid replacement,* page 676.)
- antimicrobial therapy (for all patients with major burns)
- pain medication as needed
- anti-inflammatory medications
- laboratory tests, such as CBC, electrolyte, glucose, BUN, and serum creatinine levels; ABG analysis; typing and crossmatching; urinalysis for myoglobinuria and hemoglobinuria
- close monitoring of intake and output and vital signs
- surgical intervention, including skin grafts and more thorough surgical debridement for major burns
- tetanus prophylaxis as ordered
- nutritional therapy.

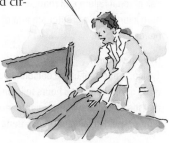

Partial-thickness burns that are over 30% of BSA or full thickness burns that are over 5% of BSA should be covered with a clean, dry, sterile bed sheet.

A closer look at fluid replacement

Fluid replacement is essential for the patient with burns because of the massive fluid shifts that occur. However, extreme caution is needed because of the risk of over-replacement (also called *over-resuscitation*).

How much?

Numerous formulas may be used to determine the amount of fluid replacement to be administered during the first 24 hours after a burn injury. Typically, these formulas use body weight and the percentage of total body surface area (TBSA) burned. One of the most common formulas used is the Parkland formula shown here:

$$\frac{X \text{ ml of lactated Ringer's solution} / \text{Patient's weight in kg}}{\text{Percentage of TBSA burns}} = \begin{array}{l} \text{Amount of fluid in} \\ \text{ml to administer} \\ \text{within the first} \\ \text{24-hour period} \\ \text{postinjury.} \end{array}$$

What is "X"?

The amount of lactated Ringer's solution used depends on the patient. For an adult burn patient, 2 ml is used in the formula. For children, 3 ml is used. However—for adult electrical burns, 4 ml is used. This is due to the high risk of renal failure and rhabdomyolysis with electrical burn injuries; so a greater amount of fluid resuscitation is needed.

Over how long?

Typically, one-half of the calculated amount is administered during the first 8 hours following the injury. (Note that the time of the actual injury—not the time of the patient's arrival in the emergency department—is used as the initial start time of the 8-hour duration.) The remaining one-half of the amount is then administered over the next 16 hours.

What fluids?

During the first 24 hours, crystalloid solutions are commonly used because capillary permeability is greatly increased, allowing proteins to leak into the interstitial tissues. After the first 24 hours, colloid solutions can be included. Giving colloids before the initial 24-hour period would supply additional protein that could leak into the interstitial tissue.

Too much or too little?

During fluid replacement, always be alert for indications of over or under fluid resuscitation. Signs and symptoms of heart failure and pulmonary edema suggest over resuscitation. Assessment findings of hypovolemic shock and low urine output suggest under fluid resuscitation.

Example: A 75-kg man with 55% TBSA, full-thickness burns presents to your emergency department 1 hour postinjury. Using the Parkland formula of 2 ml / 75 kg / 55% TBSA, you get a total of 8,250 ml to administer for the first 24-hour period. Divide that in half to get the amount to administer in the first 8 hours postinjury—4,125 ml. If you divide that amount by 8 hours, you get a rate of 516 ml/hour. Oh—but wait! Didn't we say that the patient arrived in your emergency department 1 hour postinjury? That means you only have 7 hours, not 8 hours, to administer the 4,125 ml of fluid. That gives you 589 ml/hour—whoa . . . that's a lot of fluid!

What to do

- Immediately assess the patient's ABCs. Institute emergency resuscitative measures as necessary. Monitor arterial oxygen saturation and serial ABG values and anticipate the need for endotracheal (ET) intubation and mechanical ventilation should the patient's respiratory status deteriorate, especially with facial or neck burns.

Listen to the lungs

- Auscultate breath sounds for crackles, rhonchi, or stridor. Observe for signs of laryngeal edema or tracheal obstruction, including labored breathing, severe hoarseness, and dyspnea.
- Administer supplemental humidified oxygen as ordered.
- Perform oropharyngeal or tracheal suctioning as indicated by the patient's inability to clear his airway or evidence of abnormal breath sounds.
- Monitor the patient's cardiac and respiratory status closely, at least every 15 minutes, or more frequently, depending on his condition. Also monitor the patient for cardiac arrhythmias. Assess his level of consciousness (LOC) for changes, such as increasing confusion, restlessness, or decreased responsiveness. (See *Electrical burn care*.)
- If the patient has a chemical burn, irrigate the wound with copious amounts of water or normal saline solution. If the chemical entered the patient's eyes, remove contact lenses if necessary and flush the eyes with large amounts of water or normal saline solution for at least 30 minutes. Have the patient close his eyes and cover them with a dry, sterile dressing. Note the type of chemical that caused the burn and any noxious fumes. If necessary, refer the patient for an ophthalmologic examination.
- Place the patient in semi-Fowler's position to maximize chest expansion. Keep him as quiet and comfortable as possible to minimize oxygen demands.

Advice from the experts

Electrical burn care

Keep these tips in mind when caring for a patient with an electrical burn:
- Be alert for ventricular fibrillation as well as cardiac and respiratory arrest caused by the electrical shock; begin CPR immediately.
- Get an estimate of the voltage that caused the injury.
- Tissue damage from an electrical burn is difficult to assess because internal destruction along the conduction pathway usually is greater than the surface burn would indicate.
- An electrical burn that ignites the patient's clothes may also cause thermal burns.
- Don't worry about determining where on the skin that the electrical flow entered and exited the patient; just document them as contact points.

- Prepare the patient for an emergency escharotomy of the chest and neck for deep burns or circumferential injuries, if necessary, to promote lung expansion and decrease pulmonary compromise.
- Administer rapid fluid replacement therapy as ordered, using multiple, large-bore peripheral catheters or a central venous catheter as indicated.

Shocking results

- Monitor the patient's vital signs and hemodynamic parameters for changes indicating hypovolemic shock or evidence of fluid overload and pulmonary edema.
- Assess the patient's intake and output every hour; insert an indwelling urinary catheter as indicated to ensure accurate urine measurement.
- Assess the patient's level of pain, including nonverbal indicators, and administer analgesics such as morphine sulfate I.V. or oxycodone orally, as ordered. Avoid I.M. injections because tissue damage associated with the burn injury may impair absorption of the drug when given I.M.
- Keep the patient calm, provide periods of uninterrupted rest between procedures, and use nonpharmacologic pain relief measures as appropriate.
- Obtain daily weights and monitor intake, including daily calorie counts. Provide a high-calorie, high-protein diet. Assess the patient's abdomen for distention and presence of bowel sounds. If he's on nothing-by-mouth status, administer enteral feedings as ordered.
- Administer histamine-2 receptor antagonists, as ordered, to reduce the risk of ulcer formation.
- Assess the patient for signs and symptoms of infection, including fever, elevated WBC count, and changes in burn wound appearance or drainage. Obtain a wound culture and administer antipyretic and antimicrobial agents as ordered.
- Administer tetanus prophylaxis, if indicated.
- Perform burn wound care as ordered. Prepare the patient for possible grafting as indicated.
- Assess the neurovascular status of the injured area, including pulses, reflexes, paresthesia, color, and temperature of the injured area, at least every 2 to 4 hours or more frequently, if indicated.
- Assist with splinting, positioning, compression therapy, and exercise to the burned area as indicated. Maintain the burned area in a neutral position to prevent contractures and minimize deformity.
- Explain all procedures to the patient before performing them. Encourage him to actively participate in his care as much as possible and provide opportunities for him to voice his concerns, especially about his altered body image.

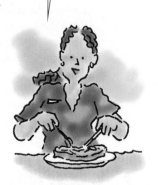

A patient with burns needs a high-calorie, high-protein diet.

Graft-versus-host disease

GVHD, also known as *organ rejection*, can occur when an immunologically impaired recipient receives a graft from an immunocompetent donor. When this happens, instead of the patient's body rejecting the donated organ . . . the donated organ attempts to reject the patient! Yikes!

100-day division

GVHD can be acute or chronic:
- Acute GVHD occurs within the first 100 days after a transplant. It's a major contributing factor to mortality after bone marrow transplantation.
- Chronic GVHD occurs after day 100 of a transplant and involves an autoimmune response that affects multiple organs. Older patients and those who have suffered previous acute GVHD face the greatest risk of chronic GVHD. Patients who develop chronic GVHD immediately following acute GVHD have the highest mortality rates.

What causes it

Causes of GVHD include impaired immune function, transplantation from an incompatible donor, or transfusion of an incompatible blood product containing viable lymphocytes.

Less than 50% of organ recipients with histocompatibility identical to the donor develop GVHD. This incidence increases to more than 60% when there's one antigen mismatch. Death in patients with GVHD is commonly due to sepsis.

How it happens

Three criteria are necessary for the development of GVHD:
1. immunologically competent cells in the graft
2. graft recognition of the host as foreign
3. inability of the host to react to the graft.

When graft cells attack

If graft and host cells aren't histocompatible, the graft cells become sensitive to the host's class II antigens and may launch an attack against the host cells. The exact mechanism by which this occurs remains unclear, although biopsy of active GVHD lesions usually reveals infiltration by eosinophils and mononuclear, phagocytic, and histiocytic cells.

What to look for

Signs and symptoms of acute GVHD include:
- rash (10 to 30 days after transplant)
- abdominal cramps and severe diarrhea
- GI bleeding
- jaundice.
  Signs of chronic GVHD include:
- skin changes resembling scleroderma that can ultimately lead to ulcerations
- joint contractures
- impaired esophageal motility.

What tests tell you

Although graft survival typically hinges on early detection of transplant rejection, no single test or combination of tests has proven to be definitive for doing this. Tests reveal only nonspecific evidence, which may easily be attributed to other causes, especially infection. Diagnosis commonly becomes a matter of exclusion and depends on the careful evaluation of signs and symptoms along with results from specific organ function tests, standard laboratory studies, and tissue biopsy.

Boffo biopsy

Tissue biopsy provides the most accurate, reliable diagnostic information, especially in heart, liver, and kidney transplants. Biopsy usually reveals immunocompetent T cells along with the extent of lymphocytic infiltration and tissue damage. Repeat biopsies help to identify early histologic changes characteristic of rejection, determine the degree of change from previous biopsies, and monitor the course and success of treatment.

Looking at the liver

Liver function studies reveal elevated levels of bilirubin, serum alkaline phosphatase, alanine aminotransferase, and aspartate aminotransferase.

How it's treated

Because GVHD may be fatal, initial interventions must focus on prevention.
   Treatment may include:
- immunosuppressive therapy with methotrexate (with or without prednisone [Deltasone]), antithymocyte globulin (Atgam), cyclosporine (Sandimmune), cyclophosphamide (Cytoxan), or tacrolimus (Prograf) for the first 3 to 12 months after a transplant
- T-cell depletion in donor marrow (selective removal of T cells from the donor graft), which has been shown to reduce the severity and incidence of GVHD; however, patients have experienced an increase in graft failure and recurrent leukemia.

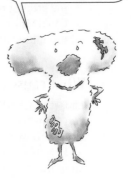

A posttransplant biopsy may reveal immunocompetent T cells, which may indicate organ rejection.

What to do

- Institute appropriate measures after bone marrow transplantation or organ transplant.
- Inspect the patient's skin closely for the development of skin erythema. Pay special attention to the soles of the feet and palms of the hands. Provide meticulous skin care if erythema occurs.
- Assess the patient's skin color for evidence of jaundice, especially the sclera of the eyes. Report any darkened urine or clay-colored stools.
- Monitor the patient's vital signs at least every 4 hours. Notify the practitioner if the patient's temperature rises.
- Assess fluid balance status. Monitor intake and output frequently. Maintain hydration status with I.V. fluids as ordered. Anticipate the need for hemodynamic monitoring to assess the patient's status.
- Administer immunosuppressive agents as ordered.
- Monitor liver function results closely for changes in enzyme levels.
- Assess the patient's bowel elimination pattern and auscultate bowel sounds. Be alert for severe diarrhea. (See *Electrolyte and acid–base imbalances*.)
- Obtain blood and stool cultures as ordered to evaluate for possible sources of infection.
- Assess the patient for signs and symptoms of sepsis.

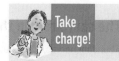

Electrolyte and acid–base imbalances

Follow these instructions when caring for a patient with GVHD:
- Be alert for the development of electrolyte and acid–base imbalances secondary to losses from diarrhea.
- Expect to administer fluid electrolyte replacement therapy based on laboratory results.
- Keep in mind that potassium is a major electrolyte that's lost with diarrhea; anticipate the need for continuous cardiac monitoring to detect possible arrhythmias secondary to hypokalemia.

Hyperthermia

Hyperthermia is defined as an elevation in the body's core temperature over 100.4°F (38°C). It may result from environmental or internal conditions that increase heat production or impair heat dissipation.

What causes it

Hyperthermia may result from conditions that increase heat production, such as excessive exercise, infection, and drugs (e.g., amphetamines).

It may also result from impairment of heat dissipation ability. Factors that impair heat dissipation include:
- high temperatures or humidity
- lack of acclimatization
- excess clothing
- cardiovascular disease
- obesity
- dehydration
- sweat gland dysfunction
- drugs (such as phenothiazines and anticholinergics).

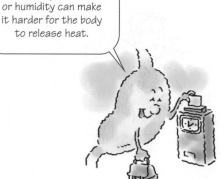

High temperatures or humidity can make it harder for the body to release heat.

The skin's role in thermoregulation

Abundant nerves, blood vessels, and eccrine glands within the skin's deeper layer aid thermoregulation (control of body temperature). The first flow chart shows how the body conserves body heat. The second flow chart shows how the body reduces body heat. Here's how the skin does its job.

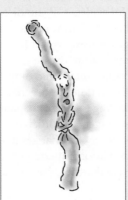

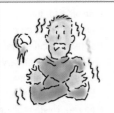

The skin becomes exposed to cold or the internal body temperature falls.

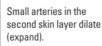

Blood vessels constrict in response to autonomic nervous system.

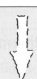

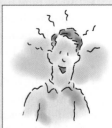

Blood flow decreases through the skin and body heat is conserved.

Now let's cool things off

Increased blood flow reduces body heat. If this doesn't lower temperature, the eccrine glands act to increase sweat production, and evaporation cools the skin.

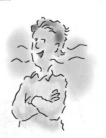

Small arteries in the second skin layer dilate (expand).

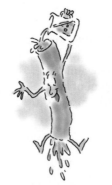

The skin becomes too hot or the internal body temperature rises.

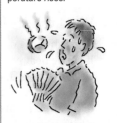

How it happens

Humans normally adjust to excessive temperatures by complex cardiovascular and neurologic changes that are coordinated by the hypothalamus. Heat loss normally happens through five routes: radiation (40%), convection (30%), evaporation (15%), conduction (5%), and respiration (10%). This heat loss offsets heat production to regulate the body temperature. However, when heat loss mechanisms fail to offset heat production, the body retains heat.

Goodbye fluid, hello hypovolemic shock

If body temperature remains elevated, fluid loss becomes excessive and may lead to severe dehydration and hypovolemic shock. If untreated, the patient's thermoregulatory mechanisms can fail. (See *The skin's role in thermoregulation*.)

The hypothalamus coordinates how the body adjusts to excessive temperatures.

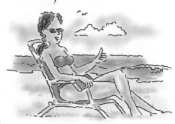

Feeling hot hot hot

Hyperthermia occurs in varying degrees:
- Mild hyperthermia (heat cramps) occurs with excessive perspiration and loss of salt from the body.
- Moderate hyperthermia (heat exhaustion) occurs when the body is subjected to high temperatures and blood accumulates in the skin in an attempt to decrease the body's temperature. This causes a decrease in the circulating blood volume, which decreases cerebral blood flow. Syncope then occurs.
- Critical hyperthermia (heat stroke) occurs when the body's temperature continues to rise and internal organs become damaged, eventually resulting in death. (See *Heat stroke in elderly patients*.)

Handle with care

Heat stroke in elderly patients

With aging, an individual's thirst mechanism and ability to sweat decrease.

These factors put elderly patients at risk for heat stroke, especially during hot summer days. Heat stroke is a medical emergency and must be treated rapidly to prevent serious complications or death. To help prevent heat stroke, teach your older patient to follow these instructions:
- Reduce activity in hot weather, especially outdoor activity.
- Wear lightweight, loose-fitting clothing during hot weather; when outdoors, wear a hat and sunglasses and avoid wearing dark colors that absorb sunlight.

- Drink plenty of fluids, especially water, and avoid tea, coffee, and alcohol because they can cause dehydration.
- Use air-conditioning or open windows (making sure that a secure screen is in place) and use a fan to help circulate air. (If the patient doesn't have air-conditioning at home, suggest that during periods of excessive heat, he can go to community resources that have air conditioning, such as senior centers, libraries, and churches. Some community centers may even provide transportation for the patient.)

What to look for

Assessment findings vary with the degree of hyperthermia. (See *Hyperthermia signs and symptoms*.)

What tests tell you

No single diagnostic test confirms hyperthermia, but these test results may help support the diagnosis:
- ABG results may reveal respiratory alkalosis and hypoxemia.
- CBC may reveal leukocytosis and increased HCT secondary to hemoconcentration.
- Electrolyte levels may show hypokalemia. Other blood studies may reveal elevated BUN levels, increased bleeding and clotting times, and fibrinolysis.
- Urinalysis may show concentrated urine, with elevated protein levels, tubular casts, and myoglobinuria.

How it's treated

Mild and moderate hyperthermia are treated by providing a cool environment and allowing the patient to rest. Oral or I.V. fluid and electrolyte replacement is administered as ordered.

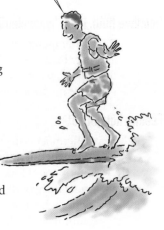

To help treat patients with critical hyperthermia, apply cool water to the skin and fan them with cool air. This breeze is all you need, dude!

Critical measures

Measures for treating critical hyperthermia include:
- removing the patient's clothing and applying cool water to the skin, then fanning the patient with cool air
- controlling shivering by giving meperidine (Demerol) or chlorpromazine (Thorazine)
- applying hypothermia blankets and ice packs to the groin and axillae, if necessary
- Treatment continues until the patient's body temperature drops to 102.2°F (39°C).

In addition to the cool down

Supportive measures for hyperthermia include:
- oxygen therapy
- central venous pressure (CVP) and pulmonary artery wedge pressure (PAWP) monitoring
- ET intubation, if necessary.

What to do

- Assess the patient's ABCs and initiate emergency resuscitative measures as indicated. Remove as much of the patient's clothing as possible.

Hyperthermia signs and symptoms

Hyperthermia may be classified as mild (heat cramps), moderate (heat exhaustion), or critical (heat stroke). This table highlights the major assessment findings associated with each classification.

Classification	Assessment findings
Mild hyperthermia (heat cramps)	• Mild agitation (central nervous system findings otherwise normal) • Mild hypertension • Moist, cool skin and muscle tenderness; involved muscle groups possibly hard and lumpy • Muscle twitching and spasms • Nausea, abdominal cramps • Report of prolonged activity in a very warm or hot environment, without adequate salt intake • Tachycardia • Temperature ranging from 99° to 102°F (37.2° to 38.9°C)
Moderate hyperthermia (heat exhaustion)	• Dizziness • Headache • Hypotension • Muscle cramping • Nausea, vomiting • Oliguria • Pale, moist skin • Rapid thready pulse • Syncope or confusion • Thirst • Weakness • Temperature elevated up to 104°F (40°C)
Critical hyperthermia (heat stroke)	• Atrial or ventricular tachycardia • Confusion, combativeness, delirium • Fixed, dilated pupils • Hot, dry, reddened skin • Loss of consciousness • Seizures • Tachypnea • Temperature greater than 105.1°F (40.6°C)

> BRRRRR!
> Reducing a patient's temperature too quickly can cause shivering, which increases metabolic demand and oxygen consumption.

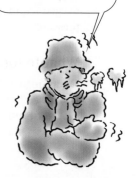

- Assess oxygen saturation and administer supplemental oxygen as indicated and ordered. Monitor the patient's pulmonary status closely, including respiratory rate and depth and breath sounds; anticipate the need for ET intubation and mechanical ventilation if respiratory status deteriorates.
- Monitor vital signs continuously, especially core body temperature. Although the goal is to reduce the patient's temperature rapidly, too rapid a reduction can lead to vasoconstriction, which can cause shivering. Shivering increases metabolic demand and oxygen consumption and should be avoided.

- Employ external cooling measures, such as cool, wet sheets; tepid baths; and cooling blankets.
- Assess neurologic and cardiac status closely, including heart rate and rhythm. Institute continuous cardiac monitoring to evaluate for arrhythmias secondary to electrolyte imbalances. Monitor hemodynamic parameters and assess peripheral circulation, including skin color, peripheral pulses, and capillary refill.
- Monitor fluid and electrolyte balance and laboratory test results. Assess renal function studies to evaluate for rhabdomyolysis.

Hypothermia

Hypothermia is defined as a core body temperature below 95°F (35°C). It may be classified as mild (89.6° to 95°F [32° to 35°C]), moderate (82.4° to 89.6°F [28° to 32°C]), or severe (less than 82.4°F [28°C]). Severe hypothermia can be fatal.

What causes it

Hypothermia commonly results from near drowning in cold water, prolonged exposure to cold temperatures, disease or debility that alters homeostasis, and the administration of large amounts of cold blood or blood products.

Likely candidates

The risk of serious cold injury, especially hypothermia, increases with youth, old age, lack of insulating body fat, wet or inadequate clothing, drug abuse, cardiac disease, smoking, fatigue, malnutrition and depletion of caloric reserves, and excessive alcohol intake.

How it happens

In hypothermia, metabolic changes slow the functions of most major organ systems, resulting in decreased renal blood flow and decreased glomerular filtration. Vital organs are physiologically affected. Severe hypothermia results in depression of cerebral blood flow, diminished oxygen requirements, reduced cardiac output, and decreased arterial pressure.

What to look for

Obtaining the history of a patient with a cold injury may reveal:
- cause of hypothermia
- temperature to which the patient was exposed
- length of exposure.

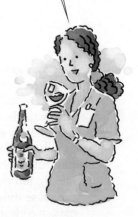

Excessive alcohol intake can increase the risk of hypothermia.

Temperature dependent

Assessment findings in a patient with hypothermia vary with the patient's body temperature:

- Mild hypothermia includes severe shivering, slurred speech, and amnesia.
- Moderate hypothermia includes unresponsiveness, peripheral cyanosis, and muscle rigidity. If the patient was improperly rewarmed, he may show signs of shock.
- Severe hypothermia includes absence of palpable pulses, no audible heart sounds, dilated pupils, and rigor mortis–like state. In addition, ventricular fibrillation and a loss of deep tendon reflexes commonly occur.

What tests tell you

- Doppler and plethysmographic studies help determine pulses and the extent of frostbite after thawing.
- Technetium-99m pertechnetate scanning shows perfusion defects and deep tissue damage from prolonged hypothermia and can be used to identify nonviable bone.

How it's treated

Treatment for hypothermia consists of supportive measures and specific rewarming techniques, including:

- passive rewarming (the patient rewarms on his own)
- active external rewarming with heating blankets, warm water immersion, heated objects such as water bottles, and radiant heat
- active core rewarming with heated I.V. fluids; genitourinary tract irrigation; extracorporeal rewarming; hemodialysis; and peritoneal, gastric, and mediastinal lavage.

Cardiac concerns

Arrhythmias are frequently seen as temperatures drop below 86°F (30°C). Those that develop usually convert to normal sinus rhythm with rewarming. If the patient has no pulse or respirations, CPR is needed until rewarming raises the core temperature to at least 89.6°F (32°C).

Measure dependent on monitoring

The administration of oxygen, ET intubation, controlled ventilation, I.V. fluids, and treatment for metabolic acidosis depend on test results and careful patient monitoring.

What to do

- Assess ABCs. Initiate CPR as appropriate. Keep in mind that hypothermia helps protect the brain from anoxia, which normally accompanies prolonged cardiopulmonary arrest. Therefore, even if the patient has been unresponsive for a long time, CPR may resuscitate him, especially after a cold-water near drowning.
- Assist with rewarming techniques as necessary. In moderate to severe hypothermia, only experienced personnel should attempt aggressive rewarming.
- During rewarming, provide supportive measures as ordered, including mechanical ventilation and heated, humidified therapy to maintain tissue oxygenation, and I.V. fluids that have been warmed with a warming coil to correct hypotension and maintain urine output.
- Continuously monitor the patient's core body temperature and other vital signs during and after initial rewarming. Continuously monitor his cardiac status, including continuous cardiac monitoring for evidence of arrhythmias.
- If using a hyperthermia blanket, discontinue the warming when the core body temperature is within 1° to 2°F (0.6° to 1.1°C) of the desired temperature. The patient's temperature will continue to rise even with the device turned off.
- If the patient has been hypothermic for longer than 45 to 60 minutes, administer additional fluids as ordered to compensate for the expansion of the vascular space that occurs during vasodilation in rewarming. Monitor the patient's heart rate and hemodynamic parameters closely to evaluate fluid needs and response to treatment.
- Monitor the patient's hourly output; fluid balance; and serum electrolyte levels, especially potassium. Be alert for signs and symptoms of hyperkalemia. If hyperkalemia occurs, administer calcium chloride, sodium bicarbonate, glucose, and insulin as ordered. Anticipate the need for sodium polystyrene sulfonate enemas. If his potassium levels are extremely elevated, prepare the patient for dialysis.

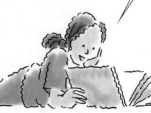

Here's a warm thought: Hypothermia helps protect the brain from anoxia, so even if the patient has been unresponsive for a long time, CPR may resuscitate him.

Hypovolemic shock

Shock is a state of inadequate tissue perfusion leading to cellular dysfunction and death. Hypovolemic shock most commonly results from acute blood loss—about 20% of total volume. Without sufficient blood or fluid replacement, hypovolemic shock may lead to irreversible damage to organs and systems.

What causes it

Massive volume loss may result from:
- GI bleeding, internal or external hemorrhage, or any condition that reduces circulating intravascular volume or other body fluids
- intestinal obstruction
- peritonitis
- acute pancreatitis
- ascites
- dehydration from excessive perspiration, severe diarrhea or protracted vomiting, diabetes insipidus, diuresis, or inadequate fluid intake.

How it happens

Potentially life-threatening, hypovolemic shock stems from reduced intravascular blood volume, which leads to decreased cardiac output and inadequate tissue perfusion. The subsequent tissue anoxia prompts a shift in cellular metabolism from aerobic to anaerobic pathways. This results in an accumulation of lactic acid, which produces metabolic acidosis.

The road to shockville

When compensatory mechanisms fail, hypovolemic shock occurs in this sequence:
1. decreased intravascular fluid volume
2. diminished venous return, which reduces preload and decreases stroke volume
3. reduced cardiac output
4. decreased mean arterial pressure
5. impaired tissue perfusion
6. decreased oxygen and nutrient delivery to cells
7. unchecked, systemic vasoconstriction and microvasodilation ensues, leading to multisystem organ failure.

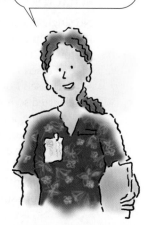

In many cases, the patient's history will reveal the cause of reduced blood volume—such as GI hemorrhage, trauma, or severe diarrhea and vomiting—and will guide your assessment.

What to look for

The specific signs and symptoms exhibited by the patient depend on the amount of fluid loss. (See *Estimating fluid loss*, page 690.)

Oh where oh where has the blood volume gone?

Typically, the patient's history includes conditions that reduce blood volume, such as GI hemorrhage, trauma, and severe diarrhea and vomiting.

Assessment findings may include:
- pale skin
- decreased sensorium

Estimating fluid loss

The following assessment parameters indicate the severity of fluid loss:

Minimal fluid loss	Moderate fluid loss	Severe fluid loss
Intravascular volume loss of 10% to 15% is regarded as minimal. Signs and symptoms include: • slight tachycardia • normal supine blood pressure • positive postural vital signs, including a decrease in systolic blood pressure >10 mm Hg or an increase in pulse rate >20 beats/minute • increased capillary refill time >3 seconds • urine output >30 ml/hour • cool, pale skin on arms and legs • anxiety.	Intravascular volume loss of about 25% is regarded as moderate. Signs and symptoms include: • rapid, thready pulse • supine hypotension • cool truncal skin • urine output 10 to 30 ml per hour • severe thirst • restlessness, confusion, or irritability.	Intravascular volume loss of about 40% or more is regarded as severe. Signs and symptoms include: • marked tachycardia • marked hypotension • weak or absent peripheral pulses • cold, mottled, or cyanotic skin • urine output >10 ml/hour • unconsciousness • narrow pulse pressure.

- rapid, shallow respirations
- urine output below 25 ml/hour
- rapid, thready peripheral pulses
- cold, clammy skin
- mean arterial pressure below 60 mm Hg and a narrowing pulse pressure
- decreased CVP, right atrial pressure, PAWP, and cardiac output.

What tests tell you

No single diagnostic test confirms hypovolemic shock, but these test results help to support the diagnosis:
- low HCT
- decreased Hb level
- decreased RBC and platelet counts
- elevated serum potassium, sodium, lactate dehydrogenase, creatinine, and BUN levels
- increased urine specific gravity (greater than 1.020) and urine osmolality; urine sodium levels less than 50 mEq/L
- decreased urine creatinine levels
- decreased pH and partial pressure of arterial oxygen and increased partial pressure of arterial carbon dioxide ($Paco_2$)

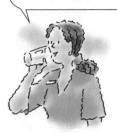

Fluid and blood replacement is crucial to restoring intravascular volume and raising blood pressure in patients with hypovolemic shock. This needs to be accomplished before attempting other methods, such as administration of vasopressor medication.

- gastroscopy, X-rays, aspiration of gastric contents through a nasogastric tube, and tests for occult blood
- coagulation studies for coagulopathy from disseminated intravascular coagulation (DIC).

How it's treated

Emergency treatment relies on prompt and adequate fluid and blood replacement to restore intravascular volume and to maintain systolic blood pressure above 90 mm Hg and/or mean arterial pressure above 60 mm Hg. Rapid infusion of normal saline or lactated Ringer's solution and, possibly, albumin or other plasma expanders may expand volume adequately until whole blood can be matched.

Treatment may also include oxygen administration, control of bleeding, and surgery, if appropriate.

What to do

- Assess the patient for the extent of fluid loss and begin fluid replacement as ordered. Obtain a type and crossmatch for blood component therapy.

ABCs and ABGs

- Assess ABCs. If the patient experiences cardiac or respiratory arrest, start CPR.
- Administer supplemental oxygen as ordered. Monitor oxygen saturation and ABG studies for evidence of hypoxemia and anticipate the need for ET intubation and mechanical ventilation should the patient's respiratory status deteriorate. Place the patient in semi-Fowler's position, if tolerated, to maximize chest expansion. Keep the patient as quiet and comfortable as possible to minimize oxygen demands.
- Monitor vital signs, neurologic status, and cardiac rhythm continuously for changes such as cardiac arrhythmias or myocardial ischemia. Observe skin color and check capillary refill. (See *When blood pressure drops.*)
- Monitor hemodynamic parameters, including CVP, PAWP, and cardiac output, frequently—as often as every 15 minutes—to evaluate the patient's status and response to treatment.
- Monitor intake and output closely. Insert an indwelling urinary catheter and assess urine output hourly. If bleeding from the GI tract is suspected as the cause, check all stools, emesis, and gastric drainage for occult blood. If output falls below 30 ml/hour in an adult, expect to increase the I.V. fluid infusion rate but watch for signs of fluid overload such as elevated PAWP. Notify the practitioner if urine output doesn't increase.
- Administer blood component therapy as ordered; monitor serial Hb values and HCT to evaluate effects of treatment.

Take charge!

When blood pressure drops

A drop below 90 mm Hg in systolic blood pressure and/or mean arterial pressure of 60 mm Hg usually signals inadequate cardiac output from reduced intravascular volume. Such a drop usually results in inadequate coronary artery blood flow, cardiac ischemia, arrhythmias, and other complications of low cardiac output. If the patient's systolic blood pressure drops below 90 mm Hg consistently and his pulse is thready, increase the oxygen flow rate and notify the practitioner immediately.

- Administer dopamine or dobutamine I.V., as ordered, to increase cardiac contractility and renal perfusion.
- Watch for signs of impending coagulopathy (such as petechiae, bruising, and bleeding or oozing from gums or venipuncture sites) and report them immediately.
- Provide emotional support and reassurance appropriately in the wake of massive fluid losses.
- Prepare the patient for surgery as appropriate.

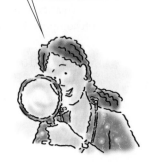

MODS isn't an illness itself. It's a manifestation of another underlying condition.

Multiple organ dysfunction syndrome

MODS is a condition that occurs when two or more organs or organ systems become dysfunctional and are unable to maintain homeostasis. MODS isn't an illness itself; rather, it's a manifestation of another progressive underlying condition.

What causes it

MODS develops when widespread systemic inflammation, a condition known as *systemic inflammatory response syndrome* (*SIRS*), overtaxes a patient's compensatory mechanisms. SIRS can be triggered by infection, ischemia, trauma, reperfusion injury, or multisystem injury. If allowed to progress, SIRS can lead to organ inflammation and ultimately, MODS. (See *Understanding SIRS.*)

Understanding SIRS

SIRS is a severe systemic response to a condition that provokes an acute inflammatory reaction. SIRS is nonspecific and can be caused by ischemia, inflammation, trauma, burns, shock, infection, or a combination of several insults.

Local tissue damage or a microorganism invasion causes a local inflammatory response, which becomes a systemic response impacting the entire body and resulting in an unregulated inflammatory response with widespread involvement of endothelial cells. It also causes a generalized activation of inflammation and coagulation.

According to the American College of Chest Physicians and the Society of Critical Care Medicine, SIRS is indicated by the presence of two or more of the following symptoms:

- temperature higher than 100.4°F (38°C) or lower than 96.8°F (36°C)
- heart rate greater than 90 beats/minute
- respiratory rate greater than 20 breaths per minute or a partial pressure of arterial carbon dioxide level less than 32 mm Hg
- abnormal WBC count (greater than 12,000/mm^3 or less than 4,000/mm^3 or greater than 10% bands).

How it happens

MODS is classified as primary or secondary:

- Primary MODS involves organ or organ system failure that's caused by a direct injury (such as trauma, aspiration, or near drowning) or a primary disorder (such as pneumonia or pulmonary embolism). Examples are renal dysfunction stemming from rhabdomyolysis or ARDS caused by gastric aspiration. As the syndrome continues, other organ systems are affected.
- Secondary MODS is due to uncontrolled systemic inflammation, with or without an infectious component. The most common infection sources include intra-abdominal sepsis, extensive blood loss, pancreatitis, or major vascular injuries. Noninfectious sources include multiple traumas, burns, or massive hemorrhage.

What to look for

The assessment findings associated with MODS typically reveal an acutely ill patient with signs and symptoms associated with SIRS. Early findings may include:

- fever (temperature usually greater than 101 °F [38.3 °C])
- tachycardia
- narrowed pulse pressure
- tachypnea
- decreased pulmonary artery pressure (PAP), PAWP, and CVP, and increased cardiac output.

As time goes by

As SIRS progresses, findings reflect impaired perfusion of the tissues and organs, such as:

- decreased LOC
- respiratory depression
- diminished bowel sounds
- jaundice
- oliguria or anuria
- increased PAP and PAWP and decreased cardiac output.

What tests tell you

No single test confirms MODS, and test results depend on the cause, such as trauma, aspiration, pulmonary embolism, or sepsis:

- ABG analysis may reveal hypoxemia with respiratory acidosis or metabolic acidosis.
- CBC may reveal decreased Hb level and HCT as well as leukocytosis.

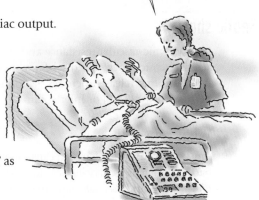

Treatment for MODS focuses on supporting respiratory and circulatory function.

- X-rays may reveal fractures, a cervical spine injury, pulmonary infiltrates, or abnormal air or fluid in the chest or abdominal organs.

Additional tests that may be performed include MRI, CT scan, and angiography.

How it's treated

Treatment focuses on supporting respiratory and circulatory function and includes:
- mechanical ventilation and supplemental oxygen
- hemodynamic monitoring
- fluid infusion (crystalloids and colloids)
- vasopressors
- measuring intake and output
- serial laboratory values
- dialysis
- antimicrobial agents.

What to do

- Keep in mind that nursing care for the patient with MODS is primarily supportive.
- Maintain the patient's airway and breathing with the use of mechanical ventilation and supplemental oxygen.
- Monitor vital signs, oxygen saturation, hemodynamic parameters, and cardiac rhythm for arrhythmias.
- Administer I.V. fluids as ordered.
- Monitor laboratory values.
- Monitor intake and output.
- Administer appropriate medications as ordered.
- Provide emotional support to the patient and family; explain diagnostic tests and treatments.

Septic shock

Low systemic vascular resistance and an elevated cardiac output characterize septic shock. The disorder is thought to occur in response to infections that release microbes or immune mediators such as tumor necrosis factor (TNF) or interleukin-1.

What causes it

Any pathogenic organism can cause septic shock. Gram-negative bacteria, such as *Escherichia coli*, *Klebsiella pneumoniae*, and *Serratia*, *Enterobacter*, and *Pseudomonas* organisms rank as the most common causes and account for up to 70% of all cases. Opportunistic fungi

Pathogens like me can cause septic shock. Shocking, huh?

cause about 3% of cases. Rare causative organisms include mycobacteria and some viruses and protozoa.

Septic shock can occur in any person with impaired immunity, but elderly people are at greatest risk.

How it happens
Septic shock is a type of distributive shock.

Endotoxins started it!
An immune response is triggered when bacteria release endotoxins. In response, macrophages secrete TNF and interleukins. These mediators, in turn, are responsible for increased release of platelet-activating factor (PAF), prostaglandins, leukotrienes, thromboxane A_2, kinins, and complement.

Compromised capillaries and more
The consequences of this immune activity are vasodilation and vasoconstriction, increased capillary permeability, reduced systemic vascular resistance, microemboli, and elevated cardiac output. Endotoxins also stimulate the release of histamine, further increasing capillary permeability.

Deepening depression
Moreover, myocardial depressant factor, TNF, PAF, and other factors depress myocardial function. Cardiac output falls, resulting in multisystem organ failure.

What to look for
The patient's history may include a disorder or treatment that causes immunosuppression, or it may include a history of invasive tests or treatments, surgery, or trauma. At onset, the patient may have fever and chills, although 20% of patients may be hypothermic.

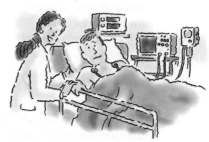

A patient with septic shock may have a history of immunosuppression, invasive tests or treatments, surgery, or trauma.

Phase facts
The patient's signs and symptoms will reflect either the hyperdynamic (early/warm) phase of septic shock or the hypodynamic (late/cold) phase.

Warm form
The hyperdynamic phase is characterized by:
- increased cardiac output
- peripheral vasodilation

- decreased systemic vascular resistance
- altered LOC (irritability/confusion)
- rapid, shallow respirations
- decreased urine output
- rapid, full, bounding pulse.

Coolin' (no foolin')

The hypodynamic phase is characterized by:
- decreased cardiac output
- peripheral vasoconstriction
- variable to increased systemic vascular resistance
- inadequate tissue perfusion
- pale and possibly cyanotic skin color
- mottling of extremities
- decreased LOC (lethargy)
- rapid, shallow respirations
- decreased or absent urine output
- absence of peripheral pulses or a rapid, weak, thready pulse
- cold and clammy skin
- hypotension, usually with a systolic pressure below 90 mm Hg or 50 to 80 mm Hg below the patient's previous level
- crackles or rhonchi if pulmonary congestion is present
- variable or reduced PAWP.

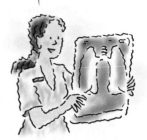

Chest X-rays that reveal the presence of ARDS indicate progression of septic shock.

What tests tell you

These findings aid in the diagnosis of septic shock:
- Blood cultures are positive for the offending organism.
- CBC shows the presence or absence of anemia and leukopenia, severe or absent neutropenia, and, usually, the presence of thrombocytopenia.
- ABG studies may reveal metabolic acidosis, hypoxemia, and low $Paco_2$ that progresses to increased $Paco_2$ (thereby indicating respiratory acidosis).
- BUN and creatinine levels are increased, and creatinine clearance is decreased.
- Prothrombin time, partial thromboplastin time, and bleeding time are increased; platelets are decreased; and fibrin split products are increased.
- Chest X-rays reveal evidence of pneumonia (as the underlying infection) or ARDS (indicating progression of septic shock).
- Electrocardiogram shows ST depression and inverted T waves.
- Amylase and lipase levels may show pancreatic insufficiency.
- Hepatic enzyme levels are elevated due to liver ischemia.
- Blood glucose levels are initially elevated and then decrease.
- CT scan reveals abscesses or sources of possible infection.

How it's treated

Location and treatment of the underlying sepsis is essential to treating septic shock. This includes:
- removing the source of infection, such as I.V., intra-arterial, or urinary drainage catheters
- aggressive antimicrobial therapy appropriate for the causative organism
- culture and sensitivity tests of urine and wound drainage
- surgery, if appropriate
- reducing or discontinuing immunosuppressive therapy
- oxygen therapy and mechanical ventilation if necessary
- colloid or crystalloid infusions first to increase the intravascular fluid volume
- administering a vasopressor such as dopamine, norepinephrine, or vasopressin.

What to do

- Assess ABCs. Monitor cardiopulmonary status closely.
- Administer supplemental oxygen as ordered.
- Monitor oxygen saturation and ABG values for evidence of hypoxemia and anticipate the need for ET intubation and mechanical ventilation should the patient's respiratory status deteriorate. Place the patient in semi-Fowler's position to maximize chest expansion. Keep the patient as quiet and comfortable as possible to minimize oxygen demands.

Vital moves

- Monitor the patient's vital signs continuously for changes. Observe his skin color and check capillary refill.
- Keep in mind that the patient's temperature is usually elevated in the early stages of septic shock and that he commonly experiences shaking chills. As the shock progresses, the temperature typically drops and the patient experiences diaphoresis.
- If the patient's systolic blood pressure drops below 90 mm Hg, increase the oxygen flow rate and notify the practitioner immediately. Alert the practitioner and increase the infusion rate if the patient experiences a progressive drop in blood pressure accompanied by a thready pulse.
- Remove I.V., intra-arterial, or urinary drainage catheters and send them to the laboratory to culture for the presence of the causative organism (prepare to reinsert or assist with reinsertion of new devices). Obtain blood cultures as ordered and begin antimicrobial therapy as ordered. Monitor the patient for possible adverse effects of therapy.

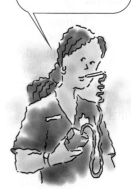

Temperature is usually elevated in the early stages of septic shock; however, as shock progresses, temperature drops.

- Institute continuous cardiac monitoring to evaluate for possible arrhythmias, myocardial ischemia, or adverse effects of treatment.
- Monitor intake and output closely. Notify the practitioner if the patient's urine output is less than 30 ml/hour.
- Administer I.V. fluid therapy as ordered, usually normal saline or lactated Ringer's solution. Monitor hemodynamic parameters to determine response to therapy.
- Be alert for signs and symptoms of possible fluid overload, such as dyspnea, tachypnea, crackles, peripheral edema, jugular vein distention, and increased PAP.
- Administer positive inotropic agents as ordered.
- Allow for frequent rest periods to minimize the patient's oxygen demands.
- Institute infection control precautions; use strict aseptic technique for all invasive procedures.
- Provide nutritional support therapy.
- Monitor laboratory test results, especially coagulation studies and hepatic enzyme levels, for changes indicative of DIC and hepatic failure, respectively.
- Provide emotional support to the patient and his family.
- Prepare the patient for surgery as appropriate.

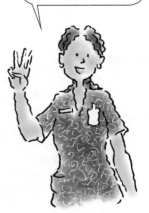

To put it bluntly, the mechanism of injury for trauma may be considered blunt, penetrating, or blast, depending on the cause of the injury.

Trauma

Trauma is any injury to human tissues and organs resulting from the transfer of energy from the environment. Trauma may be intentional or unintentional. Multiple traumas involve injuries to more than one body area or organ and are the leading cause of death in persons younger than age 45.

What's your type?

The type of trauma determines the mechanism of injury:
- blunt trauma—most common mechanism of injury; includes accelerating, shearing, and crushing forces. Examples include assaults, falls, car crashes, and sports injuries.
- penetrating trauma—includes both low-velocity wounds (such as stab wounds, impalements) and high-velocity wounds (such as gunshot wounds)
- blast trauma—Explosive devices may cause barotrauma to air-filled organs such as the lungs and stomach. Fragments and objects in the area may create secondary projectiles, whereas the wind may cause surrounding structures to collapse. It's important to remember that blast injuries may result in both blunt and penetrating trauma.

What causes it

Trauma may be caused by weapons, automobile crashes, physical confrontation, falls, or any other unnatural occurrence to the body.

How it happens

Traumatic wounds include:
- abrasion—The skin is scraped, with partial loss of the skin surface.
- laceration—The skin is torn, causing jagged, irregular edges; the severity of a laceration depends on its size, depth, and location.
- puncture wound—when a pointed object, such as a knife or glass fragment, penetrates the skin
- traumatic amputation—Part of the body (a limb or part of a limb) is removed.

What to look for

Assessment findings will vary according to the type and extent of trauma. A conscious patient with multiple injuries may be able to help focus the assessment on areas that need immediate attention, such as difficulty breathing or neurologic symptoms.

Primary assessment

During the primary assessment, the patient is assessed for life-threatening problems involving his airway, breathing, circulation, disability, and exposure (ABCDEs). (See *Primary assessment of the trauma patient*, page 700.)

Sport some life support

Monitor cardiac rhythm, initiate CPR, and administer drugs and electrical shock therapy (defibrillation and synchronized cardioversion) as appropriate for cardiac arrhythmias.

Secondary assessment

After completing the primary assessment and treating life-threatening conditions, perform a secondary assessment. This includes taking a history and performing a physical examination.

Skip to the important stuff . . .

During an emergency, you won't have time to obtain all of the patient's regular history. Focus on the most important information, including:
- signs and symptoms related to the present condition
- allergies to drugs, foods, latex, or environmental factors
- medication history, including prescription and over-the-counter medications, herbs, and supplements
- past medical history
- last meal
- events leading to the injury or condition.

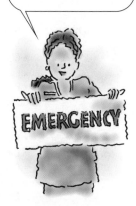

During an emergency, there's not much time for gathering health history. Focus on the most essential information, and fill in the details later, when the patient is stabilized.

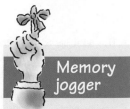

Memory jogger

To help remember what information to obtain during assessment of the trauma patient, use the acronym

SAMPLE:

- **S**igns and symptoms
- **A**llergies
- **M**edications
- **P**ast medical history
- **L**ast meal
- **E**vents leading to injury.

Primary assessment of the trauma patient

This chart shows what to look for (ABCDEs) and what to do during the trauma patient's primary assessment.

Parameter	Assessment	Interventions
A = airway	• Airway patency with cervical spine precautions	• Position the patient. • To open the airway, make sure that the neck is midline and stabilized and then perform the jaw-thrust maneuver. • Institute cervical spine immobilization until X-rays confirm the absence of cervical spine injury.
B = breathing	• Respirations (rate, depth, effort) • Breath sounds • Chest wall movement and chest injury • Position of trachea (midline or deviation)	• Administer 100% oxygen with bag valve mask. • Use airway adjuncts (such as oral or nasal airway, ET tube, esophageal tracheal combitube, cricothyrotomy). • Suction as needed. • Remove foreign bodies that may obstruct breathing. • Treat life-threatening conditions (pneumothorax, tension pneumothorax).
C = circulation	• Pulse and blood pressure • Bleeding or hemorrhage • Capillary refill, color of skin and mucous membranes • Cardiac rhythm	• Administer CPR, medications, and defibrillation or synchronized cardioversion. • Control hemorrhaging with direct pressure or pneumatic devices. • Establish I.V. access with two large bore I.V. catheters and start fluid therapy (isotonic fluids and blood). • Treat life-threatening conditions such as cardiac tamponade.
D = disability	• Neurologic assessment, including LOC, pupils, and motor and sensory function	• Identify areas to investigate during the secondary assessment.
E = exposure and environment	• Injuries and environmental exposure (extreme cold or heat)	• Institute appropriate therapy (warming therapy for hypothermia or cooling therapy for hyperthermia). • Undress the patient completely to identify all injured areas but prevent dropping their core body temperature.

... then fill in the blanks

When the patient's condition is stabilized, fill in the other components of the normal health history. Remember to include a history of blood transfusions and tetanus immunization if the patient has an open wound.

Illicit or otherwise

Question the patient about alcohol and drug use. Patients in substance withdrawal may exhibit behavioral changes and be more difficult to manage. Determine the frequency of substance use to assess whether the patient may experience withdrawal postoperatively.

he know from head to toe

After completion of the secondary assessment, you then perform a rapid head-to-toe examination that concentrates on areas relating to the patient's chief complaint rather than a body-systems examination because it's quicker. The head-to-toe examination includes assessing the patient's general appearance and vital signs, head and neck, chest and back, abdomen, perineal area, and extremities.

systems go

When the patient is stable, perform a body-system examination according to your facility's policy and procedure. A thorough assessment helps systematically identify and correct problems and establishes a baseline for future comparison.

What tests tell you

The diagnostic tests performed are based on the body system affected by the trauma. For example, a patient with a blunt chest injury would require a chest X-ray to detect rib and sternal fractures, pneumothorax, flail chest, pulmonary contusion, and a lacerated or ruptured aorta. Angiography studies would also be performed with suspected aortic laceration or rupture. Diagnostic tests for a patient with head trauma may include a CT scan, cervical spine X-rays, skull X-rays, or an angiogram.

Here are some other diagnostic tests that may be performed on the patient with multiple trauma:

- ABG analysis is used to evaluate respiratory status and determines acidotic and alkalotic states.
- CBC indicates the amount of blood loss.
- Coagulation studies are used to evaluate clotting ability.
- Serum electrolyte levels may indicate the presence of electrolyte imbalances.

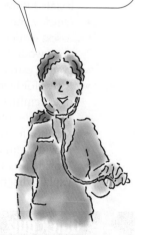

You may choose to perform a head-to-toe examination when assessing a patient with multiple traumas because it's quicker than a body-systems examination.

How it's treated

Trauma care basics include:

- triage
- assessing and maintaining ABCs
- protecting the cervical spine
- assessing the LOC
- preparing the patient for surgery and/or transport to a higher level of care.

Taking type into consideration

Management of traumatic wounds usually depends on the specific type of wound and degree of contamination. Treatment may include:

- controlling bleeding, usually by applying firm, direct pressure and elevating the extremity

- cleaning the wound
- administering pain medication
- administering antibiotic therapy
- surgery.

Additional treatment is based on the body system that's affected by the trauma and the extent of injury. For example, treatment of a blunt chest injury may include maintaining a patent airway; providing adequate ventilation; maintaining fluid and electrolyte balance; and inserting a chest tube for pneumothorax, hemothorax, or tension pneumothorax.

What to do

- Assess ABCs and initiate emergency measures if necessary; administer supplemental oxygen as ordered.
- Immobilize the head and neck with an immobilization device, sandbags, backboard, and tape. Assist with cervical spine X-rays.
- Monitor vital signs and note significant changes.
- Monitor oxygen saturation and cardiac rhythm for arrhythmias.
- Assess neurologic status, including LOC and pupillary and motor response.
- Obtain blood studies, including type and crossmatch.
- Insert two large-bore I.V. catheters and infuse normal saline or lactated Ringer's solution.
- Quickly and carefully assess for multiple injuries.
- Assess wounds and provide wound care as appropriate. Cover open wounds and control bleeding by applying pressure and elevating extremities.
- Assess for increased abdominal distention and increased diameter of extremities.
- Administer blood products as appropriate.
- Monitor for signs of hypovolemic shock.
- Provide pain medication, as appropriate.
- Provide reassurance to the patient and his family.
- Explain diagnostic tests and treatments.

Quick quiz

1. Your patient has hemophilia and experienced a major bleeding event. To replace clotting factors, you would expect to give:
    A. albumin.
    B. FFP.
    C. whole blood.
    D. packed RBCs.

Answer: B. FFP is the product of choice for replacing clotting factors. Albumin serves as a plasma volume expander and packed RBCs contain no clotting factors. Although whole blood does contain clotting factors, the amount is not enough for this patient.

2. Hypertonic solutions cause fluids to move from the:
    A. interstitial space to the intracellular space.
    B. intracellular space to the extracellular space.
    C. extracellular space to the intracellular space.
    D. intracellular space to the interstitial space.

Answer: B. Because of their increased osmolality, hypertonic solutions draw fluids out of the cells and into the extracellular space.

3. Your patient has partial- and full-thickness burn injuries to his anterior chest, anterior abdomen, and entire right arm. Using the Rule of Nines, the percentage of total BSA involved can be estimated at:
    A. 18%.
    B. 27%.
    C. 45%.
    D. 50%.

Answer: B. The anterior chest and abdomen constitute 18% of the BSA, and the entire right arm is 9%, for a total of 27%.

4. Which nursing intervention is the most important when treating a patient with hypovolemic shock?
    A. Assess for dehydration.
    B. Administer I.V. fluids.
    C. Insert a urinary catheter.
    D. Obtain blood for a CBC.

Answer: B. Although all of these interventions should be done, hypovolemic shock is an emergency that requires prompt and rapid initiation of I.V. fluids to maintain cardiac output and support intravascular fluid volumes.

5. Signs of septic shock include:
    A. clear, watery sputum.
    B. severe hypertension.
    C. hypotension.
    D. increased urine output.

Answer: C. Hypotension is a sign of hypodynamic septic shock, along with pale and possibly cyanotic skin color; mottling of extremities; decreased LOC; rapid, shallow respirations; decreased or absent urine output; absence of peripheral pulses; or a rapid, weak pulse.

6. Signs and symptoms of transfusion-related acute lung injury as a result of a blood transfusion include:
    A. abdominal cramping and tachycardia within 2 hours of transfusion.
    B. urticaria and fever within 5 minutes of transfusion.
    C. chest tightness and jugular vein distension within 1 hour of transfusion.

  D. hypotension and severe respiratory distress within 6 hours
      of transfusion.

Answer: D. Signs and symptoms of transfusion-related acute lung
injury include severe respiratory distress within 6 hours of transfusion as well as fever, chills, cyanosis, and hypotension.

7. Your patient has signs of bruising across his abdomen after a
motor vehicle crash. Which of the following assessments should be
immediately reported to the physician?
  A. A decrease in Hb from 11.2 to 10.9 g per dl
  B. Bloody urine output
  C. Hyperactive bowel sounds
  D. Complaint of generalized pain in the abdomen

Answer: B. Bloody urine may indicate a ruptured bladder. Hb
changes are minimal, bowel sounds are still active and within norms,
and pain would be expected in this condition.

Scoring

☆☆☆ If you answered all seven questions correctly, way to go! You are
      multitalented when it comes to multisystem issues.

  ☆☆ If you answered six questions correctly, good work! This last quick
      quiz must not have been too traumatic for you.

    ☆ If you answered fewer than six questions correctly, don't go into
      shock. You can always review the chapter again.

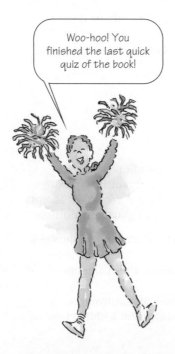

Woo-hoo! You
finished the last quick
quiz of the book!

Suggested References

Aiken, L. M., Williams, G., Harvey, M., Blot, S., Kleinpell, R., Labeau, S., . . . Ahrens, T. (2011). Nursing considerations to complement the surviving sepsis campaign guidelines. *Critical Care Medicine, 39*(7), 1800–1818.

Brown, J., Cohen, M., Minei, J., Maier, R., West, M., Billiar, T., . . . Sperry, J. L. (2012). Debunking the survival bias myth: Characterization of mortality during the initial 24 hours for patients requiring massive transfusion. *Journal of Trauma and Acute Care Surgery, 73*, 358–364.

Campion, E., Pritts, T., Dorlac, W., Nguyen, A., Fraley, S., Hanseman, D., & Robinson, B. R. (2013). Implementation of a military-derived damage-control resuscitation strategy in a civilian trauma center decreases acute hypoxia in massively transfused patients. *Journal of Trauma and Acute Care Surgery, 75*, S221–S227.

Casa, D., Kenny, G., & Taylor, N. (2010). Immersion treatment for exertion hyperthermia: Cold or temperate water? *Medicine and Science in Sports and Exercise, 42*(7), 1246–1252.

Chapman, M., Moore, E., Ramos, C., Ghasabyan, A., Harr, J. N., Chin, T. L., . . . Banerjee, A. (2013). Fibrinolysis greater than 3% is the critical value for initiation of antifibrinolytic therapy. *Journal of Trauma and Acute Care Surgery, 75*, 961–967.

Ciomartan, T. (2014). What is the best fluid for volume resuscitation in critically ill adults with sepsis? The jury is still out, but a verdict is urgently needed . . . . *Critical Care Medicine, 42*, 1722–1723.

Dellinger, R. P., Levy, M. M., Rhodes, A., Annane, D., Gerlach, H., Opal, S. M., . . . Moreno, R. (2013). Surviving Sepsis Campaign: International guidelines for management of severe sepsis and septic shock, 2012. *Intensive Care Medicine, 39*(2), 165–228.

Elinoff, J., & Suffredini, A. (2014). Exploring the boundaries of systemic inflammation. *Critical Care Medicine, 42*, 1735–1737.

Faulds, M., & Meekings, T. (2013). Temperature management in critically ill patients. *Continuing Education in Anaesthesia, Critical Care & Pain, 13*(3), 75–79.

Foster, K. (2014). Clinical guidelines in the management of burn injury: A review and recommendations from the organization and delivery of burn care committee. *Journal of Burn Care & Research, 35*(4), 271–283.

Goodwin, C. (Ed.). (2011). *Advanced burn life support manual*. Chicago, IL: American Burn Association.

Kautza, B., Cohen, M., Cuschieri, J., Minei, J., Brackenridge, S., Maier, R., . . . Sperry, J. L. (2012). Changes in massive transfusion over time: An early shift in the right direction? *Journal of Trauma and Acute Care Surgery, 72*, 106–111.

Looney, M., Roubinian, N., Gajic, O., Gropper, M., Hubmayr, R., Lowell, C.A., . . . Toy, P. (2014). Prospective study on the clinical course and outcomes in transfusion-related acute lung injury. *Critical Care Medicine, 42*, 1676–1687.

Marshall, J. C., Dellinger, R. P., & Levy, M. (2010). The Surviving Sepsis Campaign: A history and a perspective. *Surgical Infections, 11*(3), 275–281.

Mora-Rodriguez, R. (2012). Influence of aerobic fitness on thermoregulation during exercise in the heat. *Exercise and Sports Science Reviews, 40*(2), 79–87.

Nunnally, M., Jaeschke, R., Bellingan, G., Lacroix, J., Mourvillier, B., Rodriquez-Vega, G. M., . . . Buchman, T. G. (2011). Targeted temperature management in critical care: A report and recommendations from five professional societies. *Critical Care Medicine, 39*(5), 1113–1125.

Opal, S., Dellinger, R. P., Vincent, J., Masur, H., & Angus, D. (2014). The next generation of sepsis clinical trial designs: What is next after the demise of recombinant human activated protein C? *Critical Care Medicine, 42*, 1714–1721.

Palmieri, T., Greenhalgh, D., & Sen, S. (2013). Prospective comparison of packed red blood cell-to-fresh frozen plasma transfusion ratio of 4: 1 versus 1: 1 during acute massive burn excision. *Journal of Trauma and Acute Care Surgery, 74*, 76–83.

Petersdorf, E. W. (2012). Genetics of graft-versus-host disease: The major histocompatibility complex. *Blood Reviews, 27*(1), 1–12.

Presciutti, M., Bader, M., & Hepburn, M. (2012). Shivering management during therapeutic temperature modulation: Nurses' perspective. *Critical Care Nurse, 32*(1), 33–42.

Raghunathan, K., Shaw, A., Nathanson, B., Stürmer, T., Brookhart, A., Stefan, M. S., . . . Lindenauer, P. K. (2014). Association between the choice of IV crystalloid and in-hospital mortality among critically ill adults with sepsis. *Critical Care Medicine, 42*, 1585–1591.

Remick, K., Schwab, C., Smith, B., Monshizadeh, A., Kim, P., & Reilly, P. (2014). Defining the optimal time to the operating room may salvage early trauma deaths. *Journal of Trauma and Acute Care Surgery, 76*, 1251–1258.

Rotta, M., Storer, B. E., Storb, R. F., Martin, P. J., Heimfeld, S., Peffer, A., . . . Mielcarek, M. (2010). Donor statin treatment protects against severe acute graft-versus-host disease after related allogeneic hematopoietic cell transplantation. *Blood, 115*(6), 1288–1295.

Savage, S., Zarzaur, B., Croce, M., & Fabian, T. (2014). Time matters in 1: 1 resuscitations: Concurrent administration of blood: Plasma and risk of death. *Journal of Trauma and Acute Care Surgery, 77*(6), 833–837.

Wheeler, K., Lane, K., Walters, S., & Matte, T. (2013). Heat illness and deaths—New York City, 2000–2011. *Morbidity and Mortality Weekly Report, 62*(31), 617–621.

Appendices and index

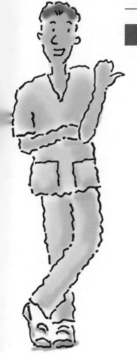

Moderate sedation

Moderate sedation, also called *conscious sedation*, is a drug-induced depression of consciousness that's used for painful diagnostic and therapeutic procedures and those procedures for which the patient must remain immobile. With moderate sedation, the patient can still respond purposefully to light tactile stimulation and verbal commands. He maintains a patent airway as well as adequate spontaneous ventilations and cardiovascular function.

In addition to the nurse trained per hospital and state requirements administering the moderate sedation, this procedure requires the presence of a doctor or at least one other nurse or respiratory therapist who can establish a patent airway and administer positive pressure ventilation to the patient, if necessary.

The patient receiving moderate sedation requires sedation monitoring before the procedure, throughout the procedure, and during the recovery period. A nurse can administer moderate sedation in the critical care unit or in a special procedure area.

For procedures requiring moderate sedation, it's imperative to prevent the patient from transitioning into deep sedation or anesthesia because he won't be able to protect and maintain his airway and may show signs of hemodynamic instability. For a patient who requires a deep sedation or anesthesia state, the presence of an anesthesia provider (anesthesiologist or certified registered nurse anesthetist [CRNA]) is required to secure a safe airway for the patient and to maintain hemodynamic stability.

Equipment

- Sedation flow record
- Positive pressure oxygen delivery system, capable of administering greater than 90% oxygen for at least 60 minutes
- Supplemental oxygen administration equipment
- Suction apparatus with connected tubing
- Suction catheter
- Pulse oximeter
- Sphygmomanometer and blood pressure cuff or automated blood pressure machine
- Stethoscope
- Cardiac monitoring equipment
- Emergency care supplies or kit with drugs and equipment to establish and maintain an airway and supplies for vascular access and a defibrillator
- Medications and reversal agents, as ordered

Preparation of equipment

Make sure that the room where the patient will be receiving the sedation has all the necessary equipment. Test all monitoring equipment to ensure that it's in proper working order before attaching it to the patient.

Implementation

- Verify the doctor's order for moderate sedation.
- Review the patient's medical record and make sure that you document the following information: any preexisting medical conditions, previous anesthesia and sedation experiences, current medications, allergies, last time the patient ate or had oral fluids, a recent height and weight, and physical examination findings, including evaluation of the airway and a cardiac and respiratory assessment.
- Ensure that informed consent for the procedure to be performed has been obtained and is included in the patient's medical record.
- Explain the procedure to the patient and his family and answer their questions.
- Ensure that the patient has had nothing by mouth except for clear liquids and prescribed medications for at least 8 hours before the procedure.
- When the patient is in the room where sedation will be administered, perform hand hygiene.
- Confirm the patient's identity using two patient identifiers and perform procedural pause to verify right patient, right procedure, and right site according to your facility's policy.
- Record the patient's vital signs including oxygen saturation and end-tidal carbon dioxide level when appropriate, level of consciousness, skin color, and respiratory status to use as a baseline.
- Apply a pulse oximeter probe, turn on the machine, and record the patient's oxygen saturation.
- Ensure that the patient has a patent I.V. access device.
- Confirm the medication dosage calculations based on the patient's weight or body surface area.
- Administer the sedation as appropriate. If you aren't administering the sedation, begin monitoring the patient.
- Continuously monitor the patient's respiratory rate, blood pressure, oxygen saturation, end-tidal carbon dioxide, head position, adequacy of chest expansion, and level of consciousness using the approved sedation-scoring tool at least every 5 minutes.
- Monitor the patient for complications and provide interventions as indicated.
- When sedation administration is complete, continue monitoring the patient according to your facility's policy—usually every 15 minutes for 1 hour or until the sedation level is at the preassessment level for two consecutive 15-minute intervals. If a reversal agent has been given, monitor the patient for at least 2 hours after the last dose.
- Document the procedure.

Complications

It's possible for the patient to become oversedated during moderate sedation. Other complications of moderate sedation include aspiration of gastric

Responding to complications of sedation

This table reviews nursing interventions for various complications of sedation.

Complication	Nursing interventions
Airway obstruction or respiratory depression	• Reposition the patient's head. • Suction. • Insert an oral airway. • Tell the patient to take a deep breath. • Stimulate the patient by rubbing his arms or legs. • Administer oxygen. • Manually ventilate with a bag valve mask device.
Oversedation	• Maintain airway, breathing, and circulation. • Manually ventilate with a bag valve mask device, if necessary. • Have drugs to reverse sedation (such as naloxone for opiates and flumazenil for benzodiazepines) immediately available and administer, as ordered, if the patient is too deeply sedated. • Monitor respiratory status until stable.
Cardiac arrhythmias	• Note baseline heart rate and rhythm. • Obtain an apical pulse for 1 minute. • Examine electrocardiogram patterns if indicated. • Ensure that the patient has a patent airway. • Monitor oxygen saturation levels. • Administer oxygen. • Administer fluids and antiarrhythmic drugs as ordered.
Hypotension	• Investigate possible causes. • Support respiratory status. • Administer fluids and vasopressors as ordered.
Hypertension	• Administer additional sedation or analgesia.

contents, respiratory depression or failure, and adverse reactions to the medication. Observe the patient for airway obstruction, respiratory depression, hypotension, and drug-specific complications. (See *Responding to complications of sedation*.)

Preexisting respiratory conditions, such as chronic obstructive pulmonary disease or asthma, and hepatic or renal dysfunction can increase the patient's risk for adverse reactions. Age and general health can also increase this risk. In general, children (because of their smaller body mass) and older adults (because of decreased renal and hepatic function and relative loss of muscle) are at greater risk. Drug interactions, such as those that occur with cimetidine and droperidol or when opioids and sedatives are used in combination, can have synergistic effects.

Documentation

Document the procedure and all of the patient's vital signs on your facility's sedation flow sheet. Also document how the patient tolerated the procedure and complications or adverse effects.

Record medications that were administered, including medications administered to manage the patient's recovery. Document I.V. fluids administered, including the type and amount. Document any adverse effects experienced in response to medications administered. Note patient teaching provided, questions asked by the patient, and your responses.

Moderate Sedation References

American Society of Anesthesiologists. (2009). *Continuum of depth of sedation: Definition of general anesthesia and levels of sedation/analgesia.* Retrieved from https://www.asahq.org/For-Members/Standards-Guidelines-and-Statements.aspx

American Society of Anesthesiologists. (2010). *Standards for basic anesthetic monitoring.* Retrieved from https://www.asahq.org/For-Members/Standards-Guidelines-and-Statements.aspx

American Society of PeriAnesthesia Nurses. (2012). *2012–2014 Perianesthesia nursing: Standards, practice recommendations, and interpretative statements.* Cherry Hill, NJ: Author.

Association of PeriOperative Registered Nurses. (2014). *Perioperative standards and recommended practices: Recommended practices for management of the patient receiving moderate sedation/analgesia.* Retrieved from http://aornstandards.org/content/1/SEC26.extract

Kodali, B. S. (2013). Capnography outside the operating rooms. *Anesthesiology, 118*(1), 192–201.

Ramsay, M. A. E. (2000). Intensive care: Problems of over- and undersedation. *Best Practice & Research Clinical Anaesthesiology, 14*(2), 419–432.

Sessler, C., Gosnell, M. S., Grap, M. J., Brophy, G. M., O'Neal, P. V., Keane, K. A., . . . Elswick, R. K. (2002). The Richmond Agitation-Sedation Scale: Validity and reliability in adult intensive care unit patients. *American Journal of Respiratory Critical Care Medicine, 166,* 1338–1344.

Studies have shown that early cardiopulmonary resuscitation (CPR) in cardiac arrest improves the patient's likelihood of survival. Chest compressions are particularly important because perfusion to vital organs during CPR depends on them. To prevent a delay in chest compressions, the 2010 American Heart Association (AHA) Guidelines for Cardiopulmonary Resuscitation and Emergency Cardiovascular Care recommend a change in the sequence of CPR. Instead of the traditional "A-B-C" (airway, breathing, and chest compressions) sequence, the guidelines recommend changing the sequence to "C-A-B" (compressions, airway, and breathing), giving highest priority to chest compressions when resuscitating a patient.

According to these guidelines, high-quality CPR is important not only at the onset of resuscitation but also throughout the resuscitation process. In their latest guidelines, the AHA also recommends integrating defibrillation and other advanced cardiac life support measures into the resuscitation process but only with minimal interruptions in CPR.

Discovering a suspected victim

If you discover a suspected victim of cardiac arrest, immediately take action. Before beginning CPR, assess the victim to determine if he's unconscious. Gently tap him on the shoulder and shout, "Are you alright?" While assessing for responsiveness, check to see if the patient is apneic or only gasping. If the patient is unresponsive and apneic or only gasping, assume that he's in cardiac arrest.

If you check for a pulse, limit your check to 10 seconds to avoid delaying chest compressions. Check the carotid or femoral pulse in an adult or child; the brachial pulse in an infant. Next, activate the emergency response system and get an automated external defibrillator (AED), if there's one close by.

If an AED isn't close by, place the patient supine on a hard surface and begin one-rescuer CPR, until other health care workers arrive. When they arrive, quickly delegate responsibilities to those team members who can assist by simultaneously performing other resuscitation tasks. Switch chest compressors after five cycles of compressions and ventilations (about every 2 minutes) to maintain quality compressions; make sure the switch takes less than 5 seconds. Moreover, switch compressors during any intervention that interrupts chest compressions, such as defibrillation or advanced airway insertion.

In adults, cardiac arrest commonly results from ventricular fibrillation, but in children and infants, it typically results from a respiratory cause. If you're alone when you discover a child or infant in cardiac arrest, perform CPR for 2 minutes before activating the emergency response system and obtaining an AED if one is nearby.

Performing CPR on an adult or adolescent

Use these guidelines when performing CPR on adults and children beyond puberty.

Start compressions.	
• Hand placement	• Place both hands, one atop the other, on the lower half of the sternum between the nipples, with elbows locked; use a straight up-and-down motion.
• Depth	• At least 2″
• Compression rate	• At least 100 compressions/minute; allow the chest to recoil completely after each compression
• Compression-to-ventilation ratio	• 30 compressions : 2 ventilations
Open the airway.	• Use the head-tilt, chin-lift maneuver, unless trauma is suspected. • If trauma is suspected, use the jaw-thrust method.
Perform ventilations.	• Give 2 breaths, each over 1 second. • Deliver sufficient tidal volume with each breath to produce visible chest rise. • If the patient is intubated, deliver continuous chest compressions with ventilations at a rate of 1 breath every 6 to 8 seconds (8 to 10 ventilations per minute).
Use the AED.	• Apply an AED as soon as it's available and follow the prompts. Minimize interruptions in chest compressions by resuming CPR with chest compressions immediately after each shock.

Performing CPR on a child (age 1 year to the onset of puberty)

Follow these guidelines when performing CPR on a child age 1 year to the onset of puberty. According to the AHA, puberty is defined as the onset of breast development in females and the development of axillary hair in males.

Integrating AED use with CPR

Ventricular fibrillation is the most common initial rhythm in witnessed cardiac arrest. Defibrillation, the treatment of choice for ventricular fibrillation, is a key to improving survival from cardiac arrest. Because the success of defibrillation decreases quickly over time, the new AHA guidelines call for rapid integration of AED use with CPR to ensure that defibrillation is performed early.

For the victim to have the best chance of survival, three interventions must occur within the first moments of cardiac arrest:
- activating the emergency medical system
- initiating CPR
- delivering defibrillation.

Start compressions.	
• Hand placement	• Depending on the size of the child, use the heel of one or two hands to compress the lower half of the sternum; if using two hands, place one hand atop the other.
• Depth	• About 2″
• Compression rate	• At least 100 compressions/minute; allow the chest to recoil completely after each compression
• Compression-to-ventilation ratio	• 30 compressions : 2 ventilations for 1 rescuer • 15 compressions : 2 ventilations for 2 rescuers
Open the airway.	• Use the head-tilt, chin-lift maneuver, unless trauma is suspected. • If trauma is suspected, use the jaw-thrust method.
Perform ventilations.	• Give 2 breaths, each over 1 second. • Deliver sufficient tidal volume with each breath to produce visible chest rise. • If the child is intubated, deliver continuous chest compressions with ventilations at a rate of 1 breath every 6 to 8 seconds (8 to 10 ventilations per minute).
Use the AED.	• Apply an AED as soon as it's available and follow the prompts. Minimize interruptions in chest compressions by resuming CPR with chest compressions immediately after each shock.

When two or more rescuers are present, one person can activate the emergency response system while another begins CPR. Keep in mind that delays in initiating CPR or defibrillation reduce the victim's chance of survival, so when using an AED within the hospital, the first shock should be delivered within 3 minutes of the arrest.

To perform defibrillation with an AED, place one electrode pad on the right side of the patient's chest just below the clavicle. Place the second electrode pad on the left side of the patient's chest to the left of the heart's apex.

Be prepared to deliver a shock as soon as the compressor removes his hand from the patient's chest and all rescuers are "clear" of contact with the patient. After the first shock is delivered, resume compressions immediately; don't delay compressions to recheck the rhythm or pulse. Continue CPR for 5 cycles, ending with compressions. Then, allow the AED to analyze the patient's rhythm and deliver another shock, if needed.

Defibrillation dosing guidelines

If you're using a biphasic defibrillators, use the manufacturer's recommended energy dose, commonly 120 to 200 joules. Use the maximum dose, if the manufacturer's recommended dose is unknown.

For monophasic AED, AHA guidelines recommend that the first shock deliver 360 joules; if ventricular fibrillation persists after the first shock, the second and subsequent shocks should deliver 360 joules. However, if your facility's AED is programmed to deliver a different dose, that dose is acceptable.

For children, begin defibrillation with 2 joules/kg; if a second shock is required, increase the dose to 4 joules/kg. Subsequent shocks should be at least 4 joules/kg; higher doses may be considered, to a maximum dose of 10 joules/kg, or 360 joules.

Advanced cardiovascular life support in cardiac arrest

When a patient experiences cardiac arrest, advanced cardiovascular life support (ACLS) interventions (such as drug therapy, advanced airway management, and monitoring) enhance basic life support measures. To improve the effectiveness of ACLS, the new AHA guidelines recommend:

- using continuous quantitative capnography to confirm and monitor endotracheal tube placement
- performing high-quality CPR
- avoiding routine use of atropine for treatment of pulseless electrical activity and asystole
- employing physiologic monitoring to improve CPR quality and detect the return of spontaneous circulation
- administering chronotropic drugs as an alternative to pacing for symptomatic and unstable bradycardia
- giving adenosine for stable undifferentiated regular monomorphic wide-complex tachycardia.

When caring for an adult in cardiac arrest, follow the latest *Adult cardiac arrest* algorithm shown on page 716.

Postcardiac arrest care

For patients that have return of spontaneous circulation and remain unconscious, institute induced hypothermia (as ordered by the doctor) to protect the brain and other organs. Current recommendations are to cool patients to 32° to 34°C for 12 to 24 hours postarrest. Methods for cooling include administration of cold saline, hypothermia blankets, and invasive cooling catheters. Patients must be monitored for coagulopathy, electrolyte imbalances, arrhythmias, and hyperglycemia. Rewarming of patients should occur slowly, no faster than 0.5°C per hour.

Adult cardiac arrest

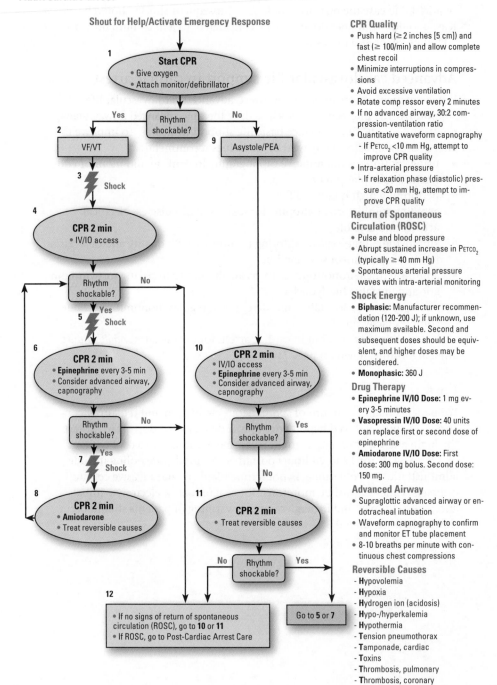

CPR Quality
- Push hard (≥ 2 inches [5 cm]) and fast (≥ 100/min) and allow complete chest recoil
- Minimize interruptions in compressions
- Avoid excessive ventilation
- Rotate comp ressor every 2 minutes
- If no advanced airway, 30:2 compression-ventilation ratio
- Quantitative waveform capnography
  - If P_{ETCO_2} <10 mm Hg, attempt to improve CPR quality
- Intra-arterial pressure
  - If relaxation phase (diastolic) pressure <20 mm Hg, attempt to improve CPR quality

Return of Spontaneous Circulation (ROSC)
- Pulse and blood pressure
- Abrupt sustained increase in P_{ETCO_2} (typically ≥ 40 mm Hg)
- Spontaneous arterial pressure waves with intra-arterial monitoring

Shock Energy
- **Biphasic:** Manufacturer recommendation (120-200 J); if unknown, use maximum available. Second and subsequent doses should be equivalent, and higher doses may be considered.
- **Monophasic:** 360 J

Drug Therapy
- **Epinephrine IV/IO Dose:** 1 mg every 3-5 minutes
- **Vasopressin IV/IO Dose:** 40 units can replace first or second dose of epinephrine
- **Amiodarone IV/IO Dose:** First dose: 300 mg bolus. Second dose: 150 mg.

Advanced Airway
- Supraglottic advanced airway or endotracheal intubation
- Waveform capnography to confirm and monitor ET tube placement
- 8-10 breaths per minute with continuous chest compressions

Reversible Causes
- **H**ypovolemia
- **H**ypoxia
- **H**ydrogen ion (acidosis)
- **H**ypo-/hyperkalemia
- **H**ypothermia
- **T**ension pneumothorax
- **T**amponade, cardiac
- **T**oxins
- **T**hrombosis, pulmonary
- **T**hrombosis, coronary

From Neumar, R. W., Otto, C. W., Link, M. S., Kronick, S. L., Shuster, M., Callaway, C. W., . . . Morrison, L. J. (2010). 2010 American Heart Association Guidelines for Cardiopulmonary Resuscitation and Emergency Cardiovascular Care, Part 8: Adult advanced cardiovascular life support. *Circulation, 122*(Suppl. 3), S729–S767. Copyright (2010) American Heart Association, Inc. Reprinted with permission.

Comparing types of shock

This chart summarizes the different types of shock, their characteristics, and their treatment.

Types	Pathophysiology	Causes	Physical findings	Treatment
Anaphylactic	• Edema • Blood vessel dilation • Bronchospasms • Fluid shifts	• Allergic reaction to antigens	• Pale, cool skin • Hypotension • Respiratory distress • Edema • Rash	• Epinephrine • Corticosteroids • Antihistamines • I.V. fluids • Oxygen
Cardiogenic	• Decreased cardiac output • Left ventricular dysfunction • Sympathetic compensation • Myocardial ischemia	• Myocardial infarction • Myocardial ischemia • Myocarditis • Papillary muscle dysfunction • Ventricular septal defect • Ventricular aneurysm • Acute mitral or aortic insufficiency	• Pale, cool, clammy skin • Decreased sensorium • Rapid, thread pulse • Rapid, shallow respirations • Mean arterial pressure <60 mm Hg in adults • Gallop rhythm • Faint heart sounds	• Vasopressors • Inotropics • Osmotic diuretics • Oxygen • Intra-aortic balloon pump • Analgesics, sedatives • Possible intubation and mechanical ventilation
Hypovolemic	• Reduced venous return to heart due to lost fluid • Decreased ventricular filling • Decreased cardiac output • Tissue anoxia • Metabolic acidosis	• Acute blood loss • Intestinal obstruction • Burns • Peritonitis • Acute pancreatitis • Ascites • Dehydration • Diabetic ketoacidosis	• Pale, cool, clammy skin • Decreased sensorium • Rapid, shallow respirations • Urine output <20 ml/hour • Rapid, thread pulse • Mean arterial pressure <60 mm Hg in adults • Orthostatic vital signs	• Prompt, vigorous blood and fluid replacement • Positive inotropics
Neurogenic	• Severe vasodilation	• Anesthesia • Spinal cord injury	• Pale, warm, dry skin • Bounding pulse • Bradycardia • Hypotension	• I.V. fluids • Oxygen • Vasopressors • Lying flat
Septic	• Activation of chemical mediators in response to invading organisms • Functional hypovolemia	• Any pathogenic organism • Primarily gram-negative bacteria	Early • Pink, flushed skin • Rapid, shallow respirations • Rapid, full, bounding pulse • Normal or slightly elevated blood pressure Late • Pale, cyanotic skin • Rapid, shallow respirations • Rapid, weak, thread pulse • Hypotension	• Antimicrobials • Colloids or crystalloids • Oxygen • Diuretics • Vasopressors

Preventing complications in the critically ill obese patient

Caring for a critically ill obese patient presents many complex challenges. This chart summarizes potential complications, their causes, and actions to take to prevent complications or intervene early.

Complication	Causes	Interventions
Atelectasis	• Immobility • Pain with respiratory effort	• Encourage early ambulation. • Provide adequate pain control. • Encourage the use of an incentive spirometer. • Provide supplemental oxygen for the first 3 postoperative days. • Use continuous positive airway pressure or bilevel positive airway pressure as ordered.
Aspiration and pneumonia	• Increased intra-abdominal pressure • Lower gastric pH • High gastric fluid volumes	• Reposition the patient every 2 hours. • Use rotational therapy as ordered. • Monitor closely for decreasing or abnormal breath sounds. • Provide oral care. • Ensure adequate nutritional intake. • Facilitate secretion removal.
Cardiac arrhythmias	• Infiltration of the conduction system by fat and fibrosis of the bundle branches	• Monitor heart rate and rhythm via continuous cardiac monitoring. • Notify the practitioner of any significant arrhythmias. • Administer medications as ordered. • Follow cardiopulmonary resuscitation and ACLS guidelines as appropriate.
Deep vein thrombosis	• Immobility • Venous stasis • Impaired coagulation • Pulmonary hypertension	• Assist with early ambulation. • Apply sequential compression devices to lower extremities as ordered. • Administer anticoagulants as ordered. • Obtain physical therapy and occupational therapy consults. • Provide assistive devices and use lifts as needed. • Learn how the patient gets out of bed at home. • Use a bariatric bed as ordered.
Hyperglycemia	• Stress	• Monitor blood glucose levels closely. • Administer appropriate therapy.

Complication	Causes	Interventions
Inadequate medication effects	• Accumulation of drug in adipose tissue • Increased glomerular filtration rate with normal renal function	• Carefully monitor clinical response and serum drug levels. • Observe for signs of toxicity and notify the practitioner. • Consult the pharmacist. • Monitor appropriate laboratory values such as creatinine clearance.
Respiratory failure	• High oxygen consumption • Decreased functional residual capacity • Decreased expiratory reserve volume • Decreased total lung capacity • Diaphragmatic fatigue	• Assist with intubation. Because intubating an obese patient is usually more difficult due to limited neck mobility, limited mouth opening, and the presence of an underbite or receding chin, assist the patient into a ramped position by elevating the upper body and head until horizontal alignment is achieved between the ear and sternal notch. • Initiate mechanical ventilation with a tidal volume of 5 to 7 ml per kg, based on ideal (not actual) body weight and add positive end-expiratory pressure, as ordered. • Position the patient in reverse Trendelenburg position at 45 degrees. • Secure endotracheal tube to prevent displacement.
Skin breakdown, pressure ulcers, and delayed wound healing	• Decreased vascularity of adipose tissue • Moisture and incontinence • Immobility • Pressure within skin folds related to tubes, catheters • Ill-fitting chair or wheelchair or improperly sized bed and equipment	• Inspect folds of the patient's breasts, back, abdomen, and perineum for signs of breakdown and infection. • Provide meticulous skin care, especially in the perineal area. • Position tubes so that the patient doesn't lay on them. • Reposition the patient every 2 hours. Be sure to also reposition large abdominal panniculus. Use rotation therapy as ordered. • Learn how the patient gets out of bed at home. • Use properly sized equipment. • Use a bariatric bed as ordered. • Use caution when moving the patient to prevent friction of skin moving on skin. • Provide adequate nutrition.

Drug overdose and poisoning

Accidental or intentional drug overdoses and poisonings can cause physical and mental changes that may require admission to a critical care unit. Managing a poisoned or overdosed patient involves interventions to prevent absorption of or further exposure to the drug or agent as well as methods to enhance elimination. Depending on the offensive substance, elimination methods may include gastric lavage, administration of cathartics, whole-bowel irrigation, administration of activated charcoal, alteration of urine pH, hemodialysis, hemoperfusion, chelation, or hyperbaric oxygen therapy. In addition, you may administer an antitoxin, antagonist, or antivenom.

Interventions for some more common overdoses and poisonings are presented in this table. Follow your facility's protocols and doctor's orders for administration of specific therapies and drugs.

Drug or substance	Signs and symptoms	Interventions
Acetaminophen	• Anorexia • Nausea • Malaise • Elevated aspartate aminotransferase (AST), alanine aminotransferase (ALT), and total bilirubin • Prolonged prothrombin time • Jaundice	• Administer activated charcoal to prevent absorption. • Obtain acetaminophen level 4 hours after ingestion and determine whether antidote is indicated. • Administer antidote, N-acetylcysteine. • Monitor daily AST, ALT, total bilirubin, blood urea nitrogen, creatinine, and prothrombin times.
Amphetamines	• Flushing • Diaphoresis • Restlessness • Irritability • Talkativeness • Panic • Seizures • Hypertension • Tachycardia • Chest pain • Cardiac arrhythmias • Palpitations • Nausea • Vomiting	• Administer activated charcoal to prevent absorption. • Place the patient in a cool, quiet room. • Institute cooling measures for hyperthermia. • Administer benzodiazepines for agitation and seizures. • Administer I.V. fluids. • Administer I.V. nitroprusside to control severe hypertension. • Administer antiarrhythmics to correct cardiac arrhythmias. • Monitor electrolyte levels and acid–base status.

Drug or substance	Signs and symptoms	Interventions
Benzodiazepines	• Respiratory depression • Lethargy • Confusion • Coma • Slurred speech • Ataxia	• Administer activated charcoal to prevent absorption. • Administer flumazenil to reverse central nervous system symptoms and respiratory depression. • Provide respiratory support.
Cocaine	• Tachycardia • Hypertension • Cardiac arrhythmias • Chest pain • Myocardial infarction • Aortic dissection • Bowel infarction • Hyperthermia • Anxiety • Seizures • Tactile hallucinations • Cerebral hemorrhage	• Administer activated charcoal to prevent absorption. • Perform whole-bowel irrigation. • Monitor cardiac enzymes. • Obtain urine for drug screen. • Place the patient in a cool, quiet room. • Institute cooling measures for hyperthermia. • Monitor for seizures. • Administer benzodiazepines for hyperactivity, hypertension, tachycardia, anxiety, and seizures. • Closely monitor cardiac rate and rhythm. Notify the doctor of any significant arrhythmias. • Administer high-flow oxygen.
Cyanide	• General weakness • Malaise and collapse • Headache • Vertigo • Dizziness • Giddiness • Confusion • Generalized seizures • Coma • Abdominal pain • Nausea, vomiting • Hypotension • Shortness of breath • Chest pain • Apnea	• Perform gastric lavage and administer activated charcoal for acute ingestion. • Provide respiratory support. • Administer 100% oxygen. • Administer crystalloids and vasopressors for hypotension. • Give sodium bicarbonate to correct acidosis. • Administer hydroxocobalamin or a cyanide antidote kit as an antidote.

(continued)

Drug or substance	Signs and symptoms	Interventions
Halogenated hydrocarbons	• Cough • Dizziness • Eye, nose, and throat irritation • Palpitations • Disorientation • Pulmonary edema • Ventricular arrhythmias • Frostbite (dermal exposure)	• Provide fresh air as soon as possible. • Closely monitor cardiac rate and rhythm. • Provide a quiet environment. • Provide rewarming as ordered for frostbite.
Heroin	• Drowsiness • Coma • Delirium • Decreased respiratory drive, shallow respirations • Pinpoint pupils • Muscle spasticity • Hypotension • Weak pulse	• Administer naloxone. • Obtain serum toxicology screen. • Provide respiratory support. • Administer I.V. fluids.
Methanol	• Blurred vision • Retinal edema • Decreased visual acuity • Headache • Vertigo • Lethargy • Confusion • Coma • Nausea • Vomiting • Abdominal pain • Metabolic acidosis • Cardiac arrhythmias	• Perform gastric lavage. • Obtain methanol level. • Administer ethanol or fomepizole as ordered. • Perform hemodialysis as necessary. • Provide respiratory support. • Administer sodium bicarbonate. • Monitor serum electrolytes and glucose levels. • Administer I.V. fluids.
Opioids	• Lethargy • Confusion • Coma • Decreased respiratory rate • Decreased tidal volume • Decreased bowel sounds • Constricted pupils • Mild hypotension • Hypothermia	• Administer naloxone. • Provide respiratory support. • Administer I.V. fluids. • Monitor for opioid withdrawal. • Closely monitor cardiac rate and rhythm. Notify the doctor of any significant arrhythmias.

Drug or substance	Signs and symptoms	Interventions
Salicylates	• Tinnitus • Tachypnea • Pulmonary edema • Lethargy • Confusion • Seizures • Cerebral edema • Hypokalemia • GI hemorrhage • Nausea • Vomiting • Hyperthermia • Dehydration • Tachycardia • Cardiac arrhythmias • Prolongation of the pro-thrombin and bleeding times • Decreased platelet adhesiveness	• Perform gastric lavage. • Administer activated charcoal to prevent absorption. • Administer cathartic. • Administer I.V. fluids for hydration. • Provide alkalization of urine by administering I.V. fluids with potassium chloride and sodium bicarbonate. • Monitor closely for signs and symptoms of pulmonary edema. • Perform hemodialysis for renal failure, cerebral edema, pulmonary edema, refractory acidosis, and high salicylate level. • Monitor serum electrolytes, coagulation studies, and arterial blood gas (ABG) results. • Institute cooling measures for hyperthermia. • Closely monitor cardiac rate and rhythm. Notify the doctor of any significant arrhythmias.
Tricyclic antidepressants	• Tachycardia • Ventricular arrhythmias • Cardiac conduction delays • Hypotension • Agitation • Sedation • Seizures • Coma • Dry, flushed skin • Decreased GI motility • Urinary retention • Metabolic acidosis	• Obtain a 12-lead electrocardiogram. • Perform gastric lavage. • Administer activated charcoal to prevent absorption. • Administer a cathartic. • Closely monitor cardiac rate and rhythm. Notify the doctor of any significant arrhythmias. • Administer sodium bicarbonate for systemic alkalization and treatment of ventricular arrhythmias. • Monitor serum electrolytes and ABG results. • Provide respiratory support. • Administer benzodiazepines for seizure activity. • Administer crystalloids and vasopressors for hypotension.

Glossary

acid–base balance: mechanism by which the body's acids and bases are kept in balance

acidosis: condition resulting from the accumulation of acid or the loss of base

advance directive: document used as a guideline for life-sustaining medical care of a patient with an advanced disease or disability, who's no longer able to indicate his own wishes; includes living wills and durable powers of attorney for health care

afterload: resistance that the left ventricle must work against to pump blood through the aorta

agranulocyte: leukocyte (white blood cell) not made up of granules or grains; includes lymphocytes, monocytes, and plasma cells

aldosterone: adrenocortical hormone that regulates sodium, potassium, and fluid balance

alkalosis: condition resulting from the accumulation of base or the loss of acid

allergen: substance that induces an allergy or a hypersensitivity reaction

anaphylaxis: severe allergic reaction to a foreign substance

aneurysm: sac formed by the dilation of the wall of an artery, a vein, or the heart

anoxia: absence of oxygen in the tissues

antibody: immunoglobulin molecule that reacts only with the specific antigen that induced its formation in the lymph system

antidiuretic hormone: hormone made by the hypothalamus and released by the pituitary gland that decreases the production of urine by increasing the reabsorption of water by the renal tubules

antigen: foreign substance, such as bacteria or toxins, that induces antibody formation

aphasia: language disorder characterized by difficulty expressing or comprehending speech

arrhythmia: disturbance of the normal cardiac rhythm from the abnormal origin, discharge, or conduction of electrical impulses

ataxia: uncoordinated actions when voluntary muscle movements are attempted

atrial kick: amount of blood pumped into the ventricles as a result of atrial contraction; contributes approximately 30% of total cardiac output

autologous transfusion (autotransfusion): reinfusion of the patient's own blood or blood components

automaticity: ability of a cardiac cell to initiate an impulse on its own

borborygmus: loud, gurgling, splashing sounds caused by gas passing through the intestine; normally heard over the large intestine

bruit: abnormal sound heard over peripheral vessels that indicates turbulent blood flow

capture: successful pacing of the heart, represented on the electrocardiogram tracing by a pacemaker spike followed by a P wave or QRS complex

cardiac cycle: the period from the beginning of one heartbeat to the beginning of the next; includes two phases, systole and diastole

cardiac output: amount of blood ejected from the left ventricle per minute; normal value is 4 to 8 L per minute

cardioversion: restoration of normal rhythm by electric shock or drug therapy

cerebral edema: increase in the brain's fluid content; may result from correcting hypernatremia too rapidly

Chvostek's sign: abnormal spasm of facial muscles that may indicate hypocalcemia or tetany; tested by lightly tapping the facial nerve (upper cheek, below the zygomatic bone)

colloid: large molecule, such as albumin, that normally doesn't cross the capillary membrane

complement system: major mediator of inflammatory response; a functionally related system made up of 20 proteins circulating as functionally inactive molecules

conduction: transmission of electrical impulses through the myocardium

conductivity: ability of one cardiac cell to transmit an electrical impulse to another cell

contractility: ability of a cardiac cell to contract after receiving an impulse

critical pathway: documentation tool used in managed care and case management in which a time line is defined for the patient's condition and for the achievement of expected outcomes; used by caregivers to determine where the patient should be in his progress toward optimal health

crystalloid: solute, such as sodium or glucose, that crosses the capillary membrane in solution

cytotoxic: destructive to cells

deep tendon reflex: involuntary muscle contraction in response to a sudden stretch that can be elicited by a hammer or finger tap on a tendon at its insertion

defibrillation: termination of ventricular fibrillation by electrical shock

dehydration: condition in which the loss of water from cells causes them to shrink

demyelination: destruction of a nerve's myelin sheath, which interferes with normal nerve conduction

depolarization: response of a myocardial cell to an electrical impulse that causes movement of ions across the cell membrane, which triggers myocardial contraction

diastole: phase of the cardiac cycle when both atria (atrial diastole) or both ventricles (ventricular diastole) are at rest and filling with blood

diplopia: double vision

distal: farthest away

durable power of attorney for health care: legal document whereby a patient authorizes another person to make medical decisions for him should he become unable to do so

dysarthria: speech defect commonly related to a motor deficit of the tongue or speech muscles

dysphagia: difficulty swallowing

enhanced automaticity: condition in which pacemaker cells increase the firing rate above their inherent rate

excitability: ability of a cardiac cell to respond to an electrical stimulus

extravasation: leakage of intravascular fluid into surrounding tissue; can be caused by such medications as chemotherapeutic drugs, dopamine, and calcium solutions that produce blistering and, eventually, tissue necrosis

granulocyte: any cell containing granules, especially a granular leukocyte (white blood cell)

hematopoiesis: production of red blood cells in the bone marrow

homeostasis: dynamic, steady state of internal balance in the body

hormone: chemical substance produced in the body that has a specific regulatory effect on the activity of specific cells or organs

hypervolemia: excess of fluid and solutes in extracellular fluid; can be caused by increased fluid intake, fluid shifts in the body, or renal failure

hypotonic: solution that has fewer solutes than another solution

hypovolemia: condition marked by the loss of fluid and solutes from extracellular fluid that, if left untreated, can progress to hypovolemic shock

hypoxemia: oxygen deficit in arterial blood (lower than 80 mm Hg)

hypoxia: oxygen deficit in the tissues

immunocompetence: ability of cells to distinguish antigens from substances that belong to the body and to launch an immune response

immunodeficiency disorder: disorder caused by a deficiency of the immune response due to hypoactivity or decreased numbers of lymphoid cells

immunoglobulin: serum protein synthesized by lymphocytes and plasma cells that has known antibody activity; main component of humoral immune response

intrinsic: naturally occurring electrical stimulus from within the heart's conduction system

ischemia: decreased blood supply to a body organ or tissue

isotonic solution: solution that has the same concentration of solutes as another solution

leukocyte: white blood cell that protects the body against microorganisms that cause disease

living will: witnessed document indicating a patient's desire to be allowed to die a natural death, rather than be kept alive by life-sustaining measures; applies to decisions that will be made after a terminally ill patient is incompetent and has no reasonable possibility of recovery

lymph node: structure that filters the lymphatic fluid that drains from body tissues and is later returned to the blood as plasma; removes noxious agents from the blood

lymphocyte: leukocyte produced by lymphoid tissue that participates in immunity

macrophage: highly phagocytic cells that are stimulated by inflammation

metabolic acidosis: condition in which excess acid or reduced bicarbonate in the blood drops the arterial blood pH below 7.35

metabolic alkalosis: condition in which excess bicarbonate or reduced acid in the blood increases the arterial blood pH above 7.45

nephron: structural and functional unit of the kidney that forms urine

neuron: highly specialized conductor cell that receives and transmits electrochemical nerve impulses

nursing diagnosis: clinical judgment made by a nurse about a patient's responses to actual or potential health problems or life processes; describes a patient problem that the nurse can legally solve; may apply to families and communities as well as individual patients

nursing process: systematic approach to identifying a patient's problems and then taking nursing actions to address them; steps include assessing the patient's problems, forming a diagnostic statement, identifying expected outcomes, creating a plan to achieve expected outcomes and solve the patient's problems, implementing the plan or assigning others to implement it, and evaluating the plan's effectiveness

nystagmus: involuntary, rhythmic movement of the eye

oliguria: low urine output, less than 400 mL/24 hours

orthostatic hypotension: drop in blood pressure and increase in heart rate that occur when the body changes position; can be caused by a loss of circulating blood volume

paroxysmal: episode of an arrhythmia that starts and stops suddenly

peristalsis: sequence of muscle contractions that propels food through the GI tract

petechiae: minute hemorrhagic spots in the skin

pH: measurement of the percentage of hydrogen ions in a solution; normal pH is 7.35 to 7.45 of arterial blood

phagocytosis: engulfing of microorganisms, other cells, and foreign particles by a phagocyte

point of maximal impulse: point at which the upward thrust of the heart against the chest wall is greatest, usually over the apex of the heart

practice guidelines: sequential instructions for treating patients with specific health problems

preload: stretching force exerted on the ventricular muscle by the blood it contains at the end of diastole

refractory period: brief period during which excitability in a myocardial cell is depressed

renin: enzyme produced by the kidneys in response to an actual or perceived decline in extracellular fluid volume; an important part of blood pressure regulation

repolarization: recovery of the myocardial cells after depolarization during which the cell membrane returns to its resting potential

respiratory acidosis: acid–base disturbance caused by failure of the lungs to eliminate sufficient carbon dioxide; partial pressure of arterial carbon dioxide above 45 mm Hg and pH below 7.35

respiratory alkalosis: acid–base imbalance that occurs when the lungs eliminate more carbon dioxide than normal; partial pressure of arterial carbon dioxide below 35 mm Hg and pH above 7.45

rhabdomyolysis: disorder in which skeletal muscle is destroyed; causes intracellular contents to spill into extracellular fluid

systole: phase of the cardiac cycle when both of the atria (atrial systole) or the ventricles (ventricular systole) are contracting

telangiectasis: permanently dilated small blood vessels that form a web-like pattern; may be the result of scleroderma, lupus erythematosus, or cirrhosis or may be normal in healthy, older adults

thrill: palpable vibration felt over the heart or vessel that results from turbulent blood flow

thrombolytic: clot dissolving

Trousseau's sign: carpal (wrist) spasm elicited by applying a blood pressure cuff to the upper arm and inflating it to a pressure 20 mm Hg above the patient's systolic blood pressure; indicates the presence of hypocalcemia

vasopressor: drug that stimulates contraction of the muscular tissue of the capillaries and arteries

$\dot{V}/\dot{Q}$ ratio: ratio of ventilation (amount of air in the alveoli) to perfusion (amount of blood in the pulmonary capillaries); expresses the effectiveness of gas exchange

water intoxication: condition in which excess water in the cells results in cellular swelling

Index

Notes

Notes

Notes

Notes